The Veterinary Book for Beef Farmers

Lee-Anne Oliver and Roger Scott

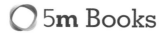

5m Books

Published by
5m Books Ltd
Lings, Great Easton
Essex CM6 2HH, UK
www.5mbooks.com

A Catalogue record for this book is available from the British Library

ISBN 9781789181197

Book layout by Servis Filmsetting Ltd, Stockport, Cheshire
Printed by Replika Press Pvt Ltd, India
Photos by Scott Mitchell Associates unless otherwise indicated

Contents

Preface

As a recent graduate I took the, then, unusual step of taking a week's holiday and using it, not for a trip to Mallorca, but, instead, a week with a vet whom I knew I could learn from. I like to think this *sabbatical* was an early nod to a belief in so called *continuing professional development*; I think it was. The vet in question was Roger Blowey. He and his wife kindly took me into their home and a few days later I left with more knowledge than I started with, an injection of confidence, a spring in my step and a copy of *The Veterinary Book for Dairy Farmers* – his parting words … 'I know this is a book for dairy farmers, and I know you're not a dairy farmer, but I think you'll find it useful.' I did.

I grew up in Northumberland in the 1970s, my father a livestock auctioneer and buyer of store cattle for my uncle's fattening unit. I had a soundtrack of not just The Who and the Rolling Stones, but one of constant dialogue on cattle and, as my father referred to it … 'the trade'. My other back drop was one of education; my mother, being a school teacher. This left me heavily influenced by all matters of knowledge transfer and, just as importantly, what to do with that knowledge. I scraped, by the skin of my teeth, into the Royal (Dick) School of Veterinary Studies and then lost the skins of several more teeth chewing my way through 5 years of difficult study. It was worth it; I became a vet.

My first job was in the Vale of York where I learnt all about beef fattening, but also all about pigs (in those days vets still farrowed sows) and of course dogs, horses and cats, in that approximate order. I then went to work as a dairy vet in Hampshire, following the aforementioned sabbatical, but I always kept an eye on … 'the trade'! (I refer of course to the beef trade.) That took up most of the 1990s, then with a young family it was time to go home to Northumberland and time to start a business of my own. I set up a one-man veterinary practice which looked after the dairy cows of the Tyne Valley and the beef cattle and sheep of the North Pennines and the Northumberland National Park. The dairy cows did not last long but like rebels, the cattle and sheep dug into the hills, and, they stayed! Thank goodness.

The practice grew and, in a milestone moment, we were joined by one Lee-Anne Oliver. Lee-Anne had also grown up in Northumberland. Lee-Anne married a local beef farmer, Nick, and in her usual expedient way, immediately started a family. After a brief spell in equine practice, Lee-Anne joined us at Scott Mitchell Associates to pursue her love of beef and sheep practice. We thought we were productive, efficient, quick and thorough. Lee-Anne raised that bar; a bar she kept raising and continues to raise to this day. When you have read Chapter 23 you will realise that Lee-Anne Oliver is an *Implementer*, the best example I have ever met, and for that the practice and its farmers are eternally grateful. Lee-Anne also did the sabbatical thing – she spent, not just a week, however, but 1 year in the diagnostic laboratories of the Scottish Agricultural Colleges in Dumfries. This proved very helpful and, not stopping at that, Lee-Anne has been an ongoing proponent of continuing professional development, studying successfully for her Royal College Certificates in not just cattle practice but also sheep; she is a recognised advanced practitioner in both species.

Along with our business partner, Colin Mitchell, Lee-Anne and I were serious about knowledge transfer and education in our chosen fields: farming and allied business management. Like many practices we were keen to lay on educational sessions for farmers and students, but we were keen to go further and formalised things somewhat with the creation of a training company, CPD Actif which we still own and run. Our next *big thing*, however, was to fill a gap that had been troubling us. We had *The Veterinary Book for Dairy Farmers* on the shelf, we also had David Henderson's excellent *The Veterinary Book for Sheep Farmers*. The next step was obvious, and 3 years later here it is, *The Veterinary Book for Beef Farmers*.

We hope this book will be useful to all farmers of beef cattle but, as the sibling books were for me, we hope this book will be useful to agricultural students, animal health students, veterinary students and, of course, young vets. We intend that this book will serve several purposes: it hopefully, in parts, will amuse you, it will be a useful reference book for quick advice and information, it will be, when read fully, an insight into the holistic nature of health, welfare, production and disease prevention rather than simply a book on disease. We also hope it will be an introduction to further holistic thinking around the business and psychological aspects of farming; areas to be brought to the fore in our humble but firm opinions. Our ultimate hope is that this book will raise the health, production and, not just the welfare, but the well-being of the cattle without whom we would not have a reason to do what we do. At times the book will appear to take a surprisingly emotive view, particularly the chapter on the newborn calf. This is intentional. If nothing else this is a heartfelt celebration of the incredible pocket of nature we have the privilege of working in, but it also aims to give out a message that we as an industry are permanently striving to uphold animal well-being and in doing so will reach out to the sectors of the public who, whether misguided or not, feel emotionally compelled to bring an end to livestock farming. We may not agree with them – we in the industry all presumably recognise and uphold the natural food chain pyramid – but to not understand the emotional drivers of those who disagree is to fail to understand, is to fail to communicate and is to fail to reach a compromise. Can we start by saying we all care, and we will all do more for animal well-being, in particular the cattle we take responsibility for? Let's not lose this industry.

Roger Scott
Tyne Green, Hexham
February 2020

Acknowledgements

We would like to thank our families: Nick and Aaron Oliver, and Alison, Helena, Alistair and William Scott for putting up with 3 years of book worming. We would also like to thank the educators, the colleagues and the allied industry connections, such as XLVets and Scottish Agricultural Colleges, who have all helped us on this journey; none of us would be anywhere without *learning from each other*.

We would both like to extend deep and sincere thanks to the farmers of South Northumberland and County Durham, our clients, who have worked with us, supported our practice, shared their wisdom and allowed us to share ours. We would also like to acknowledge our own wonderful team at Scott Mitchell Associates who since small beginnings in 2001 have worked as a team and built a veterinary practice that cares.

Lee-Anne Oliver and Roger Scott
Tyne Green, Hexham
February 2020

Abbreviations

AHDB	Agricultural and Horticultural Development Board	CHAWG	Cattle Health and Welfare Group of Great Britain
AHVLA	Animal Health and Veterinary Laboratories Agency	CHeCS	Cattle Health Certification Standards Scheme
AI	artificial insemination	CIA	critically important antimicrobials
AMA	American Marketing Association	CJD	Creutzfeldt–Jakob disease
AMR	antimicrobial resistance	CL	corpus luteum
AV	artificial vagina	CNS	central nervous system
BAL	broncho-alveolar lavage	COWS	Control of Worms Sustainably
BBSE	bull breeding soundness examination	CP	crude protein
		CPD	continuing professional development
BCMS	British Cattle Movement Service		
BCS	body condition score	CSFV	classical swine fever virus
BDV	border disease virus	CT	computerised tomography
BEPP	bovine erythropoietic protoporphyria	CTA	critical thinking appraisal
		DCAB	dietary cation–anion balance
BHB/BOHB	beta-hydroxybutyrate	DDD	defined daily dose
BLUP	best linear unbiased predictor	DLWG	daily liveweight gain
BRD	bovine respiratory disease	DM	dry matter
BSC	balanced scorecard	DPF	dorsal patella fixation
BSE	bovine spongiform encephalopathy	DSS	decision support systems
		DUP	digestible undegradable protein
BSP	bovine spastic paresis	EBL	enzootic bovine leucosis
BSS	bovine spastic syndrome	EBV	estimated breeding values
bTB	bovine tuberculosis	EHEC	enterohaemorrhagic E. coli
BVD	bovine viral diarrhoea	ELISA	enzyme linked immunosorbent assay
BVDV	bovine viral diarrhoea virus		
BZ	benzimidazoles	EMA	European Medicines Agency
CAP	Common Agricultural Policy	EPEC	enteropathogenic E. coli
CBPP	contagious bovine pleuro-pneumonia	epg	eggs per gram
		ERDP	effective rumen degradable protein
CCN	cerebrocortical necrosis		

ET	embryo transfer
ETEC	enterotoxigenic E. coli
EUROP	EU and UK Beef Carcase Classification Scheme Scale
FAnGR	UK Farm Animal Genetic Resources Committee
FAT	fluorescent antibody test
FB	foreign body
FCE/FCR	feed conversion efficiency/rate
FECRT	faecal egg count reduction test
FMD	foot and mouth disease
FME	fermentable metabolisable energy
FSC	foetal stomach contents
FSH	follicle stimulating hormone
FWEC	faecal worm egg count
GHG	greenhouse gases
GnRH	gonadotrophin releasing hormone
GSHPx	glutathione peroxidase
HND	higher national diploma
IBK	infectious bovine keratoconjunctivitis
IBP	infectious balanoposthitis
IBR	infectious bovine rhinotracheitis
IFNγ	interferon gamma
IgA	immunoglobulin A
IgG	immunoglobulin G
IPVV	infectious pustular vulvo-vaginitis
IVF	in vitro fertilisation
IVFT	intravenous fluid therapy
IVP	in vitro embryo production
JD	Johne's disease
KO%	killing out percentage
KPI	key performance indicator
LH	luteinising hormone
LSD	lumpy skin disease
LV	levamisoles
MAP	Mycobacterium avium paratuberculosis
MCF	malignant catarrhal fever
MCP	microbial protein
MDA	maternally derived antibody
ME	metabolisable energy
MIC	minimum inhibitory concentration
ML	macrocyclic lactones

MOET	multiple ovulation embryo transfer
MP	metabolisable protein
MRL	maximum residue limit
NDF	neutral detergent fibre
NSAID	non-steroidal anti-inflammatory drug
OPU	ovum pick up
ORT	oral rehydration therapy
PBE	pre-breeding examination
PBS	phosphate buffered saline
PCR	polymerase chain reaction
PCU	population correction unit
PD	pregnancy diagnosis
PG	prostaglandin
PGE	parasitic gastroenteritis
PI	persistently infected
PME	post-mortem examination
PNS	peripheral nervous system
PWSS	peri-weaning scour syndrome
QMS	Quality Meat Scotland
RFM	retained foetal membranes
RSV	respiratory syncytial virus
RTS	reproductive tract scoring
RUMA	Responsible Use of Medicines in Agriculture Alliance
SAC	Scottish Agricultural Colleges
SAR	suspected adverse reaction
SBV	Schmallenberg virus
SCC	somatic cell count
SCFA	short chain fatty acids
SICCT	single intradermal comparative cervical tuberculin test
SOP	standard operating procedures
SPC	summary of product characteristics
SQP	suitably qualified person
SRM	specified risk materials
TB	tuberculosis
TBF	tickborne fever
TI	transiently infected
TMR	total mixed ration
TNZ	thermoneutral zone
TP	total protein
TRP	traumatic reticuloperitonitis

TST	targeted selective treatment	VMD	Veterinary Medicines Directive
UV	ultraviolet	WHD	white heifer disease
VIA	video image analysis	WHO	World Health Organization
VIDA	Veterinary Investigation Diagnosis Analysis	WLD	white line disease
		WMD	white muscle disease
VLA	Veterinary Laboratories Agency (UK)	ZN	Ziehl–Neelsen
		ZST	zinc sulphate turbidity

Part I

An introduction to the beef industry

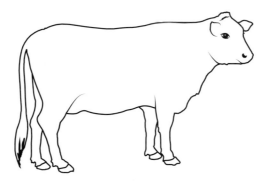

Chapter 1

The beef industry in the UK

'For hundreds of thousands of years, we have hunted animals and for tens of thousands of years we have farmed them so we can eat their meat' (Fearnley-Whittingstall, 2004, p. 12). In the UK during 2018, approximately 2 million cattle were slaughtered for beef (AHDB, 2019). Beef is the third most widely consumed meat in the world, accounting for 25% of total meat consumption after pork and poultry, each representing 38% and 30%, respectively (Raloff, 2003).

As farmers or veterinarians, we have a responsibility for the health, welfare and well-being of all animals in our care, while, at the same time, food production is an industry and needs to be profitable and sustainable – these objectives are compatible but have to be well managed.

In the UK, beef supplies come from suckler herds and from dairy herds. In 2019, the supply was roughly equal from each.

WHAT IS A SUCKLER HERD?

A suckler herd is a domestic herd of breeding cows each of which is intended to produce a calf every year, and, crucially, rear that calf; a calf that will either itself go on to be a breeding female or bull, or, as in the majority of cases, be slaughtered for meat. Initially, the calf remains with its dam who suckles the calf, hence the term 'suckler herd'. A pedantic point but cows *suckle*, calves *suck*. The calf will be weaned, typically at 5–9 months of age, allowing the cow, hopefully now pregnant again, to divert her resources to incubating the next calf before calving again at the same time, the following year.

Once weaned, the exact fate of the calf will vary depending on the farm location and the availability and cost of forage, feed, housing and bedding. Some female calves, and the odd male, may be reared and retained in the herd as home-bred replacements or sold as future breeding animals; the majority, however, go for meat.

MEAT PRODUCTION FROM THE SUCKLER HERD

The weaned calves may be reared and grown relatively slowly from pasture alone, or they may remain housed and be fed a high energy diet for faster rearing. They may stay on the same farm, or move between farms at weaning, or they may move for the *finishing (fattening) period*. Some beef cattle will be slaughtered as young as 14 months, while others may be as old as 36 months before they are ready to go to slaughter.

Cows and bulls that have been culled from the herd will also enter the human food chain if considered fit for human consumption. In the UK, this was not the case between 1996 and 2005, during the bovine spongiform encephalopathy (BSE) (Chapter 28) crisis when cattle over 30 months of age were not allowed to enter the food chain.

There were estimated to be around 45,000 suckler herds in the UK in 2011, with an average herd size of between 30 and 50 cows and with the Limousin or Limousin-cross being the predominant breed of cow (CHAWG, 2012).

Suckler herds tend to be grazed on marginal land or poor land, neither of which is suitable for dairy cows or arable crops. In fact, the hills and uplands are home to 40% of the beef cows in England, and 85% in Wales. The beef cattle often co-graze this land with sheep.

The number of suckler cows in the UK has been declining in recent years. The negative impact of the BSE crisis in the late 1990s was followed by a partial recovery of numbers until 2005. Up until 2003 farm subsidy payments made under the EU Common Agricultural Policy (CAP) were based on *production*. In 2003, however, CAP reform was introduced and, in a process called decoupling, the subsidy was not related to production but instead to the area farmed. This prompted a decline in suckler cow numbers – there was no headage incentive to keep them – and this decline has continued with current predictions, in 2020, that the decline will continue, although the exact effect of the UK leaving the EU is still to be seen.

HOW DOES THE DAIRY HERD PRODUCE BEEF?

As of 2020, around 50% of beef in the UK comes from the dairy sector: from purebred dairy bull calves, beef-cross heifer and bull calves, and cull cows (and bulls).

In the UK, the majority of dairy cows are of Holstein or Friesian breeding, or, as is fairly standard now, a hybrid of the two, namely the Holstein-Friesian, typically referred to as 'black and white'.

Certain cows within the dairy herd – those with higher production potential – will be selected to be bred to dairy bulls, usually using sexed semen, so they can produce female calves which will become replacement cows in the future. The average life of a dairy cow in the UK is 3–4 lactations or around

5–6 years of age (CHAWG, 2018). The short productive life span of these dairy cows means the replacement rate is quite high. It is estimated that 60% of dairy cows are bred to dairy semen to breed a replacement dairy cow.

On farms where 'black and white' sexed semen is used for artificial insemination (AI) then the vast majority of calves will, as expected, be female. If, however, conventional semen is used, or natural service by a bull employed, approximately one-half of the calves born will be male, the vast majority of which will enter the food chain as they have no other obvious use.

Purebred dairy male calves can be left entire or castrated. Entire males have better feed conversion efficiency (FCE), they produce a leaner carcase and they yield a higher harvest of meat in a shorter time than do castrated males. They do, however, require suitable facilities and are usually housed through to finishing. Castrated males, on the other hand, are a more flexible option.

The 'black and white' male beef animal has, in the eyes of the meat industry, a poorer conformation and a higher feed cost per kilogramme of carcase than a beef/dairy-cross male animal. They have, consequently, a lower market value. For many years, the male 'black and white' calf was seen as very much a by-product of the dairy herd, many calves were even shot soon after birth as it was not seen as financially viable to rear them. Owing to consumer pressure, however, and the fluctuating requirements of the milk buyer contracts, an increasing number of purebred dairy calves are now reared on machine-fed artificial milk, or, sometimes, natural cow's milk depending on said market, and these cattle contribute significantly to the UK beef market, either as intensively reared beef or *rose veal*.

VEAL

The legal definition of veal is: *meat from cattle aged less than 8 months old at slaughter*. Historically veal, or specifically *white veal*, was produced from calves kept in crates with no room to exercise, fed a milk-only, low iron diet and in receipt of limited sunlight. Veal crates were, fortunately, banned in the UK in 1990, and in the EU, in 2007.

The UK now produces *rose veal*, a delicate pink meat usually produced from entire male dairy-bred calves, with a permitted slaughtering age of between 8 and 12 months. There are few calves reared for veal production in the UK because of the lack of demand from consumers; veal makes up just 0.1% of meat consumed each year in the UK.

The farms that do rear calves for veal in the UK exceed the basic welfare standards required within EU law. They are reared in straw-bedded, loose housing and are fed a diet of milk and forage, a ration which is unrestricted in its iron content. The main market for this veal is restaurants, with very few sales through the supermarkets. However, this is slowly changing as myths around veal production are dispelled.

The dairy cows that are not selected to breed future dairy female replacements are often mated with a bull of a beef breed such as the Belgian Blue, Angus, Limousin or Hereford. The resultant calves, both male and female, are intended for beef production. Some of the female calves may, however, be purchased by suckler farmers to be breeding cows within their herds, although this has been a declining market in recent years, with farmers currently preferring to breed their own beef cow replacements from beef-bred animals rather than dairy-cross. Given the levels of dystocia sometimes encountered, and also the lack of milk yield, in some of these beef-bred cows, this practice does, however, get questioned and is not followed by all.

The relationship between the dairy and suckler herd in the UK beef industry is depicted in Figure 1.1.

There is a lot of support and advice available from within the industry to help in the production of meat from beef-cross dairy calves. This is now seen as an additional source of income for the dairy herd – not only does the farmer have a lactation's worth of milk to sell, they also have a calf that now has value.

A beef-bred calf, in 2020, is worth approximately £180 more at 2 weeks old than its equivalent black and white counterpart. With an unattractive sale price, calves from the dairy herd destined for meat are sometimes taken through to slaughter on the farm where they are born. Alternatively, they can, of course, be sold at any stage to a specialised unit, the lesser price tag prevailing. Calves may be sold to specialised calf rearers at as young as 1 week of age, or are sold post-weaning, or, just before finishing.

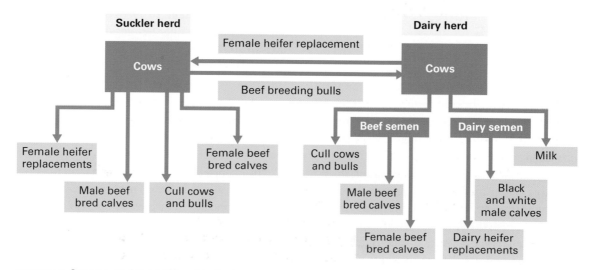

FIGURE 1.1 Structure of the UK beef industry

Bull selection is crucial when breeding a dairy cow to produce a beef-cross calf. Choosing the breed of a beef bull is the first decision: this largely depends on the market; the buyer will undoubtedly dictate what they want. There is a large amount of information available from breeding companies to support these decisions. This information is based on carcase data fed back from the abattoirs at the point of slaughter and it provides very accurate estimated breeding values (EBVs) linked to a predicted financial return. In addition, from a management point of view, EBVs should also be used to select an easy calving bull. This can significantly reduce calving difficulties, and the otherwise inevitable cost of vet visits, increased calf mortality and morbidity, reduced cow fertility and reduced milk yield.

For traceability purposes, some abattoirs request the name of the sire, and therefore the sire needs to be purebred and registered. In 2011, only 23% of sires were recorded on passports (Pritchard, 2013) at the time the calf is registered but the vast majority of carcases in the UK are DNA-tested at slaughter to determine their parentage. This has enabled a large amount of information to be recorded and fed back into the system, mainly to develop carcase trait EBVs. EBVs are discussed in Chapter 9.

CULL COWS

At times viewed as a by-product there is currently, once again, much value in the cull cow (and bull). Dairy and suckler cows at the end of their productive life enter the food chain. Cull cattle, from the beef and dairy sectors contribute 20% of the beef produced in the UK. Producers have the option to fatten these cows themselves or to sell them to another unit for finishing, accepting a lesser value but saving the cost of the additional space and feed needed to finish the animal. As with any fattening animal there is money to be made in ensuring it reaches its potential. To get the most value from a cull animal requires an understanding of what

the market wants and the prices likely to be paid, versus the costs of feed, forage and housing to get them to the condition dictated. Younger cows will have a better feed conversion ratio and are likely to yield profitable weight gain. Some very old cows, or those with health issues, may not fatten. Cattle failing to perform in the first month should be sent to market straight away so as not to waste any more time or money.

BEEF – THE MEAT PRODUCT

Cattle are slaughtered only at approved abattoirs if the meat is to be sold for human consumption. Non-approved abattoirs exist in the UK but are rare and the meat from them can only go to the owner of the animal and cannot be sold or supplied to anyone else. Approved abattoirs are highly regulated with respect to animal welfare and to meat quality and hygiene.

Regulatory standards have increased over the years and there has been consolidation of the abattoir sector with the loss of many smaller, rural abattoirs. In 1985, there were 1000 operational abattoirs in the UK. In 2007, there were only 277. Over the same time period, there has been a decline in the number of butcher's shops with consumers instead choosing to purchase their meat from the supermarket. In 1985, there were 21,000 butcher's shops selling 26% of all beef and lamb sold. In 2007, there were fewer than 6800 butchers shops selling 10% of all beef and lamb sold in the UK. That decline has continued.

In the early 1990s, the UK was a net exporter of beef. However, the BSE crisis in 1996 led to a ban on the exporting of beef, for 10 years. Exports resumed in 2006 but did not recover. During 2018, the UK exported 15–17% of its annual production, equating to around 100,000 tonnes of beef (AHDB, 2019). The majority of exported beef is now in the form of cuts rather than whole carcases. Some cow carcases are, however, exported; somewhat surprisingly they are often processed abroad and then returned to the UK as prepared meat. Cuts with low domestic value are generally exported as they are more valuable in other countries. This is certainly the case with offal: 48,000 tonnes were exported in 2015, double that of 2009 (BMPA).

The UK, in 2018, imported 35% of the beef and veal it consumed, approximately 290,000 tonnes. The dominant supplier was the Republic of Ireland (AHDB, 2019).

THE BEEF SUPPLY CHAIN

The beef supply chain consists of the following.

- **The producer** (the farmer) – there may be one producer for the entire life of the animal or multiple.
- **The meat processor** – this is the producer's customer and may be a cattle buyer in a market, or an abattoir if selling *deadweight,* direct to slaughter.
- **The retailer** – these are mostly supermarkets, but, in some cases, the traditional butcher.
- **The consumer** – the person who eats the meat, at home or in a cooked food outlet.

Each part of the supply chain has its own objectives. The key to obtaining a good market price for cattle is to find out what the market wants, decide on a target specification and try to meet it as accurately and consistently as possible.

CARCASE CLASSIFICATION

The UK and EU uses the Beef Carcase Classification Scheme also known as the Union Scale. Here three main areas are assessed: the conformation of the carcase (flesh coverage and overall shape), fat coverage and weight.

The conformation aspect is scored on the EUROP scale where EUROP stands for E – excellent, U – very good, R – good, O – fair and P – poor. U, O and P are further subdivided into + and – scores, see Figure 1.2. The more flesh coverage

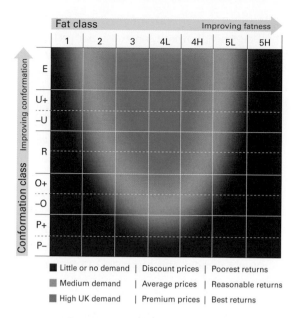

FIGURE 1.2 Carcase classification

and the rounder the shape of the carcase the higher is the score on the EUROP scale. Angular cattle will yield a carcase score typically R or O while very angular cattle such as culled Friesian-Holstein cows will typically score P, but not always.

The fat classes are an assessment of fat coverage of the ribs, loin and tail head. Rather like the body condition score scale, a very fat animal will be classified as a 5, a lean animal as a 1, although both 4 and 5 are subdivided into low and high, L and H.

The third part of the classification is the easiest – that is the weight in kg.

The carcase receives its overall grade from a qualified meat classifier once the animal has been killed, gutted and trimmed. It is possible to estimate the carcase grade in the live animal; this is quite an art, but with a good eye and experience it is an invaluable tool to ensure that animals are reared to the specification requested and therefore achieve the best price.

The grade affects how much the producer is paid per kilogramme of carcase. There is more demand and therefore higher prices paid for cattle in the

E, U and R grades with a fatness score of 3 or 4. It all depends, however, on consumer preferences dictating a retailer's requirements. A traditional butcher will require, and pay more for, a slightly fatter animal than a supermarket. Carcases that will be processed into other products, for example, pies, do not have to have good conformation, and again a fatter carcase will be acceptable especially as the bulk buying supermarkets do not seek them out.

- The killing out percentage (KO%) is the carcase weight as a proportion of the liveweight. The KO% is affected by gut fill, breed, finishing system, gender and eagerness of carcase trimming.
- Meat yield differs from KO%. Meat yield is the percentage of saleable meat from a carcase. The better the conformation, the more saleable meat there will be to sell. The fatter the carcase, the less meat there will be to sell.

The EUROP grid visual classification of carcases is largely subjective and actually correlates fairly poorly with saleable meat yield. Further developments are being made into the use of video image analysis. This analyses the cross-sectional area, fat and lean meat composition of a carcase and is a more accurate predictor of saleable meat yield. At a more research-based level computerised tomography (CT) scans are being used in the same way and are very accurate.

PEDIGREE ANIMALS IN THE BEEF SUCKLER INDUSTRY

A small number of pedigree herds exist in the UK within each breed to provide purebred bulls for not just the suckler herd industry but the dairy herd too. The best pedigree herds usually work on having a high health status and produce high genetic merit animals to supply superior genetics to the industry. A large proportion of pedigree bulls are sold at auction at dedicated bull sales. These bulls may go on to work on a traditional suckler or dairy farm, or they may be purchased by a breeding company who collect and extend the bull's semen for selling domestically and/or internationally.

Bulls can sell for a lot of money, in excess of 100,000 guineas (one guinea is worth £1.05), with the average price of a Limousin bull sold at auction being around £7000, in 2019. Some pedigree breeders are heavily criticised for producing bulls that look 'magnificent' at bull sales, but that are overfed and have poor fertility and short longevity once they 'get to work'. Many bulls are purchased solely on how they look rather than taking into account their proven genetic merit as indicated/identified by their EBVs. This is not the case with all pedigree breeders, or all breeds, and with more genetic information (*genomics*) and with a higher accuracy of EBV becoming available, the situation is sure to change.

Breed societies

Each breed of cattle has its own breed society. These societies are in charge of deciding on the breed standards; they promote the breed, they maintain a herd book or family tree, and they collect data and assess specific traits of the breed. Each breed society has its own sales which are an opportunity to view and purchase purebred registered male and female animals of that specific breed. Agricultural shows are also a showcase for pedigree cattle, with many different breeds represented. Knowing the traits of each breed allows farmers to select the genetics that are best suited for their specific farming system.

REFERENCES

AHDB (2019) *The UK Cattle Year Book*. Agriculture and Horticulture Development Board, Stoneleigh.

BMPA (n.d.) Imports and exports. British Meat Processors Association. Available at: https://british

meatindustry.org/industry/imports-exports/beef-veal/.

Cattle Health and Welfare Group of Great Britain (CHAWG) (2012) First annual report, September 2012. Available at: http://www.eblex.org.uk/wp/wp-content/uploads/2013/06/cattle-health-and-welfare-report.pdf.

Cattle Health and Welfare Group of Great Britain (CHAWG) (2018) Fourth report, September 2018. Available at: https://projectblue.blob.core.windows. net/media/Default/Beef%20&%20Lamb/CHAWG/CHAWG-Fourth-Report-2018.pdf.

Fearnley-Whittingstall, H. (2004) *The River Cottage Meat Book*. Hodder & Stoughton, London.

Pritchard, T. (2013) Selection opportunities from using abattoir carcass data. Conference paper, British Cattle Conference, January 2013, Telford.

Raloff, J. (2003) Food for thought: global food trends. Science News. https://www.sciencenews.org/blog/food-thought/global-food-trends.

Chapter 2

Appraising a national beef industry

A SWOT analysis is a well practised, valuable exercise designed to identify the internal strengths and weaknesses, as well as the external opportunities and threats of a project, an organisation or an industry, see Table 2.1. In this chapter the UK beef industry will be subjected to an example SWOT analysis – some of the analysis will apply to the global beef industry, some not, and different countries will undoubtedly have different SWOT analyses to the UK regardless of the global commonalities. The principle of the SWOT analysis is simply to list the internal strengths of the entity, the internal weaknesses, then the external opportunities and finally the external threats. Quite often this exercise is done on a white board or piece of paper divided into four quadrants as in Table 2.1.

SWOT ANALYSIS OF THE BEEF INDUSTRY IN THE UK

Strengths

Quality and versatile product

Beef contains many valuable nutrients. Iron and zinc are notable and important within the human diet. Beef contains *haem iron* – an organic iron complex readily absorbable in the human gut, which also facilitates iron uptake from other sources, namely green vegetables. Globally anaemia is the biggest nutritional deficiency:

between 2% and 5% of men and non-menstruating women are anaemic, it is even higher in menstruating women. Anaemia can be easily treated by eating more red meat. Similarly, the consumption of beef also provides zinc and improves uptake from other sources in the diet.

Beef also contains Vitamins B and D, selenium and copper.

Beef is, of course, a terrific source of protein, which provides essential amino acids used as building blocks for healthy new tissue and muscle mass. It also helps with satiety so is used in weight loss programmes. Lean beef is considered an important part of a healthy balanced diet.

Over the last 10–15 years, genetic improvements in the cattle population and new butchery techniques have resulted in the reduction of the percentage of fat in red meat; it is now typically only 5%. Beef also contains non-saturated fats which are considered to be a health benefit, cardio-protectants which help the heart muscle, anti-tumour factors, and properties that delay the onset of diabetes.

Many early studies that prompted the advice to limit red meat intake did not distinguish between unprocessed red meat and processed meat such as sausages and bacon. More recent studies have distinguished between the two and the negative effects are now cited as specifically correlated with high intakes, only of processed red meat (Binnie et al., 2014).

Consumers today are willing to spend money

TABLE 2.1 SWOT analysis of the beef industry in the UK

Weaknesses	Threats
Low margins	Resistance to antimicrobials
Length and complexity of the supply chain	Bovine tuberculosis
Reliance on subsidies	Changing markets
Cash flow	Veganism and flexitarianism
Poor integration of the supply chain	Alternative protein sources
Lack of an accurate means of calculating anti-microbial usage	Alternative land use
	Climate change
Lack of collaboration	
Lack of succession	
Lack of labour	
The water footprint	

Strengths	Opportunities
Quality and versatile product	Increase in demand
Health and welfare	Efficiency drive
UK land usage	Research and development
The brand	
The production of organic matter	

on added value products to save time and deliver a better eating experience. Beef is a versatile product and can be developed to satisfy consumer preferences, although, on the downside, over time there has been a decline in sales of the Sunday beef roasting joint. Instead, ready meals and marinades now offer opportunities for quick, easy, nutritious tasty meals at the end of the working day. Industry levy boards have focused resources into developing and marketing these options to today's consumers via multi-media campaigns.

Health and welfare

The extensive nature of the UK suckler herd production system is valued by the consumer for its perceived animal health and welfare benefits. Cows spend a good proportion of the year outside with calves at-foot, the animals are seen to be allowed to express their natural behaviours and to consume a 'natural diet' – very important realities, very important public perceptions.

UK land usage

The total UK agricultural area is 17.4 million hectares, 66% of this is grazable, and of this 38% is rough grazing which is only suitable as grassland; it cannot be ploughed and is unsuitable for dairy cows. Extensive beef production in the form of the suckler cow herd utilises these areas which are otherwise redundant and turns them into a valuable food protein source. At the same time, this unimproved grassland acts as a carbon store, and in some cases is used as flood prevention for more populated areas of the UK. Flooding is a growing problem.

The rural landscape seen today is a result of the farming methods employed over the years. Many see that farmers take responsibility for the maintenance of our landscape and for the condition of wildlife habitats; 'custodians of the countryside' as they are often described. This is thought to be part of the underpinning of the rural tourism industry. There are distinct differences in the grazing behaviours of sheep and cattle that affect sward heights, the viability of different grass and floral species, and soil structure. The interaction maintains a delicate balance and they are not interchangeable. This is important in maintaining the biodiversity and recreational value of the uplands of the UK. In addition, the farming community forms a considerable proportion of the rural population so maintains local businesses and services in these rural communities.

The brand

British beef has its own strong brand. Many supermarkets exclusively sell British beef and shout about it! Scottish beef, a subsidiary of British beef has an even stronger brand, and Welsh beef is strong too, although Welsh lamb is the real Welsh winner!

British beef is seen by some (mainly the British!) as the best in the world and part of our national heritage. Furthermore, it appears it is seen throughout the world as having been produced with very high standards of welfare and food safety in comparison to some other countries, although this is not always evidence based – just one of those all important perceptions, which is, however, probably and hopefully right.

Growth promoters are not fed to beef cattle in the UK, unlike in the USA.

Some native British breeds particularly the Hereford and Angus, have been marketed to consumers as *niche products* and therefore receive a premium as a result. Supermarkets have aligned themselves with specific breeds of cattle, again as a means of promoting a niche product to consumers.

Quality control

Assurance schemes exist to ensure safe, traceable food. Assurance schemes set out specific requirements that producers must adhere to and who are inspected on an annual basis. Although many farmers see the requirements as onerous and unjustified there is no doubt that assurance schemes have provided reassurance to consumers – farmers should remind themselves of the importance of that.

The production of organic matter

Faeces and urine produced by cows are a valuable source of organic matter and nutrients for the land, whether applied by the cows directly or indirectly spread as manure or slurry. Inorganic fertilisers are available but are tightly regulated and not environmentally popular. They contribute nutrients but no organic matter or improvement in soil structure. The use of inorganic fertilisers on grassland in Britain has been in decline since the late 1980s.

Weaknesses

Low margins

The Stocktake Report produced by the Agricultural and Horticultural Development Board (AHDB), a statutory levy board in England (not the whole of the UK), is an analysis of the physical and financial performance of hundreds of English farms. The Stocktake Report analyses the economic margins for beef and sheep enterprises only and does not take into account any alternative sources of income, such as environmental stewardship and area-based payments. The farms are classified into average, bottom third and top third, according to their *full investment net margin*. In 2016, the bottom third and average farms were making a negative full investment net margin per cow of £–445.51 and £–155.76, respectively. The top third had a positive full investment net margin of £26.53 per cow (AHDB, 2016). This was an improvement on 2015 where the bottom, average and top thirds all demonstrated a negative figure.

Length and complexity of the supply chain

The value paid for any stock, whether it be prime beef, cull cows, heifer replacements or bulls, is *dictated by the market*, and is a balance between supply and demand. The primary producer, traditionally, has limited influence over what value is paid for their produce. 'Price takers, not makers' is a phrase frequently heard within farming circles.

The implications of this are that as costs rise for the primary producer, such as cattle feed or fertiliser for example, they cannot 'pass on' this additional cost to the purchaser. In these conditions the margin falls. It is perceived by some, primary producers among them, that the convoluted supply chain that exists fails to share margin in a fair way, which in turn fails to build confidence and damages the long-term viability of this supply chain.

Reliance on subsidies

A form of subsidisation has been paid to farmers in the UK since the early 1900s, pre-EU membership. This may have been through grants and improvement schemes or subsidising feed and fertilisers. There have been many different forms of subsidisation over the years to ensure food supply is maintained, most notably after the two world wars. The biggest changes were noticed when the UK joined the European Economic Community in 1973, which saw the introduction of the CAP. The main reason for such government intervention policies was (and still is) considered to be to encourage agricultural productivity to ensure farmers have a satisfactory and equitable standard of living, and to stabilise agricultural markets and farmers' incomes. This is a slightly different emphasis from that made after the Second World War when the reason and the priority was to simply feed the people of the country!

The subsidisation of the farming industry has long been disputed within the industry itself and by the general public. This debate will remain controversial but for this exercise it will suffice to say that many consider the subsidisation of UK farming as a weakness, but many see it as a strength; the additional farm income has undoubtedly kept farmers in business, but would withdrawal of the subsidy make farming unsustainable, or would it drive a more efficient industry?

Cash flow

A typical UK spring-calving suckler farm has only two influxes of money per year: one mid-winter when the subsidy is paid, and the other in the autumn when the spring-born calves are weaned and sold. This is an extreme description as the sale of cattle may be spread over 3–4 months and there may be income from other sources, such as lamb sales on a mixed beef and sheep farm, or environmental payments. Either way, careful budgeting and cash flow management is required to maintain a successful enterprise.

Poor integration of the supply chain

As already stated, in 2019 50% of prime beef came from the dairy herd and 50% from the beef suckler herd. The contribution from the dairy herd is anticipated to rise to 70% by 2030.

This speculative increase in dairy beef is largely due to the ability of the dairy herd to produce what the retailer wants. The retailers are seeking a consistent product to minimise the range in eating quality experienced by the consumer. This requires fat cattle to be a consistent fat class, conformation, age, breed and weight at slaughter. The dairy industry seems to find this easier than the suckler industry.

The supply chain also needs to be transparent with known parentage, full medical history and traceability. Dairy farmers typically rely on AI, selecting sires based on EBVs and specification of the buyers rather than visual appearance. Service dates are recorded and, as a result, anticipated calving dates are available allowing the calf rearers and producers a solid prediction of future supply. Data collection is commonplace on dairy farms where calving interval, conception rates, mastitis incidence and cell counts have all been recorded and all been used to influence decision making for years. It is an easy transition for dairy farmers to collect disease incidence and calf growth rates to identify non-conforming animals at an early age. This is in stark contrast to many, but not all, suckler herds. The beef industry needs to become more integrated and there is much that suckler herds can do to maintain or increase their share of beef production in the UK simply by adopting these basic data recording requirements.

Lack of an accurate means of calculating antimicrobial usage

In 2017, antibiotic usage for beef cattle was an average 19 mg/kg liveweight. This was, however, calculated on just 6% of the national beef herd as at that stage there were significant limitations to the availability of such data.

The beef industry set a target of 10 mg/kg by 2020. To truly assess progress, however, a valid means of calculating antibiotic usage in beef cattle needs to be developed. The dairy, poultry and pig industry have accurate methods of recording and reporting antibiotic usage; for comparison the pig industry in 2017 used 131 mg/kg of antibiotics so in comparison the beef industry is estimated to be a relatively low user of antibiotics (RUMA, 2018).

Lack of collaboration

Collaboration between farmers has, historically, been a rarity in the industry. Yes, there have been cooperatives and initiatives but simple things like sharing equipment, machinery, labour and expertise could benefit all involved. An example would be collaboration between a spring-calving suckler herd farmer and an arable farmer. The latter could supply low-cost outwintering ground for the suckler farm in return for improved soil health.

Farming is, perhaps, an unusual industry in that the majority of farmers sell at least some of what they produce to other farmers and not just to the next stage in the supply chain, be that the wholesaler or retailer, or the consumer. An obvious example would be the supply of store cattle to a fattening unit. They are all working towards a common goal of producing food for the end user but at a business level are potentially driving deals with each other and to some extent competing with each other ultimately! This may be one reason, among others, why collaboration has traditionally been underutilised as a workable cost cutting strategy.

Lack of succession

The whole farming industry, not just beef farmers, has an ageing workforce and a lack of succession planning. Industry market research suggested that out of 700 farm businesses surveyed, less than one-half had a succession plan in place. A succession plan is needed for the smooth and successful transition of a farm between generations. This is not as easy as it sounds: equity within the farm business may be required for the older generation to retire, and it may not be as easy as just gifting the farm to the next generation. Financing the next generation's ownership of the farm is difficult with soaring land prices and rent. The equitable distribution of inheritable assets among children can also be difficult. This is clearly an area that requires specialist advice.

Lack of labour

During the 1950s and 1960s mechanisation resulted in a depletion of farm workers, leaving a core number of staff employed on a farm to satisfy the minimum labour requirements. Often seasonal workers are employed at harvest or lambing time to ensure the job gets done; the reduced profitability of many enterprises and the ever-increasing onerous legal responsibilities of being an employer has resulted in less permanent, and, instead, more casual farm workers in recent times. Owing to the long and unsociable hours and the lack of guaranteed income, the number of casual farm workers is also in decline – a clear limiting factor for many enterprises.

The water footprint

The water footprint, rather ludicrously named, is defined as a measure of the amount of water used to produce a standard unit product or service. It takes approximately 19,000 l of water to produce 1 kg of saleable beef in the UK (AHDB, 2013). As it happens, the UK's wetter climate facilitates grass growth without the need for irrigation, but, in warmer climates, the figure may be higher. Thus, the production of beef, generally, has a considerable requirement for water; 5–20 times more than crop production. Water is a valuable resource and thought needs to be given to how it can be used more efficiently.

Opportunities

Although there are considerable challenges for the industry that we have briefly highlighted and discussed there are many opportunities for British beef.

Increase in demand

The average consumption of meat globally in 2014 was 43 kg per capita per annum; the average representing a range of 100 kg/head/year in the USA down to 5 kg/head/year in India (Ritchie and Roser, 2017). Of this 2014 figure the average annual consumption of beef globally was 10.1 kg per head (Drysdale, 2016). With some sources predicting a world population of up to 9 billion in the next 10 years, then, if per capita consumption remains constant, this could equate to an overall increase in beef consumption of 42% (Drysdale, 2016). The challenge would then be to increase production of a safe, healthy, high welfare, sustainable, affordable supply of beef with minimal environmental impact but while still remaining profitable.

Efficiency drive

Can we produce more from less? The aim is to produce more meat from fewer breeding cows, less land, and less planetary resources. Improvements in fertility, health, nutrition, genetics, grazing utilisation and grassland management will result in improved efficiency. There is a vast amount of research into genetic improvement in beef cattle and this is seen by industry leaders as the main driver of efficiency. Genetic improvement has indeed been seen to result in dramatic improvements in efficiency of production in other livestock species, and if effective recording schemes are established to measure and monitor it, it will be a tool of great benefit to the beef industry too.

An example of genetic improvement is the development of the Stabiliser cattle breed. This breed is a hybrid of Hereford, Red Angus, Simmental and Gelbvieh genetics. The breed aim is to minimise costs and to increase the output of consistent, high eating quality beef from forage-based systems through various improvements including health, fertility, temperament, aggressive grazing, food conversion efficiency, easy calving and good mothering. Significant breed improvements have been made from analysing feed efficiency outcomes and selecting for feed efficiency. The UK Farm Animal Genetic Resources Committee (FAnGR) in 2015, demonstrated a saving of 12% in feed cost and about a 20% reduction in greenhouse gas (GHG) emissions by identifying the most feed efficient breeding animals upon which to base a breed – so far, an encouraging success story.

The use of genomic testing in the dairy industry is transferable to beef cattle and presents an opportunity for genetic gain. Genomic testing involves identifying genes in the animal DNA that underlie production traits. Production traits or EBVs are more commonly recorded from the performance of the offspring of an animal. With genomics these traits can be predicted from a blood or hair sample of a young animal before the animal has any offspring of its own. This greatly increases the rate at which genetic improvement can be planned and made.

Research and development

With those conducting research and development continuing to strive to help producers become more efficient, innovation needs to be implemented on farm. Knowledge transfer is required as well as a willingness by producers to adopt new knowledge, new approaches and new technology. This is not easy in an ageing, fragmented, low margin industry.

Despite a drive to reduce costs, and veterinary advice comes at a cost, vets can provide expertise and advice on a whole range of topics to improve efficiency and profitability. Vets should give value for money and provide more benefit than they cost. A vet is not best placed to do this through firefighting work alone. It is rare that the cost of a vet for an ill animal or obstetrical emergency is value for money; the damage is already done. The aim is, rather, to identify in advance where problems may arise and implement preventative measures to ensure they do not.

Threats

Antimicrobial resistance

Antimicrobial resistance (AMR) occurs when microorganisms such as bacteria, viruses, fungi and parasites change in ways that render the medications used to cure the infections they cause ineffective. (WHO, n.d.). The medications referred to are not just antibiotics but antifungal, antiviral and antiparasitic drugs also.

AMR is clearly seen as a serious threat to global public health and one that requires action. WHO recommendations aim to preserve the effectiveness of antibiotics that are important for human medicine by reducing their unnecessary use in animals.

It is, consequently, highly likely that vets and farmers cannot rely on antibiotics to prop up poor husbandry and management systems. It is possible, in the not too distant future, that beef will have to be produced without the use of any antibiotics. Although bacterial resistance to antibiotics always grabs the headlines, the term antimicrobials, as stated, includes not just antibiotics but antifungals, antivirals and antiparasitic drugs too. The emergence of resistant populations of endo- and ectoparasites, for example, is an ever-increasing problem that we face right now. It is only going to get worse if action is not taken.

Bovine tuberculosis (bTB)

Bovine tuberculosis is a notifiable infectious disease in the UK, and in certain parts of the country a high proportion of animals are infected. England is classified into *high-risk* and *low-risk* zones with a boundary around the high-risk area called *the edge* area. Statutory testing and culling are carried out to eradicate the disease. Movement restrictions and the subsequent testing regimes hamper normal trade for infected herds. (See Chapter 28 for more detail.)

Since 2011, the annual incidence of bTB within England has remained fairly constant but what is of concern is the increasing number of cases in the edge area over recent years, resulting in previously uninfected herds becoming infected. In effect, the disease is spreading across the country. This is a significant threat to those in the edge and low-risk areas and they may have to adjust to running their enterprises around bTB restrictions, something they have not previously had to do.

Changing markets

The political environment has the potential to influence trade and subsidy payments and it is not known whether this is yet a threat or opportunity. The level of uncertainty it provokes is not healthy for the industry and prevents further investment and planning. Businesses have little or no control over the outcome of political decision making yet have to deal with the consequences.

Vegetarianism, veganism and flexitarianism

Much research has been carried out by the beef industry to understand the personal motives behind vegetarianism, veganism and flexitarianism and for the rise in consumption of plant-based food products. The motivators for becoming vegan in descending order of popularity are: animal welfare, to improve personal health, environmental impact of meat production, food security and sustainability, attractiveness of vegan products as an alternative food, proof of food identity and the accuracy of the labelling of meat products (AHDB, 2018).

Market research carried out in 2018, suggested that 91% of UK households buy red meat leaving 9% that do not. Of the UK population 2% claim to be vegans and 2% flexitarians. Given these, thus far, relatively small numbers of red meat abstainers, many blame disproportionate media coverage for the drive towards meat reduction in the diet, and the quick response of food manufacturers and retailers in their development of meat alternatives. These meat alternatives can be categorised into two categories. The first category is plant-based foods where the protein substitution is not designed to mimic meat and vegetables; here, typically, legumes are used as the alternative to meat. The second category is *pseudo-meat* where the product is plant-based but manufactured to have an appearance and eating experience similar to meat. Many of the meat-alternative products are consumed by both meat eaters and non-meat eaters.

The number of people who choose to limit their meat consumption for whatever reason will, according to the statistical analysis, almost certainly continue to grow.

Alternative meat sources

Fish, lamb, pork and poultry are all traditional alternative sources of protein in a meat-eater's diet, and they are each in competition with each other to be the consumer's choice. Lots of different factors will influence this choice: price, perceived health benefits, medical campaigns, taste, convenience and previous experiences. What makes someone choose beef instead of chicken, pork or lamb? This is a continuous area of market research and marketing effort to ensure beef still has a place on the plate of the UK public.

Cultured meat or 'clean meat' cultured in a laboratory environment using foetal calf serum is an area of development. The main limiting factor is cost: 1 kg of cultured meat currently costs US$800 to produce (AHDB, 2018) although with new technology the cost is rapidly decreasing. The production of meat without the source being animals is on the horizon and is an additional threat to traditional beef production.

Alternative land use

Of UK agricultural land 38% is marginal grazing unsuitable for dairy cows or crop production. This land is the home of the suckler cow and of sheep. However, this once low value landscape is being fought over for operations other than farming. This in turn increases the price of this land. These alternative uses include:

- field sports such as deer, pheasant and grouse shooting
- forestry
- public access and recreation
- mineral extraction – coal, stone, lead and copper
- water supply – the uplands provide water catchment areas for lowland water supplies
- power generation – predominantly wind and hydro-electric power farms, some solar farms
- military training.

Climate change

Climate change in relation to cattle rearing is a highly emotive subject and has been scrutinised and publicised widely by the media. In simple terms cattle are blamed for their contribution to the production of GHGs. Let us look at the facts.

GHGs are defined as any gaseous compounds in the atmosphere that are capable of absorbing infrared radiation, thereby trapping and holding heat in the atmosphere. By increasing the heat in the atmosphere, GHGs are responsible for the well documented greenhouse effect, which ultimately leads to global warming. Global warming is then responsible for the rise in average temperatures on the earth's surface, the melting of the ice caps, the rise in global sea level, more extreme weather systems and changes in the ecosystems of the planet.

Methane, carbon dioxide and nitrous oxide are all recognised GHGs. They each vary in how they behave as greenhouse gases. For example, they all deteriorate in the atmosphere at different rates and they each have different infrared absorbancies. For standardisation the gases are classified in terms of 'carbon equivalents', which takes their different attributes into consideration.

Agriculture is a known source of GHGs. In the UK, agriculture contributes 7% of all GHG emissions (EBLEX, 2009a): 3.1% of all UK GHG emissions were attributed to livestock. Of the emissions from agriculture generally, 37% is methane produced from fermentation in the rumen of sheep and cattle, 67% is nitrous oxide, which comes from using arable crops as animal feed, and fertiliser on grassland, and 1% is carbon dioxide.

Extensive livestock systems are thought to have a higher carbon equivalent cost per kilogramme of meat produced as there is less efficient digestion in the rumen, and lower quality forage generates higher methane emissions, and the animal has a slower growth rate so takes longer to reach slaughter.

Grazing land utilised by hill sheep and suckler cows *stores carbon*; this land is then known as a 'carbon sink' or a 'carbon trap'.

A ruminant fed a diet with a higher proportion of cereal rather than forage produces less methane *but GHGs are generated in the production of the cereal feed.*

Beef from the dairy herd is considered less of a problem as the carbon equivalent cost is *shared between beef and milk production* whereas in the suckler herd the carbon cost is solely borne by the beef alone.

Beef imported into the UK is mostly of suckler herd origin rather than dairy. This combined with the carbon cost of the extra transportation means that importing beef increases the overall carbon footprint of beef consumption in the UK.

The GHG emissions from livestock farming are actually declining and for two reasons. First, there are less cattle and sheep as numbers decline due to economic pressures. This merely transfers production and therefore emissions to other parts of the world and is not considered a strategy to achieve global GHG reduction targets. Second, efficiency has improved: 5% fewer prime animals were required to produce each tonne of meat in 2008 compared to 1998 (EBLEX, 2009a).

The carbon equivalent cost per kilogramme of meat produced declines as systems become more efficient. Good, simple farming efficiency is now the main strategy employed to decrease the carbon equivalent cost of beef production in the UK.

REFERENCES

AHDB (2013) Water use, reduction and rainwater harvesting on beef and sheep farms. Available at: https://media.ahdb.org.uk/media/Default/Imported%20Publication%20Docs/Water-use-reduction-and-rainwater-harvesting-on-beef-and-sheep-farms.pdf.

AHDB (2016) *Stocktake Report AHDB Beef and Lamb.* Agriculture and Horticulture Development Board, Stoneleigh.

AHDB (2018) *Consumer Insights.* Agriculture and Horticulture Development Board, Stoneleigh.

Binnie, M., Barlow, K., Johnson, V. and Harrison, C. (2014) Red meats: time for a paradigm shift in dietary advice. *Meat Science* 98(3), 445–51.

Drysdale, R. (2016) Beef from the dairy herd: is integration the answer? The Trehane Trust, Nuffield Farming Scholarships Trust.

EBLEX (2009a) The English Beef and Sheep Production Roadmap – Phase 1. Change in the air. Agriculture and Horticulture Development Board, Stoneleigh.

EBLEX (2009b) In the balance? The future of the English Beef Industry. Agriculture and Horticulture Development Board, Stoneleigh.

Farm Animal Genetic Resources Committee (FAnGR) (2015) Report on how beef genetics can help increase the profitability of UK beef farmers. Department for Environment Food & Rural Affairs, London.

Ritchie, H. and Roser, M. (2020) Meat and dairy production. Available at https://ourworldindata.org/meat-production.

RUMA (2018) Targets task force: one year on. Available at: https://www.ruma.org.uk/wp-content/uploads/2018/11/RUMA-TTF-1-year-on-Full-Report-FINAL.pdf.

WHO (n.d.) Available at https://www.who.int/news-room/fact-sheets/detail/antimicrobial-resistance#:~:text=Antimicrobial%20Resistance%20(AMR)%20occurs%20when,spread%2C%20severe%20illness%20and%20death.

Chapter 3

General health and welfare in the beef herd

HEALTH

Stark statistics from the UK national beef herd suggest there are improvements needed in many areas to improve health and welfare. These changes will also improve the efficiency of the beef enterprise. For example, the CHAWG report published in 2012 reported that 1 in 13 beef calves were dying on farm, and collectively in the beef and dairy industry, 240,000 adult cattle also died each year from unknown causes. In England alone, 306,499 livers were condemned at slaughter as a result of liver fluke damage with an estimated loss of £1,225,996.

Fertility, as well as health, is another important area of efficiency. In 2017, the average calving interval in England and Wales was 420 days; 55 days longer than the target of 365. If improvements in fertility could be made to achieve a 365 day calving interval, then 15% more calves could be produced from the same number of cows.

There is more that vets and farmers can do together to improve health, welfare, fertility and productivity, and there is a wide range of support available to help facilitate this activity. For example, there are cattle health schemes for a wide range of diseases that help farmers to monitor, control and eradicate disease, and obtain accredited disease-free health status for their herd. Government funding has been available in England, Scotland and Wales for regional and national bovine viral diarrhoea (BVD) eradication programmes.

Breed societies, the National Fallen Stock Company, the British Cattle Movement Service (BCMS) and abattoirs are all working together to provide health related data for the industry as a whole. There is support at farm level from private vets and the AHDB to help with on-farm data collection and to establish regional health and disease incidence benchmarking groups.

Farm assurance schemes have enforced veterinary-led annual health reviews and antibiotic auditing. Auditing of all medicine usage has increased and as a result data and advice is now available from The Responsible Use of Medicines in Agriculture Alliance (RUMA), Control of Worms Sustainably (COWS) and AHDB.

Farmers have a legal responsibility for their animals' welfare, and a duty to provide for their needs. But what does this actually mean?

The Five Freedoms are the five basic requirements of animals in order for them to have an acceptable quality of life. They are:

1. freedom from hunger and thirst
2. freedom from discomfort
3. freedom from pain, injury and disease
4. freedom to express normal behaviour
5. freedom from fear or distress.

The Five Freedoms were developed in the 1960s and 1970s and released by the UK Farm Animal Welfare Council (now known as the Farm Animal Welfare Advisory Committee) in 1979 and further consolidated in 2009 (FAWC, 2009). The Five Freedoms are based on the avoidance of unnecessary suffering and the provision of needs. This is now considered the most basic of welfare standards and a more holistic approach is required with an animal's quality of life being assessed as either 'a life not worth living', 'a life worth living' or 'a good life'. This assessment takes into account the animal's whole life from birth through to death, and to have lives worth living it is necessary, overall, to minimise negative experiences but to also provide positive experiences. This method of welfare classification relies on a judgement made by a person acting on behalf of the animal's interests, it is a reflection of how we feel when experiencing a physical or social environment and is therefore largely dictated by us.

The biggest welfare concerns for beef cattle, specifically highlighted by the European Food Safety Authority, relate to respiratory disease, the mixing of cattle, lack of ventilation, feeding high concentrate and low roughage diets and the employment of poor floor surfaces, such as slatted sheds.

The importance of measuring and monitoring welfare outcomes for the delivery of good or improved animal welfare is increasingly recognised. In the UK, welfare scoring or welfare audits are carried out in the pig and dairy industry but not routinely in the beef industry. The assessments take into account different aspects of the animals themselves, and their environments and management both on-farm and at slaughter. Points are scored for up to 50 different aspects of the animal's life and are compiled to form a final welfare score.

For example, a pig welfare assessment in the UK is mandatory under Red Tractor assurance schemes. It is carried out by a trained vet from the Pig Veterinary Society, two to four times a year, and objectively assesses a sample pen of finisher pigs; the number of pigs examined is a reflection of the number of pigs finished per year. The vet scores the number of lame pigs, the number of cases of tail damage, the number of body marks, the number of pigs that require removal to a hospital pen, how dirty the pigs are, and the level of environmental enrichment provision and the extent of its use.

Welfare assessments do exist for beef production but are not required by all beef assurance schemes. If the animal-based 'welfare outcomes' of the pig industry were extrapolated to beef animals then welfare assessments could include: incidence of lameness, body condition, cleanliness, hair loss lesions and swellings. On a beef suckler farm, further information on methods of castration and dehorning, and the incidence of dystocia would also be useful in the assessment of welfare.

The welfare of farmed animals has progressively become a significant focus of public attention. Although mandatory UK welfare cattle codes ensure basic standards are met, farm assurance schemes exceed these standards in order to reassure the public that the scheme sourced meat they eat is from animals reared within high standards of welfare throughout their life, including the lead up to and execution of slaughter.

Gaining an understanding of an animal's behavioural and physiological needs is the cornerstone that enables farming systems that promote positive welfare to be developed. It is essential that a stockperson can recognise, specifically, an animal in pain. Pain is relatively subjective; it is described as an unpleasant sensory and emotional experience associated with actual or potential tissue damage. Neural pain pathways in mammals are similar to those of humans who are, of course, also mammals, so it can be assumed that pain is experienced in the same, or a similar way. However, the perception of what is painful varies among the population of farmers and vets (Leslie and Petersson-Wolfe, 2012). This has been demonstrated by assessing the responses of individuals to the severity of pain associated with various conditions on a 10-point scale, 1 being non-painful to 10 being extremely painful. For example; a study of veterinary respondents rated mastitis as an average pain level of 7 comparable to a foot abscess or limb fracture. There were notably different responses between male and female vets, and older versus younger graduates (Huxley and Whay, 2006). This clearly demonstrated the variability in the human assessment of animal pain even within highly trained individuals.

There are both physiological and behavioural responses to pain. A physiological response may be an increase in heart rate whereas a behavioural response may be to move away from the stimulus or to vocalise when anticipating or experiencing pain. Cattle are fairly stoical animals and for their survival in the wild they have evolved not to outwardly show pain or disease as presumably it is a perceived sign of weakness which could attract predation or exclusion from the group.

There are signs, although somewhat non-specific, of pain that farmers and vets need to be aware of (Hudson et al., 2008):

- decreased motion/locomotion
- decreased interaction with other animals in the group
- decreased feed intakes, indicated by a hollow flank from poor rumen fill
- looking at the source of pain, for example, flank watching with abdominal discomfort
- change in posture, lying recumbent, lowered head
- trembling, sweating or an increased respiratory rate
- teeth grinding (bruxism)
- poor coat condition from decreased grooming.

Acute pain (short last) differs from chronic pain, the latter being consistent and unrelenting. Chronic pain results in one of two scenarios: (1) hyperalgesia – a lowered pain threshold so that *low-pain* stimuli now cause notable pain to the animal; (2) allodynia in which normally *non-painful* stimuli are perceived as painful (Hudson et al., 2008).

The control of chronic pain in farm animals is difficult due to the lack of licensed long-term pain relief medicines. Euthanasia should be considered where pain cannot be adequately controlled.

There are many modes of pain relief (analgesia) and if a painful procedure is anticipated the analgesic should be administered in advance and allowed time to work. As many modes of analgesia as possible, should be used. For example, during dehorning or castration, a local anaesthetic infiltrated at the site of surgery and a non-steroidal anti-inflammatory (NSAID) can be used. In addition, a mild sedative can also provide some analgesia, as well as making the procedure less stressful for the animal, farmer and vet, and also, importantly, reducing the risk of injury to the animal and personnel (see Chapter 28).

GENERAL HEALTH AND THE CLINICAL EXAMINATION

The external appearance of an animal gives us a wealth of information about its general health and well-being, be it in the short or long term. Is its body language telling you something? Is its coat or posture revealing a problem?

The head and neck

Starting at the front! The nose of the normal animal is wet or moist with nothing emerging from the nostrils other than a small amount of clear discharge. The skin of the nose, or the naso-labial plane, as it is called in cattle, should be intact with no ulceration or peeling. Excess salivation or regurgitation of rumen contents should not be evident. The mouth can be examined relatively easily in the placid animal by holding the nose and placing a hand in the gap between the incisors and the molar teeth to lever open the mouth. The tongue can be grasped but this is usually met with resentment. Abnormalities in the mouth would include lodged food, ulcers, bleeding, a bad smell or skin peeling from the tongue. It is important to look underneath the tongue as this is a common location for foreign material to get stuck, such as sticks, wire or bale wrapping. The teeth should all be present and in appropriate alignment.

The eyes of the normal animal are bright and alert with both eyelids symmetrical when the animal is viewed from the front. There should be no discharge from the eyes. In the sick animal the eye may appear sunken – this is an indication of moderate to severe dehydration. There should be little or no tear wetting or staining of the face. The ears should be freely mobile and again symmetrical when viewed from the front; some asymmetric movement of the ears is a normal function of auditory behaviour, but a one-sided persistent dropping of an ear is a significant finding.

When examining the area under the jaw, throat, neck and belly of the animal any lumps, bumps and swellings should be noted as potentially abnormal.

General condition, body condition score, rumen fill and abdominal shape

The general condition of the whole body can be assessed and measured on a scale of 1–5; what is known as the body condition score (BCS) scale, discussed further in Chapter 10. Alongside the BCS, rumen fill can be assessed also. The rumen occupies the left side of the abdomen and the back end of this large vat extends backwards beyond the last rib to sit in the left flank. When it is full it packs out the hollow of the flank under the vertebrae – the hollow known as the sublumbar fossa. An animal that looks empty, that is with poor rumen fill, will not have been eating. This is sometimes difficult to determine if the cow is heavily in-calf. A calf can inevitably fill up the abdomen to some extent and leave the cow looking full even though the calf sits low in the abdomen – the abdominal contents inevitably get pushed up a bit. Conversely, a large rumen can hang low in the abdomen without necessarily filling the sublumbar fossa and such a cow can look heavily pregnant without being so and can look rather empty in the sublumbar fossa at the same time as looking rather rotund.

The gastrointestinal tract (gut)

The rumen (Figure 3.1) should turn over (have a muscular contraction) approximately once a minute. This can be felt by pressing firmly on the sublumbar fossa and waiting or it can be heard using a stethoscope placed in the sublumbar fossa. A stethoscope is also useful to listen for excessive gas present in the gastrointestinal system. An air-filled stomach or piece of gut will 'ping' when listened to with a stethoscope while flicking the immediately adjacent area with a finger and thumb of the other hand.

The skin and coat

The quality of an animal's skin and coat, its outer layer, the integument, is an indication of its long-standing health or lack of. A dull, dry, thin or patchy coat can be a sign of ill health. The skin should be supple and smooth and covered in hair. The animal should not be itchy, scabby or scaly. The skin should feel warm but not hot and should not be sweaty under normal conditions.

The udder

The udder of the normal cow is an even colour across all four-quarters, each of which being approximately the same size. The normal udder is soft, supple and non-painful when palpated (felt). In the lactating animal each teat can be 'fore milked' ('stripped') (briefly milked) and the consistency of the milk assessed; normally it is white and without blood or clots although the freshly calved cow produces colostrum, which is more yellow and thick. Occasionally the fresh calved cow has blood in the milk. While not ideal this bursting of a small blood vessel is relatively normal but does need to be distinguished from abnormal milk in the udder, which can accompany infection, and will generally make the cow ill and the milk appear abnormal in other ways, such as appearing watery or clotty.

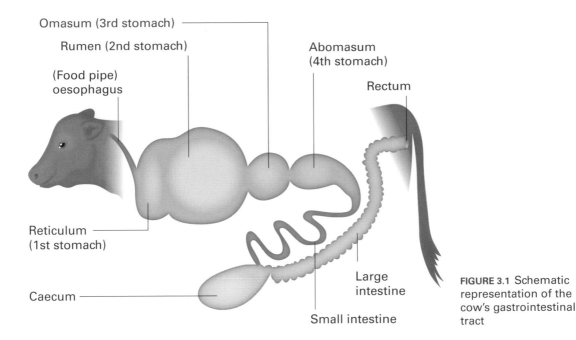

Omasum (3rd stomach)

Rumen (2nd stomach)

(Food pipe) oesophagus

Abomasum (4th stomach)

Rectum

Reticulum (1st stomach)

Caecum

Large intestine

Small intestine

FIGURE 3.1 Schematic representation of the cow's gastrointestinal tract

The external genitalia, perineum, tail and anal region

In the case of the male animal, the prepuce (sheath) and testicles should be examined, or perhaps, in some cases, more safely, inspected from a slight distance! The prepuce may be wet with urine but the hairs on the prepuce should be free from white crystalline deposits as this can be an indication of urinary crystals or stones (calculi). The penis is not routinely examined as it is difficult to extrude from the prepuce. There should be two testicles, symmetrical and freely movable within the scrotum. The skin of the normal scrotum is soft, scab free and pale pink in a light skinned animal, dark in a heavily pigmented breed.

The tail should have tone as should the anus. There should be no faecal or urine staining of the back end of the animal in the area around and beneath the anus, the area known as the perineum. There should be no discharge from the vulva apart from when the female is in season (oestrus, bulling) – at this time a clear or bloody discharge is normal. The skin of the vulva should be free from ulceration or sores. The lining of the vulva should be the colour of cooked salmon, not white (anaemic) and not brick red (toxic).

Gait

The animal should be examined for lameness by walking along a smooth flat surface in a straight line. Leg and foot conformation are important and any swelling on the limbs should be noted. The pelvis and legs should be symmetrical when viewed from behind.

Temperature

The temperature of cattle is assessed by inserting a thermometer into the rectum. The thermometer should be lubricated and gently inserted but deviated to one side so the sensor is in contact with the lining of the rectum and not the lumen of the rectum which may give a falsely low reading especially if there is air present, for example, if the animal has just been examined internally. A high temperature is indicative of heat stress or disease.

TABLE 3.1 The normal range of temperature, respiratory rate and heart rate of three different ages of cattle

	Temperature	Respiratory rate	Heart rate
Newborn calf	38.5–40.5°C (101.3–104.9°F)	–	100–130/minute
Calf 1 year and under	38.5–39.5°C (101.3–103.1°F)	30–50/minute	80–110/minute
Cow	38.0–39.0°C (100.4–102.2°F)	10–30/minute	50–80/minute

Source: Hulsen (2006).

A raised temperature is part of the cows immune and inflammatory response. A low temperature can be a sign of hypothermia or the advanced stages of disease where peripheral circulation is compromised or the body systems have begun shutting down.

Heart rate

The heart can be listened to (auscultated) on the left and right side of the chest just behind the point of the elbow using a stethoscope. The heart beats should be clearly audible, no murmurs should be present and there should be a fairly even rhythm and normal frequency (Table 3.1).

Respiratory rate

Otherwise, and actually more correctly, known as the breathing rate, an elevation here can be an indication of pain and/or disease, not always necessarily specific to the respiratory system. The pattern of breathing is also important. Is there more effort on inspiration or expiration? Is there a noise audible (without a stethoscope)? A stethoscope can be used to listen for noise or sometimes the absence of noise – an equally significant finding.

THE CLINICAL EXAMINATION

It is often said that to recognise the abnormal one must first recognise that which is normal. Repeated inspection and examination of normal animals helps with the subsequent recognition of something out of the ordinary; something not quite right.

Any animal that appears to be ill or injured should be cared for straight away. A basic inspection or basic examination may reveal the problem. The solution to the problem may already be known and can, in which case, be implemented. It may be that animal requires some first-aid style intervention. If there is any doubt over the best course of action a veterinary surgeon should be contacted immediately.

A veterinary surgeon will perform a full examination, which includes an internal examination of the cow. This involves inserting a lubricated gloved hand into the rectum. The vet then feels the contents of the abdomen indirectly through the wall of the rectum. Such an internal examination allows examination, albeit a limited one, of the left kidney, a portion of the gastrointestinal tract, the bladder, the internal reproductive tract (uterus, ovaries and cervix of the female, a calf, or in the case of the male, the accessory sex glands). Faecal consistency and the shape of the pelvis can also be assessed. A veterinary surgeon may also perform a vaginal examination by cleaning the vulva and inserting a clean, gloved hand through the vulva to assess the cervix, vagina and any discharge, retained foetal membranes or any calf or aborting foetus that may be stuck or on its way out. Figure 3.2 shows the basic equipment required for a full clinical examination.

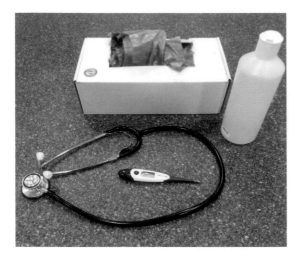

FIGURE 3.2 Equipment needed to carry out an examination of a bovine animal: lubricant, thermometer, stethoscope and rectal gloves

Blood testing

A blood sample can be taken from the tail vein or neck vein (jugular) of a cow but, according to UK law, only by a veterinary surgeon. Most commonly the tail vein is used. With practice it is a quick, relatively easy procedure. Blood is sampled into tubes, Figure 3.3, that contain different anticoagulants,

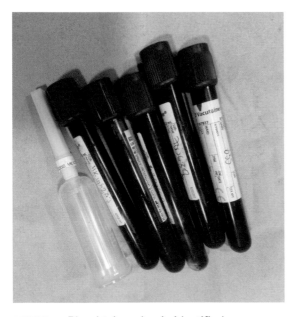

FIGURE 3.3 Blood tubes clearly identified

indicated by the colour of the tops, the choice of which depending on the tests required. The tubes used are evacuated to facilitate easy collection of blood. They should be labelled with the identification of the cow immediately to avoid any confusion.

Isolation

Sick or injured animals may require isolation for their own well-being, that is to protect them from bullying, but, also, in the case of contagious disease, to prevent further spread. Every farm should have a contingency plan for sick animals and that should include the provision of appropriate hospital pens, which are easily accessible for the frequent checking of sick patients. The pens need to be clean, dry, draught free and well bedded. Good light and easy access to feed and water are also essential. They should not share air space with other non-sick animals nor should their effluent reach them.

FEEDING THE RUMINANT

The rumen is, in effect, a large fermentation vat that is reliant on the mutually beneficial relationship between the cow and the microbes within it. The diet consists of fibre, protein, starch, sugars and oil; it is digested and fermented by the rumen microbes to produce carbon dioxide, methane, microbial protein and short chain fatty acids (butyric acid, propionic acid and acetic acid).

The carbon dioxide and methane are released as gas. The microbial protein passes through the rumen and is broken down and absorbed in the small intestine. The short chain fatty acids (SCFA) are absorbed into the bloodstream and processed in the liver to release energy. The proportions of SCFA produced depends on the constituents of the diet. A more fibrous, especially long-fibre, diet, such as hay, will lead to more acetate production, whereas readily digestible forages, such as grass or silage, tend to lead to a higher proportion of propionate production. Increasing the concentrate to forage ratio significantly increases propionate production.

For the microbes in the rumen to work effectively, the rumen environment needs to be suitable for their survival. The pH is crucial, the rumen should stay between pH 6 and 7 (Grove-White, 2004). Rumination or chewing the cud increases saliva production. This is where food that has already been partially chewed and swallowed is regurgitated and chewed again; the more fibre there is in the diet, the more rumination and saliva production will take place. Saliva contains bicarbonate, which is alkaline and neutralises the acidity of the stomach, so maintaining a stable pH.

A diet high in starch (cereals) and low in fibre will result in an acidic suboptimal ruminal pH where the microbes are unable to function efficiently. This is more commonly the case in very energy-dense diets used in beef finisher systems.

To maintain consistent ruminal conditions any dietary changes should be done gradually so the microbial population can adjust. Feeding times should be consistent and periods of time without any food should be avoided.

The digestibility of the feedstuffs influences the rate of digestion. Root crops and cereals are highly digestible and pass through the rumen quickly, whereas hay and straw are less digestible and have a slower transit time.

Energy and protein

The two key components of ruminant nutrition are energy and protein (Figure 3.4).

- Metabolisable energy (ME) is quoted in ration formulations often as MJ/kg DM – megajoules per kilogramme of dry matter (DM). It comprises fermentable ME (FME), such as carbohydrates and fibre, available to rumen microbes, and non-fermentable energy, such as oils and volatile fatty acids, which are a source of nutrition for the ruminant itself but not the microbes.
- Similarly, metabolisable protein (MP) is a combination of digestible undegradable protein

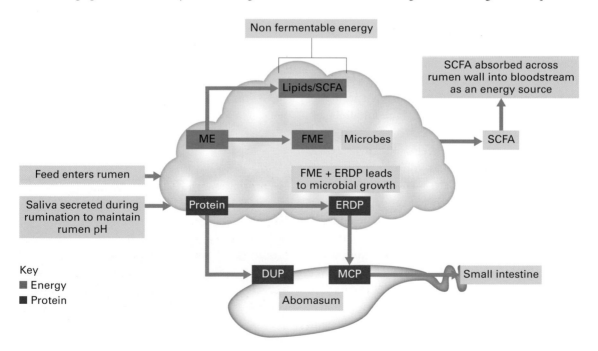

FIGURE 3.4 Energy and protein metabolism in the rumen

(DUP) fed directly to the animal, and the microbial protein (MCP) (the microbe itself!) assimilated by the microbe from its enjoyment of dietary effective rumen degradable protein (ERDP) and by using FME as the necessary energy source for building the microbial protein.

Water

Water is essential for life, and for rumen function. Clean fresh water should be available at all times – for all ages of cattle. There should be sufficient room for 10% of the cattle in a group to be able to drink at the same time.

A dry suckler cow will consume between 14 and 40 l of water per day. According to BRP+ Better Cattle Housing Design guidelines a suckler cow in early lactation drinks between 50 and 70 l per day (AHDB, 2018). Studies suggest that the temperature of the drinking water does not affect intakes (Robertson, 2018), but water supplies and troughs do, however, need to be protected from freezing which does of course drastically affect intake.

The water provided needs to be clean. A glass of water from a cow trough should appear nearly that out of a household tap, free of contamination, discoloration and smell. Figure 3.5 is a glass of water from the non-tippable trough in Figure 3.6; heavily contaminated and not fit for human or animal consumption.

Unlike temperature effects, tainted or rancid water *will* decrease intakes. Most of the research carried out into bacterial contamination of water is related to zoonotic pathogens – pathogens that affect both animals and humans, for example, *Salmonella* spp., *Escherichia coli, Cryptosporidium parvum* and *Campylobacter spp. Salmonella* can survive in water for up to 54 days and *C. parvum* for 6 months at 5–15°C (Robertson, 2018). *Bacillus licheniformis* is a cause of abortion and stillbirth in cattle and has been found in high levels – up to 5 million colony-forming units per gram – in contaminated water troughs (Stevenson, 2017).

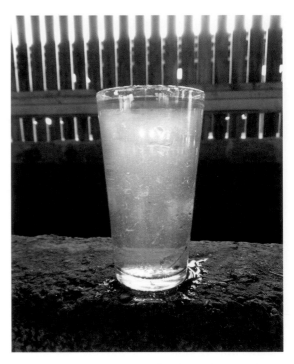

FIGURE 3.5 Dirty water sampled from the trough pictured in Figure 3.6

Contamination from bits of forage dropping out of cows' mouths, and faeces and urine, is inevitable but can be minimised if thought is given to trough height and design. Water troughs should be cleaned out regularly; tipping troughs are a great concept and can be cleaned out easily (Figure 3.7a and 3.7b).

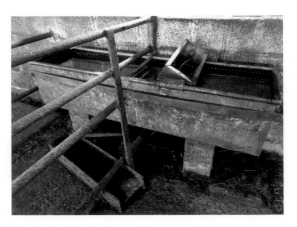

FIGURE 3.6 A metal non-tippable trough

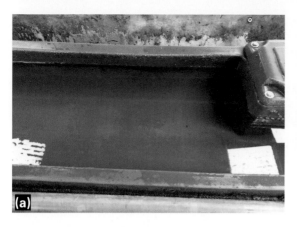 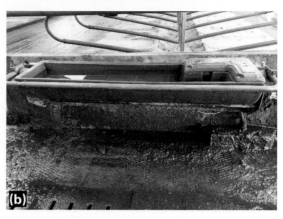

FIGURE 3.7 (a and b) A durable plastic tippable water trough

REFERENCES

AHDB (2018) *Better Cattle Housing Design BRP+*. Agriculture and Horticulture Development Board, Stoneleigh.

FAWC (2009). *Farm Animal Welfare in Great Britain: Past, Present and Future*. Farm Animal Welfare Council, London.

Grove-White, D. (2004) Rumen healthcare in the dairy cow. *In Practice* 26, 88–95.

Hudson, C., Whay, H. and Huxley, J. (2008) Recognition and management of pain in cattle. *In Practice* 30, 126–134

Hulsen, J. (2006) *Cow Signals. A Practical Guide to Dairy Farm Management*, 1st edn. Roodbont Publishers, Zutphen.

Huxley, J.N. and Whay, H.R. (2006) Current attitudes of cattle practitioners to pain and the use of analgesics in cattle. *Veterinary Record* 159, 662–668.

Leslie, K.E. and Petersson-Wolfe, C.S. (2012) Assessment and management of pain in dairy cows with clinical mastitis. *Veterinary Clinics of North America: Food Animal Practice* 28, 289–305.

Robertson, J.F. (2018) Water: the good, the bad, and the ugly. *Cattle Practice* 26(2), 105–112.

Stevenson, H. (2017) Bacillus licheniformis abortion in cattle. *Cattle Practice* 25(3), 207.

Part II

The health and management of the beef herd

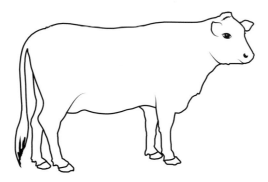

Chapter 4

The health and management of the neonatal calf

THE LEAD UP TO BIRTH

In the relative safety of its mother's uterus the calf receives all its needs for its, as yet, unborn life: obvious needs such as warmth and protection but more refined needs such as oxygen, water, electrolytes (minerals), sugars (carbohydrate), amino acids (protein) and lipids (fat), all via the structure known as the *placenta*. The placenta is a unique, temporary, organ that forms only during pregnancy. Here an extension of the calf's circulation, the umbilicus, intertwines with an extension of the cow's circulation in the 'buttons' that line the pregnant uterus. These buttons are part cow, the *caruncle*, and part placenta, the *cotyledon* (Figures 4.1 and 4.2). An extraordinarily efficient transfer of these vital supplies takes place across this subtle interface that separates the calf's blood from the cow's blood – little more than the thickness of two capillary walls. The transfer is an exchange – as well as supplying all these things, the mother's blood also extracts carbon dioxide and certain waste products back out of the calf's blood as the calf, at this stage, has no access to air for the lungs to do their own exchange with.

At birth this extraordinary lifeline is abruptly cut as the umbilical vessels are stretched, and, eventually snapped, in the course of the calf being born. In the first instance it is the obtaining of oxygen and the removal of carbon dioxide that are the calf's biggest priorities. The calf's brain rapidly detects this requirement – interestingly it is the build-up of carbon dioxide that most registers with the brain receptors rather than the lack of oxygen, but both do count. The brain then instinctively fires off the electric nerve impulses to the chest muscles and the diaphragm to take that all important, and for the farmer, if present, eagerly awaited first breath. This, however, is not just as straightforward as that. The lungs up until this

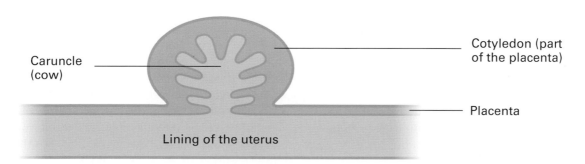

Caruncle (cow)

Cotyledon (part of the placenta)

Placenta

Lining of the uterus

FIGURE 4.1 Diagram of one of multiple caruncle and cotyledon units that line the uterus

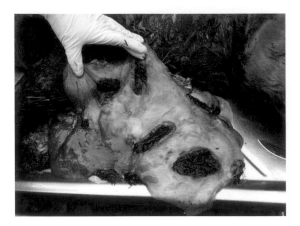

FIGURE 4.2 Bovine placenta post-calving showing red circular cotyledons

point have been fluid soaked and not the air filled 'sponges' they need to be. It is a 'good squeeze' that helps here – as the calf is squeezed out through the birth canal a lot of this fluid is pressed out into the mouth and either swallowed or dribbled out. The inflation of the lungs is then made that little bit easier (the calf born by caesarean does not get this little squeeze and misses out a little on nature's helping hand). But something else helps this inflation process, enough for the caesar calf to get away with not getting the squeeze, and that something is 'surfactant'.

Surfactant is a detergent-like chemical produced by cells in the lung in the very last stages of pregnancy – it cleverly bubbles up on first inhalation and helps the air chambers of the lungs inflate. The high surface tension of these air bubbles helps them stay intact and keep the chambers inflated. Well known to paediatric units, it is lack of surfactant that hinders breathing in premature babies and the same applies to other animals.

In the lead up to giving birth various hormonal/chemical signals get sent around the cow's body, and the calf's body too, thanks to the permeability of the placenta. These hormonal changes are complicated and not fully understood but in part at least involve the mature placenta/uterus releasing a natural prostaglandin, which 'knocks out' the corpus luteum on the ovary. Bearing in mind that it is the corpus luteum that produces

progesterone and that a constant supply of progesterone is necessary for pregnancy then it is this event that marks the beginning of the end of pregnancy (further information in Chapter 10), but clearly a sequence of other events is kicked off too: the release of *relaxin* – a muscle relaxing hormone to soften and dilate the birth canal, the release of *prolactin*, a hormone that stimulates milk production, and the release of *corticosteroids* and *thyroxine* (in the case of the last two, from the calf itself), which stimulate the birthing process to commence.

EUTOCIA (NORMAL BIRTH)

All things normal a calf should be born front feet first with the nose only slightly behind the feet.

The calf will ideally be born within 2 hours of the onset of straining. Straining for more than 1 hour without progress warrants further investigation (Chapter 17).

As the calf falls from the standing cow, or, as the cow stands up from a 'recumbent' (lying down) labour then the umbilical vessels will stretch, narrow and snap, usually without concern. A normal calf should then breathe within 30 seconds of birth – this may start deeply and erratically initially but after a few minutes should settle down to around 45–60 breaths per minute (Grove-White, 2000).

Calves born falling from the standing cow will often have burst out of the 'sac', that is the foetal membrane which wraps around the calf and holds all the fluid in. There are actually two membranes or sacs – the amniotic sac and the allantoic sac (Figure 4.3).

Sometimes a calf does not burst out of the sac and this is slightly more likely in a recumbent delivery where the calf gently slides out rather than drops out. Here the mothering instincts of the cow hopefully save the day; the cow licks the membranes clear of the nose allowing the calf to breath. Calves born to heifers or less instinctive mothers are more at risk. Figure 4.4 shows a newborn calf

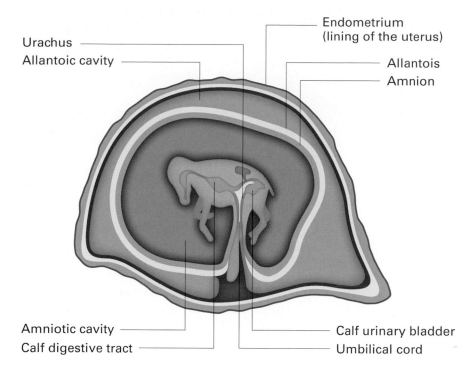

Urachus
Allantoic cavity

Endometrium
(lining of the uterus)

Allantois
Amnion

Amniotic cavity
Calf digestive tract

Calf urinary bladder
Umbilical cord

FIGURE 4.3 Diagram showing the uterus and foetus within the foetal membranes: outer allantoic and inner amniotic sac

minutes after an uneventful birth taking its first few breaths.

DYSTOCIA (DIFFICULT BIRTH)

Difficult births, whether it be an awkward presentation or a strenuous pull with the calving aid, is covered further in Chapter 17. Dystocia may result in the death of the calf immediately before, during or after calving. The calf may survive but suffer bruising from the trauma and may be deprived of

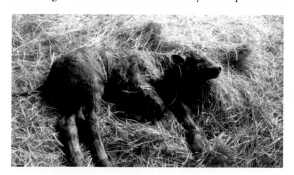

FIGURE 4.4 Newborn calf

oxygen. A calf suffering complications at birth is predisposed to disease later in the neonatal period.

SITTING, STANDING, SUCKING

The time taken from birth to the calf sitting up (Figure 4.5, sternal recumbency) and holding its own head up is considered a good predictor of calf survival. Typically calves with an unassisted, stress-free birth sit up 2–6 minutes after birth; calves which have been assisted typically take 6–12 minutes. Calves taking over 15 minutes to sit up are significantly less likely to survive past 7 days of age (Schuijt et al., 1994).

The calf should stand, locate its mother's teats, latch on and suck ideally within 1 hour of birth. This is all instinctive behaviour and should happen on its own. If not, then the calf can be assisted, with a towel used as a sling under its chest and abdomen, and helped to find its mother's teat – this needs care for personal safety, and patience.

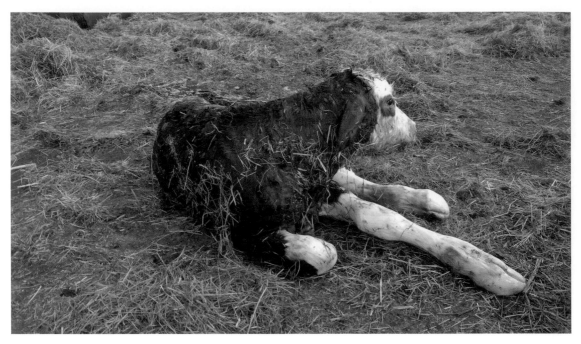

FIGURE 4.5 Calf with head up in sternal recumbency soon after birth

MATERNAL BEHAVIOUR

The hormonal changes described above are undoubtedly partly responsible for the protective mothering instincts of the cow at calving. Adrenaline is thought to massively augment this behaviour. Quiet cows can become wild and wild cows can become wilder; by wild we mean 'prepared to kill' to protect their newborn. So, any handling of the freshly calved cow, but more so her calf, carries with it great risk of personal injury. Is intervention necessary? Is it too dangerous? Have you got a stick for protection? Have you got good handling facilities? Have you got someone to help you? It may not be worth it. If an intervention is not necessary, then not only is your effort 'unnecessary' but it may even *interfere with the natural process*. For example, a calf that was going to suck may end up being tube fed so removing its stimulus to suck and so hampering its development. The interference may damage the cow–calf bond, see Figure 4.6. But when intervention is necessary, intervention is necessary.

EAR TAGGING

Calves should be tagged in the regulatory manner and to identify the calf – this is an excellent opportunity to take a tissue sample for BVD testing which should be standard practice in the interests of BVD eradication (see Chapter 15).

COLOSTRUM

Nature is full of miracles, one of them unquestionably being colostrum. Once famous as being the stuff to make the best scones from, colostrum is now famed for far more important reasons.

What is colostrum?

Colostrum is the first milk secretion of the mammary gland at the end of pregnancy – a secretion evolved through the developmental history of mammals to provide a source of all

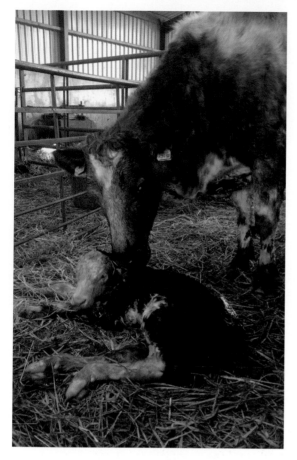

FIGURE 4.6 Newborn calf and its mother

the nutritional and immunological needs of the newborn mammal, in our case, the calf.

Is colostrum not just milk? It is similar but with some important differences. The key difference is that colostrum is particularly rich in a special family of proteins called antibodies. Antibodies, correctly known as immunoglobulins, are the proteins produced by the immune system that specifically target, attach to and inactivate 'enemy chemicals', such as those on the surface of viruses, bacteria and, perhaps surprisingly, some tumours. For the immune system to produce immunoglobulins it needs to be stimulated or triggered to do so. This happens naturally when animals are exposed to bugs (pathogens) but can be unnaturally induced using vaccines. Immunoglobulins are unable to pass the placental barrier. This means

that the newborn is severely lacking in this type of protection or 'immunity'. That is where colostrum comes in. The mother's bloodstream contains an array of immunoglobulins that reflect her historic exposure to bugs over the years. These immunoglobulins manage to get into the colostrum – made possible by a temporary slackening of the gaps between the cells lining the mammary gland. This slackening tightens up over the first couple of days of lactation and by day 3 the process largely stops – that is when colostrum has pretty much reverted back to being milk again. It is this phenomenon that explains why sometimes colostrum contains a little blood thus giving it a pink tinge or, sometimes, a blatant red colour. Often blamed on a 'knock' this is simply red blood cells leaking into the colostrum along with the immunoglobulins and is considered normal, and usually nothing to worry about although mastitis should at least be considered (McGarth et al., 2016).

What else is different about colostrum?

Compared to milk, colostrum contains less lactose but more fat, protein, Vitamin A, Vitamin E, calcium, phosphate, sodium, magnesium, hormones, growth factors, enzymes, and immune stimulants (McGarth et al., 2016). Colostrum is also an important source of Vitamin C as the calf's liver does not start making Vitamin C for the first 3 weeks. As it happens normal milk also contains Vitamin C at similar levels – so it is not a difference between colostrum and milk, but it is important. Interestingly – humans (and guinea pigs!) never learn to make Vitamin C so they rely on a life-long dietary supply – colostrum and milk therefore providing a decent start.

So, apart from the intriguing lack of lactose, colostrum can be seen to be a very dense source of nutrition to the soon to be hungry newborn, and the value of the hormones and growth factors is also easily imagined. The lower lactose level may seem inappropriate but it is lactose that, by the phenomenon of osmosis, draws water into milk; this works well for regular milk but to keep colostrum concentrated and rich it benefits from a little less water being drawn into it – so, less lactose, less dilution by water. By day three the lactose levels are rising, and the amount of water being drawn into the colostrum in turn rises – the result is 'milk'; relatively watery in comparison (McGarth et al., 2016).

Colostrum is a little more acidic than milk. This may be to compensate for the initial lack of acid production in the newborn stomach (abomasum) – it is, after all, acidity in the stomach that, among other things, is one of the first lines of defence against ingested bugs.

How does the immunoglobulin in colostrum get into the calf's bloodstream without being digested?

You would be right to expect the immunoglobulins to simply get digested by the calf; even if they did not, how would they get into the calf's bloodstream intact? Sure enough, that does not normally happen with protein – when an animal eats protein the protein has to be digested down to amino acids, which are small enough to pass through the small gaps in the gut wall. Once in the animal's bloodstream the liver can then use the raw amino acids as building blocks to re-make the many proteins needed for body structure and function. In the case of the newborn two things make this possible. First, the digestive system in the newborn is not immediately geared up to digest protein and, second, the gaps in the gut wall are intentionally wide for the first few hours of life. The result is that entire immunoglobulins and other proteins survive the digestive tract and pass straight into the calf's bloodstream. That means the calf is suddenly equipped with a supply of antibodies for immediate protection against the new outside world.

Passive immunity as opposed to active immunity

Active immunity is the process described earlier where the cow's immune system produces antibodies in response to exposure to pathogens or vaccines. Passive immunity, also described above, is the passing on of antibodies in the colostrum from mother to young, also known as passive transfer. Because the cow has lived in the environment that the calf is being born into then there is a good chance that the bugs the calf is likely to meet have already stimulated an immune response in the cow. So, the passive immunity enjoyed by the calf is hopefully helpful and relevant to its situation. This goes wrong when the calf is born into an environment that the cow or heifer has not been familiar with, for example, a move to a new environment just before calving. The other thing that can go wrong is when the scale of the challenge is just too great for the calf and the modest amount of antibody transferred from the colostrum simply is not enough and the pathogen exhausts and exceeds the number of antibodies.

How much immunity does get transferred?

This depends on several factors.

1. Age of the dam. Compared to older cows, heifers do not produce antibody rich colostrum because they are not as good at making colostrum (or milk for that matter) (it may be slightly related to their relative lack of exposure to bugs in their relatively shorter life but this is not thought to be particularly the case) (Potter, 2011).
2. Health and nutrition of the dam. A cow needs to be healthy and well fed to produce colostrum and consequently milk (Figure 4.7) (Potter, 2011).
3. Immune history of the dam. A dam well vaccinated or well exposed to bugs will produce a larger range of different antibodies.
4. 'Downer cow' (Chapter 17). The ability of the cow to present its teats to the calf for successful sucking is compromised if she is recumbent through injury or illness.

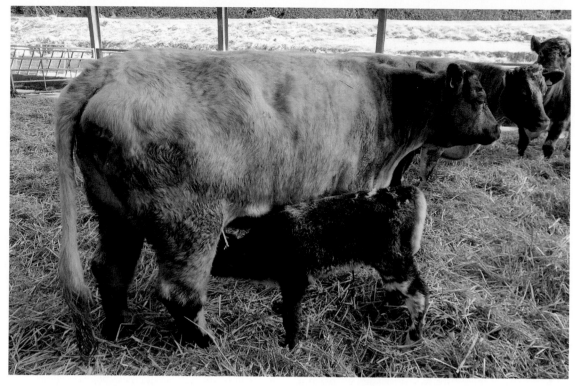

FIGURE 4.7 Beef Shorthorn cow in good health with calf suckling contently

5. Oversized or swollen teats that will not fit in the calf's mouth.

6. Painful teats or udder from mastitis (inflamed udder) or mammilitis (inflamed teat) will deter suckling for obvious reasons.

7. Poor mothering behaviour. This is a more common problem with heifers than cows. It can also be a problem with nervous dams, or in the presence of 'over interference' from stockpersons or the 'wrong smell' on the calf or 'mis-mothering' (the mother ending up with someone else's calf).

8. Calf too old when takes its first feed. The ability of the calf to absorb immunoglobulins drops off after 6 hours so the first feed ideally needs to be by then and certainly before 24 hours by which time absorption will have largely ceased (Potter, 2011).

9. A small first feed. A related factor to be aware of is that the first feed speeds up the closing of the gaps in the calf gut wall. Consequently, the first feed ideally needs to be a good one and it does not want to be too long to the next feed as time may run out even faster. This knowledge affects how we advise on supplementary feeding (see 'How do we supplement colostrum?', below).

10. Calves slow to suck because of illness or protracted or difficult/traumatic delivery are more likely to experience a delay to first feed and will subsequently have measurably lower immunoglobulin levels (Potter, 2011).

11. Beef versus dairy. Beef cows have higher levels of immunoglobulin in their colostrum. This may be attributable to superior production or it may be related to the lower yield of the beef cow reducing the extent to which a large volume of milk could feasibly dilute the antibodies as may be the case in the high yielding dairy cow (Potter, 2011).

12. Length of dry period. A cow needs a reasonable

gap between drying off and calving to have time to produce sufficient good quality colostrum, at least 3 weeks as a bare minimum, preferably longer.

How much colostrum is enough?

The newborn calf ideally requires 100–200 g of immunoglobulin depending on the size of the calf and the level of infectious challenge the calf faces. This equates to 3–4 l of a good quality colostrum; good being defined as colostrum with an immunoglobulin concentration of at least 60 g/l. It would be fair to acknowledge that in nature these targets will often not be met but these are ideals that are suited to less natural, potentially more contaminated environments as typically found on farm. When it is clear or likely that intake will be well below target, for example when a calf has failed to stand, when the calving was long or difficult or when the farmer simply knows the calf has not sucked following observation or when the experienced farmer can tell that the 'belly's empty', then supplementation is advised.

How do you supplement colostrum?

So, we are agreed; any chance a calf has not had sufficient colostrum then more should be given before it is too late.

The first and best option is to make use of the dam's own colostrum if she has some and has plenty. Obviously the first intervention would be to try to 'latch' the calf on to the teat simply by helping the calf. This is one of the many great skills of the experienced and diligent stockperson. The patience and care involved is admirable, the skill at not getting kicked impressive, the bravery of being kicked and persevering even more impressive (some would say foolhardy!). Where this is not possible then the next step is to milk the cow

– also dangerous – and in the case of the beef cow that is almost certainly going to be by hand as it usually is even in the case of the freshly calved dairy cow too. While often seeming low down the priority list, when battling with a fresh calved cow and calf in the middle of the night, the teats should ideally be cleaned to reduce bacterial contamination of the calf's first meal – particularly important to reduce the chance of *E. coli* infection. This can be done with antiseptic teat wipes, or even a baby wipe – a re-sealable bag of these can easily live in the calving kit box. The colostrum should be collected in a clean jug. Keep transferring smallish amounts into a separate clean container that is out of kicking distance of the cow. This could be a clean oesophageal feeder bag hanging off a secure hook. There can be few worse frustrations than having a full jug of colostrum kicked out your hand at a time where tempers may already be a little frayed! Once enough colostrum is collected then the calf can then be fed it using a bottle or an oesophageal feeder (see below). Where the intention is to store the colostrum and use it later, for example, for the second feed, or in the case of a high yielder, for another calf or two, then the colostrum can be safely stored in a fridge at 4°C for up to 7 days. In this time some drop in antibody level will occur but hopefully nothing too significant. Alternatively, colostrum can be frozen in plastic bags or containers and kept until needed. Defrosting such colostrum needs to be done gently and slowly, for example, by simply leaving it out at room temperature if there's no great hurry or for a faster result in a dish of warm, not hot, water. Heating colostrum in water exceeding 38°C or in a microwave can cause a denaturing of the antibodies. Some people do seem to get away with using a microwave oven, but it needs doing very carefully and on the slowest defrost setting and with frequent agitation of the container to avoid 'hot spots'. Be warned even then there is some belief that the microwaves alone, even used gently, can denature the antibodies.

Using colostrum from a different mother

This is a tempting solution when you have a cow with surplus colostrum, for example, because of a naturally high yield or maybe because she has lost her calf. If you do this there are a few things to consider. Is her colostrum free of infectious agents? We mentioned *E. coli* that results simply from faecal contamination but there are other bugs that specifically inhabit colostrum in their own sneaky pursuit of infecting the vulnerable newborn. Such infectious agents include, Johne's bacterium (MAP) (Chapter 17), *Mycoplasma bovis*, *Salmonella* spp. (Chapter 12). Were you to take colostrum from a cow on the same farm then the risk of introducing new disease is less but the threat remains from cows that are carriers of these bugs as opposed to those who are not. For this reason, it can be well worth ensuring at least some of your cows are screened for safe colostrum donation. In an ideal world of course, you would screen all your cows. If you have no choice but to source your colostrum from another farm it would, similarly, be safer to use a farm that is assured disease-free in as many of these bugs as possible or at least has a screened donor cow or two.

Another good reason for using colostrum from your own cows on your own farm is that they will tend to have antibodies against the range of local diseases that your farm has – a range that may be slightly different from your neighbour's farm.

How good an option is artificial colostrum?

Artificial colostrum is not a licensed veterinary medicinal product and is not, therefore, subject to strict regulatory approval. So, beware! How nutritious is it? In particular what is the fat and protein content? How much, if any, immunoglobulin does it contain? The main immunoglobulin in colostrum is a type called immunoglobulin G (IgG). The level of IgG should be stated on the label and you need to be able to trust that claim. An independent study of artificial colostrum IgG found levels to vary from 6–52 g/l. Even the best of these fed at the recommended rate would only deliver 30 g of IgG (Corke, 2012). Remembering from earlier that a calf needs 100–200 g of IgG we can see that most artificial colostrums are far from ideal and should only be relied on as a top up to real colostrum or when you simply have no alternative but to use them. To be fair, manufacturers are trying all the time to improve levels, and better products are appearing on the market. Always enquire as to the IgG level and judge whether you trust the manufacturer as best you can.

Is there a test for colostrum quality?

A refractometer and a colostrometer are two devices that can be used to assess the quality of the colostrum before it is administered to a calf. Obviously in the suckled calf situation not every cow's colostrum can be tested but if a cow is milked out for whatever reason it is worth just checking. A colostrometer is like a fishing float that is put into a full bucket or container of milk, how well it freely floats indicates how much immunoglobulin the colostrum contains. There is a colour coded scale on the side of the glass float; if the green zone is visible the colostrum contains more than 50 mg/ml of IgG. More scientifically it is actually a hydrometer, a device that measures the non-specific characteristic of specific gravity. The IgG levels of the colostrum affect the specific gravity, but so do other factors, so there is a small degree of variability in the results. One factor we can control is temperature. Colostrum will have a higher specific gravity at cooler temperatures, so it is recommended a colostrometer be used only in warm milk.

A Brix refractometer, see Figure 4.8, is traditionally used to measure sugar in wine production but values are correlated with IgG levels in colostrum too. This technique requires only a small

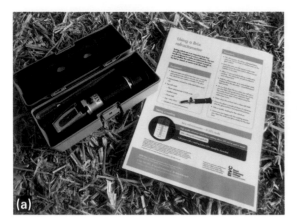

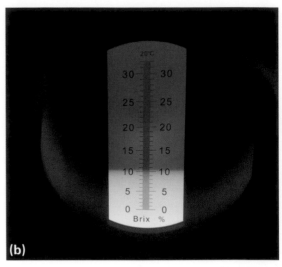

FIGURE 4.8 (a) A Brix refractometer and instructions; (b) view through the eye piece of a Brix refractometer

drop of colostrum rather than a bucket, making it easier to use in a suckler cow situation. The milk is placed on a small chamber and then looking down the refractometer through the eye piece the number on the scale associated with the colour change from white to blue can be read. A brix value of 22% corresponds to 50 mg/ml IgG.

Refractometers and colostrometers are cow side tests for colostrum IgG quality. Laboratory tests accurately measure IgG content, for example the radial immunodiffusion test.

It is possible to blood sample calves to assess the level of passive transfer of immunoglobulins. The zinc sulphate turbidity (ZST) is effective for calves less than 5 days of age and is carried out in a laboratory. Total protein (TP) levels in blood are also an indicator of passive transfer of immunoglobulins but blood proteins are affected by inflammation and dehydration so should only be measured in healthy calves. The advantage of TP is that it a relatively simple test and can be carried out at the veterinary practice rather than being posted away to a laboratory resulting in a time delay before results are available. ZST and TP are seldom carried out on a single animal. They are usually used as part of a herd level investigation into calf management.

THE OESOPHAGEAL GROOVE

The reticulum, rumen, omasum and abomasum are the four stomachs of the adult ruminant. In the calf it is really only the abomasum, the fourth stomach, that is developed and functional. It is only when the calf starts to eat a significant amount of solid food that the other three stomachs develop. So, when a young calf sucks milk what happens to it? You would understandably expect the milk to make its way sequentially through the first three stomachs eventually reaching the abomasum. What actually happens is quite complex. As milk passes down the oesophagus towards the first stomach a reflex is triggered which stimulates the rather extraordinary formation of a furrow or a nigh on cylindrical groove in the wall of the reticulum and the rumen which channels the milk straight from the oesophagus to the omasum. This groove functions like an extension of the oesophagus hence its name, the oesophageal groove (Ash, 1964). The omasum is a tiny little stomach so upon reaching it the milk rattles straight through it landing where it needs to be in the abomasum. The abomasum is actually the true stomach – analogous to any other animal's stomach and it is in here that the milk is properly digested. First it forms into a clot, thanks to the effect of the acid, and it is then digested by stomach enzymes.

Bottle or oesophageal feeder?

The taking shape of the oesophageal groove is very much a reflex reaction. Just like the sight of food stimulates a dog to salivate it is the soft teat in the mouth of a calf that stimulates the oesophageal groove to form. So, when a calf feels the soft, warm teat of a good quality milk bottle in its mouth it is highly likely that the oesophageal groove will form, and the milk happily end up in the abomasum. Unfortunately, when the hard, cold tube of an oesophageal feeder, is rammed into a calf's mouth the result is not quite the same. It is highly likely the groove will not take shape and the milk will end up in the fore-stomachs. In reality this is not a significant problem in the newborn as the fore-stomachs as mentioned are very small and non-functional and the milk still manages to quickly get to where it is needed (Lateur-Rowet and Breukink, 1983). As the days pass the problem potentially becomes more serious – the rumen becomes capable of fermenting any milk that inadvertently lands in it thus causing digestive upsets, such as bloat. This is a real problem when older calves are being bottle fed or, similarly, machine-fed and where the atmosphere is not quite right for relaxed sucking. For example, the calf house is noisy, the teats are hard or cold, the milk is cold or does not taste right, the stockperson is shouting or the calf is being bullied.

THE NAVEL AND UMBILICAL CORD

The navel is the opening in the body wall where the umbilical cord enters the body of the young mammal from having originated at the placenta. The umbilical cord is the main supply route to the calf from the cow's placenta, it contains the umbilical arteries that take blood from the calf to the placenta, the umbilical veins that take the 'enriched' blood from the placenta back to the calf, and additionally the curious 'urachus'. The urachus is a narrow tube that connects the calf's bladder to one of the fluid bags that surrounds the calf in the uterus, to be precise the allantois, see Figure 4.9.

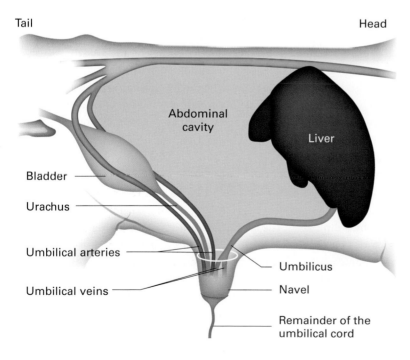

Tail

Head

Abdominal cavity

Liver

Bladder

Urachus

Umbilical arteries

Umbilical veins

Umbilicus

Navel

Remainder of the umbilical cord

FIGURE 4.9 Anatomy of the umbilicus

At birth, as the young newborn falls away from the mother, or as the mother stands up and moves away from the young the umbilical cord stretches and eventually snaps. This normally happens quite near to the navel leaving a variable amount of cord attached to the navel but usually most of it still left attached to the placenta which at this stage is nearly always still inside the mother's uterus.

Various things can go wrong here, and they do, but fortunately not too often – remember, nature generally gets most things right! Nonetheless, what can go wrong?

Bacteria can find themselves invading the abdominal cavity via the portal that is the navel or by travelling straight up the umbilical cord, which can continue to act as a bit of a fast track to the calf's body.

To reduce the environmental load of bacteria and the onslaught the calf has to contend with, the environment needs to be as clean and dry as practically possible. Dirt equals bacteria and wetness gives the bacteria a transport medium. So, plenty of dry, clean bedding needs to be provided and wet things like placentas, calving fluids and tipped over calving buckets all need removing or sorting out.

To help further, the navel and remaining umbilical cord needs to be treated with a disinfectant/drying agent as soon as possible after birth. The aim is to kill any bacteria present but also to cause the remaining umbilical cord to dry and shrivel up so as to close the tubes in the cord and stop the cord acting as a conduit for bacteria. In cases where the calf is slow to rise, especially in the case of the bull calf, where the naval becomes saturated with urine, multiple applications of antiseptic/drying agent may be required.

Navel disinfectants can be applied by a dip cup or a spray. A spray is preferred as a dip cup can become contaminated with enough organic matter and bacteria to stop it being effective, in which case transmission of bacteria could occur from one calf to the next (Figure 4.10). Whichever method is used the cord needs to be saturated and certainly the neck of the navel but, depending on how

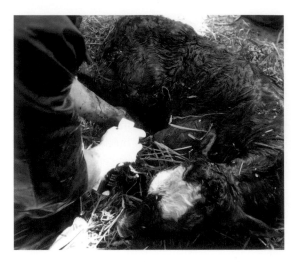

FIGURE 4.10 Applying iodine to the navel of a newborn calf

aggressive the agent is, care may be needed not to saturate more of the body wall than is necessary as the skin could be damaged.

There is currently no evidence to suggest that one navel disinfectant is any better than the rest. Commonly 10% iodine is used but 2% chlorhexidine has been trialled and was found to be equally effective and less irritant. Given the blatantly caustic nature of iodine for both the hand stained farmer and the poor calf then it is very tempting to recommend that chlorhexidine be trialled and compared with the familiar method. Chlorhexidine can be purchased in an alcohol base (Hibitane™) so the drying effect of alcohol-based iodine, or *tincture* as it was traditionally known, can still be enjoyed.

CASTRATION

The original definition of castration is 'the removal of the testicles from a male animal or person'. The alternative definition is the removal of power, vigour or vitality. Either way it can be an emotive subject and remains an area of potential criticism for the farming industry at a welfare and ethical level; an issue that we should, therefore, be sensitively aware of and take very seriously. So why do we still practice this ancient, and some would say, archaic, procedure?

It is obviously partly about fertility, but it is also a lot about *testosterone*. Testosterone is a natural reproductive hormone that is produced in large quantities by the testicles – assuming the male animal still has its testicles or is, in other words, 'entire'. Females do have some testosterone at a low level, obviously not produced in the testicles – they do not have testicles – but in the ovaries. Testosterone, in either sex, stimulates growth, bone strength and mass, muscle strength and toughness, and 'androgenisation'. Androgenisation is the development of 'male like characteristics' – this is a big feature in males, obviously, but also occurs to a varying extent in females. Here we are talking about blatant characteristics like the aforementioned size, mass, muscularity, strength and resilience to injury. Less obvious characteristics, until they are pointed out that is, are the rather more subtle effects, such as voice change, and a tendency to apathy, sluggishness and docility, sometimes interspersed with bouts of explosive aggression and fighting. Sound familiar? Sounds like some farmers we all know. OK and some vets too.

In meat industry terms androgenisation represents:

- tougher meat – more fibrous (more 'connective tissue'), more grained
- less intramuscular fat, referred to as 'marbling', and, less intermuscular fat and subcutaneous fat cover for those that want it for the long celebrated flavour and cooking characteristics it affords
- bigger, more muscular carcases and higher carcase yield (KO%)
- 'dark cutting beef' – an increased likelihood of this undesirable meat characteristic (see Chapter 7)
- male *taint* of the meat (although in cattle this is much less of a problem than in pigs for example).

So why castrate cattle?
- To achieve better meat and carcase characteristics.

- To reduce fighting and stress among groups of entire bulls.
- To reduce risk of aggressive behaviour towards personnel – farmers, hauliers, vets and abattoir workers.
- To reduce the size and power of cattle for handling and restraint purposes.
- To prevent unwanted sexual behaviour among groups of bulls and unwanted pregnancies in any accessible females.

Why not castrate cattle?
- Welfare issues – it is known to be painful both during the procedure and afterwards – potentially for days afterwards. There is also the risk of complications to the surgery, which depending on the method employed, could include haemorrhage, infection, herniation and 'guttie'.
- Ethical issues – 'animal rights' in other words. Should we be doing something to an animal that is not essential or necessary?
- Beneficial effects of testosterone – namely growth promotion and improved food conversion efficiency (FCE). The increase in body mass and muscularity results in bigger carcases, higher yield (KO%) and better cutting characteristics (cutability). The growth promoting effects also result in more food being converted into bone and muscle and less being stored as fat, be it abdominal, cod (groin), subcutaneous, intermuscular or intramuscular (marbling). Is this good? Commercial marketplaces value lean meat far more than fatty meat – it is more attractive to many modern consumers and to the manufacturing industry, but not to the traditional cook or gourmet industry who rate the supposedly improved flavour and cookability afforded by fat. This presents an interesting ongoing argument however; both sides claim flavour test results in their favour. Independent taste tests vary but it seems that agreement has been reached on yearling bull-beef having similar eating results to 2-year-old castrated males.

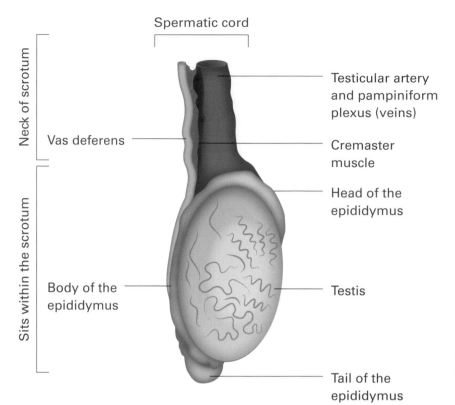

Spermatic cord

Neck of scrotum

Sits within the scrotum

Vas deferens

Body of the epididymus

Testicular artery and pampiniform plexus (veins)

Cremaster muscle

Head of the epididymus

Testis

Tail of the epididymus

FIGURE 4.11 There are two testicles within a single scrotum, this schematic diagram is of the right testis

The anatomy of the testicles

A full appreciation of the anatomy of the testicles is both interesting (well it is to vets!) and helpful for a better understanding of not only the castration process but vasectomy too, see Figure 4.11.

Castration techniques

Rubber ring

Also referred to as 'elastration' after the trade-name of the original rubber bands and applica-tor – Elastrator™ (Figure 4.12). Here a rubber ring is applied around the neck of the scrotum cutting off the blood supply to the entire structure – the scrotum and all of its contents. This complete inter-ruption of the blood supply causes the entire struc-ture to die, shrivel up and drop off after a few weeks. The procedure is very cheap, reasonably simple to

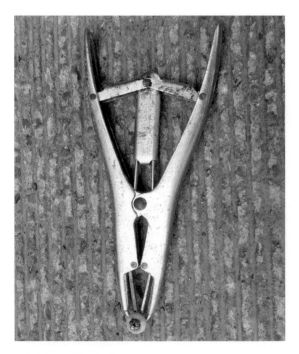

FIGURE 4.12 Elastrators

do and, done properly, very effective with a high success rate. In the UK welfare codes state that rubber ring castration should only be employed at less than 7 days of age. Ideally this should be carried out in the first 48–72 hours of life. The procedure is painful and the opportunity for criticism here is that there is no requirement for analgesia; surely an issue for further consideration. That said, pain studies have concluded that it appears less painful at the time than the other methods of castration, but, the downside, they also concluded that the pain lasts for longer (Stafford, 2007). Done at this young age this may inhibit sucking behaviour and, if carried out very young, that is, in the first 24 hours of life, then colostrum intake could be detrimentally affected – probably a sound reason not to rubber ring calves in the first day of life.

How to perform the rubber ring castration procedure

First talk to your vet about the use of pain relief for the procedure. This may simply be an injection of a suitable and licensed NSAID. These drugs, despite the name, are more for pain relief than the anti-inflammatory effect suggested in the name. Check the minimum age at which the product can be used. You may wish to consider using local anaesthetic – this will involve placing 1–2 ml around each cord on each side of the scrotum and massaging the site a little to spread the agent around. Your vet will advise on this procedure; they may wish to demonstrate the technique and advise on the exact product and dose rate. While this will slow the procedure up the pain relief afforded is well worth it and certainly demonstrates an intent within the industry to address the welfare implications.

Rubber ring castration procedure

1. With the help of an assistant sit the calf up on its rear end taking care not to get kicked, especially in the face. You may wish to tie the back legs together with a soft suitable rope or get a third person to hold them.

2. Ensure both testicles are gently 'encouraged' down into the bottom of the scrotum using thumb and fingers, best if they are warm – that is both the hands and the testicles!
3. Use the applicator to stretch the ring open.
4. Pass the applicator over the scrotum.
5. With both testicles definitely in the bottom of the scrotum, but nothing else, such as extra skin, nipples or worst of all, the penis, then release the ring.
6. Check again that both testicles are below the ring but nothing else.

Tetanus or blackleg infection is a possibility (Chapter 12). A thorough approach to prevention would be vaccination of the cow (dependent on good colostrum intake). The vaccine used on the cow would most likely be a multivalent clostridial vaccine that also covers other clostridial infections. Failing that, especially if the farm has a history of tetanus, then tetanus antitoxin could be administered – speak to your vet.

'Burdizzo' style bloodless castration

Bloodless 'Burdizzo-style' castration involves crushing the spermatic cord of each testicle, separately, through the scrotal skin.

Pain studies suggest that the procedure is, as with the rubber ring, painful. Again, to overcome

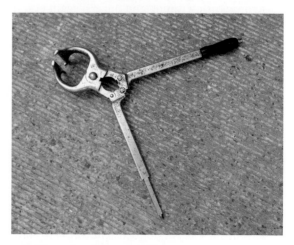

FIGURE 4.13 Burdizzo castrators

this welfare problem you should discuss with your vet the use of local anaesthetic and NSAID injection. UK welfare codes state that this procedure must not be carried out on cattle over 2 months old unless performed by a veterinary surgeon using appropriate anaesthesia.

This procedure carries little risk of infection as there is no wound and the scrotum should not drop off – the testicles shrivel up internally but persist as small fibrous walnut-like structures.

How to Burdizzo castrate

1. Give the NSAID injection at least 1 hour before the procedure.
2. For small calves they can be sat on their rear end as described above for the rubber ring technique. Larger calves can be stood up and restrained at the head end with a yoke or halter and at the rear end using tail elevation and a knee in the flank to hold the calf against a solid partition or wall.
3. Inject 2 ml of local anaesthetic into the neck of the scrotum over the left cord and repeat over the right cord. Rub the area to spread the anaesthetic around. A further 1 ml of anaesthetic can be injected into each testicle also. Wait 10 minutes for the anaesthetic to work.
4. The operator gently 'encourages' the first, say the left, testicle down into the bottom of the scrotum using thumb and fingers, again best if both hands and testicles are warm. If the calf only has one testicle, or none for that matter, mark the calf and arrange for a veterinary assessment – the testicles may be undescended, and castration will be more difficult.
5. Pull the cord of the left testicle to the left-hand side of the neck of the scrotum. Make sure only cord, and only one cord, is pulled across – take care not to pull anything else down from higher up, namely the penis – sounds odd but this can happen, especially in calves with poorly descended testicles where the neck of the scrotum is short or non-existent.
6. Clamp the cord through the skin but go across

as little scrotal skin as possible so as to minimise unnecessary damage to the skin and other structures. Hold the clamps shut for 5 seconds. The clamps are best held in the U-shape orientation, that way the lip on the edge of the lower jaw helps to hold the cord in position and stop it slipping outwith the jaws.

7. Repeat the procedure 3 cm lower down the neck/cord on the same side.
8. Now repeat steps 5, 6 and 7 but on the right-hand side with the right cord pushed to the right-hand side of the neck of the scrotum. Stagger the clamping positions as shown in the diagram and again cross as little skin as possible as shown in Figure 4.14. The idea is to leave enough non-crushed skin for the scrotum to survive the procedure, unlike in the rubber ring technique.
9. It is not possible to know immediately after clamping whether the procedure has been

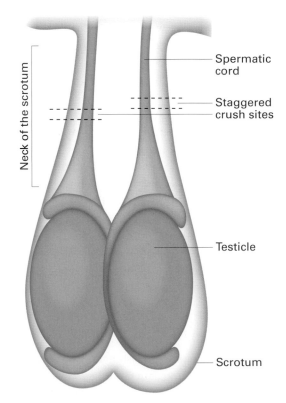

FIGURE 4.14 diagram to show crush sites for Burdizzo castration

effective or not even though notches in the cord should be palpable. It is essential therefore that all calves castrated by this method are examined 6 weeks later to check that the procedure has been effective; the testes will still be present but they will have shrivelled up. If a relatively smooth, plump testicle is felt than the animal should be assumed to be fertile and if a further attempt at castration is required a vet should be called – the procedure here becomes difficult because of scar tissue formation in the neck of the scrotum.

Surgical castration

Surgical castration, sometimes called 'open castration', is now only permissibly done by a vet and using anaesthetic. There is no legal age beyond which it is disallowed but for the safety of the animal and of the operators, the younger it is done, the better. Like all other methods of castration, it too is painful, so NSAID should be given at least 1 hour beforehand and local anaesthetic must be used. The vet will cut into the scrotum and free up the testicle from its various attachments. The surgical plan then is to break the cord to enable removal of the testicle. This is usually done by multiple twists and then gentle but forceful traction until the structures snap. The additional problem here is that the traction on the testicles causes deep abdominal pain in addition to the local pain so there is a strong case for sedation – this also requiring veterinary supervision. A method that avoids traction is to use a surgical instrument called an emasculator. This tool crushes and seals the cord as well as cutting it – it helpfully stops any bleeding, but they are not always effective. The other method your vet may employ is to knot or ligate the cord – this is the most effective way of stopping bleeding but carries the highest risk of infection due to the extra handling of tissue by the operator and, in the case of ligation, leaving some foreign material in the site – namely the ligature material such as 'catgut' or some synthetic equivalent.

Surgical castration is the most certain method of castration. When the farmer sees two testicles lying on the floor, he or she can be pretty sure that the animal is fully castrated. But remember, as with all methods of castration, a sexually mature male will still have some live sperm in what is left of 'the pipeline' so is still potentially capable of delivering one last fertile mating.

There are a number of potential complications with surgical castration.

- **Haemorrhage**. The large vessels that supply the testes are physically severed. The elastic nature of the vessels and the technique employed is usually enough to prevent haemorrhage, but it will sometimes nevertheless occur, sadly. Dripping of blood for up to 6 hours post-surgery is considered acceptable but a continuous stream of blood from the surgical site requires rapid veterinary attention.
- **Infection**. Antibiotics are not routinely administered for surgical castration on farm by most veterinary surgeons. The risk of infection is minimal in a clean environment. Calves should have the opportunity to lie on clean dry straw after the operation. Surgical castration should not take place at a time of year where there is a risk from fly strike or if for some reason a clean dry environment cannot be provided.
- **Herniation**. Owing to the close association between the abdomen and the testicles then it is possible for fat and on rare occasions loops of intestine to protrude from the surgical incision – this requires rapid veterinary attention.
- **Tetanus or blackleg**. As with any open wound there is a risk of clostridial infection. In older calves any protection from the colostrum of vaccinated dams is likely to have waned so tetanus antitoxin should be administered at the time of surgery if there is a risk, for example, previous cases in that building or on that farm.

Undescended or retained testicles

A male animal is born with two testicles, very rarely none, but almost never 'just one'. The problem is they may be retained in the abdomen or simply not fully descended into the scrotum. This problem is quite common. Most commonly the testicles are simply undescended and still in the groin, or *inguinal*, as medics say. These can sometimes be encouraged far enough down for a vet to proceed with surgical castration; use of rings or bloodless clamps should never be employed in these circumstances. Inguinal testicles may still descend given more time. Over the years various hormonal injections have been tried to encourage descent but with little or no success. Less often one or both testicles are abdominal – these can only be removed with full blown abdominal surgery – rarely justifiable? These animals are unlikely to be fertile as the high temperature inside the abdomen usually prevents sperm production – remember sperm production likes the cooler temperatures found outside the abdomen in the pendulous well cooled scrotum. The problem is that it's rather dangerous to assume that the animal is sterile – an unwanted pregnancy could be very inconvenient and costly. So, what do you do with bulls with abdominal testicles? The safest thing to do is to keep them separate from sexually mature females until they are slaughtered. Certainly, do not pass them on to someone else unless they fully understand the situation, and certainly do not pretend they are castrated! Once these bulls reach sexual maturity, they may not (or may) be fertile but they will have testosterone which, unlike sperm, is not temperature sensitive. So, make no mistake about it, these animals turn into bulls – be ready for them!

Castrate or not?

So, do you need to castrate your bulls? Think welfare, think cost–benefit, think about your preferred marketplace. If you decide you do indeed want to proceed with castration then think about which technique, think safety, think about pain relief, think about the time of year and think which of the potential complications you are prepared to risk and which you are not.

HORNED AND POLLED BREEDS

Domestic beef cattle of European origin (*Bos taurus*), as opposed to the tropical Zebu/Brahman type breeds (*Bos indicus*), either have horns (the most common state) or not. Cattle that do not have horns are referred to as being naturally polled. Of course, the other reason for not having horns is being 'unnaturally polled', that is, if they have been removed – done when the horns are small and unformed a process known as *disbudding*, or done when older and the horns have taken shape – known as *dehorning*. Other causes of horn removal would be traumatic fracture of the horn or disease of the horn producing tissue such as cancer or fungal infection.

The trait of being polled or having horns is determined by only one pair of genes. In this situation, where a trait is controlled by only one simple pair of genes, then one gene in the pair is inherited from the dam and the other from the sire. If an animal inherits two genes that are the same, then the genetic state is described as homozygous; where the two genes are different the state is called heterozygous. For these horn determining genes, if you can call them that, the polled gene (P) is dominant to the horned gene (p). If an animal has two polled genes (PP), or one polled and one horned gene (Pp), it will be polled. Only if an animal has two horned genes (pp) will it have horns. However, if it is heterozygous polled (Pp) it may pass either the polled or horned gene on to its offspring. The only situation when an animal will be horned is when it possesses two recessive horned genes (pp), in other words 'homozygous horned'.

The true polled breeds are cattle that have, as far as we know, pretty much always been that way; examples would be Red Poll, Aberdeen Angus, British White and Galloway. Some breeds, however, have developed 'polled strains' by out-crossing with these more traditional polled breeds; examples of these newer polled breeds would be Guernsey, Polled Jersey, Polled Shorthorn, Polled Hereford, the Austrian Pinzgauer, the Australian Murray Grey and the South African Bonsmara to name but a few. Of interest to sheep breeders would be to know that the polled bulls used for this cross breeding were described as 'muley bulls'.

Quite why cattle, sheep and even wild animals, such as yaks and buffalo, have the genetic capability to be polled is unclear. From an evolutionary perspective it is fairly obvious that having horns is useful for these herbivorous grazers to defend themselves against carnivorous predators and in the case of males as fighting weapons when competing for females but having the genetic potential to be polled may simply be one of nature's unintentional events.

Reasons to remove or 'breed-out' horns

Why early cattle breeders bred for polled cattle or why techniques were developed to remove horns include the following reasons:

- handler safety
- reduce injuries to other cattle – fighting or accidental – from the point of view of welfare, vet costs, carcase quality and hide quality
- easier to handle in yokes, crushes, narrow races and confined spaces
- more room for cattle at feeding troughs, silage faces and water sources.

Conversely, why did the breeding of polled cattle not totally take over? One reason may be the rather desirable appearance of some horned breeds but perhaps more likely is the widely held belief that polled status is negatively correlated with milk production and growth rates although research suggests this not to be the case, evidence for this is lacking (Goonewardene et al., 1999). The only evidenced undesirable trait linked with polling is spiral deviation of the penis in Polled Herefords (Blockey and Taylor, 1984).

The anatomy of the horn

The horns of animals from the family Bovidae ('horn bearers'), which includes bison, African buffalo, water buffalo, antelopes, gazelles, sheep, goats, muskoxen and domestic cattle all follow the same pattern of developmental anatomy.

The horns in Bovidae develop from two sources.

- An extreme thickening, hardening and proliferation of the skin on the head to form a hard shell of keratin (horn). Like any skin it is underlain with blood vessels and nerves for nourishment and sensation.
- A bony protrusion of the skull underneath the horn, bone which helps to form the spike like shape of the horn and to form a secure base. Like much of the skull the bone is aerated with a cavity – presumably to keep the weight of the skull to a manageable minimum while not losing too much strength.

The development of these two structures seem closely linked but not entirely. It is thought that some of the keratin (horn) formation may be under separate genetic control, which explains how some naturally polled animals have what are known as 'scurs' – small elevations of keratin in the site of the would be horn – but without the bony protrusion beneath.

Horns start to develop in the unborn foetus but do not develop significantly until after the point of birth; a balance needs to be struck here – yes the development of protection as quickly as possible but 'no thanks' to the presence of horns while passing through the birth canal.

Disbudding

Disbudding is the procedure designed to halt the development of the horn in the young animal with, at that stage, still undeveloped horns. The aim is to damage the skin and underlying tissue in the horn bud (the area of horn development) sufficiently so as to prevent any further significant development. By damaging the skin and subcutaneous tissue the keratin formation does not occur and the signal to the underlying bone, whatever that signal may be, is also broken. The result, done properly, is no keratin, no bony protrusion and no scurs. In reality the result is sometimes incomplete – there may be some bony protrusion, some horn or at least a little scur but these effects are normally insignificant unless you are a particularly demanding breeder of show cattle where anything less than perfect is not good enough!

There are two methods of disbudding: chemical cautery and thermal cautery; cautery being the medical term for burning.

Chemical cautery disbudding

There are many commercially available disbudding pastes designed to be used in calves less than 1 week of age (Defra, 2003). They typically contain either sodium hydroxide or calcium hydroxide – both caustic alkalis. The method of application is similar for all these pastes:

1. Trim away hair from around the horn bud with scissors.
2. Remove dirt and dust from the horn bud.
3. Apply petroleum jelly to the skin area around the horn bud but not the horn bud itself.
4. Wearing gloves, apply the chemical paste to the horn bud only, ensuring it does not run out of the area or come in contact with the calf's eyes.
5. Isolate the animal from other animals, including its mother, until the product has dried. Not doing this poses the risk of burns to other animals, especially their mouths if the paste is licked, or the cow's teats and udder when the sucking calf inevitably rubs its head on these structures.
6. Do not attempt if the calves are wet or likely to be rained on as the chemical will run and cause wider burning – most worryingly the eyes.

Although there is little pain exhibited at the time of application, treated calves exhibit a painful response within 1 hour and for typically 4 hours after application (Stafford et al., 2011). It has been suggested that local anaesthetic and an analgesic should be used in the same manner as with thermal cautery (Winder et al., 2017). It was the initial belief that chemical cautery was non-painful, and therefore did not need analgesia, that made the idea so popular, but the realisation that it too is painful has raised debate once more. At present the UK Cattle Welfare Codes dictate that chemical cautery should be carried out only in the first week of life. Hopefully in time the advice will extend to the requirement of local anaesthesia and an injection of analgesic, typically an NSAID. The disbudding sites are prone to flystrike and preventative fly preparation may be required.

Thermal cautery disbudding

In this procedure a very hot iron (or copper) is used to physically burn the skin and underlying tissue of the horn bud. The iron is specially made to be a shape that somewhat envelops the bud into the indentation on the end of the iron. The iron can be a free iron that is heated in a fire or a gas furnace, it may be an integrated iron that has a built-in gas burner or it may be electrically heated. The free irons tend to get the hottest, the electric ones the least but naturally this can vary as a result of various factors such as how hot the fire or furnace is, how long the iron has been left in, how well tuned the gas jet is, what type of gas is being used (propane burns hotter than butane), and how long the electric iron has been left on for. The gap between burnings is also significant – the irons need time to reheat after use. The temperature of the iron then dictates how long it needs to be applied to the horn bud to do sufficient damage to the tissue.

1. Check that the calf is under 2 months of age otherwise seek veterinary assistance.

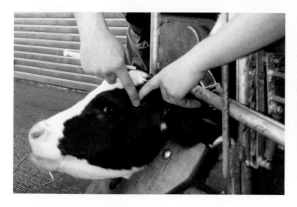

FIGURE 4.15 Administration of local anaesthetic to the cornual nerve

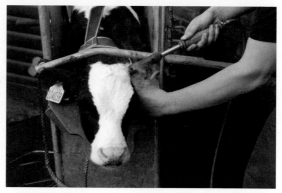

FIGURE 4.17 Disbudding with calf adequately restrained using a dis-budder with built-in gas burner

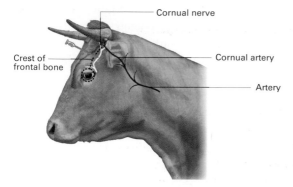

FIGURE 4.16 Needle-showing injection site for local anaesthetic to perform a cornual nerve block

2. Inject analgesic, for example, NSAID, as per veterinary directions, and 1 hour in advance.
3. Administer local anaesthetic to each cornual nerve, see Figures 4.15 and 4.16.
4. Clip the hair off the horn bud.
5. Remove dirt and dust.
6. Wait at least 10 minutes for the anaesthetic to work.
7. With the calf appropriately restrained – apply the iron to the bud until the skin blackens, this typically takes 3–5 seconds, see Figure 4.17.
8. Have a sponge and bucket of cold water at hand in case you burn yourself, your assistant, some other part of the calf or if you think you have overheated the calf's head during the procedure.

Thermal cautery disbudding is extremely painful and stressful without both local anaesthesia and injectable analgesia. The pain continues for 8 hours afterwards hence the need for additional analgesia as the local anaesthetic wears off after 90 minutes (Stafford et al., 2011). UK welfare codes state that local analgesia must be used and that the calf must be under 2 months of age. Best practice, however, demands that additional analgesia be used. Many vets are now, admirably, advocating and practising the use of sedative analgesia at the time also. This involves giving an intramuscular injection 5 minutes before the local anaesthetic is given. This provides not only sedation but additional analgesia also. This sedation and analgesia reduce the stress of the local anaesthetic injection, and of course the cautery itself. This reduction in stress in turn reduces the growth set-back that otherwise results. Evidence exists that analgesia at the time of disbudding does indeed reduce pain score and significantly reduces the impact on growth rates.

Complications of disbudding

- Under cauterising. Here the horn grows regardless of the procedure – wholly or more typically partially. Sometimes the resulting horn is inconsequential but sometimes the vet may be needed to rectify the situation – that's right – the show calf scenario!

- Fly strike. It may be worth using an approved insect repellent or insecticide.
- Infection. Sometimes infection appears to result but quite often this may simply be pus formation as a response to the dead skin as opposed to primary infection. Seek vet advice if this occurs, antibiotics may be needed.
- Overheating the head with the iron. This can cause a sterile (non-infectious) meningitis resulting in deranged behaviour and possibly seizures. This is obviously a very serious situation that requires vet intervention and a review of the disbudding procedure. The calf will need steroid treatment or some other form of anti-inflammatory and analgesia, it may need intravenous fluids and nutritional support and it may need anticonvulsant therapy. Most of these calves do survive with treatment but it is clearly to be avoided in the first instance.

How to perform local anaesthetic block for disbudding

Local anaesthetic, 2–4 ml, is placed adjacent to the cornual nerve lying just under the frontal bone palpable through the skin, Figure 4.16. The superficial temporal artery runs adjacent to the nerve, it is important that local anaesthetic is not injected into the vein by mistake. The operative should draw back on the syringe to ensure no blood enters the syringe before injecting.

Dehorning

UK welfare codes deem that once a calf is over 2 months old the procedure is called dehorning (Defra, 2003) (Figure 4.18). Dehorning must be carried out by a vet who will almost certainly employ sedation and analgesia as well as local anaesthetic. The removal of larger horns involves using either proprietary dehorning shears, a saw or a serrated surgical wire, Figure 4.19. The procedure is archaic and potentially painful, stressful and distressing for all involved. It is entirely avoidable and is therefore rarely employed these days. Hopefully it will very soon become a thing of the past. It does raise the question as to why it is sometimes needed? The answer is usually laziness or poor planning, but some producers seem to think it better to give the animal the 'set-back' when it is a little older. The general consensus among vets and producers, however, is that it is certainly the other way around.

DENTITION OF THE NEWBORN CALF

Anyone who has had their hand inside a calf's mouth during an assisted calving or while administering colostrum with a stomach feeder will know that calves are pretty much born with teeth! Why? It seems pretty tough on the cow, but it may be a means of hanging on to the teat. It is also in preparation for the fact that the eating of solid food will start surprisingly soon – as little as a few days old. The deciduous (temporary) incisors and premolars erupt at birth or within a few days, the molars erupt from 6 months onwards (Frandson, 1986).

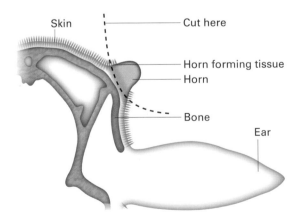

FIGURE 4.18 Cross-section of the head behind the ear demonstrating the close association of the horn bud to underlying structures

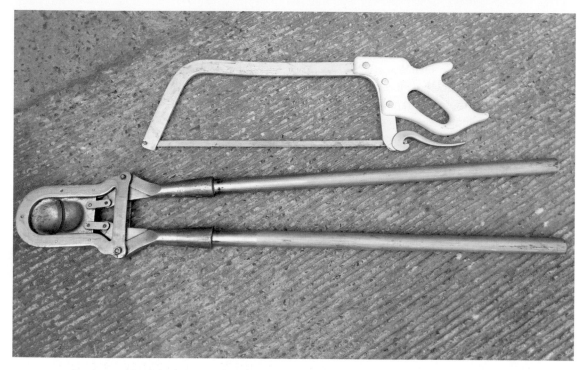

FIGURE 4.19 Tools used in dehorning cattle; saw and shears

THE ENVIRONMENT OF THE NEWBORN CALF

The concept of 'a good birth'

Life is full of shocks. But the act of being born must surely rank as one of the biggest shocks any animal will ever face. Oddly, fortunately, and, probably quite cleverly though, it is one none of us, and presumably no animal, will have any subsequent recollection of. Whether any individual is subconsciously affected by this shock is, however, a very different question. They say there are two inevitabilities in life – one version being 'death and taxes', the other that 'you are born and that you die'. We talk about the fact that death is inevitable so all you can hope for is *a good death*. So, yes, we hope for animals to have a *good death* but likewise we should be hoping that any animal should have *a good birth* too?

So, one minute the calf is floating in warm fluids, all its nutritional needs being pumped effortlessly straight into its body, the soothing pulse of its mother's heart reverberating all round, and not a worry in the world. Next thing it knows, it is being squeezed by a muscular bag, the uterus it was once so comfortable in, squeezed so hard in fact it starts to get expelled out through a surprisingly small birth canal that is so tight it compresses its chest so hard it forces all the fluid out of its lungs. The wet floppy calf then falls out of the birth canal with a great big thud, especially if the mother is on her feet, and, what started as just bruised ribs, can then become a bash to the head as it hits the ground and maybe sore legs as they too flap heavily against the ground. Then what? The supply of oxygenated blood through the placenta has stopped and the calf's brain is telling it that it needs oxygen. Fortunately, the calf's instincts kick in and it takes its first breath at a point where the desperation for air cannot get any worse. The calf takes this momentous breath but finds itself choking on fluid in its throat, it may even be suffocating thanks to a sheet of placental membrane draped over its nose. Our now battling calf instinctively shakes its head, the fluid moves, but the membrane is still there. Fortunately, the mother, this giant saviour stood over the calf, licks the membrane away from the nostrils and the air flows. Great – oxygen! And equally importantly the calf is now getting rid of carbon dioxide. The need for oxygen is fairly obvious, getting rid of carbon dioxide, however, is less so. The body produces carbon dioxide all the time – waste gas resulting from the burning of the energy component of food. Carbon dioxide starts initially in the body as a liquid – dissolved in the blood as carbonic acid. Too much of this is not a good thing. The build-up of this acid in the blood and other body tissues is known as acidosis. The brain responds to excess carbonic acid in the blood by triggering hard breathing during which the acid is encouraged to vaporise out of the blood as carbon dioxide as the blood passes through the capillaries of the lungs.

Thermal regulation in the newborn calf

Let us say the calf is outside, and that it is a cold wet night …

Having got through the issues of being squeezed, physically traumatised and then breathing for its life to get rid of carbon dioxide, the calf then has to stay warm. Mammals are homoiotherms; animals who have to hold their body temperature within strict outer limits – typically in and around the 30–40°C range. Why? Homoiotherms have body chemistry that requires sufficient levels of energy, that is, heat, to enable the chemical reactions to proceed; reactions that are often assisted by 'catalysts', in the body these catalysts are known as enzymes, life-critical molecules that help drive these chemical reactions. Enzymes are, however, very temperature sensitive – rather like enzymatic biological washing powders need warm water to work, so too do bodily enzymes. In the case of the

calf, its core temperature sits at nearly 40°C – just right for its own chemical reactions. We measure an animal's temperature most easily with a rectal thermometer; the rectum is not quite as warm as the body core and normally sits in the range of 38.1–39.2°C (Roland et al., 2015). The calf, like other homoiotherms will use various techniques to maintain this temperature – thermoregulatory mechanisms as they are known – to cool the body down when too hot or to warm up when too cold (as is the case for our calf born on this cold wet night).

In parts of the world where environmental temperatures are below 40°C the calf will lose heat when it is born. The evaporation of foetal fluids from the wet coat will be the main cause of this cooling effect, known as losing the 'heat of vaporisation' and any environmental air flow, that is, wind, breeze, draught, will speed up this chilling effect. Once the coat is dry, however, the cooling effect of evaporation stops and the body temperature starts to stabilise a little, unless of course it is particularly cold or windy, and unless of course the calf is in a rain or snow shower or lying on wet ground, in which case the cooling effect continues. The cow will often lick the calf, presumably instinctively, and presumably to help remove as much moisture from the coat as quickly as possible to help negate the cooling. Studies in New Zealand did indeed find that calves born in ambient temperatures of less than 10°C and in wet, windy weather conditions had a significantly lower rectal temperature and took longer to stand and suckle then calves born in warm, dry weather. So, it is clear that keeping the body chemistry warm is a real necessity for these all important basic bodily functions; the life-critical ability to stand and obtain colostrum from the cow. The optimal ambient temperature for newborn calves has been estimated at 16–20°C based on studies of calves up to 60 kg in weight (Roland et al., 2015). In temperatures lower than this the calf will lose heat to an extent that is detrimental to its health and survivability. We know that animals lose heat from their surface and more so if wet. The surface area of the animal is, therefore, important. Smaller animals tend to have a greater surface area/mass ratio than larger ones. Baby whales stay warm better than baby mice. There are other reasons though. Subcutaneous fat helps to insulate. Again, whales have a lot of this. This also helps make an animal rounder rather than complexly irregular in shape; seals are a good example here, but so is curling up in a ball regardless of what species you are. A thick coat is the remaining big factor – bears do well here, humans badly although for what is presumably evolutionary reasons some human babies are born surprisingly hairy, hair they subsequently lose only to regrow again at puberty.

Our calf does not fare too well so far, it is not particularly big, it is not round, it has very little subcutaneous fat and unless it is a hill breed it has not got much of a coat.

So, what does it do? Its thermoregulatory measures kick in. The hair once dry may stand on end – a way of making the coat thicker – a process called piloerection. It may shiver – this generates heat from movement and from the burning of energy in the cells of the muscle. Along with other animals something a little more special is also going on here. Calves have a supply of special fat called brown fat or brown adipose tissue to give it its full name. This special fat of the newborn and of animals that live in cold climates is particularly 'hot' when burnt – think coal as opposed to poorly seasoned logs. This fat oxidises to create chemical energy for, say, shivering, but extra heat also for no reason other than to simply warm up the body – an example of non-shivering thermogenesis. Calves have quite a good supply of this brown fat, about 2% of their body weight, whales and bears have more.

Other non-shivering thermogenesis measures that kick in are things like the aforementioned curling up in a ball to effectively reduce the virtual surface area to mass ratio albeit temporarily, and nuzzling, huddling, seeking shelter and moving round a lot. Another measure is to non-specifically raise the metabolic rate of the body – whether burning brown fat or not this increased chemical activity, especially oxidation, will raise body temperature. Small animals need to have a higher metabolic rate for at least this reason if not for others. A shrew would need several feet of fur and inches of subcutaneous fat to maintain its body heat were it to share the same low metabolic rate of an elephant. The imbibement of colostrum provides energy for oxidation and is a great help in getting this metabolic rate up to where it needs to be. A calf's temperature is known to increase after its first meal.

All this keeping warm is not ideal, it uses energy, this means that some energy is diverted away from the luxuries of growing and building body tissue. This in turn, from a farming perspective, means the food conversion rate is reduced as is liveweight gain. There are also the welfare considerations of being cold especially when things get really bad. There is a defined temperature range within which a calf does not have to expend energy simply to stay warm. This is called the thermoneutral zone (TNZ). The lower critical temperature is the start of this zone. This temperature varies for all the previously mentioned reasons – if a calf is wet and if air speed is high then the calf will need to work to stay warm at a higher temperature than if it is dry and sheltered. The TNZ therefore varies – the lower critical temperature can be as high as 18°C for a very wet calf in a wind right down to an unbelievable 0°C for a dry calf in still air (but remember – no calf is born dry – this fact is memorable only for healthy, hairy well fed calves that are at least a few days old).

Nature versus human intervention

The calf does plenty to help itself. What can we do to help? Helping good mothering, or should we say 'not interfering with good mothering' helps. Hoping for a licked, un-smothered calf that takes its colostrum quickly and abundantly is the aspiration. When climate is against us though, especially in the less robust breeds, housing makes sense. Housing is known to reduce wetting from the rain

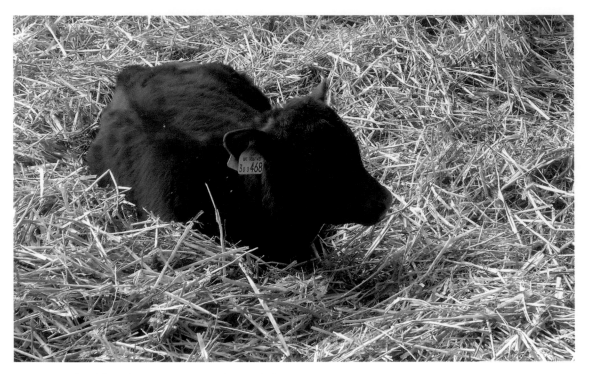

FIGURE 4.20 Beef Shorthorn cow in well-bedded clean pen

and snow and reduce air speed. Deep straw alone (Figure 4.20), has been shown to reduce ground air speed, which we know to be best kept below 0.2 m/s – in other words, do not just block the wind, avoid draughts, at least at calf level. This does not mean block ventilation though – this is essential to reduce some of the drawbacks of housing, which include the potential increase in humidity, noxious gases, dusty air and microbes. Ground drainage and ventilation should aim to keep relative humidity down. As for the noxious gases – these include carbon dioxide (a result of other animals burning energy), carbon monoxide (a result of faulty oxidation), ammonia (typically from the breakdown of urea in urine), methane (from the belching cows) and hydrogen sulphide (from the biological breakdown of faeces).

We mention belching cows – there are plenty of reasons why cows suffer less with the cold – the obvious ones such as being bigger, thicker coats, often more fat but a big factor is their possession of a functional rumen – a vat full of bugs fermenting

forage – this produces a huge amount of energy – 3500–4000 BTU per hour – another reason why housing with cows provides calves with warmth.

The thermoregulation implications of a bad calving

The assisted bad calving has an effect on thermoregulation and the consequential knock-on effects. For reasons not fully understood a hard calving leaves the calf 36% less able to stay warm through thermogenesis – peripheral vasoconstriction, shivering, standing, moving, colostrum intake and behavioural responses are all reduced. The calf will be colder, it has a reduced ability to absorb what colostrum it does manage to get (that is not just nutrient deprivation but antibodies as well) – probably because blood flow is diverted away from the gut and sent instead to the life critical areas such as the brain, lungs and heart and to the areas of inflammation caused by the traumatic birth.

So, what else can we do to help? Avoid difficult calvings for one thing. That is all about dam and sire selection, and having personnel who are well trained in assisting deliveries and know when to call for help. Once born such calves need additional support in the form of a heated bed, for example, infrared heat lamps if not a coat, bedded boxes, deep straw and obviously freedom from wetting and air flow.

The stark reality is this – cold calves cost money, and worse still when their temperature falls as low as 30°C they are going to die, and they do die when they reach 27°C. Cold calves are a welfare concern.

Overheating in the newborn calf

What about the other end of the extreme? We have not talked about overly hot calves. This is a problem in some countries and in some weather spells. The upper critical temperature is defined as the ambient temperature at which an animal has to actively do something to stay cool enough to stay within its preferred physiological limits. In complete contrast to the cold calf – here wetness and air speed are good things – they help with the loss of the heat of evaporation. The overly hot animal will flatten its coat to reduce insulation, it will sweat to wet its coat, it will keep still, it will stop eating, it will drink, it will maximise its surface area by sprawling out, and it will pant to increase evaporation from the respiratory system, and to pass cooler air over the hard plate to aid in cooling the brain. The brain fails at 45°C, body enzymes stop working, and the blood starts to clot – the calf dies.

Animals can acclimatise to some extent. The misplaced Hereford living in the hot American planes will be more adjusted to heat (and indeed cold) than the Hereford living in Hereford! Such acclimatisation usually takes the form of self-regulation of metabolic rate although changes in behaviour, coat and subcutaneous fat may also play a part.

REFERENCES

Ash, R.W. (1964) Abomasal Secretion and emptying in suckled calves. *Journal of Physiology* 172, 425–438.

Blockey, M.A. and Taylor, E.G. (1984). Observations on spiral deviation of the penis in beef bulls. *Australian Veterinary Journal* 61, 141–145.

Corke, M.J. (2012) Immunoglobulin content of colostrum supplements for calves available in the United Kingdom. *Cattle Practice* 20(2), 106–109.

Defra (2003) *Code of Recommendations for the Welfare of Livestock. Cattle.* Defra, London.

Frandson, R.D. (1986) *Anatomy and Physiology of Farm Animals*, 4th edn. Lea and Febiger, Philadelphia, PA. (Esp. chapter 19. Anatomy of the digestive system, pp. 312–314).

Goonewardene, L.A., Price, M., Liu, M., Berg, R. and Erichson, C. (1999) A study of growth and carcass traits in horned and polled composite bulls. *Canadian Journal of Animal Science* 79, 383–385.

Grove-White, D. (2000) Resuscitation of the newborn calf. *In Practice* 22, 17–23.

Lateur-Rowet, H.J.M. and Breukink, H.J. (1983) The failure of the oesophageal groove reflex, when fluids are given with an oesophageal feeder to newborn and young calves. *Veterinary Quarterly* 5(2), 68–74.

McGarth, B.A., Fox, P.F., Mcsweeney, P.L.H. and Kelly, A.L. (2016) Composition and properties of bovine colostrum: a review. *Dairy Science & Technology* 96, 133–158.

McKinnon, B.R. (1998) Beef quality corner – 'dark cutters' livestock update. Virginia Cooperative Extension.

Potter, T. (2011) Colostrum: getting the right start. *Livestock* 16, 25–27.

Roland, L., Drillich, M., Klein-Jobstl, D. and Iwersen, M. (2015) Invited review: influence of climatic conditions on the development, performance, and health of calves. *Journal of Dairy Science* 99, 2438–2452.

Schuijt, G. and Taverne, M.A.M. (1994) The interval between birth and sternal recumbency as an objective measure of the viability of newborn calves. *Vet Record* 135, 111–115.

Stafford, K. (2007) Alleviating the pain caused by castration of cattle (guest editorial). *The Veterinary Journal* 173, 245–247.

Stafford, K.J. and Mellor, D.J. (2011) Addressing the pain associated with disbudding and dehorning in cattle. *Applied Animal Behaviour Science* 135, 226–231

Winder, C.B., LeBlanc, S.J. Haley, D.B., Lissemore, K.D. and Ann Godkin, M. (2017) Clinical trial of local anaesthetic protocols for acute pain associated with caustic paste disbudding in dairy calves. *Journal of Dairy Science* 100, 6429–6441.

FURTHER READING

Ahmed, P.O., Miller, M.F., Boggs, D.L., Comerford, J.W. and Reagan, J.O. (1989) Effects of late castration and feeding on bovine muscle quality. *Journal of Muscle Foods* 1, 59–69.

Hudson, C., Whay, H. and Huxley, J. (2008) Recognition and management of pain in cattle. *In Practice* 30, 126–134.

Potter, T.J., Hallowell, G.D. and Aldridge, B. (2012) Head and ocular surgery in farm animals. *In Practice* 34, 518–522.

Wieland, M., Mann, S., Guard, C.L. and Nydam, D.V. (2016) The influence of 3 different navel dips on calf health, growth performance, and umbilical infection assessed by clinical and ultrasonographic examination. *Journal of Dairy Science* 100, 513–524.

Chapter 5

The health and management of the young calf to weaning

In the relatively natural world of the beef suckler herd, the calf remains with its mother until weaned; typically, at 5–9 months of age. During this period, the calf is either housed or grazed, or both, alongside the cow.

MILK FEEDING

Nutritionally the calf is solely dependent on milk from its mother until 2–3 months of age. During this time, it will be inquisitive and seek to try the forage, grass or concentrates that its mother is being fed. These provide the first steps towards adult nutrition, but little in the way of actual nutritional value for the calf.

The supply (volume of yield) and quality of the milk from the cow are the main dictators of the calf's growth rate in these first few months. These in turn are dependent largely on the cow's own nutrition – not just at the time, but throughout the period referred to as the dry period, the weeks leading up to calving when the cow's previous lactation has ended, and continuing into the first few weeks post-calving when her next lactation has begun. An adult Angus/Friesian cross-bred cow will produce approximately 14 kg of milk per day and between 60–75% of the milk of the whole lactation will be produced in the first 60 days post-calving. A 1 kg increase in milk intake per day results in a 9 kg increase in calf weight at 150 days of age (Lowman and Lewis, 1992).

As well as the cow's nutrition there is a genetic component to a cow's milk yield; some cows are 'milkier' than others, there is a genetic variation between breeds and within breeds. A maternal EBV measurement called '200-day milk (kg)' has been established. This measurement represents the number of kilogrammes of calf weaned rather than the kilogrammes of milk produced at 200 days – calf weight at weaning, as already stated, is largely attributable to the milk production of the dam. The concept of EBVs is discussed in Chapter 9.

A cow's milk supply will be impaired by factors such as poor body condition, an insufficient duration of dry period, a difficult calving (dystocia) and any concurrent disease (notably mastitis). Consequently, these impingements will indirectly impair the calf's growth rate.

The calf's own health will also affect its growth rate, and, as detailed in Chapter 4, the main factor contributing to calf health is the level of colostrum intake in the first 24 hours after birth and the quality of that colostrum. A shortfall here puts calves more at risk from infections, such as septicaemia, navel ill, joint ill, scour and pneumonia.

The suckled calf has a limited ability to compensate for its own poor pre-weaning growth rates. Calves that are weaned at suboptimal weights will never catch up; the time taken to reach slaughter weight will always be longer.

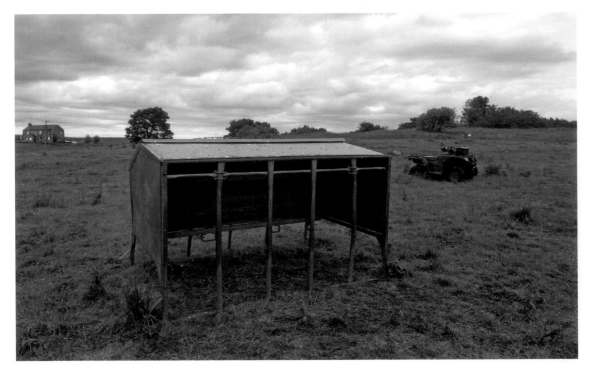

FIGURE 5.1 Calf creep feeder out at grass

CONCENTRATE (CREEP) FEEDING

The creep feeding of suckled calves is the process of allowing them access to concentrate feed that their mothers cannot access, see Figure 5.1. In the field, this is done using a 'calf creep' – a trough or area which can only be accessed through gaps that are too small for the cow but through which the calf can pass easily. In the shed, for example, narrow gaps in gates allow calves through to a separate straw-bedded area where they can feed and lie away from their dams if they choose.

Creep feeding is used to fill the deficit in energy that the cow's milk supply alone cannot satisfy, but is also needed in order to obtain the growth rates required in today's beef production systems, see Table 5.1.

Once calves are familiar with the availability of the creep feed their consumption of it will increase and their consumption of the dam's milk will decrease. This results in a reduced demand on the cow, which in turn allows her to maintain her body condition better than if she was being heavily drawn upon by the calf.

The benefits of creep feeding can be seen at weaning: heavier calf weights, less stress as the calves have already become familiar with their new feed substrate, and less of a 'growth check' as their rumen microbes are already acclimatised to concentrate feed.

For spring-born calves it is recommended that creep feed is introduced 6–8 weeks pre-weaning. In bull-beef production, the recommendation is that creep feed begins 12 weeks pre-weaning. Autumn-born calves may be fed creep feed from the time of housing at around 6 weeks old, right through the winter until turn out in spring. The timing of creep feed introduction will also depend on the cow's condition, and her grazing/forage availability. By the time of weaning a spring-born calf will be receiving approximately one-half of its nutrition from milk. An autumn-born calf, older at weaning and fed creep for longer, may only be

TABLE 5.1 Theoretical feed requirements for a suckled calf to make daily liveweight gain (DLWG) of 1.1 kg/day (Lowman and Lewis, 1992)

Calf weight (kg)	Milk for maintenance and 1.1 kg DLWG (kg)	Assumed milk yield of cow (kg/day)	Assumed hay intake (kg fresh weight/day)	14% CP (crude protein) concentrates required (kg/day)
50	8.6	10	–	–
100	10.9	9	0.5	0.2
150	13.5	8	1.0	1.1
200	16.4	7	2.0	2.0
250	19.8	6	2.5	2.9

relying on milk for 20% of its total nutritional requirements (Lowman and Lewis, 1992).

When introducing creep feed, it should initially contain a high proportion of digestible fibre, such as sugar beet pulp. Gradually this can be decreased and levels of starchier feeds, such as barley, can be increased. Acidosis of the rumen is a significant risk where calves gorge themselves on starchy creep feed – this lowering of rumen pH causes significant digestive upset and should be avoided. Creep should either be available *ad lib* so the calves have continual access to it and have no need to consume large amounts in one go, or, alternatively, the creep feed should be limited to 1–1.5 kg per head per feed. A creep feed should typically have a metabolisable energy (ME) of 12.5 MJ ME/kg DM and ideally 14–16% crude protein (CP).

NUTRITION OF THE ARTIFICIALLY REARED CALF

Not all calves reared for beef production are from suckler herds: an increasing amount of UK beef production is fulfilled by beef-sired calves from dairy herds where the calves are not reared on their dams, but, instead, artificially. Heifer replacements for some suckler herds are also sourced from dairy farms and will need to be artificially reared.

Given the potential relevance to the beef herd it seems appropriate, here, to cover the management of the beef-cross dairy calf from 7 days old until weaning at approximately 6–8 weeks of age,

generally referred to as the first part of the rearing period, see Figure 5.2.

Calves are fed milk either from buckets with teats, see Figure 5.3, or through milk machines. Milk machines can mix and warm milk and

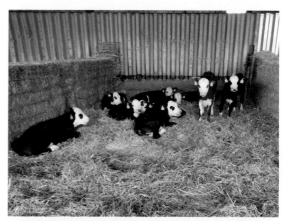

FIGURE 5.2 Beef-cross dairy calves pre-weaning

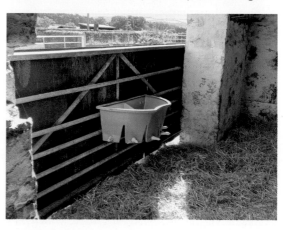

FIGURE 5.3 Milk fed to calves via a multi-teat bucket

regulate the feeding rate of the calf. Each method is equally good, as long as it is done properly. An *all-singing, all-dancing* machine that is poorly calibrated and dirty will cause far more problems than it solves!

As with the suckled calf, disease incidence, mortality rates and growth rates achieved in the rearing period rely on the calf having a good start in the first few hours of life, particularly with regards to the amount, quality and timeliness of colostrum intake.

Beef-bred dairy calves are sold or moved between units at variable ages; 7–10 days, 8 weeks, or even as growers or finishers, depending on the production system of the farm. Each move is stressful for the calf, the younger the calf the more susceptible they are to the effects of stress and disease; the fewer changes the better.

If calves are to be bought in from dairy herds, at 7–14 days of age, they should be/have been:

- from as few herds of origin (sources) as possible
- BVD free (either tested by tissue tag or from a BVD-free accredited herd)
- vaccinated with an intranasal pneumonia vaccine (see Chapter 26)
- properly fed an adequate quantity and quality of colostrum at birth
- ideally fed the same milk powder and rearing pellets as fed on the destination farm
- free from signs of clinical disease: bright, alert, no nasal discharge, normal respiratory rate, no coughing, no lameness, no navel infection and no scour.

The artificially reared calf has a shorter time period to develop a functional rumen than the suckled calf. A calf on a milk-only diet uses its abomasum (the fourth stomach) as its main stomach for digesting the milk. The reticulum, rumen and omasum are the first three stomachs (see Chapter 3, Figure 3.1) – and at this stage, are undeveloped in the young milk-fed calf. The milk bypasses these stomachs via the *oesophageal groove*, which is a furrow-like groove that diverts the milk and which

assumes its shape as a calf sucks (see Chapter 4). If the calf's normal feeding routine is upset, then the oesophageal groove may fail to function, and milk may enter the rumen. When this happens the milk ferments in the rumen and this causes bloat and scour. For these reasons the quiet, stress-free routine and feeding management of the milk-fed calf is crucial; they should be fed a consistent milk product (either powdered milk replacer or actual cow's milk but never alternating between the two) at the same time every day, at a consistent temperature and in a quiet manner.

When milk enters the abomasum in the presence of the digestive enzyme renin, the milk protein – called casein – will clot. The milk clot moves on at a controlled steady rate and is then digested in the small intestine.

As the milk-fed calf matures to become a fully functional *ruminant* by 4 months of age the abomasum goes from being 80% of the calf's total stomach volume in its first week of life to just 5% of the stomach volume in the older ruminant. Ruminants are entirely reliant on the vast fermentation vat that is the rumen.

To help the development of the rumen, calves should, from a very young age, be fed an alternative feedstuff in addition to their milk diet. Initially, the rumen cannot digest fibre, so highly digestible concentrate feeds are used instead; products referred to as 'starter feeds' or 'starter pellets'. The fermentation of the sugar and starch from starter feeds in the rumen produces *volatile fatty acids*, which are known to stimulate rumen development. It was long believed that it was fibre that achieved this; this is no longer considered to be the case.

Calves destined to be reared artificially should still be fed colostrum for the first 4 days of life before then transitioning to milk. After this, they will be fed either whole milk from the bulk tank or powdered milk replacer. There are advantages and disadvantages to each. The relative cost of whole milk versus replacer largely depends on the bulk tank milk market value at the time. Historically, waste milk was fed to calves; milk from mastitic cows or milk withheld from the tank due to antibiotic residues. This subjected all calves to antibiotic residues within the milk and infection pressure from any pathogens carried in the milk, this practice is now considered to be unacceptable and is legislated against in many farm assurance schemes.

Milk replacer, if fed correctly, is a reasonable alternative to real milk. It also has the benefit of not being at risk of carrying the Johne's disease bacterium which could otherwise infect the calf and therefore affect the herd's Johne's disease status (see Chapter 17). Real whole milk will, however, unlike replacer, contain antibodies, albeit in variable amounts, and these will help fight local infections within the gut lumen. Whole milk is also less likely to be incorrectly made up!

There is much debate over how much milk an artificially reared calf should be fed. From a financial aspect, the sooner a calf has a solid diet, the cheaper it is to feed – milk is more expensive than concentrate. For this reason, calves were traditionally fed a restricted milk diet – this meant they ate more solid feed and could be weaned sooner. The undernutrition of artificially fed calves has, however, been noticed and brought under scrutiny in recent years. Feeding a higher volume of milk, or a more concentrated milk replacer, has been trialled, and improved calf health has been observed; the calves have faster growth rates in the first few weeks of life, and heavier weaning weights, but they do take longer to achieve the intake level of concentrate feed that is advised before they can be weaned (a minimum of 1.5 kg per head per day). The result is a rearing period that costs more. Furthermore, care needs to be taken when increasing the amount of milk fed; a higher growth rate means higher protein requirements. If there is a mismatch between energy and protein fed, that is, plenty of energy but insufficient protein, then calves will lay down fat rather than lean tissue – an undesirable effect. Feeding large quantities of milk was once thought to cause nutritional scour but it is *fluctuations* that are the issue.

Clean fresh water should always be available to the calf, even the very young calf – a need that is often overlooked. Water, like concentrate, seems to be essential for the development of the rumen. Clean fresh straw in racks (not just bedding) should also be available for calves to pick at from birth; while the growth of the rumen seems unlinked to fibre provision, the development of the small papillae on the lining of the rumen *is* stimulated by this fibre. So, the old belief in fibre benefitting rumen development is not wrong after all!

An artificially reared calf should double its bodyweight from birth to 50 days, for example, from 40 kg to 80 kg. This represents a daily liveweight gain (DLWG) of 0.8 kg per day. Weigh tapes can be used in young calves to monitor weight, see Figure 5.4. The chest girth measurement is closely correlated to weight. A good target chest girth measurement for a beef-bred dairy calf at weaning is 96 cm, equating to approximately 80 kg.

HOUSING AND THE ENVIRONMENT FOR THE SUCKLED CALF IN THE REARING PERIOD

Calves that are sucking their mothers are usually run in groups. There are visible social interactions: they play together, sleep together and feed together, and this applies whether at grass or in a housed environment.

HOUSING AND THE ENVIRONMENT FOR THE ARTIFICIALLY REARED CALF IN THE REARING PERIOD

Artificially reared calves are often reared in pens – individually, in pairs, or in small groups. It was thought that calves kept in single pens, and in sight of other calves, were less likely to suffer from disease. It has subsequently been shown, however, that as long as the husbandry is good, the calves are of the same age, and the calves are in groups of no more than 12, then they are less stressed and have

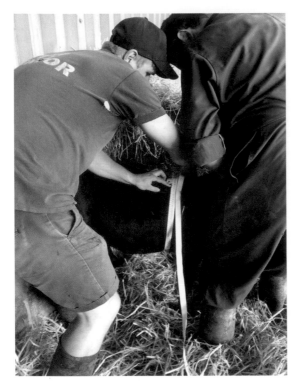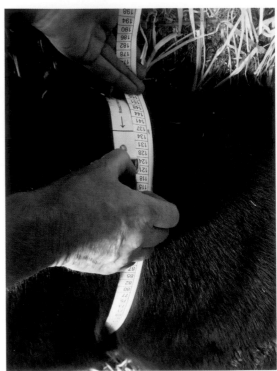

FIGURE 5.4 Routine weighing (using weigh tapes) of beef-cross dairy calves

higher solid feed intakes pre-weaning than similar calves individually penned (Miller-Cushon and DeVries, 2016).

Calf hutches or 'igloos' are popular for artificially reared calves, especially where existing buildings are not suitable or where the investment in a new calf shed is not feasible. Calf hutches and igloos can easily be moved, cleaned and disinfected and they are conducive to an all-in-all-out system. They can, however, be labour intensive, hard work in bad weather and very hot in the summer.

Whether grouped or individually housed, space allowances specified by welfare assurance schemes should be adhered to, see Box 5.1. It is stated in UK welfare guidelines, and should be obvious, that housed calves need adequate space to turn, lie down and exhibit normal behaviour.

The group size for calves and youngstock is largely determined by the age distribution within the group. For a home-bred rearing system, if calving is rapid, then calves can be kept in groups

of up to 12 with little age variation between the oldest and the youngest in the group; this markedly reduces the transmission of disease. Irrespective of the age difference of the calves during the rearing period, no group should contain more than 12 calves as this has been established as incurring a higher risk of disease, see Figure 5.5.

Whether a calf is sucking its dam or is artificially reared, there are five crucial factors to consider in its environment.

1. **Ventilation**. The breathing of constantly fresh air is required to prevent respiratory disease. An indicator of air freshness is a lack of urine (ammonia) or faeces smell, and an absence of dust. Cobwebs are a sign of poor ventilation. It could be assumed that new sheds are well ventilated and old sheds not; this is often not true. A new high and wide shed built onto the side of another building can be the poorest ventilated of all, while a single narrower high-pitched slate

The Welfare of Farmed Animals (England) Regulations 2000, schedule 4 states:

The width of any individual stall or pen shall be at least the height of the calf at the withers, measured in the standing position, and the length be at least equal to the body length of the calf, measured from the tip of the nose to the pin bones.

No calf should be confined in an individual stall or pen after the age of eight weeks.

Individual stalls or pens should have perforated walls which allow calves to have direct visual and tactile contact.

For those kept in groups the space allowance for each calf should be at least 1.5 square metres for a calf less than 150 kg and 2 square metres for a calf weighing between 150 and 200 kg. 2 square metres is required for a calf of 200 kg liveweight or more.

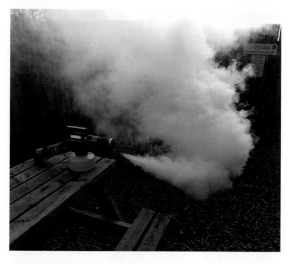

FIGURE 5.6 Fogger

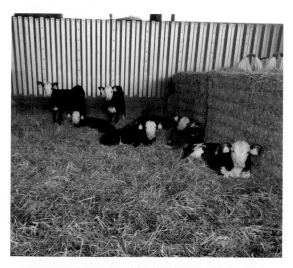

FIGURE 5.5 Eight pre-weaned beef-cross dairy calves housed together in a well-lit, well-bedded, clean, dry pen

roof may in fact operate a better *stack effect* than many new buildings thanks to its outlets through the slates. The stack effect (Chapter 6) should not, however, be the sole means of ventilating housing for artificially reared calves as they simply do not generate sufficient heat to cause the air to rise. Consequently, mechanical ventilation is often required. This differs from the suckled calf situation where the dams housed with their offspring generate a lot of heat and the stack effect is naturally created. Smoke bombs or 'foggers', see Figure 5.6, are commonly used to assess ventilation by watching how long the smoke takes to clear and what direction it travels in. Air flow should not be greater than 0.5 m/s and can be measured with a wind speed gauge, see Figure 5.7. There is a risk with high air flows that the shed is draughty. Low-level draughts from high hung doors are of concern for calf housing. Flaps on the bottom of the doors or straw bales to block gaps may be the solution. Ventilation is discussed further in Chapter 6.

2. **Humidity**. Overstocking, poor drainage, broken water troughs, overflowing gutters and inadequate ventilation all contribute to humidity. Calves do not thrive in humid environments – humid air feels colder in winter, and moisture

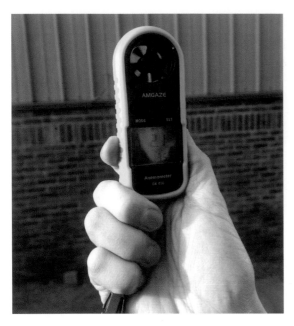

FIGURE 5.7 Wind speed gauge

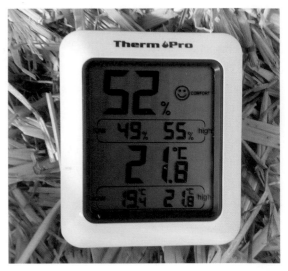

FIGURE 5.8 A combined temperature and humidity meter in a calf shed (humidity 52%, temperature 21.8°C)

harbours pathogens. For suckled calves there is also the moisture output from their dams to consider, and this is considerable. Milk preparation areas should be situated outside the calf housing. Pens that house machine-fed calves can be designed so that the milking machine is on a concrete plinth which has good drainage and can be kept clean. Humidity and temperature monitors are readily available at low cost. Figure 5.8 shows typical humidity and temperatures of a calf house, at calf level, in mid-July. Relative humidity should not exceed 70%.

3. **Bedding**. Calves require a clean, dry area in which to lie down. Cows suckling calves may be housed in cubicled or slatted sheds. If this is the case a 'creep area' should be provided for the calves to lie together, away from their dams, on clean dry bedding, not slats. The bedding is typically straw, but paper waste is now commonly used in areas of the country where straw is either in short supply or expensive to transport. An adequate depth of dry bedding is vital in colder weather to limit air flow around the calf and so keep it warm. As a ready indicator it should be comfortable for a person to kneel on

the bedding without any discomfort; the knees of that person's trousers or waterproofs should not be wet when they stand up.

4. **Temperature**. Every calf house should have a room thermometer. In the first month of life, calves are comfortable in an ambient temperature of between 10°C and 15°C. At 1 month old, calves can withstand temperatures down to 6°C. Cold temperature will affect the calves' behaviour: they will huddle together, trying to seek out the warmest, least draughty, part of the shed and over time, they will grow hairy coats. They will also use energy to keep warm rather than for growth. Deep straw beds for nesting and calf jackets are two ways to keep calves warm. Calf jackets may not be suitable for the suckled calf but are useful to have if a calf is poorly and needs some additional insulation. For more information on thermoregulation in the calf see Chapter 4.

5. **Hygiene**. In suckled calf systems, sheds should be cleaned and disinfected after turnout; water troughs should be kept clean and regularly rinsed out. For artificially reared calves, attention to the milk preparation area, equipment, buckets, milking machine and pens is required.

A standard operating procedure (SOP) detailing the cleansing and disinfection routine should be established, displayed and followed by all those involved in the calf shed. Recommended is a pre-wash routine to remove milk residues from the equipment, followed by washing with a chlorinated alkaline detergent solution at a temperature of 54–57°C; this kills bacteria and lifts milk proteins. A further scrub to remove residues and a rinse with water above 49°C is required before a final rinse using an acid sanitiser to prevent the attachment of further bacteria. The equipment should be allowed to dry on raised racks before use (AHDB, 2018). If *calf jackets* are used, they should be washed between calves – a dirty wet jacket will do more harm than no jacket at all. Maintenance of the building is required to ensure surfaces are smooth and devoid of cracks and crevices which may harbour pathogens and make cleaning and disinfection more difficult. Calves do not have a fully developed immune system – like human babies, they are susceptible to disease. Whether a calf succumbs to disease is a balance between the pathogen load and the level of immunity. Calf scour is the predominant disease affecting these young calves and the vast amount of these cases are avoidable with good hygiene, good colostrum management and nutrition.

ANTIBIOTIC USAGE IN BOTH THE SUCKLED AND ARTIFICIALLY REARED CALF

Antibiotic usage is under strict control, and, increasingly so, measurement as described in Chapter 19. Antibiotics should not be used to prop up poor management and husbandry, such as insufficient trained labour or poor farm infrastructure. Tactical use of antibiotics and supportive therapy will still need to be employed at times, but the aim is to prevent disease occurring in the first place. Vaccination plays a role here: in an ideal world, the ultimate combination of preventative measures would remove the need even for vaccines but inevitably, so often, vaccines are still needed to bolster the animal's own natural immune system rather than using unnatural antibiotics that have consequences for the rest of the animal kingdom, humans included.

Vaccination in both the suckled and artificially reared calf

- Scour vaccines are discussed in Chapter 11.
- Clostridial vaccines are discussed in Chapter 12.
- Pneumonia vaccines are discussed in Chapter 13.

REFERENCES

AHDB (2018) *Better Calf Housing. BRP+.* Agriculture and Horticulture Development Board, Stoneleigh.

Lowman, B. and Lewis, M. (1992) Feeding the beef suckler herd. In: *BCVA Summer Meeting*, Wye College, pp. 9–27.

Miller-Cushon, E.K. and DeVries, T.J. (2016) Effect of social housing on the development of feeding behaviour and social feeding preferences of dairy calves. *Journal of Dairy Science* 99, 1–12.

Chapter 6

The health and management of growing cattle

WEANING THE SUCKLED CALF

At weaning, depending on its age, on the provision of creep feed and on its mother's milk supply, a calf will be consuming between 20–50% of its nutrient intake as milk.

As described in Chapter 5, consumed milk, in the pre-ruminant calf bypasses the reticulum, rumen and omasum, via the oesophageal groove, and enters the abomasum where it clots, moves steadily on and is then digested in the small intestine. When a calf is weaned and milk consumption ceases, the reticulum, rumen, omasum and abomasum start to function in an adult ruminant manner.

Over its lifetime a suckled calf will have eaten some of the same forage as its mother, grazed some grass and probably been fed some creep feed. This gradual exposure to different food substrates allows the rumen wall to develop in strength, the rumen microbes to establish and the papillae (small finger-like projections lining the rumen wall) to develop. The papillae are essential to increase the surface area for the absorption of volatile fatty acids – the predominant energy source for the ruminant. By the time calves are weaned, the rumen will be adequately developed and ready to cope with fermentation and rumination.

'Creep feeding' involves allowing calves access to feed that their dams cannot reach. As well as increasing weaning weights, and minimising the post-weaning growth check, creep feeding prepares the rumen for the cessation of the milk diet.

Fresh water is essential to rumen development. Ensuring young calves always have access to clean water is essential.

Unlike milk which ends up, ideally, in the abomasum, water drunk from a bucket or trough enters the rumen. Although largely water, milk, through a poorly understood mechanism, triggers the oesophageal groove bypass reflex. It is recommended that suckled calves are at least 5 months old when they are weaned. Calves can be left on their mother up until no less than 5 weeks before the cow is expected to calve again. The cow ideally needs to be dry (not lactating) for a minimum of 5 weeks so she can prepare an adequate store of colostrum for her next calf. There are occasions where autumn-calving cows suckle calves up until they are just about to calve again. This technique is used to prevent the cow getting mastitis when she is dry (not lactating), and to stop the cow from getting too fat after a summer at grass; this is, however, a trade-off against good and plentiful colostrum supply for the next calf. Knowing now the supreme importance of colostrum then the ideal system would address mastitis and cow condition through means other than curtailing the dry period.

Given that lactation is an energy drain on the cow, those that are thin and struggling to gain condition can benefit from having their calves weaned early. As well as helping the cow gain condition this will also help with her colostrum production which would otherwise really suffer.

Weaning is a stressful process for the calf and the cow. The calf will experience a loss of maternal contact, a change in social structure, possibly a new environment and, to some extent or more, a new diet. Any stress will affect its growth rate. Cows and calves vocalise their distress, pace back and forth, and make attempts to get back to each other. Consequently, weaning is a high-risk period for physical injury to cattle, for injury to personnel, and for stress-induced diseases, such as pneumonia in the calf and mastitis in the cow.

There are several methods used to wean calves.

1. **Abrupt weaning**. Calves are removed from their dams and kept completely away from them. The cows and calves cannot see, hear or smell each other, the idea being to get it over and done with as quickly as possible and not drag out the hope of re-uniting.
2. **Fence-line weaning**. Cows and calves are separated over a fence line for 7 days before complete separation. Calves can no longer suckle their dams, but they can see, hear and smell them, and have nose-to-nose contact.
3. **Gradual weaning**. Cows and calves are separated for an increasing number of hours every day; after 7 days they are no longer allowed any contact with each other.
4. **Antisucking devices**. 'Nose flaps' or 'nose plates' are attached to the noses of calves to prevent them from sucking their dams for 7 days before complete separation of the cow and calf.

There is no firm evidence as to which is the best method of weaning suckled calves. Research suggests (Enríquez et al., 2010) that abrupt weaning has the least effect on liveweight gains when compared to fence-line weaning or antisuckling devices. When weaning is carried out over a prolonged period, or calves can still see or hear their dams, it prolongs the period of stress and adversely affects liveweight gains. Other studies report that calves subjected to fence-line weaning achieve better average DLWG over a 10-week period post-weaning than those that are abruptly weaned; it was considered in this study that the calves abruptly weaned are not able to compensate for the initial losses in weight gain.

It is thought that a calf's response to weaning will largely depend on its intake of concentrate feed prior to weaning and how much milk its mother was producing. Recommendations for weaning include the following.

- Cows should be removed from calves rather than the other way around so that the calves remain in the environment they are familiar with.
- Calves should be weaned in good weather.
- Other management tasks should be avoided at the time of weaning, for example, dehorning or castrating.
- Calves should be left in the same environment and social groups.
- Pneumonia vaccination should be completed well in advance of weaning.

WEANING THE ARTIFICIALLY REARED CALF

In contrast to the suckled calf, a conscious effort needs to be made to ensure that the artificially reared calf has had access to adequate food substrates to allow for the development of the rumen before it is weaned (see Chapter 5). The artificially reared calf will be weaned at around 6–8 weeks of age and will have full rumen function by 4 months of age.

Weaning should not be solely determined by age. Calves should be eating a minimum of 1.5 kg/head/day of a high-quality starter feed or starter pellet.

As with suckled calves weaning should not coincide with any other stressful procedures, this includes the mixing of strange stock. Calves that are sick with scour or pneumonia should not be weaned until they are back to full health.

Abrupt weaning involves less time and management, but growth checks are larger. Gradual weaning by decreasing the milk fed day by day over a 7–14 day period reduces the chance of growth checks. Once artificially reared cattle are weaned the aim is to achieve a DLWG of greater than 1.1 kg/day.

PRODUCTION SYSTEMS

What a calf is fed after it is weaned largely depends on the production system. Many systems exist and thoughts on production systems are changing as the industry moves to an integrated supply chain, smaller carcases and a younger slaughter age. Many different systems of production exist.

- **Weaned suckled calf production**. Calves are sold soon after weaning (sometimes on the day of weaning). This is a common scenario on marginal hill farms where there is limited shed space and insufficient straw to house spring-born calves over the winter months. Some calves are not fed any creep feed pre-weaning. They are often purchased and then transported to areas of the country where there is straw and cheap feed. They are often mixed with calves from other farms and introduced to an unfamiliar growing ration. This is a very stressful system for calves; dietary upset, trauma and pneumonia are highly likely. The check in live-weight gain is likely to be considerable.

- **'Store' suckled calf production**. This system is used for weaned, spring-born calves, approximately 7 months old at housing, see Figure 6.1. These cattle are fed a low-cost diet over the winter months; they are 'stored', that is, they are not expected to gain weight, but only maintain themselves. Then, in the spring, their growth rates can be maximised cheaply through grazing. Even though calves only need to maintain their condition over the winter months, they do still need to be fed sufficiently

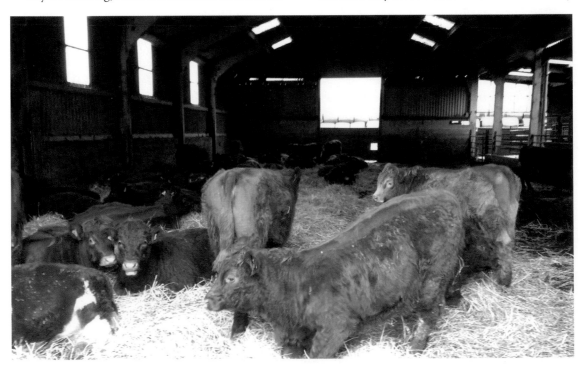

FIGURE 6.1 Weaned castrated male Luing calves housed in a well-bedded, clean, dry shed

for at least 1 month post-weaning for the rumen to fully develop. If the rumen is not allowed to develop in muscularity and increase in surface area, then the calf will not be efficient in converting grass to liveweight gain when turned out in the spring.

- **Dairy beef production**. Beef-cross dairy calves are weaned at 8 weeks and then gradually introduced to the growing diet. They may remain on the same farm from birth through to slaughter or they may be moved from their birth farm to a rearing unit, for the growing period, and maybe a finishing unit for fattening. Every move constitutes a change in environment, in diet, in social grouping and these are all stressful for the calf.
- **Intensive beef production**. Entire (non-castrated) bulls, beef-bred or black and white bull-beef, will be required to deliver consistently high growth rates from weaning to slaughter. Again, similar to beef-bred dairy calves, this may take place on one holding or multiple holdings. The calves are fed for maximal growth rates and slaughtered anywhere from 13–18 months of age.

NUTRITION IN THE GROWING PHASE

Once calves have been weaned, they enter what is known as the growing phase. This is when cattle grow their *frames*, that is, their skeletons.

Typically, the ration in the growing phase consists mostly of forage or grazed grass, with the addition of a supplementary feed containing protein, energy, vitamins and minerals. Good quality grazing or forage will substantially reduce the costs of the growing period. The amount of feed required will depend on the ME of the forage, the grazed grass quality and the intakes thereof. Feeding too much starch in the growing period is to be avoided as it will result in early fat deposition rather than the growth of lean muscle and, more importantly at this stage, bone.

The breed or type, however, significantly affects the length of this growing phase.

Traditional breeds such as the native breeds of the UK and upland Europe tend to be of smaller frame and grow relatively slowly but, to achieve this, only require a modest forage based ration to do so. Once grown, however, these cattle need only a short finishing period as they fatten quickly and easily once their small frames have taken shape. Examples would be the Hereford, the Beef Shorthorn, the Galloway and the Welsh Black. These cattle are often described as being *early maturers*.

Continental breeds of low mainland Europe on the other hand tend to be larger framed and grow relatively quickly to achieve these large frame sizes. This, however, can require more intensive feeding, typically involving cereal provision in addition to high quality forage. Although the growing phase is relatively quick it is still relatively expensive to achieve as these cattle are big to start with and they eat a lot of this more costly ration. When the relatively fast and furious growing phase is over these cattle enter the finishing phase which conversely takes relatively longer and as with any finishing ration also needs to be energy rich. This longer energy demanding finishing period does produce a large finished product but comes at relatively high expense. Examples would be the Charolais and the Limousin. These cattle are described as *late maturers*.

The feed conversion rate (FCR), the number of kg of feed needed to generate 1 kg of body weight, decreases as cattle get older and/or bigger. Take a calf at 12 months of age, for example: 5 kg of DM intake will result in 1 kg of liveweight gain. At 24 months of age the same calf would need to eat 16 kg of DM to produce the same 1 kg of liveweight gain (AHDB, 2016a). This phenomenon contributes to the relatively high cost of farming late maturing cattle to their optimum potential.

Regardless of breed, bull-beef cattle, largely due to their high testosterone levels, tend to fall into the same characteristics as larger framed continental cattle, better suited to high energy diets to exploit their potential for fast growth rates. Gender, in general, does indeed affect growth rates and fat deposition. Bulls have higher growth rates and are typically leaner than heifers and castrated males. Heifers deposit fat at a younger age than males. Bulls and castrated males may have a shorter growing period compared to heifers, while heifers will get fat if left too long on a finishing ration. The FCRs are also different between genders; bulls being higher than castrated males and heifers, and in that order.

The growth rates and FCR of an *individual animal within a breed or type* will be affected by its own individual *genetics*. This is the basis of EBVs. There are EBVs for both *200-day growth rates* and *400-day growth rates*, and for *fat* and *muscle* depth (see Chapter 9).

So the influence of cattle type, breed, gender and genetics, and consequently their preferred ration, is reasonably simple to grasp but to add extra layers of complication, diets can be manipulated to try to change these patterns and the *intended target carcase weight* and *intended target growing period*, as dictated by the market perhaps, will also bear an influence on how the farmer tries to work with these patterns.

So, for example, where a maximum carcase weight limit prevails, things may be a little different. A late maturing, Continental animal will struggle with a restricted finishing weight; they want to get big; they do not want to fatten!

And an example of a dictated target growing period would be where markets specify the number of days cattle must be at grass. Here, once again, the need for late maturers to enjoy energy-dense rations for both growth and finishing may not be met, and these cattle may not grow to their potential or fatten; this system may suit the early maturing types.

To complicate matters further the market may also dictate the maximum permissible number of movements between holdings, and, not the weight at slaughter, but the *age*. It is not easy being a beef farmer! The production system needs thinking about very carefully and not all production

systems are suited to all farms. But most of all it is worth remembering that staying as close to nature as possible is normally the best route for health and welfare, and ultimately, therefore, production.

Grazing

Grazed grass is, under normal circumstances, the cheapest feed of all. On many farms, however, cattle are turned out to pasture and there is little management of the grass quality, the growth or how to get the best from it. It must be acknowledged, however, that marginal hill grazing, see Figure 6.2, often used in suckled beef production, is not suitable for improvement or, in the UK, is not usually allowed to be improved under the rules of the environmental stewardship schemes.

For a farm that lends itself to grassland improvement and management, however, productivity and profitability can be greatly improved by understanding grass growth – and by measuring, managing and monitoring it.

The amount of grass – often referred to as pasture cover – is measured as kilogrammes of DM per hectare. Defined very crudely, the value is determined by the height of the grass and its water content, which varies depending on the time of year. Pasture cover can be measured using a plate meter, an electronic device that is placed in the grass sward, or with a sward stick, see Figure 6.3. A representative area of the field should be measured and up to 30 measurements taken by walking a 'W' path across the field.

The 'welly boot test' is a less accurate measure of sward height; the optimal sward height for growing cattle on a rotational grazing system is 10–12 cm. This can be marked with a pen on the side of a wellington boot and sward height can be assessed while walking around the field.

Grass growth is affected by the nutrients available to the grass, by moisture, by altitude, by aspect, by soil temperature, by light, by day length, by grass type and by seasonality.

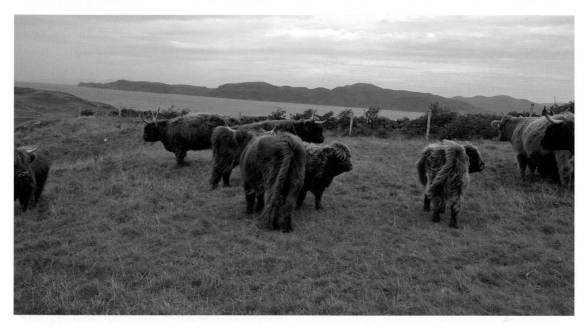

FIGURE 6.2 Highland cows and calves grazing unimproved marginal land

Under-grazing will result in mature stemmy grasses, which are undesirable to cattle, and in the accumulation of dead leaves at the base of the sward, so limiting the exposure of new leaves to sunlight. Over-grazing will result in a short sward height which, if below the growing point (the minimum height for the plant to thrive) will significantly limit grass growth.

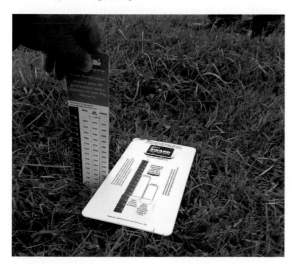

FIGURE 6.3 Sward stick used to measure pasture cover (kg/DM/hectare of grass)

Good utilisation of grass is the key to an efficient grazing system.

- **Set-stocked grazing**. Calves are turned out into a field of a set area, and left there, achieving grass utilisation of only 50%. The grass becomes trampled, contaminated with faeces and urine, and consequently under grazed; this grass becomes old and stemmy, which perpetuates its lack of appeal.
- **Paddock grazing**. The most effective utilisation of grass is achieved through paddock grazing. This involves moving stock frequently, often daily, between small paddocks, and basing the movements on close regulation of the sward heights. In this system, 80% utilisation can be achieved (AHDB, 2016b).
- **Rotational grazing**. An intermediate option between the two systems is rotational grazing whereby cattle may be moved weekly, or, as required, again on the assessment of the sward heights, see Figure 6.4.

Paddock grazing and rotational grazing do require some infrastructure, such as electric

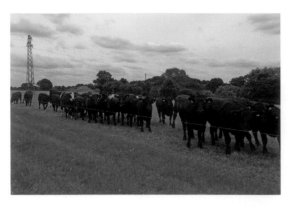

FIGURE 6.4 Rotational grazing of weaned beef-cross dairy calves

fencing and the provision of water. A set of weigh scales is also important for accurate calculations of the calves' requirements.

Paddock grazing calculations

Once the pasture cover (grass kg/DM/hectare) is known, it is possible to calculate how many cattle of a given weight can be allocated to a specific area.

> For example: a field is 1 hectare and there is 2500 kg/DM/hectare of grass.
> There needs to be 1500 kg/DM/hectare left on the pasture for regrowth (referred to as residual), thus there is 1000 kg/DM/hectare available to graze.
> A growing animal (of, say, 350 kg) needs to eat 3% of its body weight in DM per day.
> 3% of 350 kg is 10.5 kg.
> The 1 hectare paddock will graze 31 growing cattle for 3 days.

There are several assumptions with this calculation.

1. The liveweight used in the calculation is correct: at least ten cattle in the group should be weighed and used to calculate the DM requirement. The key to ensuring all cattle in the group are nutritionally satisfied is to ensure they are as uniform as possible in weight, age and breed.

2. The sward is of good quality. Ideally, a good clover content, dense cover, plenty of leaf and few weeds.

Growing cattle can achieve between 1–1.5 kg of DLWG from well-managed grazing alone. If they are gaining less than 1 kg per day then there is a flaw in the system or something else is wrong and investigation is required.

With paddock grazing, a cattle group allocation plan is needed, along with good monitoring of grass growth using *predicted grass growth rates*. Grass growth rates may be static or even negative at certain times of year – during drought, for example.

Understanding soils is as important as understanding grass but the subject is outside the scope of this text. This is only an introduction to grazing strategies and grazing management. There is much science behind it, and it should not be entered into lightly or without knowledge, understanding and planning.

Minerals

Cattle require *macro-minerals* and *micro-minerals*. Macro-minerals are those required in large amounts such as calcium, phosphorus, magnesium, chloride, potassium and sulphur. Micro-minerals – often referred to as trace elements – are required in smaller amounts and include copper, zinc, selenium, cobalt, iodine, manganese and iron.

Any ration formulation needs to have the correct balance of minerals: too much and toxicity is likely, too little and animals will become deficient. A knowledge of how minerals interfere with each other, in the gut, is also needed.

Trace elements play a vital role in forage digestion, reproductive performance, the immune system, the development of bones, muscle and teeth. Therefore, a deficiency in any of the trace elements displays as specific clinical signs. Reduced feed intake and reduced feed conversion ratios are common signs of trace element deficiency, which is

TABLE 6.1 Trace element mineral requirements for beef cattle (mg of mineral required per kg of DM consumed) (Paterson and Engle, 2005)

Mineral	Growing-finishing cattle ration inclusion requirement (mg per kg DM)
Cobalt	0.1
Copper	10.0
Iodine	0.5
Iron	50.0
Manganese	20.0
Selenium	0.1
Zinc	30.0

why in the growing diet, especially when cattle are grazing with no supplementary feed, their trace element requirements must be satisfied by some means as they are highly at risk of being deficient.

A guide for mineral inclusion is included in Table 6.1. All other supplementation needs to be taken into account. For example, if the cattle have received a trace element bolus, this needs to be acknowledged.

THE PREVENTION OF BOVINE RESPIRATORY DISEASE

Calf pneumonia, enzootic calf pneumonia and bovine respiratory disease (BRD) are all names for essentially the same condition. In summary, it is infection of the respiratory system with a pathogen that causes an immune response, damage to the tissues within the respiratory system, and associated clinical signs, possibly mortality. This can occur at any age but is commonly, but not exclusively, seen in calves during their first housing season.

There are multiple infectious agents that cause BRD; these are covered in more detail in Chapter 13. BRD is still a major source of economic loss and has an adverse effect on animal welfare. It can affect calves from a few days old through to adulthood. Concurrent infection with BVD, lungworm or tickborne fever may decrease calves' defence against infection and exacerbate the clinical signs.

Various studies exist that have attempted to quantify the economic loss incurred by BRD. Costs result from reduced liveweight gain, mortality, veterinary and medicine costs, and labour. For a suckled calf, the cost of BRD is estimated to be £82 per affected calf (Bryson, 2000). This is merely an indication and will be variable depending on the age of the animal and the severity of the disease.

The hidden cost of subclinical disease means it is almost impossible to know the true cost of a BRD outbreak. Slaughterhouse studies suggest that far more calves suffer from BRD than are detected and treated by stockpersons. It is estimated that average daily growth rates are reduced by up to 202 g in the worst affected calves (Penny, 2015). These calves take considerably longer to fatten, stay in the system for longer, endure a higher risk of mortality, and yield a carcase which may be downgraded at slaughter (due to the chronic BRD affecting the tissue of the ribcage and surrounding area).

The calf's own natural defences

The lining of the calf's respiratory tract has its own defence mechanisms: a mucous membrane lining that prevents the adhesion of microorganisms, and fine hairs that provide a constant 'conveyor belt' flicking and moving any particles, including microorganisms, from the lungs up and out of the respiratory tract. In the lining of the lungs, there are also a high number of white blood cells and special proteins that are able to destroy micro-organisms if they get that far. Within 4 hours, healthy animals can clear 90% of inhaled bacteria from their lungs (Griffin et al., 2010).

Disease occurs: (1) when these defences are compromised, which occurs when the animal is stressed, exhausted, has become chilled, over-heated, dehydrated, starved, or has concurrent disease; and/or (2) when there is an overwhelming bacterial challenge by a high number of micro-organisms in the environment, when cattle are mixed, or when there are a lot of infectious animals in an air space and environmental conditions allow microorganisms to persist. Building design largely controls this environment; the correct environment is a major factor in preventing respiratory disease, see next subsection.

Environment

Ventilation

In the UK it is estimated half the naturally ventilated cattle buildings are inadequately ventilated for the weight and number of livestock they house. Fresh air is required to maintain oxygen levels and to remove bacterial pathogens, gases and dust which may challenge the respiratory system's defence mechanisms. Cattle sheds with a lack of fresh air are smelly and are often dark. Air inlets and outlets are required to allow for fresh air to enter an air space and old air to be removed.

Air speed needs to be measured at calf head height, that is, 20–40 cm above the bed level (Chamberlain, 2015). The rate at which old air is replaced with new air is partly related to the air speed which should be between 0.2 and 0.5 m/s. A higher air speed at animal level will subject it to a draught and cause chilling.

There has been a vast amount of research into building design and computer models exist to calculate the heat, gas and moisture production of the animals and therefore the air flow and air exchange that is required to manage the air quality. Ventilation requirements may well be known, but implementing the necessary building alterations to achieve them may require considerable investment. The adaptation of an existing building may be necessary rather than starting afresh with a new build.

Put simply, cattle housing should provide the animals with a clean, dry bed, protection from the weather and a plentiful supply of clean air.

In the 1970s, the theory of natural ventilation through *convection* was established and became known as the 'stack effect'. The heat produced from an animal's own metabolism (which is significant in a growing ruminant) warms the air surrounding it, air which then rises and escapes from the building through outlets above in the roof. This creates negative pressure which draws in the outside air through side inlets. The larger the temperature difference between the inside and outside of the shed, the more pronounced is the stack effect and the more air is consequently drawn into the shed. This stack effect is not reliant on the wind, it is effective on a still day, but buildings are, however, generally better ventilated if they are positioned at 90° to the prevailing wind. The air within a building should change at least four times an hour. Any air flow created from open doorways and from wind generally is, theoretically at least, an added bonus but cattle should still be protected from rain, snow, strong sunlight and those all important troublesome draughts.

For the stack effect to work, the positioning of the inlets and outlets, and their design, are vital to its success. Figures 6.5 to 6.9 demonstrate different inlet and outlet designs. Some common problems are as follows.

- Insufficient numbers or size of cattle in a shed to heat the air sufficiently. Very young calves (not housed with their dams) cannot generate enough heat to create the stack effect; mechanical ventilation may well be the only solution to achieve well-ventilated calf housing.
- Adjoining buildings that interfere with, or even completely block, inlets.
- Insufficient outlets to allow warm air to escape

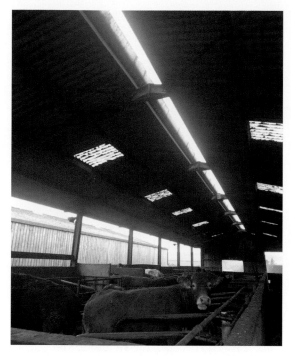

FIGURE 6.5 A chimney ridge allows an outlet for rising warm air – the edges are baffled to allow air out without allowing rain in

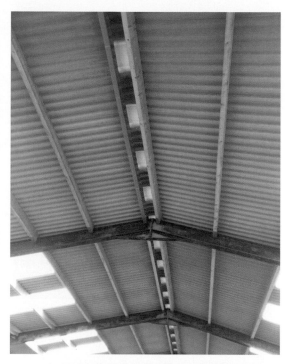

FIGURE 6.7 The ridge has been sheeted and small gaps left to provide outlets for the rising warm air

– this can result in condensation and increased moisture within the shed so allowing microorganisms to persist (Figure 6.10).
• Cold surfaces and moisture which remove heat from the air. Tin clad roofs and concrete walls have poor thermal properties.

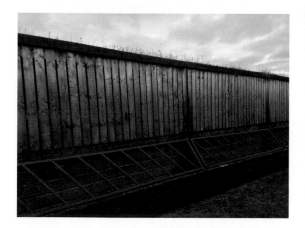

FIGURE 6.6 The gaps in space boarding provide inlets for air to enter a shed

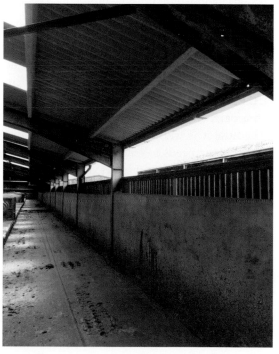

FIGURE 6.8 Air inlets sited above cow height prevent animals experiencing cold draughts

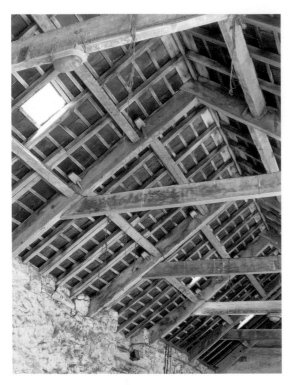

FIGURE 6.9 It may be an old shed, but this roof provides natural outlets for air through the gaps in the structure

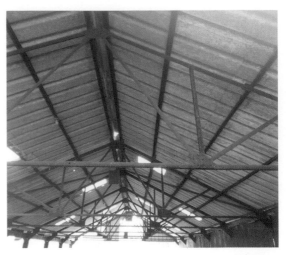

FIGURE 6.10 An asbestos roof with no overhead outlet for warm air to escape, preventing the stack effect

- The inlets should be on at least both sides of the building and be four times the size of the outlet area. Why have the inlets bigger than the outlets? The simple theory is that the air inside the building is in an expanded state because it is warm, therefore a larger volume of cold air needs to enter the inlets to replace this expanded air as it leaves through the roof. Does physics not dictate that this would actually mean an ever-accelerating flow of cold air into the building driving an ever-accelerating expansion and exit of warm air? The building would eventually take off like the house in the Wizard of Oz! This is, in reality, seemingly not the case of course – a simpler explanation would be that larger inlets offer no resistance to inflow so can never be a limiting factor in the upward ventilation flow. Suffice to say, for whatever reason, make the inlets bigger than the outlets!

- There needs to be a temperature gradient of at least 2°C between the air inside and the air outside for the stack effect to work. This is not always the case.
- The stack effect is influenced by extreme building dimensions. A very wide shed may impede the effect and may require additional inlets on the gable ends. A low roof will fail. If the pitch of the roof is very steep, or very shallow, this will also affect the flow of air and compromise the stack effect.
- Additional inlets such as doors or canvas side-curtains which are manually operated need to be considered carefully in any assessment. How often they are adjusted will depend on the climatic conditions. Is there not, therefore, a risk that there will be times when they are not altered in changing climatic conditions and therefore actually risk poor ventilation for that period?

The diet of housed animals will greatly influence their heat, moisture and gas outputs. It is estimated that the heat output from growing cattle achieving 2 kg DLWG will be 2.5 times greater than those fed a forage-based maintenance diet.

Most naturally ventilated sheds end up being

ventilated by a combination of stack effect and *cross draught* – not ideal.

Cross draught is the terminology used to describe air exchange in a shed resulting from wind alone. Wind speed needs to be at least 2 m/s to create this movement of air. Neighbouring buildings can interfere with wind speed and create a 'wind shadow' equal to five times the height of the building. As wind can come from any direction, or not at all, cross draughts cannot be relied upon to ensure good shed ventilation.

With the unpredictable nature of natural ventilation factors, mechanical active ventilation systems have been introduced; they can be either negative pressure systems or positive pressure systems.

Negative pressure systems rely on a closed unit and fans that extract air from the building, resulting in fresh air being drawn in. Widely used in parts of the USA, these have not been a success in the UK (Chamberlain, 2015).

Positive pressure systems are more common; air is blown into the shed with a fan thus forcing 'old' air out through any available outlets. The fresh air needs to reach the calf and a ventilation tube with spaced out holes in it runs the length of the shed. The fan pushes the air through it.

Moisture

Humidity is the concentration of moisture within the air. *Relative humidity* (RH) (usually expressed as a percentage) is a measure of the water content of the air compared to the maximum amount of water that the air could carry. The ability of air to carry water increases as it gets warmer so relative humidity falls as air temperature rises.

Conversely, as air temperature falls, relative humidity will rise to the point that condensation occurs. So, when humidity is high to start with, but temperatures then fall, condensation is seen on the inside of the shed roofing sheets and on the cattle's backs. This is not desirable as viruses and bacteria survive in moisture and bacteria may even multiply. A threshold of below 75% RH is considered

necessary for microbial desiccation. This is rarely achieved in UK winter conditions and can be discounted in the UK as a means of controlling bacterial load in the environment (Chamberlain, 2015). Nevertheless, the higher the RH the worse the situation is for cattle. Every attempt should be made to keep sheds as dry as possible – both the floors and the air.

The *lower critical temperature* of an animal rises if they are wet, so a dry bed to lie on is important. This may involve some structural changes such as altering the slope of the shed floor or improving the drainage. It may be just simple maintenance that is required, such as cleaning out guttering and mending any leaking water troughs. The building should not be washed out when cattle are in it.

The moisture output of cattle is influenced by their diet. Cattle fed a low DM diet will have watery faeces and more urine and this obviously adds to the moisture in the shed.

In poorly ventilated housing, condensation on the cattle's backs can occur, as can sweating in humid, hot, still air conditions. These all add to the moisture content of the air and building. Wet weather outside also affects moisture inside the shed, due to a general increase in humidity.

Temperature

Animals that are in temperatures outside their *thermoneutral zone* (see Chapter 4), that is, the environmental temperature range where they are most comfortable, have to utilise energy to maintain their body temperature rather than to grow. They will also be stressed and more susceptible to disease. The thermoneutral zone for yearling cattle is 5–16°C.

Every building that houses cattle should have a climatic thermometer. Temperature data logger readings from UK sheds have shown there will be occasions where an occupant will be below its lower critical temperature. This is more of an issue for pre-ruminant animals that have no heat generated from fermentation within the rumen and therefore have higher thermoneutral zones.

In these cases, wind speed and air flow need to be moderated. Deep straw beds limit air flow around the calf and prevent heat loss, and calf jackets are useful in very small calves.

Occupant numbers

As respiratory pathogens are generally airborne, having multiple cattle in the same air space increases the risk of disease. The risk is increased further if groups are regularly changed and if there is an age difference between calves in the same air space; young naïve calves are constantly introduced to the pathogen load of the older recovering calves. This may maintain a subclinical level of disease; studies monitoring the growth rates between *continuous stocking* systems and *all-in-all-out* stocking systems showed that growth rates for the all-in-all-out system were considerably higher (Chamberlain, 2015). Batch housing is easier in seasonally calving herds, and this system can be adopted in growing units with some forward planning. A period where the building can be cleaned, disinfected and rested between batches is desirable.

As already stated, the development of disease depends on the level of bacterial/viral challenge and the level of immunity in the animal. The correct building design will reduce the replication of microorganisms and clear them from the shed, and thus reduce the challenge.

Respiratory disease vaccination

Vaccines are an additional tool to improve an individual's, but more importantly a population's, immunity against respiratory disease. Within the UK, in 2020, there are a number of licensed vaccines available for some of the major respiratory pathogens, see Table 6.2.

Despite the importance of *Mycoplasma* as a cause of calf BRD, there are no commercially available vaccines for this bacterium. The production of

TABLE 6.2 Vaccines available in the UK used to increase immunity against common BRD pathogens

Infectious agent covered by vaccine	Vaccine route of administration
RSV	Intranasal and injectable
IBR	Intranasal and injectable
M. haemolytica	Injectable
H. somni	Injectable
Pi3	Intranasal and injectable

autogenous vaccines (see Chapter 26), manufactured on a farm-specific basis, is possible; anecdotally there are positive reports on their efficacy.

BVD and lungworm (see Chapter 15) are common concurrent diseases that predispose calves to BRD; both diseases require their own control programmes, which may also involve vaccination. Some calf BRD vaccines contain a BVD component designed to protect calves from the immunosuppressive effects of the virus, which can be a contributory factor in BRD outbreaks. If a herd is using BVD 'check tests' (that detect antibodies and therefore exposure to the virus) to monitor for the disease, this needs to be considered when designing a BRD vaccination programme. A 'check test' is routinely carried out in calves aged between 9 and 18 months old. If they have been vaccinated with a respiratory vaccine containing a BVD component then they will have antibodies to BVD triggered by vaccination rather than by natural exposure, and this will result in a false positive result.

In the absence of up to date diagnostics, vaccination programmes are usually based on a knowledge of which respiratory agents have been detected on the farm in the past. This is possible if previous diagnostic testing has been carried out and that information is still available. Even with this information, however, the disease profile of the farm may change over time, and not all the causal agents may have been identified. Furthermore, there are many infectious respiratory agents and not all of them can be vaccinated against.

Sometimes a vaccination programme is designed and implemented in the *anticipation* of disease. This will take into account the age of cattle, the system they are reared in, the age variation within the group, the degree of mixing of the cattle, the shared air space and the BVD risk. Assumptions based on the patterns and common presentation of each respiratory infectious agent are used to make a 'best guess' at what vaccine is appropriate. This may be influenced, be it appropriately or not, by convenience of administration, timing of administration, and cost.

For example: *M. haemolytica* associated BRD is commonly seen in the autumn in spring-born calves that have been recently housed. Infectious bovine rhino (IBR) is seen in fattening cattle and is more common when groups of cattle are mixed. Respiratory syncytial virus (RSV) can be seen in all ages of cattle, but autumn-born calves housed in the first few weeks after birth are at risk. To protect these calves at the point of housing, when they may only be a few days or weeks old, often requires an intranasal vaccine as the only option. It is impossible to give respiratory disease protection to a calf younger than 8 weeks of age using injectable vaccines. This is because two injections are required, 4 weeks apart and the first vaccine dose cannot be given until calves are 2 weeks old. Full immunity will not develop until 2 weeks after the second dose of vaccine. There are anecdotal reports of pneumonia vaccines being administered to dams 4–6 weeks pre-calving to generate an immune response in the mother which is passed to the calf via the colostrum. The calf is protected from birth and can then receive a full course of vaccine when it reaches a suitable age. However, this is an untested, uncertain, off-licence application and should not be carried out without first seeking advice from a vet.

It is important that any vaccination programme is regularly reviewed and modified as required. To assess whether a vaccination programme is effective, the following measurable parameters are worth measuring and recording: morbidity,

mortality, DLWG, number of days to slaughter, and antimicrobial usage.

Promoting immunity

Vaccination primes the immune system to respond rapidly to a challenge from the infectious agent in question. Stress has an immunosuppressive effect and every attempt should be made to decrease the level of stress that a calf is subjected to. This should be taken into consideration when scheduling management tasks, most of which are stressful, especially in relation to the timing of vaccination and the expected time of disease outbreak.

Calf stressors (factors associated with stress)

- **Housing**. Housing is stressful, but for most farms is inevitable at some point in the autumn or early winter. It also inevitably involves a *dietary change* – from grass to conserved forage and additional feed constituents. Attempts should be made to house cattle when they are dry, and to avoid any other management tasks on that day. Once housed, calves should be allowed to settle in for at least 2 weeks before making any other changes.
- **Worming**. On many farms, calves at grass, whether it be their first or second grazing season, are wormed before housing. Many anthelmintics, however, have a persistent action against gut and lung worms so can be administered well in advance of housing so as to minimise the stress at the actual point of housing (see Chapter 26).
- **Vaccination**. Vaccination against BRD is needed in time for the risk period, which is usually from housing time onwards. It is therefore best that calves are given the full course of BRD vaccine in advance of this time rather than at point of housing – tempting though the latter is. The other benefit is, once again, that the vaccine is not adding to the stress of housing and it is worth remembering that

non-stressed animals respond better to vaccination – another reason not to do it at point of housing.

- **Castration and dehorning**. These tasks are extremely stressful for the cattle. These procedures can be avoided by applying elastrator rings soon after birth and using a caustic horn paste (or even better, having polled cattle) (see Chapter 4).

- **Heat stress**. Clipping the backs of cattle prevents them from getting too hot and sweating which creates additional moisture in the shed. Clipping, however, should not be required if the cattle housing is adequately ventilated.

- **Clipping**. This, although intended to reduce heat stress, is, in itself, a stressor!

- **Mixing**. Mixing cattle increases the risk of an outbreak of BRD for two reasons: (1) calves are stressed by a change in social group structure; and (2) calves within a group establish a stable microbial population to which they have a level of immunity, but when calves are mixed they are exposed to new pathogens that they have no immunity to. The age range within housed cattle in the same air space should be as small as possible.

- **Weaning**. Weaning is stressful. It is discussed further in Chapter 5 and this chapter. It should not be carried out at the same time as any other management tasks.

BRD cases are not just seen in housed cattle. Extreme fluctuations in the weather will cause the respiratory system to become compromised and calf immunity to dip, resulting in disease. In these cases, it is not necessarily the transmission of microorganisms from another calf but rather a multiplication of the commensal bacteria (such as *Pasteurella*) that naturally exist in a calf's nasal cavity and upper airways. BRD outbreaks are, consequently, seen when warm temperatures drop suddenly or cold temperatures rise abruptly.

If vaccination is used as part of a BRD control strategy, then the calf's immune system needs to be in full working order to ensure a strong immune response is generated – here stress reduction is crucial. Calves should not be subjected to any other of the above listed management tasks/stressors within a week of vaccination, before or after. The nutritional status of the calf is also important for an effective immune response to be achieved; calves deficient in vitamins or trace elements such as Vitamin E, copper or selenium will be immuno-compromised to some extent. Animals infected with parasites – fluke, gut worms, lungworm or *Coccidia* – will also fail to elicit a strong immune response. Finally, vaccines should be administered in accordance with the product data sheet, unless advised otherwise by a vet.

MONITORING PERFORMANCE FROM WEANING THROUGH THE GROWING PERIOD

Monitoring is essential to check animal health and performance, to assess whether any changes are needed, and to ultimately ensure full potential is reached.

$$\text{DLWG (kg/day)} = \frac{\text{end weight (kg)} - \text{start weight (kg)}}{\text{age (days)}}$$

A start weight is essential. This is usually the weaning weight (in an artificially reared calf or a suckled calf). Weigh scales are the most accurate method of monitoring weight gain and ideally calves should be weighed monthly to identify trends and highlight problems soon enough to make changes. This may be relevant to an individual calf underperforming due to underlying disease, or a nutrition related problem affecting the whole group.

The 'gold standard' is to weigh monthly, but there are several compromises available. Often calves are only weighed on farm at weaning and then at the auction mart at point of sale. An individual weight at the auction mart is desirable but not always possible. For instance, some auction marts will weigh groups of calves before they enter the sales ring and average the weight across the group. This allows at least for a rough DLWG from weaning to sale to be calculated. If a weaning weight is not available, then an assumed birth weight and sale weight can be used instead. Each of these compromises adds a layer of inaccuracy, but it is at least some data to make reasonably *informed decisions.*

Calf mortality and the incidence of calf BRD are important key performance indicators (KPIs) which must be monitored. Each KPI has an agreed interference value. When the *parameter* being measured exceeds the pre-agreed *interference value* it is not acceptable, and investigation and action is required to improve it. Suggested interference values are:

- < 2% calf mortality
- < 3% incidence of BRD.

Antibiotic audits are a useful tool to assess the number of treated cases of BRD. If medicine records are up to date, they can provide a useful insight into the number of calves treated and how many needed repeat treatments. Calf mortality should also be recorded and monitored – and a post-mortem examination is invaluable in confirming, rather than guessing, the cause of death.

Calf weight gains, the incidence of BRD and calf mortality are easily measurable and can be compared with previous years' data on the same farm. They can also be benchmarked against other farms running similar rearing systems.

REFERENCES

AHDB (2016a) *Feeding Growing and Finishing Cattle for Better Returns. Beef BRP Manual 7.* Agriculture and Horticulture Development Board, Stoneleigh.

AHDB (2016b) *Planning Grazing Strategies for Better Returns. Beef and Sheep BRP Manual 8.* Agriculture and Horticulture Development Board, Stoneleigh.

Bryson, D.G. (2000) The calf pneumonia complex – current thoughts on aetiology. *Cattle Practice* 8(2), 103–107.

Chamberlain, T. (2015) Environmental aspects of pneumonia control in-calf units on British dairy farms. *Livestock* 20(6), 306–314.

Enríquez, D.H., Ungerfeld, R., Quintans, G., Guidoni, A.L. and Hötzel, M.J. (2010) The effects of alternative weaning methods on behaviour in beef calves. *Livestock Science* 128(1), 20–27.

Griffin, D., Chengappa, M.M., Kuszak, J. and Scott McVey, D. (2010) Bacterial pathogens of the bovine respiratory disease complex. *Veterinary Clinics of North America: Food Animal Practice* 26, 381–394.

Paterson, J.A. and Engle, T.E. (2005) Trace mineral nutrition in beef cattle. Nutrition Conference, University of Tennessee, USA.

Penny, C.D. (2015) The control of bovine respiratory disease (BRD) – are we making progress? *Cattle Practice* 23(2), 314–319.

FURTHER READING

Morris, S.T. and Kenyon, P.R. (2014) Intensive sheep and beef production from pasture – a New Zealand perspective of concerns, opportunities and challenges. *Meat Science* 98, 330–335.

Robertson, J.F. (2000) Building designs to optimise health. *Cattle Practice* 8(2), 127–130.

Chapter 7

The health and management of finishing cattle

The finishing period is the final stage before slaughter where cattle have finished growing their frames, their skeletons, and increase their muscle mass and lay down fat. Historically, it was referred to as the *fattening period*, but, terms such as *fat stock* and *fattening* are, these days, viewed as unappealing to the consumer, so the term 'finishing' is more often used now.

NUTRITION

The finishing stage should be a relatively short period of high growth rates. Liveweights may increase by 100–140 kg in some breeds, such as the continentals. For native-bred heifers, in contrast, that are small and finish quickly, increases of only around 60 kg will typically be made.

It takes four times more energy to lay down 1 kg of fat tissue than 1 kg of lean tissue (AHDB, 2016). Over-fattening cattle is a costly mistake. Apart from the inefficiency of production, the fat is trimmed off by the processor and binned!

Typically, the energy content of the finishing ration is increased and the protein component is decreased.

CHARACTERISTICS OF BEEF

The UK industry is moving towards a more integrated supply chain, which will more closely connect the consumer to the producer. Theoretically the consumer, or at least the intermediary (wholesaler or retailer) dictates what characteristics of beef they require, and the producer has to respond accordingly. At least that is what should happen! There are various responses in the production system that can make a difference.

How can nutrition impact on the characteristics of beef?

- Fat colour: white fat is present in carcases of cereal-fed cattle while cattle fed grass or forage-based diets have more yellow coloured fat thought to be attributable to retinoid pigments in the grass.
- Shelf life: beef from cattle finished on grass has a longer shelf life than beef from cereal-fed cattle. This is attributable to the higher level of antioxidants, including Vitamin E, in the grass-fed beef animal. Adding additional Vitamin E to a cereal-based diet will, however, have the same effect.

Meat characteristics, such as tenderness and flavour, are largely influenced by processes carried out post-slaughter.

- Tenderness is important to the consumer and various post-slaughter techniques have been developed to improve it. In the live animal, age, gender and animal genotype all have some effect on tenderness, albeit a small effect. Most cattle for prime meat production are slaughtered at a young age (<30 months) so there is little variation there. There is a link between fatness and tenderness. As an animal fattens, it initially lays down subcutaneous fat and *intermuscular fat*, and then *intramuscular fat*. First, the intramuscular and subcutaneous fats in carcases protect the muscles from the cold during refrigeration and this prevents 'cold shortening', which induces toughness. Second, intermuscular fat dilutes the fibrous protein component with this softer tissue, that is, fat, making it a less 'chewy' eating experience (Moloney et al., 2001).

- Flavour is difficult to measure, such subjective judgements are often the findings of a taste panel whose opinions are generally a reflection of experiences they have had in the past. Although there is a perception that 'grass-fed is best', in many taste studies there seems to be no suggestion that grain-fed or grass or forage-fed cattle taste any better than each other. What is widely agreed, however, is that flavour increases with fat content and varies notably with the *cut*, the part of the carcase.

- *Dark cutting beef* is the phenomenon where stress or aggression or any increased activity before slaughter depletes the glycogen energy stores in the muscles – this is not a good thing. Glycogen in the muscles at the point of death is desirable as this energy store continues to fuel metabolism in the muscle post-mortem which, in the absence of oxygen (the animal is no longer breathing), causes the production of lactic acid. Lactic acid keeps the muscle pH down which is thought by some to preserve the pinkness in the muscle. Where this process fails to take place, the muscle goes relatively alkaline and the meat appears brown. It is also known that this muscle retains more water and makes the meat relatively flaccid and translucent. The meat appears a darker colour to the consumer, who simply does not like the look of it, and the meat inspector (who knows that!) rejects the carcase. (McKinnon Bill, 1998; Beer, n.d.)

FINISHING ON GRASS

Native-bred heifers and castrated males can be finished on grass alone, providing the grass quality is good. The energy demand to fatten Continental breeds, however, means they are difficult to finish on grass alone, and supplementary feeding outside is helpful if practical to do so. The land needs to be dry enough to avoid poaching and to enable feed to be taken out to the field without damaging the sward. Lameness can be an issue if the land becomes poached and cattle are standing in wet ground for long periods of time. For the welfare of the cattle they need to have a dry area to lie. For safety and managemental reasons, entire bulls should be finished inside.

MAXIMISING DM INTAKE

Maximising DM intake (DMI) is essential for finishing cattle. Rations need to be formulated to provide the correct balance of energy, protein, fibre, minerals and vitamins. They also need to be palatable so that the cattle will eat them.

Freshness

Feed that has become heated, or is old and smelly, is not appealing for cattle to eat. So, feed troughs need to be cleaned out regularly. Mouldy or *butyric* silage will also reduce intakes and can cause digestive upsets.

Moisture

Cattle will eat less of a very dry or fibrous feed. To add moisture to a total mixed ration and, consequently, improve this palatability factor, a liquid feed such as molasses can be added.

Trough and feeder design

There needs to be plenty of space along the feed barrier, if cattle are expected to feed all at one time.

The positioning of the vertical and horizontal bars of the feed barrier is important too. Hair loss and callus formation on the back of cows' necks is a sign that they are having to reach for food, or that the feed barrier is set too low.

Concrete feed troughs should have a smooth floor, pleasant for mouthing and licking, and not be rough or pebbled.

Group structure

Each group of cattle should be as uniform as possible – if there is large variation in the size, sex, breed and age of cattle in a pen it is difficult to formulate and feed a ration to suit all. Although every group of cattle will have its own social standings, minimising the size difference between animals in a group will reduce bullying and reduce the incidence of submissive cattle being pushed out from the feed.

Ration consistency

A consistent pH in the rumen is essential to sustain viable and healthy populations of rumen microbes. To ensure this, the diet needs to be consistent and any changes in ration carried out over a reasonably extended period, say 10 days.

Finishing rations can be high in starch and low in fibre, and this can cause rapid fermentation and dramatic drops in pH. Clinically, this can present as *ruminal acidosis* where the cattle are visibly sick. Even at subclinical levels of acidosis, however, where the animal does not show visible signs of disease, the rumen is not fully functioning and feed conversion will be compromised – this is well known in the dairy industry as subacute ruminal acidosis (SARA). A diet with good fibre content will help here, it helps rumination and salivation, and helps maintain a stable pH.

Where a total mixed ration (TMR) ration is not a feasible option, and forage and cereals are fed separately, it is important that cattle are not fed too much concentrate in any one feed – no more than 2 kg per meal is recommended and it may need to be split into twice or even three times a day feeding. There needs to be adequate trough space so all cattle can feed at once and the greedy/dominant characters do not gorge on the feed.

Concurrent disease

Gut worm, liver fluke, chronic pneumonia, liver abscessation and lungworm are all typical examples of diseases that will decrease an animal's appetite, DM intake and feed conversion during the finishing period.

Water

Cattle do not eat if they are thirsty so clean fresh accessible water should always be available to maintain DMI. Conversely the actual water requirement of the cattle will in turn depend on the animal's DMI; the higher the DMI the more water they will need to drink. Ambient temperature will also affect water intakes. Table 7.1 displays water requirements for non-lactating beef cattle at varying ambient temperatures relative to their DMIs.

There should be enough water sources available for at least 10% of housed cattle to drink simultaneously at any one time. Troughs should be placed where they are at low risk of being contaminated by faeces or urine, where they are protected from freezing in cold weather, and where there is sufficient access for all stock (Defra, 2003). Water sources should be checked at least twice daily to ensure they are not blocked, overflowing or contaminated.

For example: a 400 kg heifer eats 2.5% of its liveweight in DM = 10 kg DMI. At an ambient

TABLE 7.1 Water requirements of non-lactating beef cattle (AHDB, 2016)

	Ambient temperature (°C)		
	<16	16–20	>20
Water requirement of non-lactating beef cattle	5.4 l/kg DM	6.1 l/kg DM	7 l/kg DM

temperature of less than 16°C she will require 5.4 l of water per kg DMI intake.

$$5.4 \times 10 = 54 \text{ l per day}$$

Assuming the ration has a DM content of 40%, she will be getting 15 kg of water from the ration. In addition, she will need to drink 39 l of water per day.

HOUSING

Within any housing system there needs to be adequate room for animals to move around and express their normal behaviours. This may involve social interaction but also allows subordinate animals to avoid confrontation from dominant aggressors in the group; a common example being those cattle with horns.

Straw-bedded systems are ideal for finishing cattle; sheds should be re-bedded and kept clean with the addition of straw as required. Every 6 weeks, or sooner if appropriate, they should be completely cleaned out of all straw and faecal material. The straw used for bedding should be stored inside (Figure 7.1), or at least under cover, to prevent it from becoming damp and mouldy. Wet straw is not bedding, it is what bedding becomes! There are a range of alternative bedding materials

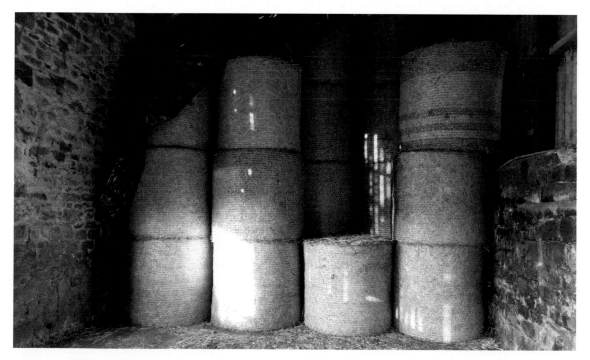

FIGURE 7.1 Straw stacked inside to be kept dry

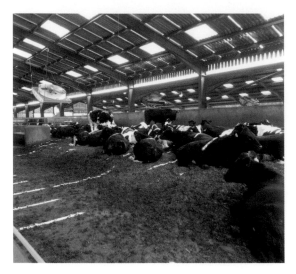

FIGURE 7.2 Finishing cattle in well-ventilated shed with fans, bedded on sawdust

for loose housing such as sand, paper or wood shavings as seen in Figure 7.2.

Any bedding material needs to be:

- non-toxic if eaten
- easily disposable and not cause undue wear and tear on machinery in the process
- affordable, cost-effective
- consistently available in sufficient quantities
- comfortable, with no sharp bits or chemical irritants
- absorptive to keep cattle dry and clean
- non-slip to ensure loafing areas do not become a hazard
- free of foreign bodies.

Slatted floors are still relatively common, although less so than they were. Slatted floors are concrete beams laid side by side with a small gap for faeces to drop between into a slurry pit situated below the animal. The slats need to be close enough together to prevent the animals' feet or claws getting trapped. They need to be even, smooth and well maintained so as not to be the cause of foot lesions.

The slat system became popular as no bedding is required, which is a cost-saving, and there

is little labour involved as cattle only need to be fed and inspected; there is no slurry to scrape, or straw to muck out, only a pit to empty periodically. It is recommended that stock so housed do have a clean, dry, lying area. In some systems, sadly, this is not provided, and cattle spend all their time either lying or standing on the slats – this is not acceptable. Slatted floors were predominantly designed for fattening and growing cattle. It is recommended that breeding cows and suckled calves are not kept on slatted pens. If they are not good enough for cows and calves then why would they be good enough for growing cattle? Yes, admittedly the issue with cows and calves may be one of foot and claw dimensions but is the comfort factor acceptable in any of these cases? Some shed designs have a slatted feed passageway and separate straw-bedded areas or cubicles for animals to lie in. This seems an acceptable compromise.

The slurry tanks under the slats are emptied as required, sometimes just once or twice a year. Noxious and potentially toxic fumes, including ammonia and hydrogen sulphide, and simple humidity can be issues in badly designed or badly constructed systems or even in the best of systems. When removing slurry from under the slats, it needs to be agitated to facilitate its removal and this can release the poisonous hydrogen sulphide; a danger to personnel and cattle alike. The authors have seen a fatal case of *hydrogen sulphide intoxication* in a cow.

The addition of silage effluent or silage itself to slurry *increases* gas production as does calcium sulphate dihydrate (typically gypsum in waste plasterboard). Cattle should be removed from a slatted shed before stirring slurry, and human operatives should work in pairs and not enter the shed while slurry stirring is in process. Only trained operatives should enter a slurry store.

Lighting

In the cattle shed, there should be sufficient lighting to inspect cattle at any time and for the cattle to exhibit normal vision-based behaviour. As a rule of thumb, in an adequately lit cattle shed, it should be possible for a newspaper to be read. Light is linked with mental health in personnel and undoubtedly helps in animal well-being too.

MONITORING THE HEALTH OF FINISHING CATTLE

Abattoir feedback

Abattoir feedback is a valuable tool for on-farm disease monitoring. Information about the cattle and the subsequent carcase as observed in the abattoir is usually provided on *kill sheets*. The findings are usually gross observations by the meat inspectors. Their primary job is to detect any conditions that are a risk to human health or not aesthetically acceptable, but, at the same time their findings are secondarily, and very usefully, reported back to the producer, or they should be. Parasites such as lungworm and fluke may be reported. Excessive carcase trimming due to bruising or injection site trauma are also important pieces of information for the producer to respond to with changes to be made on-farm.

A common finding is the presence of liver abscesses. These are an indication of acidosis: this occurs when rumen bacteria are absorbed through the damaged rumen wall and travel along the main blood vessel to the liver where they then establish an infection.

Faecal scoring

Faecal scoring is the examination of the faeces of cattle to gain an appreciation of digestive health. One parameter to look out for is the proportion of water in the faeces: do the faeces form a healthy *pat* or does the animal essentially have diarrhoea? Diarrhoea is defined as abnormally watery faeces.

There are many infectious and non-infectious causes of diarrhoea. Non-infectious causes include digestive upset due to an imbalance in the diet, over supplementation with minerals, such as magnesium sulphate, or certain toxins in the feed such as fungal mycotoxins. The colour of the faeces is important too – dark, blackened faeces can be a sign of digested blood from an upper gastrointestinal bleed while fresh red blood suggests bleeding further along the gut as the blood has not had time to be digested. For animals on a finishing ration, there should be no undigested material passing through into the faeces. If undigested material is present, it indicates that food is either indigestible, for example, whole grains, or that there is insufficient transit time in the gut for the digestion of all food particles to occur. This is often a problem with the simple physcial composition of the ration or with the energy:protein ratio being suboptimal (Hulsen, 2006). Faeces can be examined in several ways: wearing a rubber glove it is possible to feel for the presence of undigested particles. Faeces can also be placed in a sieve and washed using a hose-pipe: less than half the material should remain in the sieve, and this is a good indication that the fibre content of the diet is adequate. The fibre strands should not exceed 1.25 cm in length – where they do it may be suggestive of poor rumen function, most likely to be associated with ruminal acidosis (Grove-White, 2004). Undigested feed will also be apparent in the sieve along with any *fibrin casts*. Fibrin casts are clumps of inflammatory cells and cells from the lining of the gut; their presence is an indication of gut inflammation from disease or acidosis. It is recommended that 12 animals are examined in this way to validate any findings and to allow meaningful decisions to be made.

HANDLING FACILITIES FOR FINISHING CATTLE

For various managements tasks, such as routine medicine administration, weighing, and veterinary examinations and procedures, cattle need to be restrained and handled. Beef cattle are less used to being handled than dairy cows, and it can be a stressful and dangerous time for all involved unless the correct techniques are employed, and appropriate facilities and equipment are available.

Why invest in properly designed handling systems?

- To minimise stress to the cattle – stress increases cortisol levels, lowers the immune system and affects carcase quality (Grandin, 2013).
- To minimise stress to the handlers – the better the handling system, the happier team members will be to handle cattle and the less likely they are to avoid an otherwise necessary intervention.
- To maximise efficiency for the handlers – the better the handling system, the fewer members of staff will be required to handle the cattle.
- To minimise injuries to the cattle – it is important to consider the welfare implications of poor handling systems, good systems are associated with fewer injuries.
- To minimise injuries to the handlers – there are health and safety regulations relating to the handling of cattle on farm that need to be considered. Employers have an obligation to the employees and other contractors on farm, for example, the AI technician, vet, state veterinary service, trading standards, assurance scheme inspectors and foot trimmers. Injuries can include being kicked or bashed by cattle, hit by gates swinging open or coming off their hinges, trapping fingers and arms between the cattle and the metalwork or in the mechanics of the crush itself.
- To prevent bruising – this is visibly present on a carcase and requires trimming which is wasteful. Bruising may result from physical contact with sticks or corners of pens, gate hinges or bars that stick out. High incidences of bruising are likely to generate a welfare investigation by the authorities.
- To save money – the easier it is to do the job, the more likely it is to get done and carried out properly, and where a vet's fees are based on time, the quicker the cattle run through a handling system the cheaper will be the bill. So, in just a few years, the cost of a new handling system may well be covered.

Cattle handling systems are commonly made up of a collection pen or corral, a race or chute, a crush or crate, a covered well-lit crush-access area and a holding pen.

Crush (or crate)

The crush, see Figure 7.3, is where the management procedure is carried out by the operatives. The animal is fully restrained by its neck. There are many designs of crushes and not all crushes will do all jobs.

Some crushes will allow full access to the side of an animal, as is required for suckling a calf, performing a caesarean section or semen testing a bull. Some crushes have a door that opens so that injections can easily be performed into the rump or neck, including intradermal skin testing for bTB. Head stocks that restrain the head can be self-locking, that is, where an animal pushes its shoulders against the head stock and it locks shut, or, it may be manually locking, where an operative pulls a handle to close the head stock on the neck of the animal when it is in position.

Squeeze crushes – either manual or hydraulic – can be set to the width of the animal to prevent it turning around when entering the crush. They can be further adjusted once the animal is in position, to limit movement and by nipping in more at lower level they can reduce the likelihood of the animal going down. They should hold the animal snuggly enough to have a calming effect but not cause it to be uncomfortably squeezed, which results in a fight against the restraint.

Whatever the crush design, it needs to be robust enough to withstand the cattle it is expected to restrain, and securely fixed not to tip over. There should be no sharp edges that could cause injury,

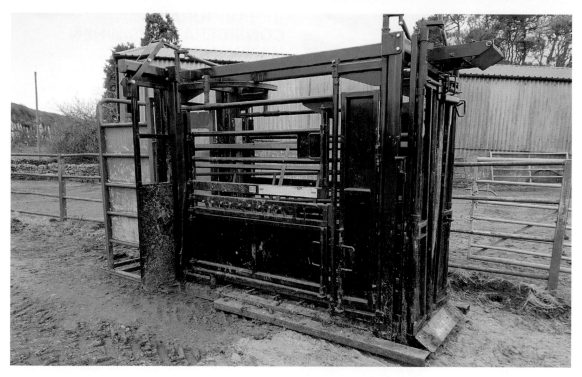

FIGURE 7.3 A Self-locking squeeze crush

nor gaps where the cattle's heads or legs could get trapped. The floor surface is important: it should not deter cattle from entering the crush, it should be non-slip and should not be abrasive to the feet – some metal-ridged floors have been known to 'grate' the soles of the cattle's feet as they repeatedly run and skid on the floor. An obvious but crucial point is that if the crush is not securely fixed to the ground (which it should be, but with some portable crushes may not be) then the floor must be an integral part of the crush box design; the authors have seen cattle pick up crushes and run with them when the crush has no floor. Cattle and personnel can die in such situations.

Head stock

The head stock, see Figure 7.4, is a cheaper alternative to a crush but is less substantial. It needs to be adequately attached to stanchions in the race or chute, which in turn need to be adequately attached to the floor. Just as a crush without its own floor is a danger if not secured so too is a head stock.

Race (or chute)

The race is a corridor from the holding pen to the crush in which the cattle line up in single file. A race should have solid sides so cattle are not distracted by what is going on around them; the sides should be high enough to stop cattle jumping out and solid and narrow enough at all points (including personnel access points) to prevent cattle turning around. Curved races allow the animal to see the way ahead, maybe the animal in front, but not the crush at the end so they are more inclined to enter the race, especially if a circular or wedge shaped holding pen with a *forcing gate* is used to guide and funnel the cattle into the race.

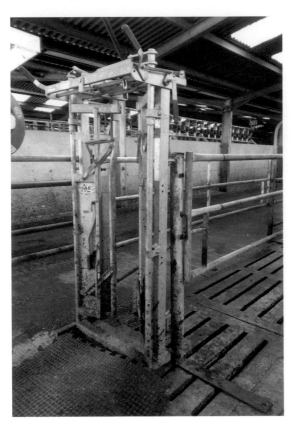

FIGURE 7.4 A head stock

Holding pen

The holding pen is where small groups of cattle are held and wait to enter the race. It may be that the handler does not have to enter the pen and that cattle can be moved through a series of gates, perhaps with the aid of forcing gates. If the handler does have to enter the pens to move cattle, there should always be an escape route – a narrow gap in the railings where a human can get out, but cattle cannot, or a stanchion in the corner to stand behind without the cattle being able to get around it. The side and gates of the holding pen should be high enough to prevent cattle from jumping out – some breeds and temperaments jump higher than others, Limousins seem to hold the high jump record!

BEHAVIOURAL CONSIDERATIONS WHEN HANDLING CATTLE

Cattle are herbivorous grazing animals, they are prey animals, they are continually surveying their environment for predators; this includes humans. They are also herd animals and are happier within a herd but have their own social standing within it. They keep their distance from certain individuals, and this is compromised when cattle are brought into tight confined spaces for handling; aggression and bullying may result, again in some breeds and temperaments more so than others. Cattle are easier to handle in smaller socially stable groups that are not so tightly packed into holding pens.

Cattle's response to a potential threat, such as unfamiliar surroundings, noises, people or other animals, elicits a 'fight or flight' response, in the case of cattle usually flight but sometimes fight, particularly in the case of the protective maternal cow. The flight response can actually help in the managed movement of cattle. Cattle like their own personal space, a distance that they are happy to stand away from a human: this area around the animal is called the 'flight zone', see Figure 7.5. A person entering this zone will make the animal move away from them. Entering it too quickly, or

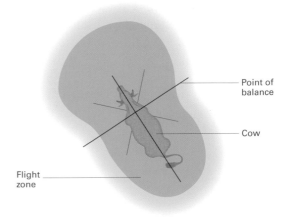

FIGURE 7.5 Diagram showing the flight zone and point of balance

too far, will elicit a more extreme fight or flight response.

For cattle that are familiar with their surroundings and handlers, the flight zone will be smaller than those that have unfamiliar surroundings and handlers. Their 'point of balance' is at their shoulder; if a person moves behind the point of the shoulder, the animal will move in a forward direction away from them, if a person moves in front of the point of balance, it will move backwards away from them. Using the flight zone and point of balance, cattle can be moved quietly, calmly and safely.

The following useful sensory facts about cattle should be borne in mind when handling them.

- Cattle are more sensitive to high pitched noises than humans. Humans hear well between 1000 and 4000 Hz. Cows hear best at 8000 Hz; they therefore hear things that humans cannot (Hulsen, 2006). Noisy pens and shouting will deter cattle from entering a space.
- Cattle cannot see immediately behind them, but they nearly can – they manage 340° vision. They are sensitive to changes in light and are perturbed by shadows, drains and puddles, all of which spell potential danger; they are less inclined to move towards blinding direct sunlight or in from the light to a potentially dangerous dark space. They can only judge distances straight ahead as they require information from both eyes, the principle of binocular vision.
- They have a smell 14 times more sensitive than humans; they often refuse to enter an area where a calving, caesarean section, surgical castration or dehorning has taken place that has not been fully cleaned and most distressing of all they are very reluctant to enter a slaughtering area. Great efforts are needed to help minimise the emotional trauma of these natural aversions.
- Cattle will remember a bad handling experience for up to 12 months (Grandin, 2013).

FOOTCARE IN FINISHING CATTLE

The foot is comprised of the outer and inner claw, sometimes referred to as the lateral (outer) and medial (inner) claw. In the front foot, the medial claw is slightly larger than the outer and it is reversed in the hind feet with the lateral claw being the larger. The larger claw is the more weight bearing. The space between the claws is called the interdigital space and runs from the front to the back of the hoof.

Cattle do not bear weight on the entire sole, instead the weight-bearing surfaces are the heel and the wall, the wall extends from the heel all round the outside (the abaxial wall) to the toe and then one-third of the way back along the inside of the claw (the axial wall) (Figure 7.8).

Anatomy of the normal hoof

White line

The wall and sole grow separately and are 'glued' together at the 'white line' – this is a point of weakness, see Figures 7.6 to 7.9.

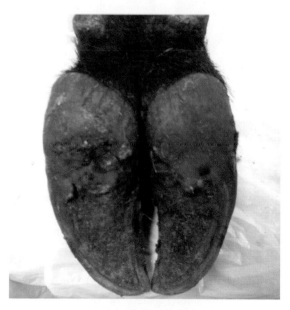

FIGURE 7.6 Solar view of the normal hoof

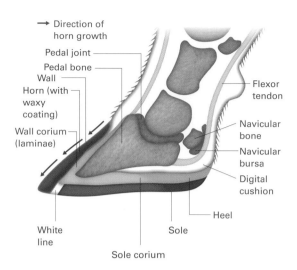

FIGURE 7.7 Diagrammatic representation of the cross-section of the bovine hoof

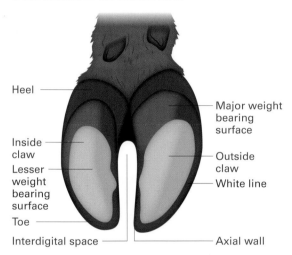

FIGURE 7.8 Diagrammatic representation of the solar view of the normal hoof (right foot)

Corium

The corium is the sensitive 'quick' that nourishes the horn. It is situated between the bone and the hoof capsule (the wall corium sometimes gets called the laminae although the laminae are really the folds of tissue within the corium) The sole corium is the quick between the bottom of the bone and the sole (Figure 7.7). The hoof capsule is not very flexible, and it does not expand or

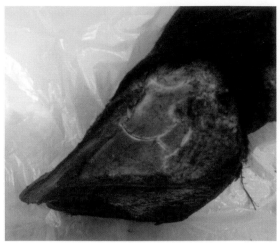

FIGURE 7.9 Cross-section of the hoof in a post-mortem sample

compress so any inflammation in the foot causes great pressure and pain in the corium. The corium is particularly tight at the toe while relatively loose towards the heel where the digital cushion introduces scope for movement, so pain from pressure, for example an abscess, nearer the toe is worse than in the heel. The sole corium manufactures the sole horn and keeps it attached. The wall corium, however, does not produce the wall horn – this is produced at the coronary band and slowly grows downwards (Figure 7.7 and 7.9).

Digital cushion

This acts as a shock absorber during weight bearing and as a 'pump' to push the blood around the foot (Figure 7.7).

Heel

Because of the flexible digital cushion, the horn over the heel is relatively thin and flexible (Figures 7.7 and 7.8).

Waxy coating

The whole hoof capsule should have a waxy coating to retain moisture in the horn and keep it fairly flexible. It can be scraped off or desiccated in very dry weather whereupon the hoof becomes brittle.

Periople

The periople is the white hairless rubbery zone of tissue that runs around the top of the hoof adjacent to the coronary band and produces the waxy coating. It is delicate and easily damaged in dry or sandy conditions resulting in the horn losing its natural moisture retaining properties.

Pedal bone

This is the bone suspended inside the hoof capsule by the laminae of the corium (Figure 7.7 and 7.9).

Pedal joint

This is the lubricant-filled sac which enables the hoof to move relative to the pastern (see Figure 7.7).

Flexor tendon

This structure channels the forces from the leg muscles to the back of the pedal bone to enable the cow to bend (flex) the foot when walking (Figure 7.7).

Navicular bone

This small bone 'bridges' the flexor tendon from the pastern to the pedal bone (Figure 7.7 and 7.9).

Navicular bursa

This is like a joint in that it is a lubricant-filled sac; it prevents friction between the tendon and the bridging navicular bone (Figure 7.7).

Hoof capsule

The horn coating each claw (two hoof capsules per foot) is an extensively modified layer of skin (technically known as the epidermis) impregnated

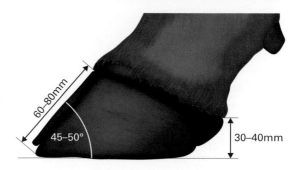

FIGURE 7.10 Normal hoof growth and dimensions

with a natural 'hardener' known as keratin. The hoof capsule provides the hard, durable structure needed to walk and stand on.

The dimensions of the hoof vary with breed, with age (smaller in heifers), between front and hind feet (front feet are more *boxy*), between individual animals, and with the effects of foot disease. Typical hoof dimensions are shown in Figure 7.10.

The rate of horn growth is approximately 5 mm/month.

FOOTCARE IN FINISHING CATTLE

Footcare is all about preventing foot disease which, in turn, is all about preventing lameness. There are both infectious and non-infectious causes of foot disease. The prevention and control of either type is slightly different but mutually beneficial.

Non-infectious causes of lameness are:

- white line disease
- sole ulcer
- bruising
- abscess
- foreign body such as a stone (or even a discarded bovine tooth!)
- fracture of the pedal bone
- heel erosion
- sand crack
- interdigital growth

- under run sole
- laminitis.

These conditions will be covered individually and in detail in Chapter 14. Here, the focus is on prevention of foot disease.

Keeping the feet as dry and clean as possible helps to stop the main causes of foot disease. Cows standing in slurry have feet that are always wet and subject to the corrosive action of the slurry which softens the horn and removes the waxy coating, so predisposing them to disease. Cows at grass have better grip, softer ground, less abrasive surfaces and less bacteria to contend with, but trauma due to stones, poorly managed gateways or feeding areas will increase bruising, and gravel can penetrate the white line or sole, ultimately causing a white line abscess and sole abscess, respectively.

Lying time affects foot health. If cows are happy to lie down when they are not eating, drinking or socialising they are taking weight of their feet and removing the pressure on the structures of the foot and the soles, also allowing free circulation of blood and fluids within the foot. Cows can rest for between 14 and 16 hours every day. This helps prevent lameness.

Using data from the dairy cow, body weight is distributed reasonably evenly over all four feet. So, in a standing 700 kg cow each foot is taking approximately 175 kg and that is at best. When walking, running or worst of all, pivoting, then one foot could at times be taking almost the whole 700 kg (Hulsen, 2006).

An adequate, clean lying area is essential, as is good cubicle design, covered later in Chapter 10. If the housing space is designed with tight corners or bottlenecks, and cows are twisting and turning on a concrete surface, this applies *shear forces* to the foot which results in white line separation which enables gravel and infection to enter the foot at that point. Rough surfaces such as poorly laid or poorly maintained concrete or tracks increase bruising to the sole. Many finishing cattle will be kept on concrete slatted floors which were designed to cut down on the need for expensive straw and are labour saving. Slats appear to be, and are highly likely to be, uncomfortable, but where they are used they need to be adequately maintained to avoid any holes or rough edges which may cause trauma.

Diet, health, bodily changes, environment and stress can all influence hoof horn quality. As the horn grows down from the coronary band, it is common to see so called 'stress lines' which are horizontal ridges of horn that run around the hoof and as time passes grow down with the hoof. These result from an abrupt change in management, health or feeding. As horn grows at approximately 5 mm per month, a rough guess can be made as to when the stressful event occurred. If nothing else in life causes a stress line, calving does. Some otherwise content cows have *a line for each calf* – a bit like the rings in the trunk of a tree.

Biotin is an element required for healthy horn growth and should be included in any ration. If a herd has a high incidence of lameness associated with claw horn lesions, the addition of biotin may help but, remember, it will not be a complete solution; the causes of lameness are multifactorial, and the adjustment of many small things usually results in a reduction in incidence rather than there being a single 'magic' bullet.

Laminitis is a non-infectious cause of lameness; it is covered in Chapter 14.

Genetics play a large part in the frame, leg and hoof conformation of cattle, and of their overall weight, all of which in turn affect weight distribution, pressure points, horn growth and ultimately the incidence of lameness. The temperament of a cow (again influenced by environmental and genetic factors) will also affect the risk she poses to herself in terms of becoming lame. Flighty cows apply more shear forces to the hoof and spend less time lying down. Common genetic conformational defects are low fetlocks, straight hocks, sickle hocks and shallow hoof angles. Very heavy animals, large cows and bulls, apply more forces to the structures of the foot and are more likely to become lame.

Infectious causes of lameness include foul of the foot and digital dermatitis; both are covered in more detail in Chapter 14. Foul of the foot is associated with bacteria that are ubiquitous in the environment, but do not just cause infection spontaneously – there needs to be damage to the interdigital skin to allow the bacteria to enter. Wet long grass can be sufficient and often cases of foul of the foot are more prevalent in early summer when the grass is long. As with the control of non-infectious hoof lesions, a clean dry environment with no stones or sharp material, will help to prevent cases.

Digital dermatitis results from the introduction of specific causative infectious agents into a herd, which then spread between cattle. Strict biosecurity is the main critical control point to stop the entry of the disease into the herd. Once the causative agents have gained entry to a herd and are circulating, hygiene and a clean, dry environment do help and are essential to its control.

It is sometimes necessary to introduce regular foot bathing into the management system to maintain good foot health. Good foot bathing procedure is essential to make sure this process is minimally stressful. Traditionally, formalin, copper sulphate and zinc sulphate solutions (each at relevant dilutions) have all been used in foot bathing. In addition, there are many proprietary products on the market each with various claims.

The primary objective of foot bathing is to clean and disinfect the hoof. For this reason, many disinfectants (providing they are non-irritant) can be used and biological washing powder is also surprisingly effective but should only be used under veterinary advice.

The foot bath solution should be sufficiently deep to cover the hoof but not extend further up the leg as repetitive exposure of the skin may cause sores or burns. For maximum effect, the feet need to be clean when entering the footbath – a pre-bath containing only clean water helps to achieve that. The area on exiting the footbath also needs to be clean and free from mud and faeces. The footbath needs to be wide enough and long enough that cattle walk through slowly and calmly, placing each foot into the solution at least once, preferably

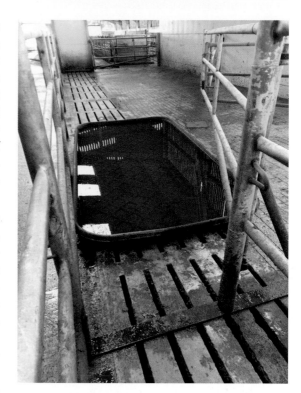

FIGURE 7.11 Wide footbath containing formalin with clean entry and exit

twice, see Figure 7.11. Regular foot bathing (a minimum of once per week) helps accustom the cows to the procedure so they do not rush through or athletically long-jump the footbath!

Foot trimming is a routine procedure or therapy used to ensure the normal dimensions of the hoof are maintained and early signs of disease are detected and addressed. Foot trimming can be undertaken by a stockperson on farm with adequate training, and many training courses are available. There are also many trained hoof trimmers and vets that provide a high-quality service. Professional foot trimmers have specialised handling equipment that makes the job safer and less stressful for the cattle, the leg and hoof need to be adequately restrained for the safety of the operator and the animal (see Figure 7.12).

Different beef farmers approach cattle footcare differently: some will examine all four feet and give a routine trim to cows at housing and again before turn out. In some herds cows are only

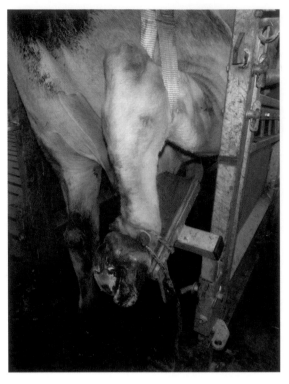

FIGURE 7.12 Adequately restrained foot for examination

TABLE 7.2 Timing of permanent tooth eruption (months) (Dyce et al., 2002)

Tooth	Age at eruption of permanent tooth (months)
Incisor 1	18–24
Incisor 2	24–30
Incisor 3	36–42
Incisor 4 (canine)	42–48
Premolar 2	24–30
Premolar 3	18–30
Premolar 4	20–36
Molar 1	6
Molar 2	12–18
Molar 3	24–30

The cows are graded 0 = a healthy normal walk, 1 = slight abnormality, 2 = lame cow where the lame leg can be identified, 3 = 'the crippled cow'. It may be difficult with unhandled fractious suckler cows or youngstock to perform such an objective assessment, but frequent assessment of the gait of every animal should be carried out and lame animals attended to promptly.

examined once they go lame. A proactive preventative approach is always better than a reactive one. Routine footcare in the suckler herd often lags behind that in dairy herds; admittedly dairy herds have a greater incidence of the problem but maybe a little more proactivity in the beef world would be wise.

MOBILITY SCORING

Mobility scoring or locomotion scoring is routinely used in UK dairy herds to monitor the incidence of lameness and to identify individuals that are lame and need treatment. This involves an objective assessment of every cow in the herd, usually monthly, as they walk past a trained observer on a level, hard, non-slip surface.

DENTITION OF FINISHING CATTLE

Permanent tooth eruption – where deciduous (temporary) teeth are replaced with permanent teeth – starts at 18–24 months of age. The incisors are replaced, starting with the middle pair, every 12 months and for this reason cattle are often aged by the number of incisors they have present, up to 4 years of age, see Table 7.2. This is not a reliable method of ageing as the eruption of teeth is dependent on the breed and stage of development, and not just age alone.

REFERENCES

AHDB (2016) *Feeding Growing and Finishing Cattle for Better Returns. Beef BRP Manual 7.* Agriculture and Horticulture Development Board, Stoneleigh.

Beer, M. (n.d.) Dark cutting beef – what is it? New South Wales Government. Available at: https://www.dpi.nsw.gov.au/animals-and-livestock/beef-cattle/management/market-information/dcb (accessed January 2020).

Defra (2003) *Code of Recommendations for the Welfare of Livestock. Cattle*. Defra, London.

Dyce, K.M., Sack, W.O. and Wensing, C.J.G. (2002) The head and ventral neck of the ruminants. In: *Textbook of Veterinary Anatomy*, 3rd edn. Sauders, Philadelphia, PA, chapter 25.

Grandin, T. (2013) *The Design and Construction of Facilities for Handling Cattle*. Animal Science Department, Colorado State University.

Grove-White, D. (2004) Rumen healthcare in the dairy cow. *In Practice* 26, 88–95.

Hulsen, J. (2006) *Cow Signals. A Practical Guide to Dairy Farm Management*, 1st edn. Roodbont Publishers, Zutphen.

McKinnon, B.R. (1998) Beef quality corner – 'dark cutters' livestock update. Virginia Cooperative Extension. Available at: https://www.sites.ext.vt.edu/newsletter-archive/livestock/aps-98_03/aps-891.html (accessed January 2020).

Moloney, A.P., Mooney, M.T., Kerry, J.P. and Troy, D.J. (2001) Producing tender and flavoursome beef with enhanced nutritional characteristics. Animal Nutrition and Metabolism Group Symposium on 'Quality inputs for quality foods'. *Proceedings of the Nutrition Society* 60, 221–229.

FURTHER READING

Blowey, R. (1993) *Cattle Lameness and Hoofcare*. Farming Press, Ipswich.

Chapter 8

The health and management of the heifer replacement

Even in a well-managed suckler herd, a percentage of cows will be culled every year. Culls can be voluntary; animals that have been selected to be removed from the herd for old age or for undesirable traits such as bad temperament, dystocia, mastitis or infertility. Alternatively, culls can be involuntary culls; those that die on farm as a result of disease or accident – they leave the herd whether we like it or not. To maintain numbers, replacement breeding animals are needed; for maximum longevity these should be heifers, hence the term 'heifer replacement'.

Heifer replacements may be home-bred or sourced from other farms. Choosing which option to take is an important decision.

There are advantages and disadvantages to each option.

The benefits of buying in breeding heifers is that there is an instant increase in herd size and a one-off known cost. It also allows new genetics to be introduced, such as changing to a breed of cow better suited to the objectives of the farm. For example, if the objective of the farm is to reduce wintering costs by *outwintering* cows a tough but smaller lighter weight breed of cow may be required to reduce poaching of the wet winter ground.

On the downside, however, although it is possible to source heifers from farms with disease-free accreditations, the only way to ensure diseases do not enter a herd is to not buy in cattle at all. This is one of the main advantages of breeding replacements – the herd's health status can be maintained. Further information on biosecurity is provided in Chapter 18.

Another advantage of breeding heifer replacements, rather than buying them in, is that it allows a complete knowledge of their life history from conception, and in some cases their mother's and grandmother's life history too. This includes information on characteristics such as longevity, fertility, disease history, growth rates, milk yield and foot soundness. This information is rarely available when purchasing heifers.

BREEDING HEIFER REPLACEMENTS

The best strategy for breeding heifer replacements is to select older cows from the herd as the dams. These older dams will have a track record and will be required to satisfy the following criteria:

- have had only unassisted calvings
- have calved every year
- calve early in the calving season
- have the heaviest calves at 200 days
- have a good temperament
- are foot sound, with good hoof and leg conformation
- are not too big in stature.

BULL SELECTION FOR HEIFER REPLACEMENTS

The sire selected to breed heifer replacements should be one with good *maternal trait* EBVs: calving ease, age at first calving, 200-day milk, longevity, scrotal size and fertility (see Chapter 9). A heifer that undergoes a difficult calving (dystocia) will take longer to recover from the birth, cyclicity will be delayed and premature culling will be more likely. It is clear, therefore, that every effort should be made to avoid cases of dystocia – appropriate bull selection is usually the answer over and above other factors.

Breeding the herd's own replacements allows bespoke selection of the sire so that herd objectives can be met. One of the reasons that some smaller herds (fewer than 50 cows) have found it difficult to breed heifer replacements is that these herds tend to run only one bull, which is selected for its terminal traits, such as growth rates or muscle depth. So not only will this bull serve his own daughters if he remains in the herd for two to three years or more, he is also likely to have weaker maternal traits, such as calving ease, and is therefore not suitable for the *siring of breeding females.*

AI may be a solution to this problem. Advances in sexed semen have made this an even more attractive option. The selected cows can be artificially inseminated. This is covered in more detail later in this chapter and in Chapter 27.

The resultant heifer calves born, those destined to be breeding females, need to be managed as such. This requires good record keeping and advance planning and organisation.

For this strategy to work, the number of heifer replacements needs to be predicted 2–3 years in advance. The number required will depend on the cull rate and the future objectives of the farm, such as if the herd size is to increase, decrease or remain the same. This may, of course, change within the 3 year timeframe, so an over-estimation is advisable. There is also a certain 'failure rate' throughout the process (see Figure 8.1): some cows will not conceive, there may be calving difficulties, cows may die, calves may die, or bull calves may still be born despite using sexed semen (it does happen). The number of cows selected to inseminate therefore needs to exceed the number of heifer replacements required. Furthermore, some of the heifer replacements reared may fail the pre-breeding assessment because of abnormal pelvises, bad temperament,

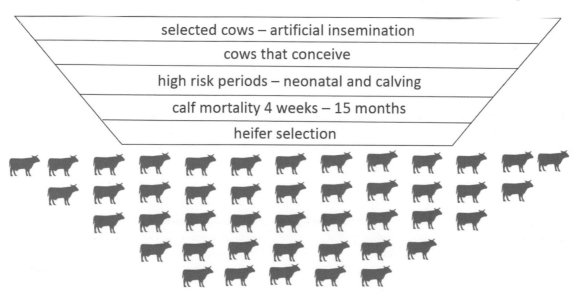

FIGURE 8.1 Diagrammatic representation of the failure rate of cows selected to breed heifer replacements to the number of heifer replacements required

or through having incomplete or abnormal reproductive organs.

WHEN TO BREED HEIFER REPLACEMENTS

Heifers are born with between 10,000 and 350,000 follicles within their ovaries. They do not develop any more, this is their total reserve. So, a cow may 'run out' of follicles in her lifetime and become infertile. Thus, for cow longevity, a large number of follicles is desirable. Follicle number is in part determined by the heifer's genetics, and, interestingly, the maternal diet can also affect the progeny's ovarian reserve (Summers et al., 2013).

Puberty has been reached when a heifer expresses oestrus behaviour and can ovulate a fertile egg (oocyte). Quite often the first ovulation is not accompanied by a display of oestrus behaviour, but the second ovulation is, and this is considered a true oestrus.

The age at which a heifer should have her own first calf is a much-debated subject. In suckler herds, heifers have traditionally calved down between 2.5 and 3 years old. The efficiency of this strategy has, however, been challenged and calving at two years of age is being increasingly adopted by many. It is definitely achievable, that has been proven, but it seems it is not popular or suitable for all farming systems.

There are guidelines to adhere to if calving heifers at 2 years old. Sexual maturity is related to weight, rather than age. Heifers need to achieve their target weights for bulling at 15 months of age which is 65% of their will-be mature weight.

To calculate this figure, the weight of a typical, average, mature cow on the farm needs to be known; cows can be considered as mature once they reach 5 years of age or more. An idea of mature cow weight can be gained by weighing 10% of the mature cows and calculating the average. Table 8.1 is a guide. Early maturing breeds such as the Aberdeen Angus and Hereford reach sexual maturity at lower weights and this makes two-year-old calvings more achievable than in later maturing breeds such as the Charolais or Limousin.

Knowing the weight that heifers need to be at mating allows a DLWG from birth to be calculated. If a weight of 455 kg is required at 15 months (450 days) and the birth weight is 45 kg, then a DLWG of 0.91 kg is required. This sort of rate is easily achievable if nutrition is well-managed.

Selecting heifer calves born early in the calving period means that it is easier to achieve target weights with them and easier to maintain the same calving period as the cows. It also means their mothers were likely to have been more fertile than their herd mates – this is a heritable trait and a desirable one too.

Many herds that adopt 2 year old calving fail to get some heifers back in-calf for their second pregnancy. The heifers often lose condition while suckling their first calf. This may not be the heifer's fault, it is usually because their nutritional needs are not being met. After calving, heifers require extra nutrition, simply to recover from the anatomical and physiological ordeal, but also to produce milk, resume cyclicity and to grow themselves. The feed requirements of these first-calvers are, perhaps surprisingly to many, approximately 10% higher than for mature cows (Lowman and

TABLE 8.1 Target body weights (kg) for first to third mating for suckler cows (Riddell et al., 2017)

Estimated mature cow weight (kg)	Heifer target body weight (kg) for mating based on % of estimated mature body weight*		
	First mating	Second mating	Third mating
	*65%	*85%	*95%
600	390	510	570
700	455	595	665

Lewis, 1992). For these nutritional needs to be met, they need preferential treatment and should be managed separately from the cows so as to prevent them from being bullied, and from being competed with for trough space and for lying space. If there is no provision on the farm for this, then a 2 year old calving system should not be attempted.

PRE-BREEDING CHECKS

When heifers intended as replacements have reached 12–14 months of age, they should be examined by a vet to assess their suitability for potential future breeding. A pre-breeding check should include the following:

1. identification of the heifer including extra management tags if required
2. bodyweight
3. confirmation of date of birth
4. BVD status: if unknown, then a blood sample should be taken to test for the presence of the BVD virus antigen, which ensures persistently infected (PI) animals are not retained as breeding animals
5. BVD vaccination compliance
6. internal veterinary examination for reproductive tract scoring (RTS): (a) ruling out of pregnancy; (b) confirmation of presence of two normal ovaries and a uterus; and (c) confirmation of normal ovarian cyclicity
7. pelvimetry – measurement of the internal dimensions of the pelvis using a pelvimeter
8. conformational assessment, for example, leg and hoof angle (problems identified at a young age will be exacerbated as body weight increases and may result in premature removal from the herd)
9. udder health assessment: heifers that have suffered from summer mastitis should not be bred
10. temperament assessment: 'wild' or aggressive heifers should not be used as replacements

The female reproductive tract

The female reproductive tract is made up of the vulva, vagina, cervix, uterus, two oviducts (Fallopian tubes) and two ovaries each with an associated infundibulum, see Figures 8.2 and 8.3. The reproductive tract sits below the rectum and above the bladder within the pelvis (Figure 8.4).

The egg ovulates from a follicle (a fluid-filled spherical structure up to 25 mm in diameter) on the surface of the ovary. The infundibulum is a pouch around the ovary that guides the released egg towards the oviduct and prevents it disappearing into the abdomen. The lining of the oviduct is covered in microscopic hairs called cilia which waft the egg along the tube towards the uterus. It is while travelling down the oviduct the egg meets a sperm swimming up the tube towards it, swimming valiantly against the tide of the wafting cilia! There will of course be many sperm, but one gets it right, sometimes two.

When they meet, fertilisation occurs. The fertilised egg then passes down into the uterus, approximately 4 days after conception, where it implants into the uterine wall. The uterus is a muscular organ comprising two horns and a body. The neck of the

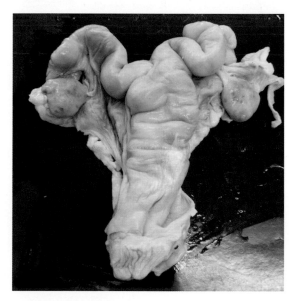

FIGURE 8.2 Post-mortem photo of the uterus and ovaries of a 2 year old heifer

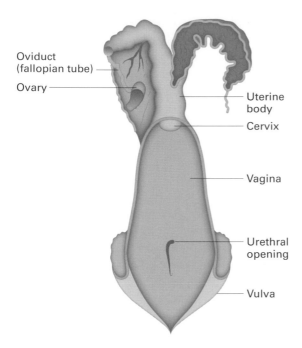

FIGURE 8.3 Diagrammatic representation of a 'bird's eye view' of the female reproductive tract

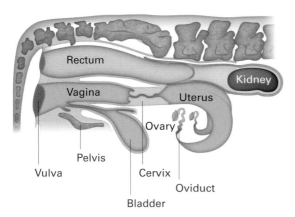

FIGURE 8.4 Diagrammatic representation depicting the location of the female reproductive tract within the abdomen

uterus is a firm tough structure – called the cervix – which seals the uterus and only opens slightly during oestrus to allow the sperm in and 9 months later dilates fully during the calving process.

Back to our fertilised egg. Once in the uterus, the cells of the fertilised egg divide rapidly, and develop into an embryo, and then a foetus and then a fully formed calf. At birth, the calf passes

from the uterus through the dilated cervix, and through the vagina and vulva to the outside world. That is reproduction!

The ovaries produce hormones – oestrogen and progesterone among others – that are released directly into the bloodstream. Oestrogen is responsible for oestrus behaviour: chin-resting, hyperactivity, bulling slime, standing to be mounted, vocalising and increased blood flow to the reproductive organs. After ovulation has occurred a structure – called a corpus luteum – forms on the ovary inside the remains of the ruptured follicle. The corpus luteum produces progesterone, which signals the state of pregnancy to the rest of the body.

The vagina links the cervix and the vulva; it is located within the pelvis, beneath the rectum and above the entrance to the bladder. The vagina is where a bull, during natural service, deposits semen that then travels through the slightly dilated cervix, into the uterine body and up the uterine horns to meet the egg. Where a female is artificially inseminated, the semen is inserted directly through the cervix with a catheter straight into the body of the uterus. The convoluted folds of the cervix make this a difficult task and it requires training and experience.

The vulva is the external part of the reproductive tract that is located below the rectum. It forms the entrance into the vagina. The opening to the urethra, the tube that passes urine from the bladder to the outside world, is located just inside the vulval lips on the floor of the vagina.

Reproductive tract scoring

The earlier a heifer achieves puberty the more oestrus cycles she will have before the breeding season. It has been shown that heifers served on their third oestrus cycle after puberty had a 23% improvement in pregnancy rate compared to those served on their first (Poock and Payne, 2013).

Assessing the size of a heifer's ovaries ultrasonographically and the number of follicles present in them is a good indicator of their pubertal status

TABLE 8.2 Reproductive tract scoring parameters (Poock and Payne, 2013)

RTS	Uterine Horns	Ovarian Length (mm)	Ovarian Height (mm)	Ovarian Width (mm)	Ovarian Structures
1	Immature, <20mm diameter, no tone	15	10	8	No palpable follicles
2	20–25mm diameter, no tone	18	12	10	8mm follicles
3	20–25mm diameter, slight tone	22	15	10	8–10mm follicles
4	30mm diameter, good tone	30	16	12	10mm follicles, CL possible
5	>30mm diameter	>32	20	15	CL present

and therefore a good predictor of how early in the breeding season they will likely conceive.

The technique to evaluate the heifer's tract pre-breeding is called RTS (Table 8.2). Heifers are examined 30–60 days pre-breeding and given a score of 1–5. Most heifers should be level 4 or above. Those scoring level 1 should not be bred from.

Pelvimetry

Pelvimetry is a technique that was developed in North America and is now used widely in UK beef suckler herds. It involves using a pair of large callipers, see Figure 8.5, inserted into the heifer's rectum to measure the internal dimensions – width and height – of the pelvis so that the *pelvic*

area can be calculated. The pelvic height is the narrowest vertical distance between the pubic symphysis and the sacral vertebrae, Figure 8.6. The pelvic width is the horizontal distance between the shafts of the ilium at the widest point (Poock and Payne, 2013). For accurate placement the vet will probably take a hand into the rectum with the callipers – *doing it blind* is tricky.

A heifer's pelvic area increases by the same amount each day between 12 months and 24 months of age. The rate of expansion decreases after 24 months. By knowing the age of the heifer in days, the pelvic area measurements can be used to calculate the predicted pelvic area at 12 months

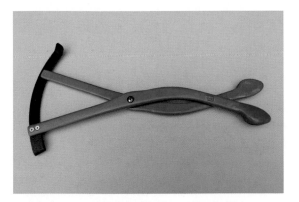

FIGURE 8.5 Callipers designed to measure the internal dimensions of the pelvic cavity of a heifer

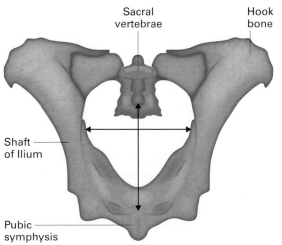

FIGURE 8.6 Diagram to show the points of measurement using the pelvimeters in the pelvis

of age. This allows for comparison across a group of heifers of different ages, see Table 8.3. From the vast number of animals that have been measured worldwide, reference ranges have been established of what is considered to be an acceptable pelvic area to allow for an unassisted calving and therefore what is unacceptable. The reference ranges differ for Continental and native-bred cattle so the correct chart must be referred to.

Pelvimetry is used to detect abnormally small or abnormally shaped pelvises (the veterinary manual examination alone will pick up abnormal shape) and then these animals can be removed

from the breeding programme. Pelvic area is a heritable trait and responds rapidly to breeding selection. For this reason, paradoxically, larger pelvic areas should not be selected either. Why? The explanation for this is that these heifers with particularly large pelvises will produce a calf that also has a large pelvis, and that in calving terms means 'wide hips'. These wide hipped calves may then be difficult to deliver even though the heifer, the mother, theoretically has a large pelvis. To add a little more to this story, the other problem that can result from breeding calves from these large pelvised heifers is that the male offspring, if used

TABLE 8.3 Pelvimetry results – heifer 2038 was subsequently not bred from due to an abnormally small pelvis

Management ID	Date of birth	Horizontal (cm)	Vertical (cm)	Pelvic size (cm2)	12 month old pelvic size (cm2)
2034	31/03/2016	13.5	14	189	176.04
2077	21/04/2016	13.5	15.5	209.25	201.96
2060	07/04/2016	13	14.5	188.5	177.43
2038	01/04/2016	12.5	13.5	168.5	156.06
2043	02/04/2016	15	16.5	247.5	235.08
2055	06/04/2016	14	16	224	212.66
2059	07/04/2016	13.5	14.5	195.75	184.68
2048	04/04/2016	13.5	15	202.5	190.62
2045	04/04/2016	14	16	224	212.12
2027	29/03/2016	14.5	15.5	224.75	211.25
2111	03/05/2016	13.5	15	202.5	198.45
2040	01/04/2016	14.5	15.5	224.75	212.06
2101	29/04/2016	12.5	14.5	181.25	176.12
2047	04/04/2016	14	15.5	217	205.12
2066	09/04/2016	13.5	15	202.5	191.97
2107	01/05/2016	14	14.5	203	198.41
2088	18/04/2016	14	16	224	215.9
2053	05/04/2016	16	16.5	264	252.39
2032	30/03/2016	11.5	14	161	147.77
2041	02/04/2016	14	13.5	189	176.58
2105	30/04/2016	14.5	15.5	224.75	219.89
2026	28/03/2016	15	14	210	196.23
2089	19/04/2016	13.5	13	175.5	167.67
2118	06/05/2016	13.5	17	229.5	226.26
2092	21/04/2016	13.5	14.5	195.75	188.46
1950	23/04/2016	16.5	17	280.5	174.93

Note: Red is an abnormally small pelvic area; amber is an adequate pelvic area; green indicates a large pelvic area.

as breeding bulls, will breed wide hipped calves that get stuck and the female offspring, if used for breeding, will simply perpetuate the problem started by her heifer mother. And one last problem, as if that is not enough – these large pelvised females tend to grow into particularly large cows, cows that may be too large for the finely tuned housing, feeding and carcase production systems already signed up to.

Calf size is still the predominant reason for dystocia, more so than pelvic area, so the use of an easy calving bull is more effective in reducing the number of assisted calvings than pelvimetry results alone.

HEIFER BREEDING MANAGEMENT

Heifers should be allowed a compact bulling period of 6 weeks and no longer, regardless of their age at breeding. Those that fail to get in-calf in that time should be culled because it is an indication that they are not as fertile as their herd mates and will continue to take multiple serves to get back in-calf. Year on year, they will fall further and further

behind in the calving period, eventually being prematurely culled due to *infertility*.

Heifers, during this 6 week period, can either be served naturally by running a bull with them for what amounts to two full cycles, or they can receive one or two rounds of AI depending on the systems of synchronisation employed, or they can enjoy both. Oestrus synchronisation, see Figure 8.7, can indeed be used to help achieve a tight calving period (see Chapter 10); any heifers that return to oestrus can be inseminated a second time or instead run with a sweeper bull. Again, only two serves are advised and if the heifer has still not conceived, she should be culled.

Heifers should not be allowed to get overfat; they should calve down at condition score 2.5. Heifers that are allowed multiple chances to get in-calf but do not have their first calf until they are over 3 years old, are often overfat at calving. Figure 8.8 shows two Beef Shorthorn heifers 15 months old managed at grass with a small amount of concentrate feeding each morning to make them easier to handle for subsequent synchronisation and AI.

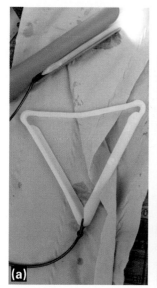 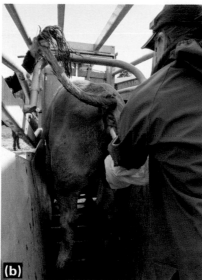 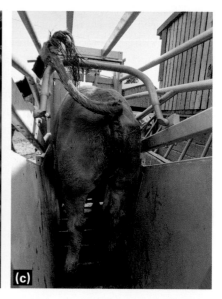

(a) (b) (c)

FIGURE 8.7 (a) A progesterone device (b, c) inserted into the vagina as part of an oestrus synchronisation programme

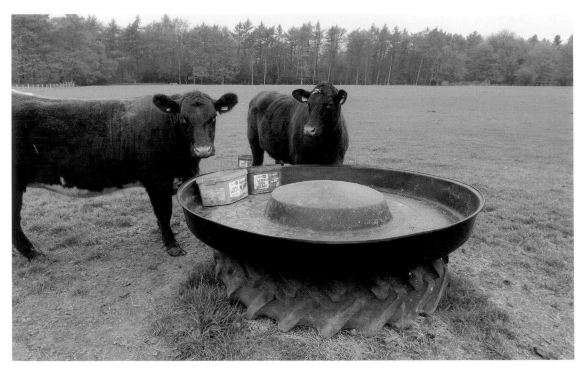

FIGURE 8.8 Beef shorthorn heifers at grass pre-calving

The anatomy of the udder

The udder is composed of four-*quarters* – two at the front and two at the back. There is no flow of milk between each quarter. Each quarter is made up of many *alveoli*, these are cell-lined pockets that largely comprise the tissue of the udder and this is where milk is produced. They are surrounded by muscle cells that contract to push milk from the alveoli into the gland cistern and then the teats, or to be precise the cavity in the teat called the *teat cistern*, see Figure 8.9. This is called milk 'let down'. The milk remains in the teat cistern until it is released by relaxation of the *teat sphincter* muscle. The teat orifice is lined with keratin, a tough protective layer which prevents the teat orifice from damage and forms a seal preventing bugs from entering the teat cistern.

There is a huge blood supply to the udder, 4000 l of blood flow through the udder to produce 1 l of milk (Blowey and Edmondson, 2010).

Development of the udder

The udder goes through four stages of development from calf to first lactation.

1. **First isometric phase**. From birth to 4 months of age, the rate of growth of the calf and udder is the same. The udder is largely a fat pad at this stage.
2. **First allometric phase**. At 4–8 months, around puberty, the udder develops very quickly. This is particularly associated with spikes of oestrogen as the heifer starts to cycle. The initial development is that of the cisterns that extend into the fat pad. As puberty is influenced by weight, not age, the timing may vary and poor nutrition early in life may have consequences for future milk production. Conversely, overfeeding at this stage means that an over developed fat pad takes the place of the future udder, also detrimental to future yield.
3. **Second isometric phase**. From 8 months

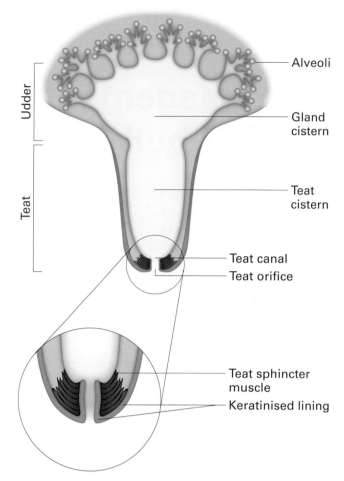

Udder

Teat

Alveoli

Gland
cistern

Teat
cistern

Teat canal
Teat orifice

Teat sphincter
muscle
Keratinised lining

FIGURE 8.9 Diagram showing the alveoli, gland cistern and teat cistern of one-quarter of the bovine udder

until conception, again, the udder develops at the same rate as the rest of the body through this period.

4. **Second allometric phase**. This is triggered by the conception of a pregnancy. In this phase, the alveoli start to develop milk-producing capabilities. Most of the development will take place from *mid-pregnancy*.

REFERENCES

Blowey, R. and Edmondson, P. (2010) *Structure of Teats and Udder and Mechanisms of Milk Synthesis*. In: *Mastitis Control in Dairy Herds*, 2nd edn. CABI, Wallingford, ch. 2.

Lowman, B. and Lewis, M. (1992) Feeding the beef suckler herd. *BCVA Summer Meeting*, Wye College, pp. 9–27.

Poock, S.E. and Payne, C.A. (2013) Incorporating reproductive management of beef heifers into a veterinary practice. *Veterinary Clinics: Food Animal Practice* 29(3), 667–678.

Riddell, I., Caldow, G., Lowman, B. and Pritchard, I. (2017) *A Guide to Improving Suckler Herd Fertility*. QMS, Midlothian.

Summers, A.F., Cushman, R.A., Moline, K.V., Bergman, J.W. and Cupp, A.S. (2013) Heifers with low antral follicle counts have low birth weights and produce progeny with low birth weights. Nebraska Beef Cattle Report, Institute of Agriculture and Natural Resources, University of Nebraska-Lincoln, pp. 11–12.

Chapter 9

The health and management of the breeding bull

In UK beef suckler herds, natural service, rather than AI, is predominantly used to impregnate heifers and cows.

The contribution of the bull in a suckler herd, the *bull effect,* is paramount. The overall aim in a suckler herd is to achieve a compact calving period of 9–12 weeks, with a low number of barren cows and few calving difficulties, and to maximise the number of kilogrammes of calf weaned per cow put to the bull (see Chapter 20); the bull plays no small part.

Temperament is important. Bulls need to be safe to be turned out to grass with the cows, and amenable to handle and house during the winter months, but even so, always treated with great respect and caution.

The bull's own health, soundness and longevity are important for welfare, performance but also because a bull is a significant financial outlay.

The cost of a bull might, as an example, be estimated as follows.

- A bull is purchased for, say, £5000.
- He sires 50 calves a year for 5 years, a total of 250 calves.
- It costs, say, £700 a year to maintain a bull (veterinary costs, medicines, feed, bedding).
- The bull has a cull value of, say, £800.
- The bull's cost is therefore £30 per calf sired.

And that is when all goes well! The cost per calf increases when there are fewer calves sired, or if there is no cull value because the bull dies on the farm or if he leaves the herd in less than the planned 5 years.

ARTIFICIAL INSEMINATION

Alternatively, AI can be used, which negates the need to have as many bulls on the farm and allows the herd to benefit from superior genetics that are otherwise unobtainable. Often a bull is still needed to 'sweep up'; to serve cows that have not conceived to AI. Where a large number of cows or heifers are to be inseminated *synchronisation programmes* are used by the vet to bring the females to the same stage in their oestrus cycle, hence the term, synchronisation. They are then inseminated at the same time, without observation of heats being necessary, this is known as *fixed time AI.* The cost of the veterinary time and drugs is approximately £50 per cow. Semen straws are an additional cost and good quality straws from proven bulls cost between £25 and £50. Conception rates to fixed time AI are around 60%.

GENETICS

The bull will be contributing half of the genetics to the output of the herd. He may be contributing half the genetics to the future breeding herd if his daughters are kept as heifer replacements and his genetics will be inflicted on the dam when it comes to her having to give birth to his progeny. Thus, buying or breeding the right bull as well as maintaining him in working order is vital for the short- and long-term performance of a beef suckler herd.

Herd performance can be altered and adjusted through changing management practices, but an animal's genetics are permanent and determine baseline potential productivity. There is always genetic variation within a population, so by selecting animals with superior performance traits for breeding, improvements can be made over time, sometimes surprisingly quickly. If the objectives of a herd are to be changed – for instance, to have smaller framed cows – then the breeding plan can be adapted by selecting a different bull with the genes for smaller frames.

The performance potential of different bulls can be evaluated and compared using EBVs. These are explained later in this chapter.

REPRODUCTIVE ANATOMY OF THE BULL

A bull has a 1 m long *fibroelastic penis* that retracts into the sheath when not erect, see Figure 9.1. The penis should be straight but has a small curve at its tip. This should not be confused with a 'corkscrew penis' where the end is truly coiled, and which prevents the bull serving a cow.

The production of sperm is called spermatogenesis and occurs within the two testicles (*testes*) contained within the scrotum. They are suspended independently of each other by the spermatic cord; this includes the various blood vessels and nerves and the all important *vas deferens* (sometimes called the ductus deferens), which connects the testes with the penis and carries sperm to the *urethra* during ejaculation (see Chapter 4, Figure 4.11). Adjacent and closely associated with the cord is the cremaster muscle which is able to contract and draw the testicles closer to the body

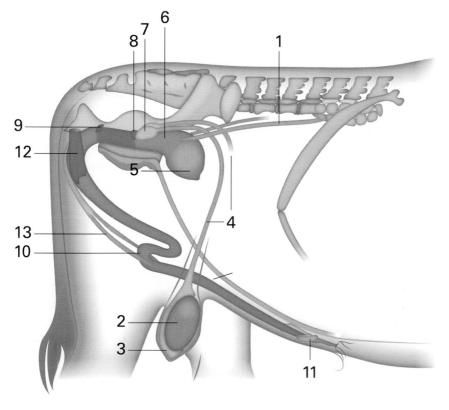

FIGURE 9.1 Anatomy of the male reproductive tract (modified from Dyce et al., 2002): 1 – ureter; 2 – right testes; 3 – epididymis; 4 – vas deferens; 5 – bladder; 6 – vesicular gland; 7 – ampullae; 8 – body of prostate; 9 – bulbourethral gland; 10 – sigmoid flexure of penis; 11 – glans penis; 12 – ischiocavernosus; 13 – retractor penis

for safe keeping in a state of danger or when it is cold. The sperm are stored, awaiting ejaculation, in a convoluted structure called the *epididymis*. This is between 5 and 8 cm long and is tightly coiled up and attached to the testicle within the scrotum.

The temperature of the testicles is strictly regulated. They function at 3–4°C less than body temperature, any alteration in temperature can affect spermatogenesis (Statham, 2010).

The numerous sweat glands on the surface of the scrotum and the ability for the bull to control the distance the testicles are away from the body largely affects their temperature. There is also a large network of veins within the spermatic cord where heat exchange occurs – hot blood on its way to the testes has the heat taken out of it by the returning coiled vein acting as a heat exchanger.

Also included in the male reproductive tract, are the *accessory reproductive glands*, Figure 9.2, which are located within the pelvis, closely associated with the urethra. The accessory glands include the *ampullae* (paired), the *vesicular glands* (paired), the *bulbourethral glands* (paired) and the *prostate gland* (singular). They each produce a fluid that combines to form seminal fluid which contains an energy supply for the sperm and a medium for it to travel in during its journey through the male and female reproductive tracts.

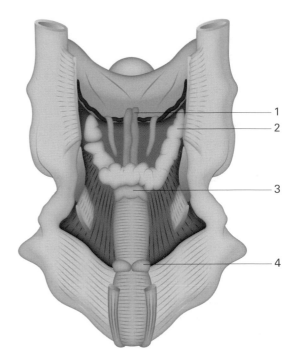

FIGURE 9.2 Plan view of the anatomy of the accessory glands (modified from Entwistle and Fordyce, 2003): 1 – ampullae; 2 – seminal vesicles; 3 – body of prostate; 4 – bulbourethral gland

LIBIDO AND COURTING

Libido, or sex drive, is driven largely by the hormone *testosterone* released from the testicles. An area of the brain called the *hypothalamus* initiates the cascade of hormones that results in the release of testosterone – the hypothalamus is stimulated by visual and olfactory stimuli. Research suggest bulls do indeed visually detect females in oestrus through the high activity and mounting behaviours that occur within a group when one female is in oestrus and this starts the ball rolling so to speak. Pheromones do play a role, but they

are usually involved further down the line when physical contact occurs, that is, sniffing. So, the primary sense used for detection of oestrus is sight – bulls need to be able to see.

Male and female contact involves the bull sniffing and licking the genital region and, thought to be a response to female pheromones, the bull sometimes exhibits the *flehmen response* (curling of the upper lip). This process seems to add to the sex drive.

MATING

The cow determines when service can occur and in the case of multiple males in a group, by which male. The bull will 'test' the situation by chin-resting on the cow's rear end and attempting to mount. She will only stand for service when she is ready; when she is in 'standing oestrus'. A cow ovulates

24–36 hours after the start of standing oestrus and the sperm needs to be in the oviduct before the egg gets there (see Chapter 10). After intromission, ejaculation occurs within a few seconds.

While libido has a strong genetic component bulls often have to 'learn' how to serve a cow (Chenoweth, 2007). Young inexperienced bulls need time with a small group of cows on a non-slip surface to perfect the technique. They are thought to benefit from watching an older bull at work.

Any pain associated with mounting, or a previous painful experience when serving a cow will inhibit a bull's performance. If a bull is presented with a cow in heat, he should serve her within 20 minutes, and ideally, within 10 minutes of introduction. Many farmers comment that they never see their bull serve a cow, yet all are in-calf: some bulls waste no energy and time courting a female and work quickly under the cover of darkness!

Libido is not routinely assessed as part of a pre-breeding examination (PBE); however, it is vital in achieving conception. To assess a bull's libido, it requires a female to be in heat and bulling observed. This can be facilitated by hormonal synchronisation of a group of cows in time for the assessment (see Chapter 10).

PUBERTY

The onset of puberty is defined as being when an entire male animal first exhibits bull-like behaviour and has the start of a small number of sperm in the ejaculate – approximately 50 million sperm per millilitre. A mature bull's ejaculate contains 400 million sperm per millilitre.

The age of puberty will vary depending on the breed. Typically, a Charolais bull will reach puberty at 7.5 months, whereas an Aberdeen Angus might take 9 months. There will also be variation *within breeds* depending on genetics and environmental factors.

FERTILITY

A fertile bull is expected to get 90% of 50 normal cycling disease-free females pregnant within 9 weeks, and 60% of these should become pregnant in the first 6 weeks (McGowan, 2001).

In the authors' experience, this is rarely achieved. Bulls are often *subfertile* and are not able to achieve this target. This is frequently mismanaged on farm by moving bulls between groups, decreasing the number of cows that a bull is expected to get in-calf or lengthening the service period to minimise the number of barren cows. None of these solutions are conducive to a productive efficient herd.

Sterility is a complete and permanent inability to breed; it is rare. Infertility, or more correctly subfertility, is defined as a *temporary inability or reduced ability* to reproduce, this scenario is more common.

To identify sterility, infertility or subfertility, a PBE of the bull is recommended 3–4 weeks before the expected bulling period. This is sometimes referred to as a bull breeding soundness examination (BBSE).

Unknowingly using a sterile, subfertile or infertile bull results in a high barren rate and the time taken to achieve the pregnancies results in a protracted calving period. The consequences do not just affect 1 year's breeding; it will take several years to bring the length of the calving period back to where it needs to be.

This is a significant and avoidable loss of production, a proactive approach using PBEs is strongly advised. In a survey in the south of Scotland where PBEs were carried out on 319 bulls, 33.4% were found to be sterile, subfertile or infertile (Eppink, 2005).

For a PBE, the bull needs to be adequately restrained using a cattle crush and halter to ensure the safety of the bull, vet and farmer, Figure 9.3.

A physical examination of a bull should include the following.

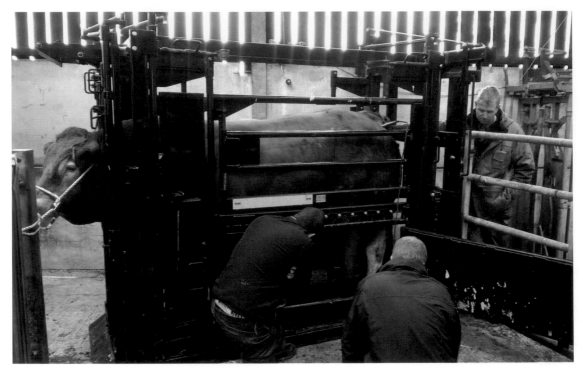

FIGURE 9.3 A bull adequately restrained for PBE

- **Eyes**. The eyes should be bright, eyelids open and no tear staining of the face, the latter of which can be an indication of in-turned eyelids resulting from irritation, a common problem, or less commonly from congenital causes.
- **Teeth**. The incisor teeth should be in line with the front edge of the dental pad on the top jaw to ensure the bull can take in food properly and maintain condition. Halitosis can be an indication of infection in the mouth, or trapped food from poor dentition.
- **Legs and hooves**. The bull should be allowed to walk and trot freely, on a clean smooth level surface, so any lameness or abnormalities in gait can be detected. The hind feet should track forward and be placed in the footprint left by the front foot, or even in front of it. Conformational abnormalities of the legs and hooves should be noted. Any swellings, sores or ulcers are significant findings (conformational defects and leg and hoof abnormalities are discussed in Chapter 16). An excessively high energy cereal-based diet will predispose a bull to laminitis and other musculoskeletal disease (see Chapter 14).
- **The brisket**. This should be examined as this area is in contact with the cow during service; any lesions can cause pain and discomfort, and disincline the bull from mounting the cow.
- **Body condition**. Condition should be noted and whether the bull has previously been examined, any change in BCS is also significant. If the bull is less than BCS 2, further investigation is required (Chapter 10).
- **Testicles**. The scrotal skin should be smooth and not 'scabby' or thickened. The testicles should move freely within the scrotum and be able to be drawn down into the scrotal sac to allow palpation of the neck of the scrotum. Within the neck of the scrotum there should be no lumps, but the spermatic cord and cremaster muscle should be palpable. The testicles should be identical in size and consistency. They should

TABLE 9.1 Scrotal circumference minimum recommendations (McGowan et al., 1995)

Age (months)	Scrotal circumference (cm)
12–15	30
18–21	32
24 or older	34 or more

be not be hard or soft, but firm with a consistency similar to a nearly ripe tomato.

- **Scrotal circumference**. An accurate predictor of sperm output in mature bulls. Large testicles are highly correlated with sperm production and quality (Table 9.1). Bulls with above-average scrotal circumference reach puberty earlier and this can be passed to female offspring. This can be an advantageous trait where bulls are being selected for maternal characteristics. By 24 months of age a bull's testicles are 90% of their mature size (McGowan, 2001). Variations of 1–2 cm year on year are acceptable and will be due to changes in body condition. Changes exceeding 4 cm indicate an abnormality. To obtain a reliable reading of scrotal circumference, the testicles need to be manipulated so they are side by side in the scrotal sac, with no wrinkles in the skin and consistent pressure applied to the measuring tape. A vet may choose to examine the testicles in more detail by using ultrasonography. This enables fibrosis or calcification within the testicles to be detected. Ultrasonography is not routinely used in a PBE.

Where bulls are fed an excessively high energy ration to obtain target weights, fat is deposited in the neck of the scrotum and around the testes. This is undesirable as it affects the thermoregulatory mechanisms and falsely elevates the scrotal circumference. Bulls fed excessively at an early age, during puberty, have poorer sperm quality than bulls fed a regular forage-based ration.

- **Accessory sex glands**. A vet may examine a bull's internal or accessory glands as part of a physical examination. This involves inserting a gloved, lubricated hand through the anus into the rectum of the bull. The prostate, the pair of ampullae and the seminal vesicles are palpable per rectum.

SEMEN EVALUATION

Semen can be collected using electro-ejaculation or an artificial vagina (AV).

Electro-ejaculation involves applying a low-level electrical pulse from a specially designed electric rectal probe, Figure 9.4, which selectively stimulates the nerves responsible for ejaculation. The bull needs to be adequately restrained, for his safety and that of the operator. The ejaculate is collected in a cup directly from the bull's penis if erect, see Figure 9.5, or indirectly from the sheath

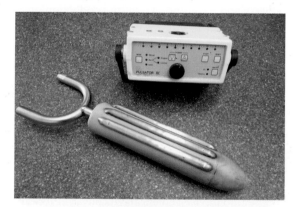

FIGURE 9.4 Bull electro-ejaculator

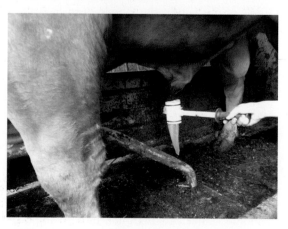

FIGURE 9.5 Semen collection via electro-ejaculation

if the bull does not extrude his penis. The majority, 95%, of bulls will provide a sample using this technique, 5% will not respond to electro-ejaculation (Entwistle and Fordyce, 2003).

Alternatively, an AV can be used. This is the most common method of collection for bulls where semen is collected for AI as larger ejaculates are produced in this relatively more natural way. A cow in oestrus is restrained and the operator allows the bull to mount the cow and then diverts the penis into the AV – a warm, rubberised, tubular container. This is a natural and representative ejaculate, but this technique is impractical when testing bulls on farm. This technique does, however, incorporate the performance of natural service so libido and the ability to physically mount a cow can be observed.

A bull is considered to have gone through puberty and have normal sperm production once he has reached 16 months of age. If a bull is evaluated before that, then semen quality may not be as good, and this fact needs to be allowed for in the assessment. In some cases, where a bull has not been running with females recently, and has therefore not been reproductively active, the initial semen sample collected may be suboptimal and is referred to as a 'rusty load'. The bull should be allowed to rest for an hour or so, and then a second collection attempted.

The amount of ejaculate and its physical appearance is relevant and recorded. A blood-stained sample or pus within the sample is an indication there is something wrong. If the sample is contaminated with urine, this may affect the motility of the sperm. The amount of ejaculate will vary depending on the bull and the method of collection.

The semen can then be examined microscopically, see Figure 9.6. This is a three-stage process and is covered further in Chapter 16. Briefly the three stages are as follows.

1. **Gross motility**. Motility of the sperm *en masse* is graded between 1 and 5 where 5 is a highly motile sample and 1 is a non-motile sample. A score of 3 or more is acceptable.

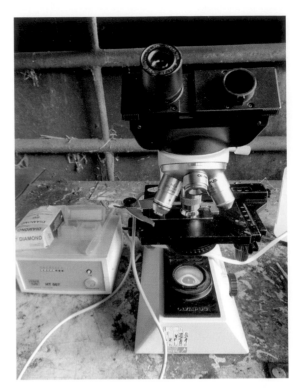

FIGURE 9.6 On-farm set-up for semen evaluation which includes a heated microscope stage to keep the semen warm

2. **Progressive motility**. The sample is diluted further and examined under a higher magnification and in more detail; this is to ensure individual sperm are moving in a progressive manner and not just wriggling around in circles!

3. **Morphology**. The final 'test' is to apply a purple-coloured stain to the semen sample and allow it to dry, see Figure 9.7. The sperm are killed, and 100 sperm are counted and examined individually to identify the ratio of normal to abnormal sperm. A sample containing more than 70% normal sperm is considered acceptable.

On their own or in combination, lameness, poor body condition, concurrent disease, over-condition, heat stress, certain medicines and a high body temperature will all affect semen quality, sometimes permanently, sometimes temporarily.

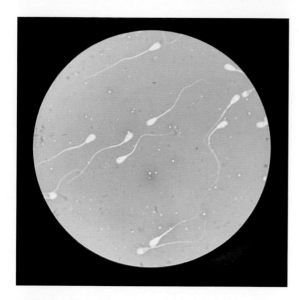

FIGURE 9.7 Stained semen examined through a microscope at high magnification

By using information from the bull's management history, and the physical examination and semen evaluation, a decision can be made on the suitability of the bull for breeding. If the bull has an unsatisfactory semen evaluation with no significant abnormalities from the physical examination, then a semen evaluation may be repeated after 10 weeks. It takes 61 days for a new cycle of sperm to be produced and 10–12 days for the sperm to travel from the testes to the epididymis (McGowan, 2001).

MANAGEMENT OF BULLS

Housing

When bulls are not in use, they should be kept in a safe, comfortable pleasant environment. Where temperament and weather permit this would be a safe, secure paddock where no risk to the public is posed. Failing that they should have their own individual bull pen, as they are liable to fight with other bulls and be a bully in a group of smaller cattle. Many smaller herds fail to achieve a compact calving period simply because they have nowhere

safe to keep the bull, so he runs with the cows all year round.

The bull should have regular contact with humans and be in visual sight of other cows or bulls. This needs to be borne in mind when deciding where to construct the bull pen.

A bull pen needs to be built to restrain a 1200 kg animal. The sides need to be high enough to prevent the bull jumping out, the hinges need to be covered to avoid the bull catching his nose ring and damaging himself, there should be provision of a personnel-escape for human safety, there should be a feed trough that can be accessed from the outside without having to go in with the bull, a self-locking yoke for restraint, a comfortable lying area, natural light, rain cover and be draught free but ventilated. The bull will benefit from having *both* a soft clean lying area and a hard, dry concrete surface to stand on; this will help keep his hooves in good condition. Access to an area to exercise is important. Strong, fit, well-exercised bulls are less likely to suffer injury during the bulling period.

Feeding

Bulls need to be turned out with cows and heifers at a BCS of 3–3.5. During a busy service period they will have little time to eat and will use considerable energy, so they have the potential to lose condition. This condition needs to be restored between service periods.

When feeding a young bull, it is important to take into account that he is still growing. Failure to do this may affect his future fertility and longevity in the herd. The ration should include appropriate vitamin and mineral supplementation. It is well documented that over feeding is, however, the bigger problem. Overfeeding bulls with concentrate feed should be avoided as it results in reduced semen quality, affects locomotion, and increases the risks of acidosis and liver abscessation.

Vaccination

Bulls need to be included in the herd vaccination protocols. The bull requires protection from disease, especially as any disease within the bulling period, or up to 8 weeks pre-breeding, will affect his fertility. The bull is a high value animal and vaccination against clostridial disease should also be considered. Advice from a vet should be sought if the vaccine datasheet does not state that it is safe to use in a male breeding animal – this is the case with some vaccines. Vaccines should not be administered during the breeding period or within 8 weeks of the start of the service period because rather like an infection, vaccines can produce a transient rise in body temperature which may reduce fertility.

Parasite treatments

Whether administering worming, fluke or ectoparasite treatments, bulls need to be included in the herd parasite control plan; their requirements will depend on grazing patterns and age. Some bulls reared in intensive systems will not have had access to grass and will have no immunity to gastrointestinal parasites so more frequent worming treatment may be required in the first grazing season. There may also be a lack of immunity to lungworm. Ticks can cause temporary infertility if the bull is naïve to tickborne fever and becomes infected. If the farm is known to have a high tick risk, then bulls should be purchased at a younger age, that is, as weaned calves, and run on the high-risk pasture to gain some immunity. Irritation from flies can also reduce fertility, and bulls are prone to lice infestation over the winter months.

Foot and limb care

Physical soundness is so important for a bull to work. A mature bull's body weight can be well in excess of 1000 kg so musculoskeletal problems

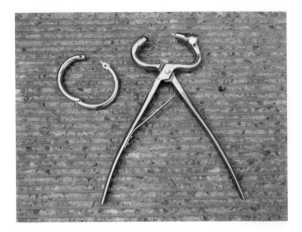

FIGURE 9.8 Bull ring and bull-ringing pliers

are a common finding, both limb and feet abnormalities. Feet should be inspected, and trimmed if required, every 6 months out, with and well in advance of, the breeding period.

Ringing

Bulls kept for breeding are commonly fitted with a nose ring to facilitate handling. This procedure involves inserting a copper ring in the septum of their nose. This should be carried out hygienically by a veterinary surgeon or trained operative using the appropriate painkiller and the correct equipment as seen in Figure 9.8.

Buying a bull

Choosing the right bull for the herd is critical, and this depends on whether he will be used to breed cattle for slaughter, or for heifer replacements.

When breeding cattle for slaughter, the aim is to satisfy customer need. This will depend on the market; a supermarket may require leaner carcases less than 400 kg while a butcher in a farm shop may seek a native-bred carcase with extra fat deposition. The choice of genetics is therefore important but then matching genetics with the feeding system is equally important to ultimately produce the carcases planned for; the right size, weight and grade at the right cost of production.

In the case of breeding heifer replacements, either to sell or retain in the herd, the qualities sought in a bull are quite different. Breeding the right type of cow for the herd, in terms of her size, preferred nutritional requirements, ability to calve, ability to feed the calf and adaptability to the environment are all crucial and half of the genetic coding for this comes from the bull and some more still from his compatibility with the female.

EBVs can be used to provide data to support breeding decisions and are discussed later in this chapter. There are two ways to buy a bull: direct from another farm, or through the open market via a bull sale. There are traditionally two main bull sale periods in the year – autumn and spring.

A bull should be purchased well in advance of when he is needed for breeding. This will allow time for an adequate quarantine period, and for vaccines to be administered. He can also have time to adapt to the farm and be exposed to the pathogens living on the new farm. He can be fed appropriately to get into condition for work rather than the inappropriate feeding he may have been given to gain so called *show condition*. Ideally, a bull intended for use in the summer should be purchased the autumn before.

It is advisable when buying a bull through a 'bull sale' at an auction mart, that the bulls are visually assessed before they are washed and dressed for sale. Many 'tricks of the trade' are used to dress cattle and some defects in conformation and some lesions could be disguised.

When purchasing a bull off-farm, there is a limited choice and often valuing a bull can be difficult when there are no contemporaries to compare him with. There are, however, advantages in that the bull can be seen in his own environment, and it gives an insight into how the bull might have been kept in terms of bedding, silage quality, ration composition, grazing and farm biosecurity. The bull's dam may also be present, as well as other siblings to give an indication of both maternal and paternal characteristics.

When a purchased bull is brought back to the farm, whether it be from the mart or from another farm, he should be isolated for a minimum of 3 weeks and vaccination programmes completed before he enters the herd (see Chapter 18). It will be unlikely that he is familiar with being kept alone so some visual contact with cattle is important. It is also an opportunity to spend some time with him too; human contact is important so that voices and smells become familiar and handling becomes less stressful for all involved. The bull should be fed a similar ration to what he is used to. This can be gradually changed over time to a preferred ration, done slowly to allow the rumen microbes time to adapt. Asking the vendor for a bag of feed to take home with the bull is recommended, perhaps in place of luck money!

Insurance

Ideally, the bull should be insured before he is transported. It is important to check the wording of the policy document – there are variations between policies and there may be exemptions for pre-existing conditions, infectious diseases or transportation. Generally, policies usually insure against mortality and loss of use, that is, permanent loss of fertility. The definition of such terminology is important; as we know it is rare that a bull is sterile (commonly insured against), but subfertility/infertility is a common problem against which insurance would be wise but is not always offered.

Before introducing the bull to the cows, he should have been subject to a PBE by a vet, including a full physical examination and semen evaluation. A young bull, 16–24 months old, should run with no more than 15–20 cows for just two cycles. The number of cows that return to oestrus after 21 days should be recorded. This should be no more than 50%. It is important that the bull is given a fair chance and that the cows are at the appropriate BCS with no history of infertility, abortion or recent calving complications; they should also be cycling when the bull is introduced. The first few services of cows should be observed to check that the bull has good technique and that there are no abnormalities of his penis.

Health

Bulls offered for sale at auction marts through breed society sales often have a 'sale card' present on their pen. In the UK these typically provide information on five major cattle diseases: BVD, leptospirosis, Johne's disease, IBR and bTB. For IBR, leptospirosis and BVD, the sale card will state the herd health status, the animal's individual status and its vaccination status. For bTB it will state the date of the last bTB test and the herd's bTB testing interval. For Johne's disease (JD), it will state the herd's risk level and the number of years since a positive animal was identified in the herd.

There are some additional disease-specific factors to be aware of as follows.

BVD (Chapter 15)

A bull should be purchased from an accredited BVD-free herd or be tested and found negative for the BVD virus itself. This confirms he is not a PI animal. This is different to an antibody test; a positive BVD antibody test indicates that the bull has either been exposed to BVD virus at some point in his lifetime or has been vaccinated against it. There is a reason for considering an antibody test as well as a virus test.

If a bull has been exposed to the BVD virus and temporarily infected, after 14 days he will be virus negative on a blood test but he can shed virus in his semen for up to 10 weeks. It takes 4 weeks from exposure to BVD virus for antibodies to be detected in the blood. Depending on the bull's antibody test result, he may require isolation for a period in excess of 10 weeks.

Johne's disease (Chapter 17)

A herd can never be accredited free of JD. The nature of the incubation period of the Johne's

bacterium (MAP) means that herds can only be classified on the basis of whether there is a low or high risk of the bacterium being present. A low-risk herd is a 'Level 1' herd. The longer the herd has achieved this low-level status, the less risk there is of a bull from this herd being infected. A blood test of an individual animal for JD does not equate to it being free of the disease. Herd status is the most important piece of information.

IBR (Chapter 15)

If a bull has tested antibody positive to IBR then he has either been vaccinated or exposed to the disease. If an IBR 'marker' vaccine has been used then there are tests to distinguish between antibodies generated in response to vaccination and antibodies generated due to exposure. Bull studs, however, do not allow entry of any animal that is IBR antibody positive, whether it is antibody from exposure or from vaccination.

If a bull has been exposed to IBR, then there is a chance he may be a carrier and shed virus at times of stress – such as at a bull sale, a new home or when mating cows. Even a bull that is vaccinated but has been exposed to the disease, can be a low-level shedder and therefore poses a risk.

Leptospirosis (Chapter 15)

Animals that have previously been exposed to leptospirosis will have antibodies present in their blood. They can also become carriers and intermittently shed bacteria in their urine, which can then infect other animals. If a bull has tested positive to leptospirosis, he may have been vaccinated or exposed to the virus. Unlike IBR, there is no way of differentiating between the two.

Campylobacter (Chapter 16)

There is a risk that *Campylobacter* spp. can be introduced to a herd from a non-virgin bull. Campylobacteriosis is a sexually transmitted disease that bulls can carry and spread from cow to cow resulting in a high barren rate due to reabsorptions and abortions. There is no blood test available to test for *Campylobacter* spp., but a sheath wash and culture can be carried out by a vet. The laboratory test has limited sensitivity and carrier animals may be 'missed'. To eliminate the risk of *Campylobacter* spp. being introduced, only virgin bulls should be purchased.

Ectoparasites and endoparasites

The quarantine procedure established for the farm should be applied to bulls, as with any other incoming livestock and that includes the use of an agreed antiparasite regimen.

ESTIMATED BREEDING VALUES

Assessing bulls by eye gives an indication of certain characteristics like *length*, conformation and soundness. But it gives no information on how easily their calves will be born, or the future performance of their offspring – their growth rates or fertility – for example. These traits are within the animal's genetic makeup. Data crunching procedures have been developed to measure these traits and are called EBVs. Some farmers have been slow to adopt the use of EBVs to help make breeding decisions; seemingly an element of distrust. They are a *tool* to be used alongside good commonsense and observation in making objective breeding decisions and they have for some time now been used successfully by progressive farmers to increase the profitability of their herd.

EBVs indicate the genetic potential of an animal for individually recorded traits. They are calculated from recorded performance data of the animal itself, data from all its known relatives, (on the same farm and across other farms), the correlation between traits (knowing how one trait affects another), and the *heritability* of the trait (heritability is the extent to which a trait is passed on from one generation to the next).

Traits for reproduction have a low heritability;

milk production has a medium heritability; growth and fat and muscle depth are highly heritable. The data is put through a *best linear unbiased predictor* (BLUP) to remove the influence of environmental factors (Hull, 2018). This involves a statistical analysis using several hundred equations to calculate an EBV. Data is submitted and EBVs are calculated either twice or three times a year depending on the breed. EBVs can be compared within breeds, but not between breeds. So, first, choose your breed.

The recording of individual animals is generally carried out by pedigree breeders. Fat depth and muscle depth is, however, measured by technicians who visit the farms and ultrasound-scan the loins of the recorded cattle between the ages of 300 and 500 days. The specifics of what is recorded varies, depending on the breed. Birth weights, calving ease, udder conformation, temperament, 100-day weights and scrotal circumference are some of the measurements required. Not all herds record for EBVs, but there is sufficient data from relatives of each animal in other herds that do record, to produce an EBV for each trait. Where there is data lacking for a trait, known correlations can be used, for example *200-day weight* is strongly correlated with *400-day weight*, and 400-day weight is negatively correlated with *calving ease*. Some data is also fed into the system via the BCMS to help develop traits for longevity and calf survival, and some data from abattoirs to ascertain the *retail beef yield* (KO%).

There are two providers of EBVs in the UK: Breedplan, an Australian company; and Signet, a UK-based provider. The traits recorded and the breed indices vary between the two, but the data is presented in a similar manner. An EBV value, the breed average, and an accuracy percentage, is stated for each trait.

An EBV is a measure of how better or worse a beef animal is in terms of its genetics, compared with an average animal of the same breed born in 1980. For example, a 400-day weight of +20 kg suggests that the genetics of the bull will result in him being 10 kg heavier at 400-days old if reared in an identical environment to an average bull born in 1980 (Lowman, 2004). Why 10 kg and not 20 kg heavier? The offspring of an animal is the sum of the genetics of its dam and its sire. So, in calculating the benefit of a +40 kg 400-day weight EBV in a bull, its offspring have the genetic potential to be +20 kg at 400-days of age. If the EBVs of both the sire and dam are known, then the genetic benefit can be calculated as the sum of half of each. For the purposes of the calculations commercial, cross-bred cows are assumed to have an EBV of 0.

EBVs offer considerable financial benefit to a herd. If a bull can increase 400-day weight at weaning by 20 kg for 40 calves per year that is potentially 800 kg of extra saleable meat per year.

Once the objectives of a herd are established then specific traits can be selected for.

There are many EBVs for individual traits being recorded between Signet and Breedplan, the most commonly referred to EBVs are included in the following table (Table 9.2).

The traits that can be used to help select animals to breed for beef carcase production, often called terminal traits, carcase traits or growth traits are:

- birth weight
- carcase weight

- 200-day growth rate
- 400-day growth rate
- muscle depth/eye muscle area
- fat depth
- carcase weight
- carcase conformation
- fat class
- average daily carcase gain
- days to slaughter.

The traits that are relevant when breeding cattle as breeding heifer replacements are:

- direct calving ease
- maternal calving ease (Signet)/calving ease of daughters (Breedplan) (%)
- birth weight
- gestation length
- 200-day milk
- mature cow weight
- scrotal size
- cow/heifer fertility calving interval (Signet)/ days to calving (Breedplan)
- age at first calving
- longevity (Signet) measured by parity (number of calves born in a lifetime)
- cow/heifer fertility calving interval (Signet)/ days to calving (Breedplan) (days).

TABLE 9.2 Individual EBV traits and their definitions

EBV trait	Definition
Birth weight (kg)	The expected birth weight. Heavier birth weights are linked to difficult calvings. Lower weights are a *positive* value. This figure is also used to calculate growth rates (200-day, 400-day) and some carcase traits.
Direct calving ease (%)	A measure of the difficulty of calving. Positive values are calves born more easily.
Gestation length (days)	A longer gestation is seen as a negative because longer gestation periods give rise to heavier calves and it is also harder to achieve a 365-day calving interval. There can be up to 14 days difference in gestation period between bulls, which is two weeks of the year that the cow is pregnant longer than she needs to be.
200-day weight (kg)	This is the equivalent of the predicted weaning weight and reflects the expected growth rate of offspring in their first 200 days. Positive values are a heavier calf.

400-day weight (kg)	This is the equivalent of the predicted slaughter weight and reflects the expected growth rate of offspring in their first 400 days. The difference between the 200-day weight and 400-day weight is the growth within the finishing period. Positive values are heavier animals. A high 400-day weight is also an indication of mature size and of note when breeding heifer replacements.
Muscle depth (mm) or eye muscle area (mm)	Deeper muscle depth is a positive trait, linked with better overall muscling of the carcase and an increase in the yield of lean meat from the carcase.
Fat depth (mm)	This is the predicted fat coverage at 400 days of age and is reflected in carcase classification. A fatter carcase is considered a positive trait, so it is depicted on the right-hand side of the breed average.
Carcase weight (kg)	The predicted carcase weight at a given slaughter age.
Carcase conformation	The predicted carcase conformation at a given slaughter age, using records of carcase conformation based on the EUROP classification system (Chapter 1).
Fat class	The predicted carcase fat class at a given slaughter age, using values based on the EUROP grid, where 1 is leanest and 5H is fattest
Average daily carcase gain (kg/day)	The predicted lifetime daily carcase gain.
Days to slaughter (days)	The predicted days to slaughter at a given weight and fat class.
200-day milk (kg)	A calf's weight at weaning is partly determined by the milk production of its dam. This EBV is the weight of the weaned calf in kg at 200 days of age. A positive value identifies an animal whose offspring will have a better than average milk yield and therefore have offspring with higher weaning weights. The value is calculated by comparing the weight gain difference between the 'grand children' calves of a given animal.
Maternal calving ease (Signet)/calving ease of daughters (Breedplan) (%)	This is a predictor of the ease of calving of the offspring of the animal. For example, the female progeny from a bull with a positive EBV will have fewer calving difficulties than those sired by a bull with a negative EBV. This identifies females that will calve easily due to their own characteristics such as pelvic size (this is different to direct calving ease which is a predictor of how easy the offspring themselves will be born).
Age at first calving (%) (Signet)	A negative value indicates female offspring of this animal are able to get pregnant at a younger age than the breed average.
Scrotal size (cm)	The circumference of a bull's scrotum is an indication of not only their own fertility, as there is more tissue for sperm production, but also the age at which their heifer calves will reach puberty. A positive value indicates a larger than average scrotal circumference and a younger age of puberty for their female offspring.
Cow/heifer fertility calving interval (Signet)/days to calving (Breedplan) (days)	This EBV predicts the ability of the offspring from this animal to get back in calf again. A negative value represents a shorter interval between calving and becoming pregnant.
Mature cow weight (kg) (Breedplan)	A positive value indicates this animal's female offspring will be heavier at 5 years of age than the breed average.
Longevity (Signet) measured by parity (number of calves born in a lifetime)	This EBV predicts the productive lifespan of the offspring from this animal. Positive values indicate a longer life.

To simplify selection, certain traits can be grouped together to make *breeding indices*. These indices are weighted by their relative economic importance into a single value to enable selection for a defined breeding objective (Moore, 2011). Breedplan has combined traits to make a *terminal index* and a *self-replacing index*. Signet combines traits to make breeding indices for *beef value*, *calving value*, *maternal production value* and *maternal value*.

- **Maternal value** (£) (Signet). This is the economic value of an animal's genetic potential to produce breeding females. It is made up of maternal calving ease, 200-day milk, age at first calving, longevity, and calving interval. A positive value indicates the animal's likelihood of breeding more productive, fertile longer-living cows (Moore, 2011).
- **Maternal production value** (Signet)/**self-replacing index** (Breedplan) (£). The economic value of an animal's genetic potential to produce both breeding females and high-quality carcases from their male offspring. Positive values indicate the animal's likelihood of breeding productive breeding heifers/cows and finished cattle with quality carcases (Moore, 2011).

Accuracy of EBVs

For some animals it is not possible to assign a reliable EBV as they have few recorded relatives and sufficient data is not available.

The BLUP *best-guesses* a value, which is often close to the breed average but at the same time has a low accuracy value. This is often the case with imported bulls for which there are no UK records available, that is until offspring statistics start to be collected.

An accuracy of less than 30% means the EBV is not reliable; accuracies above 60% are acceptable. Accuracy increases over time as more data is fed into the system. So very young bulls may have a low accuracy to start with, but as more offspring are recorded the accuracy will increase, and the EBV value will likely change. AI bulls and off-spring from AI bulls have a high accuracy as more offspring are born in the same period than can be achieved by a bull through natural service. Accuracies over 90% are only achieved in bulls 6 years and older, and those used in pedigree herds via AI (Lowman, 2004).

For maternal traits – such as longevity, age at first calving, maternal calving ease – it can take a long time for accuracies to increase as the progeny of the animal have to have offspring of their own, that is, two generations, before there is sufficient data for collection.

Terminal trait EBVs (200-day and 400-day weight, carcase value, and so on) often have higher accuracies sooner, as they require only one generation before data is available to process (Moore, 2011).

Using EBVs

The EBV figures calculated by Signet and Breedplan are displayed in charts to give an overall view of a bull's relative performance for each of the traits recorded.

The charts look slightly different depending on the EBV provider, but the principles are the same. The central line is the breed average. Bars to the right indicate the trait is above the breed average, the further to the right, the better. Any values to the left of the middle line are below the breed average. There may be scenarios where traits with negative EBVs are selected for. For example, if the objective is to decrease the fat on a carcase, a negative EBV for fat depth may be desirable (a negative EBV in the case of fat depth equates to being leaner than the breed average).

Figure 9.9 illustrates the EBVs for a Limousin bull born in 2011 which has been used widely for AI. He has a high accuracy for nearly all traits. The EBVs of this bull are above average for carcase traits such as age to slaughter, carcase weight, 200-day and 400-day weight. However, birth weight, direct

	EBV	Accuracy	GEBV	
Birth weight	4.60	97%	n/a	
Calving ease	−5.40	97%	n/a	
Maternal calving ease	−0.80	53%	n/a	
Gestation length	−1.00	99%	n/a	
Calving value	−2.00	99%	n/a	
200 day growth	35.00	97%	n/a	
400 day growth	75.00	96%	n/a	
Muscle depth	4.40	91%	n/a	
Fat depth	−0.30	88%	n/a	Lean
Beef value	43.00	97%	n/a	
Scrotal circumference	0.50	90%	n/a	
200 day milk	0.00	89%	n/a	
Docility	4.10	81%	n/a	
Age to slaughter	n/a	90%	−30.00	✓
Carcase weight	n/a	93%	30.25	✓
Fillet	n/a	92%	0.23	✓
Striploin	n/a	92%	0.15	✓
Rump	n/a	92%	0.27	✓
Topside	n/a	94%	0.92	✓
Silverside	n/a	91%	1.11	✓
Knuckle	n/a	92%	0.50	✓
Retail value	n/a	92%	26.71	✓

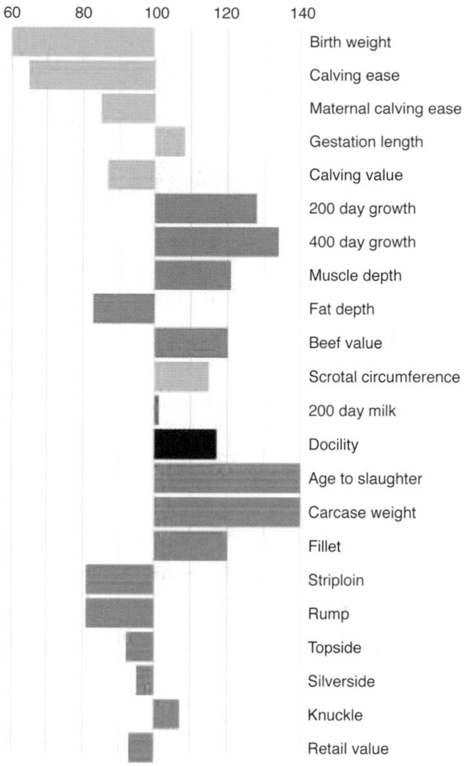

FIGURE 9.9 EBV values for an example Limousin bull

calving ease and maternal calving are all negative traits. This bull's female offspring and any females it is bred to, are more likely than the average Limousin cow to have assisted calvings.

EBVs are available online, free of charge, for pedigree bulls of all breeds. They are a useful tool when making a new bull purchase and should be combined with a visual and physical assessment to get the best result.

REFERENCES

Chenoweth, P.J. (2007) Bull libido/serving capacity. *Veterinary Clinics of North America: Food Animal Practice* 13(2), 331–344.

Dyce, K.M., Sack, W.O. and Wensing, C.J.G. (2002) The pelvis and reproductive organs of male ruminants. In: *Textbook of Veterinary Anatomy*, 3rd edn. Sauders, Philadelphia, PA, ch. 30.

Entwistle, K. and Fordyce, G. (2003) Semen-assessment and standards. In: *Evaluating and Reporting Bull Fertility*. Australian Association of Cattle Veterinarians, Indooroopilly, pp. 50–53.

Eppink, E. (2005) A survey of bull breeding soundness evaluations in the south east of Scotland. *Cattle Practice* 13, 205–210.

Hull, J.J. (2018) Understanding estimated breeding values (EBVs) – a simple practitioner's guide. *Cattle Practice* 26(1), 29.

Lowman, B. (2004) Estimated breeding values for beef cattle. *In Practice* 26, 206–211.

McGowan, M. (2001) Bull selection and management – the veterinarian's role. *Cattle Practice* 9(3), 173–178.

McGowan, M., Galloway, D., Taylor, E., Entwistle, K. and Johnston, P. (1995) *The Veterinary Examination of Bulls*. Australian Association of Cattle Veterinarians, Brisbane.

Moore, K. (2011) Utilising maternal trait EBVs of beef bulls. Technical Note TN641. SAC, Edinburgh.

Statham, J. (2010) Differential diagnosis of scrotal enlargement in bulls. *In Practice* 32, 200–206.

Chapter 10

The health and management of the suckler cow

FEEDING THE SUCKLER COW

Around 75% of the total variable costs of a suckler herd are feed costs, and 80% of these are attributed to the adult females. The cost of feeding calves is of relatively little significance (Lowman and Lewis, 1992).

Of the feed eaten by a suckler cow in any 12 month period, 73% is for her own maintenance, 20% for milk production and 7% for the demands of pregnancy (Lowman and Lewis, 1992).

By far the cheapest feedstuff for the cow is grazed grass – estimated to cost £0.06/kg DM. By comparison, concentrate feed costs are over £0.25/kg DM (2019 prices). To make the most of the cheapest feed, cows should gain condition in the summer and store fat. They can then use the 'fat store' to support them over the winter, so decreasing the reliance on expensive purchased feeds and conserved forage.

SUCKLER COW NUTRITION

Ration formulations usually start by calculating the animals *DM requirement* as a percentage of their liveweight. Knowing a reasonable estimate of the weight of the cows is an essential requirement. Weighing all the cows in a group and taking an average is desirable but in a non-automated system may be time consuming. Weighing a minimum of ten cows and calculating an average would suffice

and is better than a rough visual estimation of liveweight.

A cow's weight may fluctuate by up to 120 kg throughout the year. A fluid-filled uterus and near-term calf will significantly distort the average aside from the effects of varying BCS. Weighing at housing to aid winter ration formulation would be good timing. The weigh scales should be calibrated before use, using, say, known tractor counterbalance weights or several 25 kg feed bags.

MID-PREGNANCY, DRY PERIOD AND PRE-CALVING NUTRITION

Dry cows require between 1.5–2% of their live bodyweight in DM/day of feed to satisfy their appetite. For example: For a 650 kg cow that equates to 13 kg DM/day. If a 25% DM silage is fed that equates to 52 kg fresh weight of silage per day.

For spring-calving herds, low quality winter forage fed ad libitum, or marginal grazing, will support the non-lactating cow's energy requirement through mid-pregnancy. If they are fed ad lib good quality silage, however, they risk becoming too fat; straw can be mixed in with the silage to provide rumen fill without providing too much energy.

Approaching calving, the proportion of silage to straw can be increased to improve colostrum quality and minimise body condition loss. Research suggests the provision of DUP, for example, soya-bean meal, may be required in late pregnancy and early lactation when a cow is lactating heavily and mobilising a large amount of body fat – this supplementation re-dresses the balance between energy and protein; the balance is important. Achieving this balance will minimise the mobilisation of muscle which is the cow's own source of protein. DUP also happens to have a positive effect on colostrum quality (Sinclair and Suttle, 2000). It is a common misconception that restricting the cow's energy intake in the last 4–6 weeks of gestation makes for an easier calving by reducing the birth weight of the calf. It does not reduce dystocia, some evidence suggests it can even make it worse through weakening the cow, and it does result in weak newborn calves, poor colostrum quality, and a delay in the return to cyclicity.

Straw diets are commonly used for dry cows, but without supplementation they are low in energy, protein and trace elements. Straw, on average, has an energy content of 6–7 MJ/kg DM and protein content of 3.5%. A straw-only diet can result in an under-supply of protein: rumen microbes require at least 9% CP in DM (Sinclair and Suttle, 2000). *Rumen impactions* are common in cows fed a high percentage of straw or low protein silage (less than 8% CP) – this is not simply due to it being dry and fibrous but also because lack of ERDP starves the rumen microbes who are then unable to do their job of digesting the otherwise indigestible fibre. In a case of impaction, the rumen becomes distended and full of dry undigested forage; after a few days this results in the death of the animal. ERDP can be added to a diet in a number of different ways, for example, urea-treated grain, ammonia-treated straw, wheat distiller's grains, beans, soya-bean meal. It is essential to seek advice from a competent impartial nutritionist to ensure the ration matches the needs of the cow and without any adverse effects; urea can cause toxicity if fed at incorrect levels. In summary, managed correctly, straw diets are utilised effectively by dry cows and adding silage to the straw is beneficial as calving approaches.

Brassica crops such as kale can be an effective outwintering feeding system for dry cows on some farms, but trace element supplementation needs to be carefully considered. Native-bred cows are better suited to outwintering than Continental breeds although for either, energy requirements can rise by 15% in cold weather conditions.

Autumn calvers are dry during the height of summer when there is an abundance of grass. The challenge is therefore to prevent them getting too fat. Delaying weaning is one mechanism and can also be useful to prevent the cows being affected by summer mastitis at drying off. A dry period of 5 weeks, however, is required, as a minimum, to ensure there is adequate production of good quality colostrum in time for calving. Grazing cows on marginal pastures or stubble or at higher stocking densities are also useful techniques to prevent cows becoming over conditioned. Mineral supplementation still needs to be adequate and catered for even in the face of limited DM intakes.

POST-CALVING AND EARLY LACTATION NUTRITION

There is a huge demand for energy and protein by the cow post-calving – twice that of the dry period. She is recovering from calving, lactating, gaining condition and will soon be conceiving her next pregnancy.

For the spring-calving cow, the cheapest way to satisfy this demand is from grazed grass, see Figure 10.1. This will meet the energy and protein requirements of the lactating cow (Sinclair and Suttle, 2000) providing that good attention is paid to grassland management and grazing systems.

For autumn-calving cows, their highest energy demand is at the end of the grazing season when grass quality is waning, and housing is imminent. It is essential that their nutritional requirements are met, and this will require some supplementation with concentrate feed. Cow condition should remain constant with *minimal dietary changes* for the bulling period and for up to 6 weeks after conception.

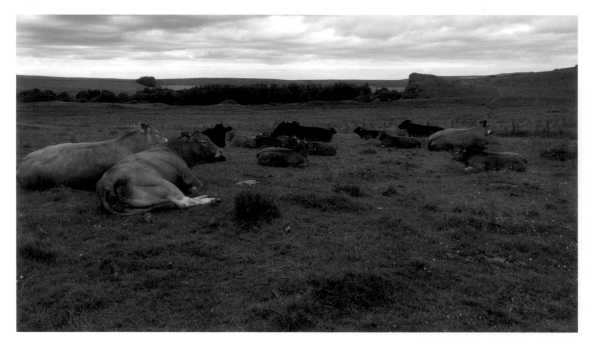

FIGURE 10.1 Cows and calves at pasture

For housed cattle, it is essential to have forage analysed so that quantity provision, and any supplementation required, for the winter months ahead, can be calculated. Silage analysis can be carried out 6 weeks post-ensiling. If winter requirements are known early in the season, then any additional energy or protein sources can be purchased comparatively cheaply rather than waiting until mid-winter when market demand is likely to have increased the cost.

FEEDING PRACTICES

Nutritionists provide expertise in ration formulation. This involves taking into account the cow liveweight, cow condition, calving and weaning dates, available feedstuffs and, of course, the costs. The ration calculated on paper is not, however, always the same as what the cow is, in reality, fed. A light-hearted theory exists that there are three rations on any farm: what the nutritionist thinks is being fed, what the farmer thinks is being fed and what the cows actually eats!

The feed presented to the cows needs to be fresh and appetising. Mouldy, heated, blackened silage will not be appealing to the cows and intakes will be markedly reduced. Furthermore, poorly conserved silage can be high in microorganisms such as *Listeria*, *Bacillus*, moulds and fungi, all of which can cause abortion, among other diseases, in the cows eating it.

Feed troughs should be regularly cleared of leftover feed and not just topped up with fresh.

Feed space also needs to be considered. If there are dominant cows within a group and there is limited feed available and/or insufficient feed space, then the more timid cows, often heifers, will get bullied out from the feed. Farm assurance scheme recommendations in the UK suggest a feed space width allowance for a 700 kg suckler cow of 70 cm on restricted feeding and 30 cm per cow when fed ad lib. Ring feeders pushed up against walls decrease feeding space. In some cattle buildings, the placement of neck rails can make it awkward for cows to reach their feed. Examining the cows for hair rubbed from the back of their necks is an indication that this is the case, and feed needs to be pushed up to the feed rail more often. Diagonal feed barriers give each cow their own space and help shy feeders gain access, whereas a single horizontal rail can be 'patrolled' by dominant cows essentially 'running the line'.

The frequency that the cows are fed will affect their intakes. If fed once a day, their intakes will not be as high as when feed is presented twice a day, even if this is just pushing the forage back up to the feed rail.

The composition of the ration is important. A TMR is defined as a homogenous mixture of all constituents of the cows' diet fed all at the same time. For example, straw, silage, minerals and barley can all be mixed in a diet feeder or mixer wagon before being distributed to the cows. Feeding a TMR ensures the same diet is fed to the cows continuously so ensuring the environment in the rumen for the microbes is consistent. With TMR, DM intake can increase by up to 10%.

If a TMR is fed then the chop length of the forages needs to be between 2.5 and 10 cm (Grove-White, 2004); a crude measurement is that the chop length needs to be equal to the width of a cow's muzzle, in other words smaller for smaller cattle.

There is a risk that dominant cows sort through the ration as soon as it is fed and pick out the 'best bits' leaving the rest for the other cows in the group. This is exacerbated if there is a chop length greater than 10 cm. If the chop length is too short, however, it will not stimulate rumination so well and the cows' rumens may consequently become more acidic through lack of buffering saliva; a balance is needed.

Concurrent disease, such as liver fluke and gut worm, and trace element deficiencies will also affect intakes.

GRASS AND SILAGE

Grazed grass is the cheapest feed on the farm and managing it well can *reduce input costs*. Grazing management should not be considered the domain of only high input lowland farms; it needs to be

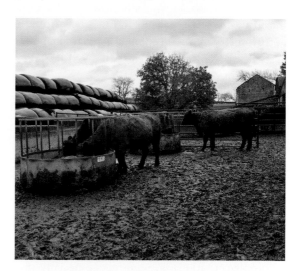

FIGURE 10.2 Cows during winter with access to baled grass silage in ring feeders

considered on all farms, especially hill farms in environmental schemes. Greater utilisation of grassland and understanding supply and demand will help drive efficiency.

Grass silage is the most commonly conserved forage fed to cattle in the UK, see Figure 10.2. Basic guidance on silage making is covered in Chapter 25. Maize silage and whole crop silage are also popular. They are attractive because they are cut and harvested at the same time and they work out cheaper per unit of ME than grass silage (Wilkinson and Chamberlain, 2017). The downside is they are comparatively unstable once the pit is opened, and high-quality arable ground is required to grow maize and whole crop, which does not always fit with beef farms tending to be on more marginal land.

There are many other forages which can be successfully fed to cattle: brassicas, chicory, forage maize, forage roots and legumes.

Forage crops can be a cheaper option to sourcing straw or buying proprietary feeds. They offer the opportunity for forage rotation and to improve soil quality, that is, its nutrient content and structure. The choice of forage crop will depend on the requirements of the livestock to be fed but also the type of land available, including its soil type. Obtaining advice from a nutritionist and an agronomist is recommended, at least for the first few years, to avoid mistakes and known pitfalls.

Some alternative forage crops have health considerations too and a conversation with the farm vet is worthwhile. Some options of note follow.

- Cattle grazing leafy brassica type crops are prone to selenium and iodine deficiency and need careful monitoring.
- Forage rape is high in calcium and low in magnesium and phosphorus, so additional mineral supplementation is required, especially for in-calf cows and cows close to calving.
- Brassicas contain high levels of readily digestible carbohydrate and are low in fibre. A fibrous forage should therefore be fed in addition, such as silage, straw or hay, for optimal rumen pH and function.
- Fodder beet (Figure 10.3), turnips and swedes are hard for cattle to eat if they do not have a full set of teeth. These crops are often fed in situ or brought in to the shed and are heavily contaminated with soil. This can increase the risk of listeriosis. High consumption of soil, which contains iron, may also result in a reduction in copper levels due to the known antagonism that occurs between copper and iron.

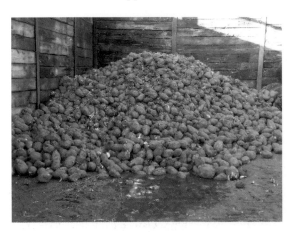

FIGURE 10.3 Fodder beet heavily contaminated with soil

- Clover, which contains a high level of protein, can predispose cattle to bloat due to the rapid breakdown of the clover protein and the associated creation of froth. Cattle should be introduced to high clover pastures gradually; they should not be hungry when introduced to these pastures so as to reduce the likelihood of gorging. Feeding some high fibre feed such as straw, hay or silage before introduction to these pastures, and while grazing, can help.
- Remember, in general, any changes in diet should be carried out gradually to avoid dietary upset.

Outwintering cattle on forage crops, see Figure 10.4, has become popular in recent years and poses several advantages.

- There is less demand on labour and machinery during the housing period.
- It is more cost-effective, especially if the alternative housing system requires bedding which happens to be expensive.
- Muck and slurry disposal are no longer a requirement.
- It requires less infrastructure, that is, shed space.
- If managed effectively stock can be healthier; a reduced incidence of lameness is a common finding.
- As part of a crop rotation/break system there are benefits to soil fertility.

Typically, cattle are allowed to strip-graze the crop behind an electric fence. Bales of straw or silage are placed at regular intervals to add fibre to the diet. The daily allowance of crop per day is dictated by the cow's requirement and the crop's DM yield. The stock must have some shelter, a wall/hedge or wall, a dry lying area and clean fresh water available at all times. Heavy poaching is not acceptable. The system needs to be suitable for the environmental conditions, soil type and breed of cow. A contingency plan should be in place for excessively wet or snowy winters to ensure the

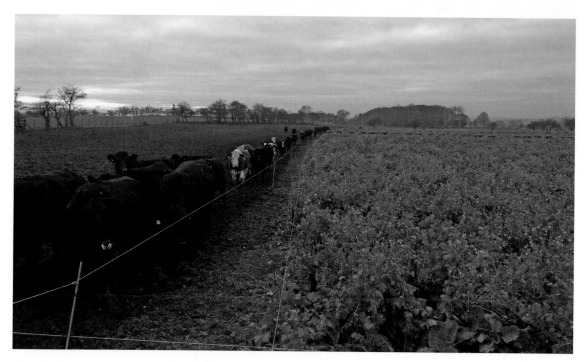

FIGURE 10.4 Cows out wintered and strip grazed on kale

cattle can be cared for appropriately and welfare is not compromised.

MINERALS

All cattle require micro-minerals and macro-minerals. Micro-minerals – often referred to as trace elements are required in small amounts and include copper, zinc, selenium, cobalt, iodine, manganese and iron.

Macro-minerals are those required in large amounts, such as calcium, phosphorous, magnesium, chloride and potassium.

Micro-minerals (trace elements)

Copper

Copper is involved in many enzyme pathways in the body. Signs of deficiency will vary depending on the animal's age and stage of production. Copper deficiency can cause poor growth,

anaemia, an enlarged heart, defects in the bone, impaired nervous system development, connective tissue disorders and a compromised immune system (Cutler and Jones, 2003).

The absorption of copper from the gut into the blood is antagonised by sulphur, iron and molybdenum. So simply knowing the copper content of the diet does not predict the cow's copper status.

Copper is stored in the liver. Blood is just a distribution system for the copper, so its levels vary, sometimes unrelated to the liver and body tissue reserves. The most accurate measure of a cow's copper level is measuring the amount stored within the liver. Although there have been techniques described on how vets can perform liver biopsies on dairy cows, it is not widely practised, and is certainly rarely carried out on suckler cows. Post-mortem liver sampling is, however, frequently carried out although the choice of animal affects interpretation.

Analysing copper blood levels is a 'second-best' option; it gives an indication on the day of sampling of how much copper is within the blood. Copper levels will fluctuate over time and a single sample will not give an indication of whether copper levels are on the rise or decline. Blood testing one individual animal is not useful in assessing the need for supplementation as copper absorption can be affected by diseases, such as gut parasites, fluke burden or JD. Ten animals from a group that have had the same nutritional management should be sampled, the results averaged to allow for outliers, and repeat testing should be done at intervals of, say, 6 months, to detect trends. This way, informed decisions can be made on copper supplementation. Effective copper supplementation can be provided through free access minerals and boluses.

Copper is passed across the placenta to the unborn calf, so it is born with sufficient copper. Copper is also present in milk, and copper absorption in the pre-ruminant is highly effective. If the cow is copper-deficient the calf will be born low in copper and will not receive copper through the milk supply either.

Iodine

Iodine is required for the production of thyroxine, a hormone manufactured in the thyroid gland that heavily influences the body's rate of metabolism. Selenium also has a role in iodine metabolism.

Leguminous plants and brassicas interfere with iodine uptake from the gut and therefore limit the production of thyroxine. Calves that are born to cows low in iodine are often premature, weak, small, and have a swelling around their throat – an enlarged thyroid gland, commonly referred to as *goitre*. The thyroid gland is enlarging in an attempt to grab more iodine and produce more thyroxine. Iodine deficiency is related to poor cow fertility and poor semen quality.

Blood testing for iodine is challenging as it gives no indication of historic intakes, only the intakes of the animal in the previous 24 hours. In the case of stillborn calves or those that died in the neonatal period, post-mortem sampling of the thyroid gland is very useful for accurate assessment of

iodine levels; further histological examination can confirm iodine deficiency.

Iodine is easily supplemented with boluses, free access mineral, plus any feed product containing seaweed, which is usually high in iodine. The old system of pouring iodine preparations onto the coat to be licked off is still practised but is poorly regulated and potentially dangerous so cannot be recommended.

Cobalt

Cobalt is converted into Vitamin B12 in the rumen by the rumen microbes. Cobalt deficiency is rarely seen in cattle as it usually exists in high levels in soil itself, plenty of which gets inadvertently eaten with grass and forage.

The risk of cobalt deficiency exists, however, and is highest in alkaline soil areas, which are high in manganese (Suttle and Sinclair, 2000). Signs of cobalt deficiency are non-specific and include inappetence, decreased growth rates in the young or weight loss at any age.

In sheep, blood B12 levels are used to make decisions about the requirement for cobalt, but it is not a reliable test in cattle (Suttle and Sinclair, 2000).

Cobalt is easily supplemented in free access mineral mixes and boluses. Cobalt toxicity is possible, but there is a large safety margin and it is rarely encountered (Cutler and Jones, 2003).

Manganese

The role of manganese is in the development of normal bone and normal reproductive function in males and females. There is little storage of manganese in the body, and absorption from the gut is variable and inhibited by calcium and more so phosphorus (Cutler and Jones, 2003). Calves born to manganese-deficient dams are often called *dwarf calves*, a condition also known as *chondrodystrophy* (see Chapter 11). Manganese can be supplemented through free access minerals or boluses.

Selenium

Selenium and Vitamin E are closely linked and are responsible for growth and fertility. Selenium is the key element in an enzyme called glutathione peroxidase (GSHPx). Both GSHPx and Vitamin E are *antioxidants* that protect cells within the body from harmful chemicals called *free radicals*.

Deficiencies of either or both are seen as white muscle disease (WMD) (see Chapter 12), poor fertility due to reabsorptions, and premature or weakly born calves. Deficiencies can be detected by blood testing live animals or testing the liver levels post-mortem. Testing for the selenium-containing GSHPx is, however, easier and cheaper than testing for Vitamin E.

When blood testing, a minimum of ten animals should be sampled and an average calculated, rather than looking at individual results.

Selenium can be supplemented through powdered mineral mixes or boluses. Long acting injections of *barium selenite* are effective in mature animals. An injectable preparation of *alpha-tocopheryl acetate* (synthetic Vitamin E) combined with *potassium selenate* is used for short-term supplementation in young animals which are at risk of, or showing, signs of WMD.

Deficiencies in the young calf can be avoided by ensuring the dam is adequately provided for. The calf is, consequently, born with sufficient selenium and continues to receive an adequate supply through the cow's milk.

High levels of selenium provided in the diet or through supplementation are toxic; acute or chronic toxicity can occur but are rarely seen in practice. *Acute toxicity* presents as blindness, staggering, collapse and sudden death. Signs of *chronic toxicity* are dullness, inappetence, weight loss, hair loss, stiffness and lameness (Cutler and Jones, 2003).

Zinc

Zinc is involved in regulating appetite and a deficiency may present as weight loss and poor growth rates. Sometimes thickening of the skin on the head and neck is seen, and sperm quality is poor. Zinc is poorly regulated and poorly stored in the body, so a regular source in the diet is required. Despite this, deficiencies are rarely seen, or should that be, rarely diagnosed?

Vitamins

Vitamins are not trace elements, but they are micro-nutrients although some vitamins are manufactured within the body so those, are not, strictly speaking, nutrients. Cattle need most vitamins to be supplied in the diet, the exceptions being C, K and the B complex.

Vitamins A, D and E are dietary requirements. They are all fat-soluble and are readily stored in the fat tissue of animals. When cows are thin and have little body fat, they have limited reserves of these vitamins and an additional supply will be required.

Vitamin E is present in green feedstuffs and forages, so grazed grass is a major source. Generally, the Vitamin E provision to cattle is far too low and it is of the opinion of some nutritionists that the inclusion rate in mineral/vitamin mixtures should be as high as 2000 IU/kg (Sinclair and Suttle, 2000).

Vitamin D deficiency occurs through lack of exposure to sunlight: so, cattle on a northern UK farm on the north face of a valley are at higher risk. Vitamin A deficiency (see Chapter 12) can be a problem when growing cattle are fed straw based diets. Vitamin A levels in mineral and vitamin mixes is usually high but deteriorates while the product is in storage; observing 'best before' dates is important.

Supplementation of adult cows with vitamins and minerals

Most proprietary mineral and vitamin mixes contain a mixture of all vitamin and minerals and are not bespoke to the cow's needs. They can be mixed within a TMR or sprinkled on top of the forage.

It is difficult to know the *bioavailability* of the minerals within a powdered mineral. European regulations stipulate that the weight of trace mineral compound in a product needs to be stated on the label, for example, 100 mg of zinc oxide. This, however, actually equates to 72 mg/kg of zinc. Thus, calculating what the mineral compound provides to the cow requires extensive knowledge of chemistry and the periodic table!

Licks and blocks are another method of supplementation but there will be individual variation in their access and uptake. The administration of rumen boluses is an effective method of supplementation but again boluses can contain multiple vitamins and minerals and are often fairly non-specific. To be fair there are boluses containing just one mineral, for example, copper or magnesium.

Some injectable preparations exist such as iodinated peanut oil containing organically bound iodine, and barium selenite, the latter for selenium supplementation.

It is easy to blame trace elements for all sorts of problems especially infertility and poor growth rates. Trace element deficiencies are, however, rarely the sole cause of these performance issues; all other avenues should be explored before a trace element imbalance wholly takes the blame.

Macro-minerals

Calcium

Cows have a vast skeletal store of calcium which can be drawn upon when blood levels of calcium are low. This is regulated by a complex hormonal system that can go wrong. The hormonal cascade requires magnesium and is influenced by the pH of the blood. Therefore, despite cows having a huge amount of calcium in their skeleton, if there is a high demand by the contracting muscles during parturition followed by a huge demand by the udder for milk production, the abundant calcium may not be in the right place at the right time and *hypocalcaemia* (low blood calcium) occurs. This results in a 'wobbly' cow which later becomes recumbent and may die, a condition known as 'milk fever'.

The recommended feeding rate for calcium in late pregnancy is intentionally low at 3.2 g/kg DM increasing to an intentionally high level in lactation at 4.5 g/kg DM (Suttle and Sinclair, 2000). Grazed grass is typically 5.4 g/kg DM (± 1.7) so may cause problems in dry cows. Cereal diets are low in calcium but root crops such as fodder beet are high – this needs to be taken into consideration when they are being fed, and at which stage.

Phosphorus

Phosphorus is needed by the cow, and also the rumen microbes. Like calcium, the cow has a skeletal reserve of phosphorus and does not rely on a daily intake.

Phosphorus is a vital component of bones, and deficiencies in growing animals can cause bone malformation which is exacerbated by a deficiency in Vitamin D. Phosphorus is required for general cellular functions and deficiency in adult animals results in poor condition, lack of appetite and poor fertility. Cows often seek out phosphorus when they are deficient, eating spoil or licking rocks (Eddy, 2004).

Calcium and phosphorus are closely interrelated in the body, especially in the bloodstream where they exist as ionised calcium and ionised phosphate – they seem to have something of a see-saw effect on each other. In the diet, however, it is the ratio between calcium and phosphate that is important, and this varies between feed types. For example, sugar beet and kale are particularly high in calcium and low in phosphate. It is generally assumed that a lactating cow on a grazed diet requires additional phosphate supplementation either through free access mineral, licks or concentrate feed. A cow in late pregnancy requires 2.3 g/kg DM per day of phosphorus increasing to 2.7 in lactation (Suttle and Sinclair, 2000).

Magnesium

There is no store of magnesium within the cow's body, so she is reliant on a daily intake of this mineral.

Magnesium is involved in the calcium hormonal mechanisms, so a deficiency in magnesium can also be associated with milk fever.

Magnesium deficiency in cows can present initially as dullness and depression, then subtle excitability and later progress into so called *staggers* namely stiffness, excitability, tremors, chewing, salivation, ear flapping, collapse, contracted muscles, coma and death (Foster et al., 2007). Staggers is considered a genuine veterinary emergency; treatment is discussed in Chapter 17.

Low magnesium levels have also been the cause of slow-calving cows, often linked with hypocalcaemia, which results in dopey calves that are slow to rise and suck.

Sodium is required for the uptake of magnesium in the gut so rock salt can aid magnesium absorption.

In contrast, high levels of potassium are inhibitive of magnesium absorption. Fields that are subjected to large amounts of slurry or pot ash fertiliser often have high potassium levels. Soil analysis of pastures can detect if high potassium is an issue. The risk of hypomagnesaemia is increased when grass growth is rapid and lush; such grass is low in magnesium compounded by the fact it passes through the gut rapidly leaving insufficient time for any magnesium in it to be absorbed from the gut. Often, adding some long fibre to the diet can help slow the progression of food material through the gut and increase the absorption of what magnesium is present.

Older cows are more at risk from staggers as they generally produce more milk – their demand for magnesium is higher. The small amount of magnesium that these older ruminants have in their skeleton cannot be mobilised as easily as it can be in the younger animal.

Magnesium requirements in late pregnancy are quoted as being 1.5–2 g/kg DM (Suttle and

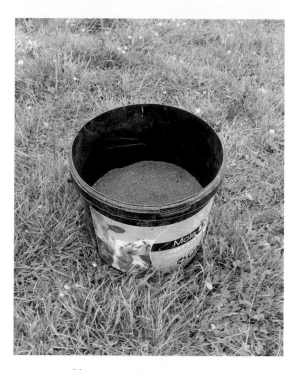

FIGURE 10.5 Magnesium lick at pasture for adult cows

Sinclair, 2000) and are usually fed to suckler cows through dry cow mineral mixed with the silage or sprinkled on top.

Pre- and post-calving licks are commonly used as a method of supplementation, and molasses that contains magnesium can be provided as a lick for cows, see Figure 10.5. Not all cows will access the licks so uptake will be variable.

Magnesium boluses will more reliably supply every animal with the magnesium it needs and should be administered 2–3 days before the period of risk. They typically last 4–6 weeks, depending on the product used; administration may need to be repeated. Magnesium chloride can be added to drinking water but must be evenly distributed in the water trough and the trough should not be allowed to run dry. Adding too much magnesium can make the water unpalatable, and for those cattle that do drink it diarrhoea is a risk – magnesium salts are generally purgative (laxative).

MONITORING COWS' DIETARY REQUIREMENTS

Body condition score

Body condition scoring is the cheapest and easiest way to monitor cow condition. It is, however, rather subjective, although it does allow for *changes* in cow body condition to be monitored, on both a herd and individual basis.

BCS is based on a 5-point scale; 1 is an emaciated cow and 5 is a very fat cow. Scores are further divided into half or even quarter scores. One BCS is equivalent to 13% of the cow's liveweight.

Research work carried out in the UK by the Meat and Livestock Commission has shown that cow condition influences two things: the cow's ability to get in-calf; and the ease with which a cow calves. Research consistently shows that over-conditioned (fatter) cows are more likely to suffer from dystocia (calving difficulty) due to fat deposition in and around the pelvis, rather than an increased calf birth weight. Dystocia is a common reason for subsequent infertility arising from trauma, and/or infection, see Figure 10.6.

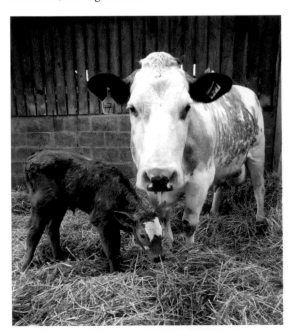

FIGURE 10.6 A cow and calf after a caesarean birth

TABLE 10.1 Effect of BCS at calving on subsequent calving interval in suckler cows (Drennan and Berry, 2006)

BCS at calving	Calving interval
1–1.5	418 days
2	382 days
2.5–3	364 days

BCS also has a direct impact on fertility. If cows are gaining condition during the bulling period, their fertility will improve even if they are in suboptimal condition to start with. Feeding an undernourished cow in the post-calving period will not, however, compensate for the negative effects of her poor condition pre-calving. The oocyst (egg) for conception in the following pregnancy is developing within the cow's ovary during the 6–8 weeks before ovulation. The viability of an oocyst is influenced by the nutrition the cow receives during this period.

Table 10.1 demonstrates a decrease in calving interval (the number of days between consecutive calvings for an individual cow) suggesting that the fertility of cows improves when calving at BCS 2.5–3 rather than 1–1.5.

Target BCSs for each stage of the reproductive cycle were established in the 1980s and are considered to be relevant to this day (Lowman and Lewis, 1992). The target scores for spring and autumn-calving herds differ as depicted in Figure 10.7 and Figure 10.8. This is influenced by the differing nutritional requirements at the different stages of the production cycle and by the need to maximise the cheaper nutritional benefit that can be provided by grazed grass.

Both systems require the cows to gain a whole condition score between turnout and housing. For a 650 kg cow this equates to 85 kg, roughly 0.5 kg per day. To achieve this, the quality of the grazed grass needs to be good. Alternatively, on marginal farms where the grazing quality is not sufficient to obtain the required liveweight gain, other options to improve body condition have to be considered; for example, choosing a breed of cow whose energy demands are less.

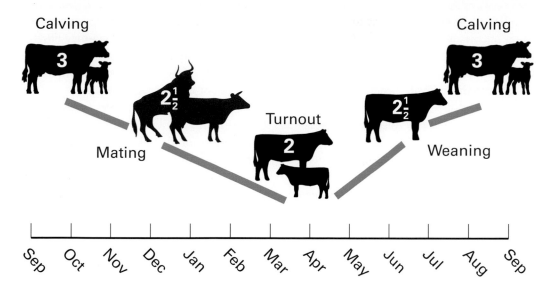

FIGURE 10.7 BCS targets for the autumn-calving herd

The energy demand of a cow depends on her maintenance requirement (calculated as a percentage of her liveweight) plus any demands placed upon her by pregnancy or lactation or, in the young cow, growth. Both liveweight and milk production are variable and dependent on the breed of the cow, with huge variation between smaller native-cross cows that produce less milk versus a large Continental cow, which has often been crossed with the Holstein for even better milk production.

The autumn-calving cow is entering a period of negative energy balance during the winter months at a time she is expected to get back in-calf. This can be reflected in disappointing pregnancy rates and a higher barren rate compared to spring-calving herds. Autumn-calving cows are also at their fattest at calving (BCS 3), which can lead to an increased risk of dystocia. This is especially the case where a spring-calving cow who failed to get in-calf is kept in the herd, 'run on' as some say, and then calves with the autumn herd. As she has failed to calve for 18 months, she is likely to have a BCS of 4 or more, which again often results in a difficult calving.

BCS should be altered gradually and any alteration in the last third of pregnancy is

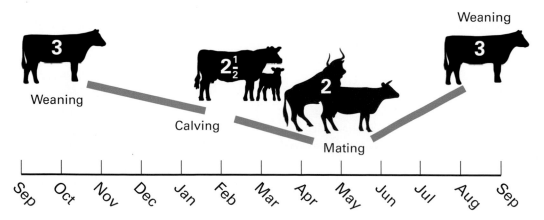

FIGURE 10.8 BCS targets for the spring-calving herd

contraindicated. In fact, attempting to increase the condition of cows at this stage will often result in the birth of heavier calves, rather than improve the condition of the cow, some call this the *parasite effect* – the calf, the 'parasite' benefits at the cost of its mother, 'the host'.

Within any group of cows there will always be a range of condition scores depending on the cows' parities, genetic variation, physiological status and health. The average condition score for the group should be the same as the target condition score, but the *range* of condition scores also needs to be considered. For instance, the average condition score may be the target of three, but there may also be a lot of cows with BCS 2 and a lot with BCS 4. The aim is to have as little variation as possible with a high percentage of individual cows hitting the target. A compact calving period facilitates this as it aids nutritional management of a group of cattle when they are all at a similar stage of production.

Although body condition scoring is used mostly to assess a group of cattle, it is important at an individual cow level also; if a cow has lost body condition unexpectedly, or is failing to gain body condition, it could be an indication of an underlying health problem that requires veterinary investigation.

Condition scoring provides the evidence upon which actions can be taken: a nutritionist can use the information to re-formulate rations. Fat and thin cows, once identified, can be separated off and treated separately and appropriately.

Body condition scoring should take place at specified times of the year to help inform management decisions. A minimum of four times each year is recommended.

1. **At housing**. This is essential as a starting point for the winter. Cows can be grouped depending on their condition and fed and managed accordingly, for example, thin spring-calving cows can have their calves weaned early.
2. **Mid-winter**. For spring-calving cows this is a safety check that they are on track to reach target condition score for calving. If not, the ration can

be altered accordingly. Groups may need to be adjusted as thin and fat cows may have gained or lost weight respectively. For autumn calvers it is useful to see how much condition can still be lost, or not, through the winter.

3. **Turnout**. For spring calvers to maximise cow fertility they will ideally be on a rising plane of nutrition for the breeding season. Thin cows can graze the best pastures. For autumn calvers the thin cows can have their calves weaned at turnout to reduce the demand on them.
4. **Weaning**. This is mainly for autumn-calving cows to check they are on track to reach target condition score at calving. Very fat cows can be housed or grazed tighter to lose some condition pre-calving.

Figures 10.9 and 10.10 shows the changes in condition score from housing to calving in a 90-cow spring-calving suckler herd. The target condition score at housing is 3 and at calving is

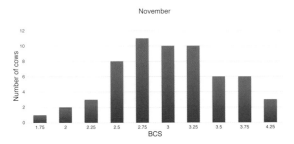

FIGURE 10.9 Condition scores from a 90-cow spring-calving herd at housing

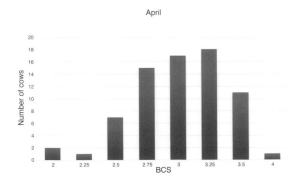

FIGURE 10.10 Condition score from a 90-cow spring-calving herd at calving.

TABLE 10.2 Detailing the bodily characteristics of BCS scores 1–5

Body condition score (BCS)	Bodily characteristics
1	Transverse processes easily palpable and visible. No fat coverage across the backbone, ribs or tail head. Skin/hair rough in appearance. Unlikely to be fertile, compromised milk production and susceptible to disease. Veterinary attention required.
2	Transverse processes visible, but with some fat coverage across the ribs and spaces either side of the tail head moderately sunken.
3	Cow in good condition. Transverse processes just palpable. Backbone no longer visible.
4	Cow over-conditioned, ribs no longer visible, fat around tail head and brisket. Transverse processes no longer palpable.
5	Fat! Fat deposits around tail head. Difficulty calving is highly likely, fertility is compromised.

2.5 (see Figure 10.8). The graphs show there was an increase in cow condition over the winter period – an unnecessary cost to the herd. If the cows had been condition scored mid-winter the increase in condition could have been noted and action taken to avoid it before it was too late.

How to perform the body condition score

The body condition of a cow is assessed by feeling what coverage of fat she has over the transverse processes in the loin area, sometimes called spinous processes (Table 10.1). The transverse processes are the bones that protrude 90° from the spine, just behind where the ribs end, just above the flanks. Animals should be handled on their left side, and the same hand of the operator used each time. Some assessment can also be done by looking at the fat coverage over the ribs, tail head, brisket, and hip bones. The conformation of the cow, stage of pregnancy or not, and gut fill, can affect the visual appearance of a cow irrespective of her body condition.

Metabolic profiles

Metabolic profiles are a set of blood parameters that can be measured and used in addition to

BCS to assess the energy and protein status of an animal and detect problems in the animal or the diet before they cause too much harm.

A metabolic profile typically includes measuring levels of the following.

- **Urea** is synthesised in the liver from ammonia, which is produced predominantly in the rumen during the process of fermentation (Otter, 2013). Low urea levels are an indication that there is insufficient feed intake or that there is insufficient ERDP in the diet (see Chapter 3). This is common in suckler cows fed poor-quality silage or straw rations with no additional protein supplied. ERDP is essential for rumen function, without it the rumen shuts down and, in extreme cases, rumen impactions and death occur. High urea can be a result of very high ERDP in the diet; this can be the case at grazing, especially early in the summer, or it can be an indication of high or adequate ERDP but insufficient FME to utilise the ERDP provided in the diet, that is, an energy:protein mismatch in the rumen.
- **Albumin** is the main blood protein, synthesised in the liver (Otter, 2013). A low albumin level in a group of animals is an indication of chronic protein deficiency. In an individual, low albumin may mean that protein is not

being made, that is, there is liver disease, or it is being lost either through the kidneys (kidney disease) or through the gut (gut disease such as Johne's disease or parasitism).

- **Globulin** is another blood protein. Albumin and globulin added together equal the total protein parameter. Raised globulin levels are an indicator of *inflammation* and *chronic disease* (Whitaker, 2004).
- **Beta-hydroxybutyrate** (BOHB or BHB) is a ketone produced by the liver when a cow is in negative energy balance, that is, when her diet is not providing sufficient energy for her daily function. The higher the level, the worse the energy deficiency is.
- **Magnesium** testing is commonly added to pre- and post-calving metabolic profiles due to the potentially serious implications of low magnesium, that is, hypomagnesaemia, staggers. Magnesium is not stored within the body so low levels indicate a low dietary intake – an issue that needs to be resolved quickly.
- **Calcium** is under hormonal control within the cow, so interpreting blood calcium levels is difficult. For this reason, calcium is not commonly assessed as part of a metabolic profile. Where, however, calcium is measured and levels are low milk fever is imminent.

When to sample?

Blood testing should not be undertaken during a period of dietary change, 2 weeks should have passed to allow the cow and her rumen microbes to get used to a new diet before any assessment is made. Cows should also not be blood tested within 2 hours of a concentrate feed as blood parameters alter and provide unreliable information (Whitaker, 2004).

In a spring-calving suckler herd, blood testing can be done *2 weeks after housing* to assess if the winter ration is providing sufficient energy and protein. A suckler cow's nutritional requirements are low at this time. By knowing the composition of protein and energy in the winter ration, any shortfalls should have been accounted for, and a metabolic profile will assess the cows' responses to the ration. BOHB, urea, globulin and albumin are the significant parameters at this time of year.

Over the winter months the cows will be condition scored. If the condition of the group, as a whole, is not behaving as expected, then additional metabolic profiles can be carried out and the diet and management adjusted in good time.

In addition, *mid-winter* is a good time to assess the cows' trace element status. Blood testing for copper, selenium and iodine can be carried out so supplementation can be provided, if required, well in advance of calving.

Cows can be blood tested again *4 weeks pre-calving* when their energy demands are higher. BOHB, urea, albumin, globulins, magnesium are the key parameters at this stage.

Ideally suckler cows should also be blood tested *2 weeks post-calving* to assess if their diet is adequate for the demands of lactation. This is not always practically possible as cows are often turned out to grass and handling is difficult. Assessing nutrition at this time allows the ration to be tweaked to ensure cows are not in negative energy balance and will resume cyclicity quicker, as well as have a good milk supply for their calves (Whitaker, 2004).

Which cows to sample?

The value of blood testing an individual cow to assess her energy and protein requirements is largely worthless; cows are fed as a group and therefore they need to be assessed as a group. Some greedy/dominant cows may be adequately provided for whereas others may be undernourished. A minimum of five cows, all average and typical of the group, should be tested; bullies, victims, and poorly cows should be excluded from the profile but may well warrant individual attention.

TABLE 10.3 Dentition of the adult cow

Tooth type	Upper jaw	Lower jaw
Incisors	0	3
Canine	0	1
Premolar	3	3
Molar	3	3

DENTITION

By the time a cow reaches 48 months of age, she should have all her permanent teeth as above, see Table 10.3. Ruminants differ from other species in that they do not have upper incisors or a canine tooth on the upper jaw. On the lower jaw, the canine teeth sit adjacent to the incisors (they look like incisors rather than the more familiar pointed canine tooth of other species) and they do not have an upper or lower first premolar (Dyce et al., 2002).

The lower incisors form a crescent shaped cutting blade, which opposes the firm mucosa covered dental pad on the top jaw. Cows graze grass not by using their incisors, but by wrapping their long tongue around swards of grass and pulling with only some slicing from the teeth. To do this effectively, they require a pasture height of greater than 10 cm. Cows can on average pull 50–60 mouthfuls of grass in an hour and chew 14–20 times a minute (Houpt, 2018).

THE OESTRUS CYCLE

The cow's oestrus cycle is 21 days long but can vary between 18 and 24 days. Heifers begin to cycle when they reach puberty, the age at which a heifer reaches puberty depends on a number of factors including breed, health status, growth rate and nutritional status (Chapter 8).

Day 1 of the oestrus cycle is considered to be the day of oestrus or 'heat', which ends in ovulation. Ovulation is when an egg is released from the ovary into the oviduct to then make its way into the uterus. The cow will show oestrus behaviour: standing to be mounted, restlessness and an increased amount of clear vulval mucus. The oestrus period lasts between 8 and 12 hours.

Oestrus behaviour is associated with the hormone oestrogen, which is secreted into the bloodstream from the ovary. Oestrogen causes specific changes in the reproductive tract during oestrus such as relaxing the cervix and increasing the blood flow to the uterus. It also causes the release of a hormone known as luteinising hormone (LH). This is secreted into the blood from a gland close to the brain called the pituitary gland. An LH surge causes the egg to ovulate from the ovary. Ovulation occurs approximately 32 hours after the LH surge.

If there are viable sperm present in the oviduct, the egg will be fertilised and the resulting embryo will travel down the oviduct arriving in the uterus approximately 3–4 days later. Where the eggs were released from the ovary, a structure called a corpus haemorrhagicum forms, and over a few days this turns into a corpus luteum (CL) which secretes progesterone.

Progesterone suppresses LH so there are no more ovulations during the presence of the CL. Meanwhile a hormone called follicle stimulating hormone (FSH) prepares waves of follicles (premature eggs) ready for the next ovulation. Follicles develop in waves: usually three waves occur during the 21-day cycle in cows, and two waves in heifers. If fertilisation did not occur and there is no embryo, the uterus releases prostaglandin (PG) into the bloodstream which causes regression of the CL from the ovary and therefore the progesterone in the bloodstream diminishes, see Figure 10.11.

As progesterone levels decline, and LH and oestrogen levels rise, oestrus and ovulation once again occur; a *cycle*.

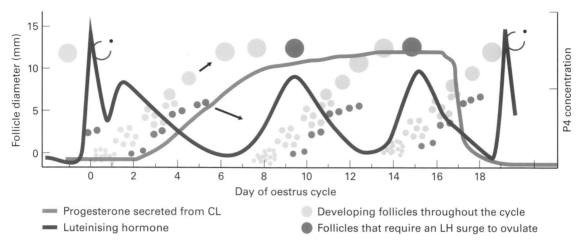

FIGURE 10.11 Graph depicting progesterone, LH and waves of follicle development in the oestrus cycle

If fertilisation was successful, then PG is not released, and the CL continues to produce progesterone, which prevents further heats and ovulations. Thus, progesterone is the essential hormone needed to maintain a pregnancy. The CL is responsible for progesterone levels up to day 150 of pregnancy; thereafter the placenta also secretes progesterone and takes over the maintenance of the pregnancy.

Post-calving the ovaries regain some activity within as little as 5 days, and follicles start to develop and produce oestrogen. There needs to be a sufficient build-up of oestrogen to stimulate an LH surge for ovulation to occur. The period when a cow is not cycling is called *anoestrus*.

The complex hormone interactions that take place during the oestrous cycle can be manipulated by artificial hormones to synchronise the oestrus cycle of a group of cows or heifers, or, to treat problem cows. There are three hormone treatments that vets frequently use: prostaglandin (PG) injections, progesterone releasing intravaginal devices or gonadotrophin releasing hormone (GnRH) injections.

As already stated, cows have their own naturally occurring 'endogenous' PG, which is released to remove a CL from the ovary and drop progesterone levels. The same can be achieved with an injection of PG – the drop in progesterone removes

the inhibition on the release of LH and FSH, which can then proceed, so causing the development of another follicular wave and ovulation.

This intervention is used as one of the ways to bring a cow into oestrus for AI. The time between injection depends on the stage of the follicular wave when the injection is administered; the timescale can vary from 3–5 days. The CL, which has not yet truly formed, is none responsive to PG for the first 6 days after ovulation, so PG will not induce a heat during this time. PG injections have been used successfully in synchronisation programmes for heifers, with poorer results in cows as PG will not work when a cow is in anoestrus. Typically, two injections are administered 11 days apart and the heifers can be served on observed heats or at fixed times of 72 and 96 hours after the second injection.

Progesterone releasing intravaginal devices are inserted into the cow's vagina for a period of 7–9 days. They release progesterone and so inhibit LH release. When the device is removed, and progesterone levels drop, there is a surge of LH and ovulation occurs. Intravaginal devices are commonplace in most synchronisation protocols. An injection of PG is recommended at least 24 hours before the device is removed to remove any naturally occurring progesterone source, that is, a CL on the ovary, otherwise progesterone levels would stay raised after device removal and stop the induction of oestrus.

A GnRH injection causes an immediate LH surge and ovulation if a follicle/egg is at the correct stage of the follicular wave. GnRH is integrated into synchronisation protocols to ensure that the semen and the fertile egg arrive in the uterus at the same time for successful conception.

GENERAL CONCEPTS AND PRINCIPLES OF SUCKLER COW FERTILITY

The industry aim is for a suckler cow to have a calf once a year. With a typical 285 day gestation she must get back in-calf within 80 days of calving to achieve this. Cows in optimal body condition have the potential to return to oestrus within 60 days and most do so within 50 days. A cow in poor body condition, less than condition score 2, will take in excess of 80 days to return to oestrus. Of importance and note is that nutrition pre-calving has a greater impact on time to first oestrus than nutrition after calving.

Block calving

Block calving, calving the group in a short, controlled period of time, typically in spring, autumn or sometimes summer, is standard practice in most suckler herds, certainly in the UK. Some herds calve all year round, this may be for a niche butcher's market or more often due to management resulting in poor reproductive performance and the need to leave the bull in all year round rather than for a short, controlled bulling period.

Block calving has a number of advantages.

- It is easier to pick out cows that are not performing reproductively.
- It is easier to spot calves in the group that are not achieving target DLWG.
- Cow condition and feeding can be more easily

managed for a group of cows at the same stage of production and having the same nutritional requirements.
- Calving supervision can be focused to a higher intensity for a shorter period of time.
- There is little variation between the oldest and youngest calf in any group which minimises disease transmission such as calf scour or BRD.
- An all-in-all-out approach to the calving field or pens can help cleanliness and minimise disease build-up and transmission.
- All management procedures can be carried out at the same time, for example, parasite control, vaccinations, dehorning and castration.

Cows should calve as early in the calving period as possible to make it subsequently easier to maintain the 365 day calving interval (Box 10.1).

Box 10.1 The 365 day calving interval

If the service period is 9 weeks, starting on 1 June and finishing on 3 August, then the calving period will extend from 5 March to 7 May every year. If a cow calves on the 5 March, she has over 11 weeks for her uterus to recover, and cyclicity to resume, before she has the chance to be served by the bull. In addition, she will be cycling when the bulls are turned out with the cows, and she is likely to have three full oestrus cycles to get back in-calf. A cow calving on the 7 May has only 24 days to recover before the breeding period starts on the 1 June. So, even if she is at the optimum condition score and returns to cyclicity 50 days post-calving, she will not cycle until 4 weeks into the bulling period and may only have one oestrus before the bull is removed. She is more likely to end up barren or at best be a late calver again next year.

Calves born late in the calving period, that are weaned with their cohorts, are lighter in body weight at weaning, they are more susceptible to disease, and growth rates are often further reduced as they are bullied away from the feed.

There are five key areas in which to improve the reproductive efficiency of a suckler herd. Each of these five points is discussed at length in this book:

1. management of bulling heifers (Chapter 8)
2. managing cow condition and nutrition (Chapter 10)
3. avoiding difficult calvings (Chapters 10 and 9)
4. bull management, fertility and soundness (Chapter 9)
5. maintaining herd health (Chapters 15 and 18).

Pregnancy diagnosis (PD)

PD can be carried out from 30 days post-conception using a rectal ultrasound scanner, see Figures 10.12 and 10.13. The embryo can be seen with a heartbeat at this stage and twins can be identified at approximately 2–3 months of pregnancy. It is possible to tell the sex of a foetus from 60 days of gestation and this can be useful in planning replacement policies. From 6 weeks a pregnancy can be detected by a veterinary surgeon manually without an ultrasound scanner – this procedure involves feeling a fluid distension, a subtle membrane slip sensation and, if extremely gentle, maybe even a pea like embryo. At 3.5–4

months into gestation, cotyledons are palpable (see Chapter 4) but the uterus still remains in the pelvis (not to be confused with a full bladder!). At 4.5–5 months of pregnancy, see Figures 10.14 and 10.15, the volume and weight of the fluid and calf pulls the uterus over the edge of the pelvis into the abdomen where it increases in size over the next few months. By 6 months, a calf is readily palpable per rectum and by 8–9 months the calf may be out of reach but the cotyledons are 6–8 cm in diameter.

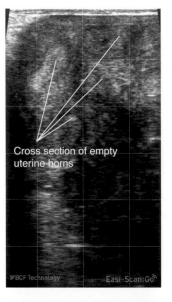

FIGURE 10.13 Ultrasound image of the non-pregnant uterus

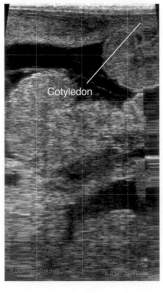

FIGURE 10.14 Ultrasound image of a 5 month pregnancy with cotyledons clearly visible

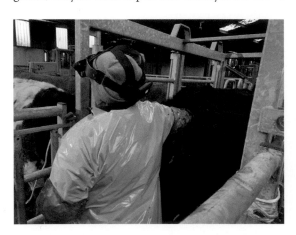

FIGURE 10.12 Vet ultrasound scanning a cow per rectum for pregnancy

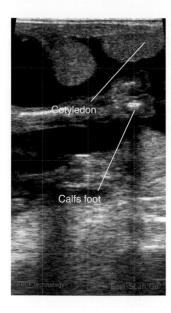

FIGURE 10.15 Ultrasound image of a 4.5 month pregnancy with calf's hoof and leg visible

The earlier in gestation that PD is carried out, the more accurate the age of the foetus can be estimated. This is useful if a service date is unknown; then an expected calving date can be calculated. Figure 10.16 displays the PD results from a winter/spring-calving suckler herd where scanning took place in early September.

There are many advantages to carrying out PD as soon as possible.

- Barren cows can be identified and culled as soon as they have weaned their calf.
- Late calvers falling outside the calving pattern can be dealt with accordingly. They may be sold with calves at-foot or their calves weaned later to prevent them from gaining too much condition.
- Any problems with fertility can be investigated more promptly.
- Twins can be identified and the dam managed accordingly.
- Cattle can be grouped and fed according to their expected calving dates.
- Supervision at calving can be targeted to the groups of cows that are expected to calve rather than observing the whole herd.
- If cows are moved from slats or cubicles to a straw yard to calve, then the calving area will be less crowded and have less faecal contamination.

Pre-calving changes in the cow

Within the last couple of weeks of gestation, the udder may become noticeably enlarged in preparation for calving. In heifers, this may occur from 5–6 months of gestation onwards, as the mammary

Animal ID	Animal DOB	Last calving Date	PD Result	No weeks in calf	Approx. service date	Approx. calving date	Days between calving & service	Comments
B15	06/05/2013	N/A	+	19	15/04/2015	24/01/2016		Maiden
B14	13/04/2013	N/A	+	19	15/04/2015	24/01/2016		Maiden
69	23/05/2007	22/02/2015	+	18	22/04/2015	31/01/2016	59	
A6	27/03/2012	28/02/2015	+	18	22/04/2015	31/01/2016	53	
33	12/02/2001	21/03/2015	+	18	22/04/2015	31/01/2016	32	
70	04/06/2007	31/03/2015	+	18	22/04/2015	31/01/2016	22	
B9	13/04/2013	N/A	+	18	22/04/2015	31/01/2016		Maiden
B11	06/04/2013	N/A	+	18	22/04/2015	31/01/2016		Maiden
82	11/05/2009	11/02/2015	+	17	29/04/2015	07/02/2016	77	1st cow to calve
90	24/04/2010	01/03/2015	+	17	29/04/2015	07/02/2016	59	
A5	14/05/2012	27/01/2015	+	16	06/05/2015	14/02/2016	99	Caesar
A1	16/04/2012	05/02/2015	+	16	06/05/2015	14/02/2016	90	
56	15/05/2005	10/02/2015	+	16	06/05/2015	14/02/2016	85	
88	24/04/2010	20/02/2015	+	16	06/05/2015	14/02/2016	75	
99	12/04/2011	22/02/2015	+	16	06/05/2015	14/02/2016	73	
64	14/06/2007	26/02/2015	+	16	06/05/2015	14/02/2016	69	
50	18/06/2004	04/03/2015	+	16	06/05/2015	14/02/2016	63	

FIGURE 10.16 Pregnancy diagnosis results for an example spring-calving herd

gland goes through its final stages of development and starts to produce colostrum for the forthcoming newborn calf. There are other physical changes underway that give an indication that calving is imminent although none of them are specific enough to indicate the exact time of parturition. Owing to the hormone *relaxin*, the ligaments surrounding the pelvis relax and the gluteal (rump) muscles sink meaning the tail head becomes more prominent. The vulva becomes swollen and floppy.

The process of parturition (giving birth, labour)

Parturition is a continual process but can be divided into three main stages of labour for ease of explanation. It is the calf that triggers parturition through the release of naturally produced steroid hormone, which then triggers a complex cascade of hormonal changes resulting in the reduction of the cow's blood progesterone levels.

First-stage labour

First-stage labour is characterised by progressive relaxation and dilation of the cervix, and, by the start of early uterine contractions. The muscle within the uterine wall is called the *myometrium* and as it contracts, it puts pressure on the calf causing it to rotate in the uterus, so it is presented the 'right way up' with its head and front feet facing the back end of the cow. If there are ineffective myometrial contractions or there is not enough room for the calf to move around, then a malpresentation may result (see Chapter 17). Throughout this time, the cervix is dilating. The last stage of cervical dilation is caused by the calf entering the birth canal and applying a mechanical stretching pressure to the cervix. The end of first-stage labour is signified by rupture of the first foetal membrane, the *allantois*. First-stage labour may last between 6 and 24 hours (Norman and Youngquist, 2007).

In some cows, and especially heifers, first-stage labour may be associated with behaviour signs: vocalisation, agitation, nesting and separation from the main herd. In experienced cows, there may be no outwards signs of parturition to this point.

Second-stage labour

Second-stage labour is characterised by the delivery of the calf. Strong abdominal contractions force the calf up into the birth canal where the calf applies more pressure to the continually dilating cervix. Stretching of the cervix stimulates the cow to release *oxytocin* hormone from the pituitary gland in the brain, and myometrial contractions strengthen in response.

In cases of dystocia, where the head and feet do not enter the birth canal, this does not occur and there is often little abdominal straining in the cow (Norman and Youngquist, 2007). This is commonly reported in cases of breach births and in uterine torsion (see Chapter 17).

The next layer of foetal membrane is now visible at the vulva – the *amnion* – which then ruptures. Abdominal contractions continue, increasing in strength and frequency. The cow will repeatedly stand and then lie down, but in the last stages of parturition she will usually lie on her side and vocalise her efforts. A big effort is required to push the calf's head from the vulva and then the rest of the body follows, with, maybe, some additional effort to pass the shoulders and, again, the hips. It is estimated that an average force of 70 kg is required to deliver a calf, 40% of the force is supplied by uterine contractions, 60% by abdominal contractions. Second-stage labour usually lasts 2–4 hours. A calf can survive up to 8 hours of second-stage labour (Norman and Youngquist, 2007).

Third-stage labour

Third-stage labour is characterised by the passage of the placenta. This has to detach from the uterine wall, and this occurs because the blood supply constricts due to the continuation of myometrial contractions. Third-stage labour normally lasts

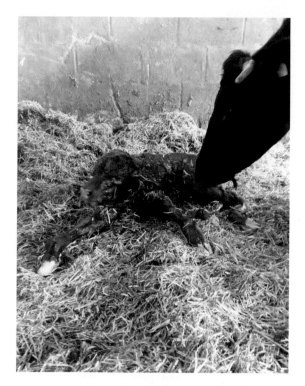

FIGURE 10.17 Newborn calf being tended to by its mother

up to 12 hours (Norman and Youngquist, 2007); during this time the cow is hopefully standing and tending to her calf, see Figure 10.17.

THE ENVIRONMENT OF THE SUCKLER COW

Housing the suckler cow

Many suckler cows will spend their winter months inside. A variety of shed designs exist to accommodate cows and, if required, their calves. Straw yards are common but expensive and there is the need to dispose of the muck generated. Cubicle housing is another method of housing; it is more common in the dairy industry but can be effectively used for suckler cows too. The design of the cubicle housing, and cubicles themselves, is important for their success. Little research has been carried out on the behaviour or requirements of the suckler cow in cubicle housing, instead, information on dairy cows must be extrapolated.

The dimensions and design of the cubicles should allow the cows to lie down and rise freely and unrestricted by bars or walls. The cubicles need to be long enough for a cow to lie fully in the cubicle, but also short enough that she defaecates in the passageway and keeps the raised cubicle clean. Brisket boards and head rails prevent cows from lying too far forward in a cubicle and help avoid this problem. Cows have a standard way of standing up: they rise up on their hind feet first and then complete the stand with their front legs. When they stand on their hind limbs, it is quite dramatic, and they lunge forward to do so. So, there needs to be adequate space in front of the cow in a cubicle to do this; 0.7–1.0 m of lunge room is recommended for Holstein cows (AHDB, 2012). Cubicles immediately facing a wall restrict cows when they want to rise and are far from ideal. When cubicles face each other, cows can share head space and the length of the lunge space of each can be reduced (Table 10.4). The position a cow lies in a cubicle (how far forward or back) is decided by the head rail initially as she enters the cubicle and then by the brisket board as she lies down. The brisket board should be no more than 10 cm high and positioned 1.6–1.8 m from the back of the cubicle.

The cubicle needs to be raised above floor height, so it does not get contaminated with slurry. The height of the kerb should be 15–20 cm, depending on the slurry removal system. Cows prefer to lie on

TABLE 10.4 Recommended cubicle length (AHDB, 2012)

Cow weight (kg)	Total length of bed (m)		
	Open fronted	Closed fronted	Head to head
700 kg	2.30	2.55	4.60 (= 2 × 2.30)

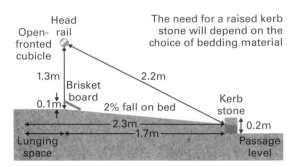

FIGURE 10.18 Suggested cubicle dimensions for an adult Holstein dairy cow

a slight incline falling from front to back, this also facilitates faeces and urine running off the back of the cubicle. A 2% incline is recommended (AHDB, 2012). The width of a cubicle needs to be such that a cow cannot turn around but can lie down without parts of her body rubbing or colliding with the metalwork. Cows in cubicles the right size should be able to lie straight. As a guide cubicle width should be 1.8 times the gap of the cow's hook bones. Figure 10.18 shows suggested dimensions of a cubicle designed for the dairy cow; the dimensions need to be extrapolated for the suckler cow.

Cows should not lie on concrete alone; they should have some bedding material on the cubicle base – straw, sand, paper waste or sawdust, or a rubber mat or cow mattress. There should be provision of 10% more cubicles than cows. This gives cows a choice of where to lie in the shed, for example, if there is a wet or cold draughty cubicle, they have the choice not to lie in it. Having choice also reduces confrontation and bullying.

Generally, a shed is designed for a number of cows, and for a cubicle shed this is largely determined by the number of cubicles installed. However, the water trough and feed trough spaces also need to be considered as DM and water intakes will be severely affected if access to either is restricted. The area for slurry is also important: in a cubicle shed, all faeces and urine will stay in the passageways until removed – ideally twice a day. A cow produces between 50–60 litres of slurry a day, and the level of slurry should not rise above

the back step of the cubicle. The more passageways there are the more slurry capacity there will be.

There should be no dead ends in a shed; cows are bullied by more dominant cows, so crossover passages are required. The more free-flowing the cattle movement is in the shed, the more the cows can exhibit their natural behaviour – this helps with everything – eating, drinking, ruminating, resting the feet, bulling behaviour and de-stressing in general. Wider passageways mean they are less likely to catch themselves on corners, bump into one another, or slip (Table 10.5). Consideration also needs to be given to the size of the machinery that will operate in the shed, for example, slurry scrapers.

Many designs of cubicle exist. The traditional type is the Newton Rigg design, which is a fixed frame attached to the floor with a fixed back leg, see Figure 10.19. They were common in the 1980s

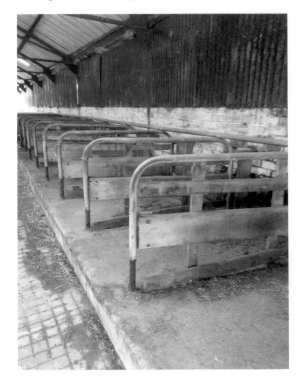

FIGURE 10.19 Newton Rigg ridged framed cubicles with wooden fillers installed in the 1980s (unsuitable for the comfort of the modern day suckler cow)

TABLE 10.5 Recommended dimensions for passages in cubicle houses (AHDB, 2012)

Passage	Recommended width of passage (m)
Crossover passage	2.4
Passageway between cubicle rows	3.0
Crossover passage with trough	3.6
Passage with feed access that cows back onto out of the cubicles	5.2
Passage with feed access that cubicles do not back onto	4.6

but have largely been replaced as cows went on to be bred with larger frames and there were issues with cows getting stuck or rubbing their legs and backs on the metalwork. To avoid these problems, cubicles attached only to a front rail and not the floor are now commonplace. This is called a cantilever design (Figures 10.20 and 10.21); there is little metalwork to obstruct the cow and it can be unbolted and repositioned after assessment of how the system is working.

Although cubicle dimensions are crucial and using a measuring tape to assess cubicle design is logical, in reality, much can be learned by just watching the cows and observing their comfort, or lack of, and their behaviours.

If there are a large number of lame cows – one needs to ask why this is? If the cubicles are not comfortable, the cows will choose to stand and not lie down, which predisposes them to lameness issues.

If cows have swollen hocks or leg sores, then they are colliding and rubbing on the metalwork associated with the cubicles or they are abraded on hard concrete; this may also present with an increase in lameness. Are the cows clean? If there are lots of dirty cows, then either they are choosing to lie in the passageways and not the cubicles, or the cows are defecating in the cubicles and then lying in it.

Cows have to learn how to use cubicles, and it is preferable that heifers have some exposure to cubicles before they have calves at-foot; one less stressor

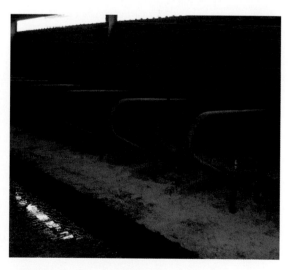

FIGURE 10.20 Cantilever loop cubicles with cow mattresses and sawdust (the lack of vertical rear bars allows cows to lie more comfortably without restricting their leg position)

FIGURE 10.21 Compromise between a loop and ridged frame cubicle and sawdust bedding (the cubicles are facing an outside wall, which can impede the cows ability to lunge forward when rising)

at the time of being a new mother. This will be less of a problem for home-bred suckler replacements that have been reared in cubicles as young calves while sucking their dams.

Cold, heat, humidity and ventilation

Cows are comfortable between a temperature range of –5 to 20°C. Below –5°C they use energy to keep warm. Above 20°C, a cow will use energy to keep cool. Above 25°C, food intakes will decrease; this is made worse by humidity and poor air movement (Hulsen, 2006). Insulated shed roofing helps retain cow-generated heat in cold weather and keep cows cool in the summer. Fans are recommended to maintain air flow in hot summer weather and help keep the flies away.

REFERENCES

AHDB (2012) Dairy housing – a best practice guide. Available at: https://ahdb.org.uk/knowledge-library/dairy-housing-cubicles.

Cutler, K.L. and Jones, I.G. (2003) The trace element nutrition of beef suckler cattle. *Cattle Practice* 11(2), 117–120

Drennan, M.J. and Berry, D.P. (2006) Factors affecting body condition score, liveweight and reproductive performance in spring-calving suckler cows. *Irish Journal of Agricultural and Food Research* 45(1), 25–38.·

Dyce, K.M., Sack, W.O. and Wensing, C.J.G. (2002) The head and ventral neck of the ruminants. In: *Textbook of Veterinary Anatomy*, 3rd edn. Sauders, Philadelphia, PA, ch. 25.

Eddy, R.G. (2004) Major metabolic disorders. In: Andrews A.H., Blowey, R.W., Boyd H. and Eddy, R.G. (eds) *Bovine Medicine Diseases and Husbandry of Cattle*, 2nd edn. Blackwell Science, Oxford, pp. 791–792.

Foster, A., Livesey, C. and Edwards, G. (2007) Magnesium disorders in ruminants. *In Practice* 29, 534–539.

Grove-White, D. (2004) Rumen healthcare in the dairy cow. *In Practice* 26: 88–95.

Houpt, K.A. (2018) *Domestic Animal Behaviour for Veterinary and Animal Scientists*, 6th edn. Wiley Blackwell, Hoboken, NJ, ch. 8.

Hulsen, J. (2006) *Cow Signals. A Practical Guide to Dairy Farm Management*, 1st edn. Roodbont Publishers, Zutphen.

Lowman, B. and Lewis, M. (1992) Feeding the beef suckler herd. *BCVA Summer Meeting*, BCVA, Wye College, 9–27.

Norman, S. and Youngquist, R.S. (2007) Parturition and dystocia. In: Youngquist, R.S. and Threlfall, W. R. (eds) *Current Therapy in Large Animal Theriogenology*, 2nd edn. Elsevier, Maryland Heights, MO, 310–335.

Otter, A. (2013) Diagnostic blood biochemistry and haematology in cattle. *In Practice* 35, 7–16.

Sinclair, K.D. and Suttle, N.F. (2000) Suckler cow nutrition: I. Management by condition score. *Cattle Practice* 8(2), 187–192.

Suttle, N.F. and Sinclair, K.D. (2000) Suckler cow nutrition: II Minerals and vitamins. *Cattle Practice* 8(2), 193–199.

Whitaker, D.A. (2004) Metabolic profiles. In: Andrews A.H., Blowey, R.W., Boyd, H. and Eddy, R.G. (eds) *Bovine Medicine Diseases and Husbandry of Cattle*, 2nd edn. Blackwell Science, Oxford, 804–815.

Wilkinson, J M. and Chamberlain, A.T. (2017) Silage for veterinary surgeons – making, feeding and understanding silage. *Cattle Practice* 25(2), 82–91.

Part III

Disease and production failure in the beef herd

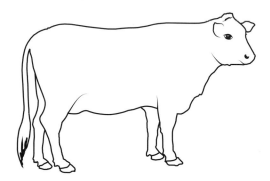

Chapter 11

Disease and production failure in the neonatal calf

DYSTOCIA – AN ABNORMAL OR DIFFICULT BIRTH

Dystocia, in the veterinary sense, is generally defined as a birth requiring human intervention. While dystocia could result simply from a cow being too unwell or finding herself in abnormal circumstances of some sort, the usual causes of dystocia fall into two categories:

1. **Malpresentations**. This is where the head and two fore limbs of the calf are not present in the birth canal, the calf is therefore abnormally positioned and manipulation is probably required to correct it.
2. **Foeto-maternal disproportion (oversize)**. The calf is simply too big for the cow or the cow is too small for the calf. Either way it is too big to push out!

Dystocia of any type is clearly detrimental to both cow and calf. In the case of malpresentations, the detrimental effects can be minimised by prompt hygienic intervention from a trained or experienced stockperson or from a vet. In the case of oversize – if it is judged that the calf will come out, but with additional force, then the experienced stockperson or vet will proceed with this carefully applied and controlled force. In its simplest guise increased force involves attaching leg and maybe head ropes to the calf and applying manual traction. Manual traction can be made easier with wooden handles on the ropes or amplified by machinery of various types. This could be something as basic as a pinch bar stuck in the ground to apply leverage to the pull on the ropes. It may be more elaborate and involve the use of a block and tackle fixed to something solid behind the cow to increase the pull on the ropes, or, more usually, it will involve the use of a proprietary calving aid (Figure 11.1).

It is important to remember how much force these various techniques can apply. For comparison, a cow during natural calving exerts a force equivalent to a weight of 70 kg, two people pulling on the calving ropes exerts a force equivalent to a weight of about 115 kg, a lever would increase this significantly, a block and tackle will double or quadruple the force depending on the design and a calving jack exerts a force of five times the strength of the operator. A calving jack can consequently apply a force in excess of 400 kg (Noakes et al., 2009). This force can cause considerable damage to cow and calf so to avoid this a calving aid or block and tackle should be used only by trained, experienced personnel and always with great care. A caesarean section is an alternative option and, in some cases, the only option if the calf is to be born alive and unharmed. Caesarean sections, however, are not without risk to the cow – complications from abdominal surgery are significant and subsequent fertility is also at risk. There are also financial considerations, the surgery is not cheap, and there also needs to be sufficient manpower and

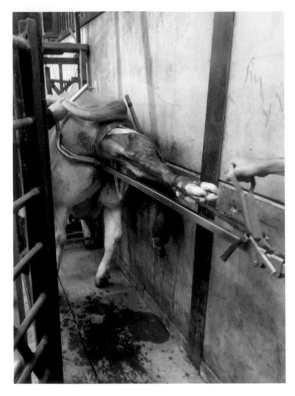

FIGURE 11.1 Calving aid used by a vet to assist calving due to foeto-maternal disproportion

suitable, safe facilities for the operation to be carried out.

The facts surrounding the devastating and all too common effects of dystocia are striking:

- 70% of perinatal losses occur before or at the point of calving rather than afterwards and are frequently a result of dystocia (Mee, 1991)
- dystocia accounts for nearly 65% of losses within 96 hours of birth (Patterson et al., 1987)
- calves that survive dystocia are almost 2.5 times more likely to become sick with infectious disease during the first 45 days of life (Toombs et al., 1994).

The simple message is that dystocia should be avoided at all costs – it clearly has a massive impact on calf mortality and morbidity and is a welfare issue for both cows and calves. The impacts on the cow's future reproductive performance, cull rate,

milk yield and economic implications are discussed in Chapter 17. A number of difficult births will always exist in the cattle population due to malpresentation but dystocia due to foeto-maternal disproportion is largely avoidable with the following strategies.

- Using EBVs or on-farm knowledge sires and dams can be selected for breeding based on their ability to have an easy calving (Chapter 9).
- Abnormally small pelvises can be detected pre-breeding using the technique of pelvimetry (Chapter 8).
- When rearing heifer replacements body weights should be measured and recorded at key stages and heifers only bred from if they reach known established targets (Chapter 8).
- Body condition scoring of cows (and heifers) should be performed and recorded and also compared to known target ranges, and ration formulation, and planning adjusted accordingly. Dystocia can result from being too fat or too thin during pregnancy – both are avoidable (Chapter 10).
- Cull cows should not be put back in-calf if there are pre-existing reasons for culling her. This 'one last chance' approach is risky and therefore not fair on the cow.
- Bulls that emerge as having a high incidence of dystocia should be retired immediately this becomes apparent.

The objectives of suckled calf production will be best achieved by driving efficiency, productivity and welfare in a climate of responsible drug usage (especially that of antibiotics). Tolerating dystocia is not compatible with these drivers.

In a normal birth the umbilicus ruptures, the calf's oxygen levels drop, carbon dioxide (CO_2) in the blood rises and the calf is stimulated to take its first breath (Figure 11.2). In the event of dystocia, oxygen drops as expected, CO_2 rises and continues to rise but the reflex to initiate the first breath is absent as oxygen levels have dropped so low the brain can no longer function normally. The calf is

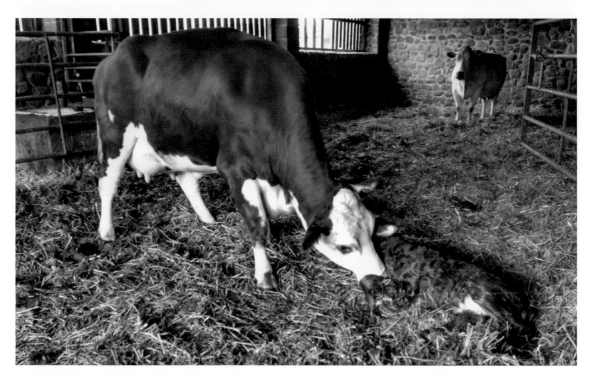

FIGURE 11.2 A healthy newborn calf from an unassisted calving

unable to breath and dies (Figure 11.3). During the period where the calf is without oxygen (hypoxia), the rising CO_2 in the blood (carbonic acid) causes acidosis. The calf's muscles also start to produce acid (lactic acid) as a result of anaerobic respiration,

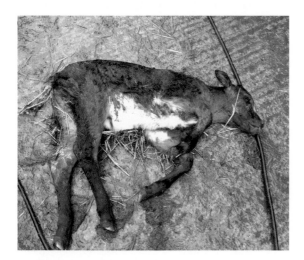

FIGURE 11.3 A calf death as a consequence of dystocia

the only type of respiration possible in the absence of oxygen. This acidosis affects organ function, the obtruded calf is rendered weak, unable to stand and unable to suck. Failure to suck means failure of colostrum ingestion, failure of passive transfer of immunoglobulins and apart from starvation then furthermore an increased susceptibility to other disease. Examining the pink conjunctiva of the eye (the mucous membrane) gives an indication of the degree of acidosis and oxygen deprivation – instead of being pink it goes brick red and in extreme cases develops a grey-blue tinge (cyanosis). If the conjunctival membrane and white of the eye is covered in red spots, small haemorrhages resulting from the bursting of oxygen starved blood vessels, then this carries a poor prognosis (Grove-White, 2000). In addition to the hypoxia and acidosis, and all that goes with it, it should not be forgotten that dystocia leaves a calf in pain, and often unable to stand as a result of mechanical damage – yet more reasons to remove dystocia from the herd.

Where a calf is born by caesarean section the calf may not have had the usual stresses and strains of birth so the CO_2 levels in the blood may not have risen to a sufficient level before delivery to stimulate the reflex to breathe (Grove-White, 2000). The calf may therefore take slightly longer to take its first breath, often to the consternation of those present.

Although dystocia is the main cause of neonatal calf mortality and morbidity, other factors contribute. Birth weight, immune function and the ability to control body temperature (thermoregulation) are three factors that are influenced by the maternal environment, before birth, in the cow's uterus. This phenomenon is called foetal programming. The cow's nutrition at different stages through gestation affects these three parameters through an influence on birth weight, organ development, adipose (fat) tissue development, metabolic rate, the appetite of the calf, the calf bonding ability and its immune function – all interrelated. It has been suggested that passive transfer of immunoglobulins in the colostrum can be influenced by pre-natal ambient temperature (Perry et al., 2019). The connections and pathways of foetal programming are complex, and research is ongoing. Hopefully outcomes of this research can be put into practice to improve neonatal calf health in the near future.

NEUROLOGICAL DISEASE

Neurological disease is any abnormality of the nervous system, be it the central nervous system (CNS) or the peripheral nervous system (PNS) – the CNS comprises the brain and spinal cord while the PNS comprises all the many nerves of the body that feed in and out of the central nervous system. Neurological disease is manifest in various clinical signs, in this case known as neurological signs. Neurological signs associated with disease of the brain include blindness, decreased levels of awareness, abnormal behaviour, star gazing, circling, head pressing (the pressing of the head against walls or corners), opisthotonos (extreme upward flexion of the neck), and seizures (convulsions, fits) to name but a few. Neurological signs associated with the spinal cord include paralysis, paresis (partial paralysis) and ataxia (wobbliness). Signs associated with the PNS include local paralysis or paresis, when limited to one or few nerves, or whole body signs when all the nerves are affected.

Neurological disease in neonatal calves is not uncommon, here follows a list of some examples.

CNS diseases of the newborn

- **Hypoxia**. A lack of oxygen during birth can cause irreparable damage to the brain in particular – it seems to suffer more than the spinal cord as its function is more complex.
- **Brain or spinal cord trauma**. Usually from a kick from the cow or being stood on, or in the case of the spinal cord, excessive traction from a calving aid.
- **Meningitis**. Inflammation of the meningeal membranes that surround, lubricate and protect the brain usually follows on secondarily to bacteria entering the bloodstream, or is sometimes a primary viral infection, as is common in humans.
- **Congenital abnormality**. A birth defect is a problem with the development of the brain or spinal cord during pregnancy.
- **Neospora**. Neospora is a protozoan parasite that is excreted in the faeces of infected dogs. When ingested by cows the parasite can cross the placenta of the pregnant cow and enter the brain of the calf resulting in abortion or the birth of an infected calf which may then have neurological abnormalities (Otter, 1995).
- **BVD**. A calf infected by its mother during pregnancy can be born a PI and may consequently present with neurological signs and/or eye abnormalities. The virus can damage the brain during its development, so called 'teratogenic effects', translated as 'monster-inducing' effects (Chapter 15).

- **IBR virus**. Although this virus is more likely to cause respiratory disease, encephalitis (inflammation of the brain) has also been reported in neonatal calves infected soon after birth (Penny et al., 2002). This scenario usually arises when naïve (unexposed) dams are purchased and then the calves are born in a herd where IBR is present. The dams have no antibodies to IBR and therefore the colostrum fails to offer any protection to calves born in the face of infection in the herd (Chapter 15).

PNS diseases of the newborn

- **Schmallenberg virus (SBV)**. This virus affects the development of both the brain and spinal cord of the unborn calf (and lamb). The calf is born typically with an enlarged abnormal brain but most notably with twisted limbs. This is another example of a virus demonstrating teratogenic effects.
- **Femoral nerve paralysis**. The femoral nerve is the main nerve supplying the quadriceps, the large muscles on the front of the thigh. Femoral nerve paralysis can be caused when calves are born backwards with excessive traction from a calving aid but more commonly when born in normal presentation but when the stifle (knee) joints catch on the rim of the pelvis and the thighs get overly stretched. This is more likely following excessive traction especially where the partially informed stockperson does what is believed to be the right thing, that is to bend the jack downwards, but on this occasion perhaps too much – so much that the calf is unable to pull round the corner so created by the edge of the pelvis without the knees catching. The condition can also be caused by excessive extension of the hip joints which can be caused by the opposite manoeuvre which is to have the calving aid too high for too long. Either way affected calves struggle, or are unable, to stand. Recovery can occur but can take up to 3 weeks. If no progress is being made in the first week the outcome is

likely to be poor; here the thigh muscles will be seen to be wasting noticeably. The calf will need artificially feeding with colostrum at birth then milk. Anti-inflammatories, particularly steroids, may help as will physiotherapy, such as massage and gentle working of the limb. Where only one leg is affected the calf fares better.

- **Sciatic nerve paralysis**. The sciatic nerve is the largest nerve in the body. It passes over the hip joint and down the back of the thigh before diverting to the front of the leg lower down. Over extension of the hip or over stretching of the spinal cord can damage the nerve. Again, the calf will struggle to stand and may demonstrate the characteristic knuckling appearance of the fetlocks. Steroids, physiotherapy and time may be helpful, and recovery can occur over 2–3 weeks.
- **Spinal cord trauma**. Trauma can result from excessive traction or from being stood on or from being jammed against a wall or crush side when halfway out the birth canal. It may be difficult to differentiate spinal cord trauma from bilateral (both sided) femoral or sciatic nerve paralysis; in cases of spinal cord damage there is often reduced rectal tone, or absence of a rectal reflex (when the anal sphincter is touched it should constrict).

In neurological disease a full neurological examination of the calf is required. Vets are trained to do this, and often further laboratory and/or post-mortem work is needed to establish a diagnosis.

CONGENITAL ABNORMALITIES

Congenital abnormalities refer to the plethora of defects an animal can be born with. The abnormality may be obvious such as an absence of eyes or the possession of two heads, or any other noticeable structural abnormality. It may be less obvious; a metabolic abnormality such as a

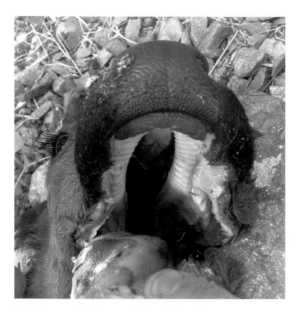

FIGURE 11.4 Calf born with a cleft palate

missing enzyme, or a functional abnormality such as malfunctioning kidneys. Occasional sporadic congenital abnormalities will occur and usually go unreported to the veterinary surgeon, but if there are a number of incidents further investigation may be warranted. Causes of birth abnormalities can be genetic, such as a one-off mutant gene or a more persistent chromosomal abnormality, or a recessive gene carried by either or both cow and bull. If the dam is exposed to certain pathogens or chemicals while pregnant this can trigger abnormalities in the development of the calf. Chemicals, medicines, plants or pathogens that cause birth defects are called teratogens.

One of the most common congenital abnormalities is the cleft palate. Here the roof of the mouth is defective, it has an opening down the middle of it which communicates with the nasal cavity, Figure 11.4. During the embryonic development of the calf the two sides of the palate failed to meet and fuse. The calf cannot suck and swallow milk properly; it pours out of their nose. Calves with cleft palate tend to have other defects in addition (Leipold et al., 1993). Euthanasia is required as surgery is difficult and expensive and fraught with complications.

Hyperextension deformities

Extension of a joint in simple terms usually means the straightening of the joint. Flexing of a joint refers to the bending of it. Hyperextension describes the phenomenon of over-straightening a joint beyond where it would usually stop. For example, some people can bend their fingers backwards until they almost reach the back of their arm – that is hyperextension. Hyperextension of joints often results from a lack of tension or strength in the muscles and tendons that flex the joint. In the calf the joint most frequently affected is the fetlock. The fetlocks will be observed as sinking towards the ground when the limbs bear weight. This is more likely seen in premature calves. With time and gentle exercise the tendons strengthen. If this is ineffective, heel blocks can be used to raise the calf's heels and take the strain off the tendon so allowing it to contract slightly. The heel block can usually be removed after 2–3 weeks.

Flexural deformities (contracted tendons)

The over flexion of joints, the over bending of joints, is a common problem in calves, of all breeds. The condition most commonly seen is where the leg is permanently bent at the carpus (knee) and the fetlock joints of the front legs or the fetlock joints of the back legs (Figure 11.5). It can be caused by teratogenic agents such as the lupin plant (Steiner et al., 2014) or it may simply be to do with the fact the calf did not have sufficient room inside the dam to stretch its legs.

The defect can be classified as mild, moderate or severe. If the calf can stand and bear weight on its toes but its heels do not touch the ground then this is a mild defect. Over time the weight of the calf will result in the tendons stretching and a normal conformation will be achieved within 1–2 weeks. A moderate defect is when the calf is able to stand on the point of the toes, but the front wall of the hoof breaks over the vertical plane perpendicular

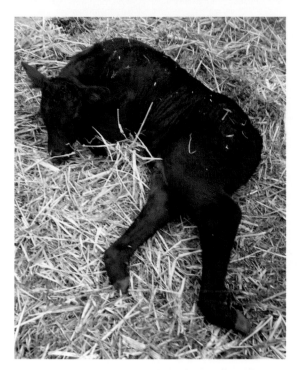

FIGURE 11.5 Flexural deformity of the fetlock of the back leg

to the floor. A severe defect is classified as the calf not bearing weight on the foot at all but standing or walking around on the skin of the fetlock or knee. In these severe cases it is imperative the calf is bedded in deep straw to prevent trauma to the skin overlying the joints. The treatment of moderate and severe contracture is rarely successful. Regular, three times a day, manual stretching of the tendons is advised, pulling the toe out to straighten the leg. Toe extensions can be fitted to magnify the amount of force directed through the tendons and to change the break over point. Casting and splinting offer limited improvement and worse still often results in further complications with rubs and sores. Surgery is an option where one or both of the flexor tendons on the back of the leg are partially severed. This usually results in hyperextension; the calf's leg is then bandaged or cast for 2–3 weeks while the tendons heal. This procedure carries a guarded prognosis.

Arthrogryposis

A condition that initially presents similarly to contracted tendons is arthrogryposis. This is a syndrome of permanent joint contracture. One or more legs are affected, the joints are fixed or fused in rigid flexion and cannot be moved, unlike the case with contracted tendons. Often a calf with arthrogryposis requires assistance at calving as the legs are in a fixed position. The bony change that has resulted in fusion of the joint is non-reversible and the calf requires euthanasia. The spine is often affected as well as the limbs – this is referred to as *crooked calf syndrome*. Classic arthrogryposis is a genetic malformation. Calves affected by SBV virus can appear similar.

Congenital chondrodystrophy (dwarfism, long bone deformity)

Calves affected by congenital chondrodystrophy are born with abnormal shortening of their bones resulting in a short, often bow-legged appearance, hence the nick name 'dwarf calves'. The condition has been reported worldwide affecting up to 10% of calves born. Some calves are unable to walk or suck and require euthanasia. Occasionally they also have domed heads and dished faces. The condition does not appear to be breed specific. It occurs in cows fed a predominantly grass silage ration in the fourth and fifth month of pregnancy when bone development is taking place in the foetus. Numerous causes have been postulated including genetic, nutritional, toxic and infectious. Current thinking from recent outbreaks in Scottish herds suggest it may be linked to a deficiency in manganese. Manganese is well documented as important in skeletal growth and development and deficiencies of the mineral have been associated with skeletal deformities (White and Windsor, 2012). The incorporation of at least 25% straw in the ration has been shown to decrease the incidence of the disease although the mechanism for this solution is not understood. Where the feeding of straw is not an option, up to 7000 mg/kg of manganese is included in the ration using a proprietary mineral supplement.

Schmallenberg virus

SBV was first detected in the hill town of Schmallenberg in Germany's upper Rhine in 2011. It quickly spread across Europe and was first diagnosed in the UK in southern England in 2012. Schmallenberg has since been diagnosed across much of England, Wales and Scotland but its main incidence is still southern England. SBV is transmitted by the *Culicoides* midge (the disease vector); direct transmission from cattle to cattle cannot occur. Although SBV virus has been found in semen there is no evidence that virus is transmitted venereally.

When cows or heifers are bitten by an infected midge between 2–4 months of pregnancy the calf may be born with certain typical deformities but not all cows infected with the virus at this time will give birth to a deformed calf (Wernike et al., 2014). Stillborn but otherwise apparently normal calves can also result from SBV infection, as can abortions, although the latter is not common. Interestingly, in the case of twins, one normal and one deformed calf can be born (Wernike et al., 2014).

SBV associated deformities include some or all of the following (Figure 11.6):

- undershot jaw
- legs with rigidly fixed and over flexed or over extended joints – as in arthrogryposis
- joints that are too flexible and bend the wrong way
- curvature of the spine in either a horizontal or vertical plane
- cavitation of the brain, and skull deformity, resulting in overt neurological abnormalities.

The nature of the deformities may result in a difficult calving and a caesarean may be required. The deformities are permanent and there is no treatment; euthanasia is required.

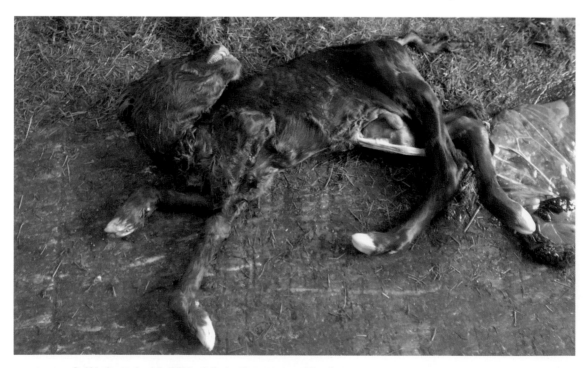

FIGURE 11.6 Calf infected with SBV while in the uterus of its dam

When a non-pregnant animal is bitten by an infected midge they may be off colour, scour and have a raised temperature for a few days, and in the case of dairy cows a milk drop may be seen. The animal has SBV virus in her blood for 5 days and any midge that takes a blood meal from an infected animal in that time becomes infected itself and can pass the virus to another cow (Davies et al., 2012).

Over time animals in a population become naturally infected and immune to SBV. Once a cow has been infected she will become immune and will not give birth to SBV deformed calves in future years. The results of studies from blood sampling herds affected by SBV suggests that once SBV has been detected in a herd, infected midges have already bitten a large percentage of the animals which are consequently rendered immune, generally between 80 and 100% of the herd. Not all of these animals will have been sick, and actually very few that have been bitten by the midge during the second to fourth month of pregnancy will give birth to a deformed calf. While this is good news, it is still fairly shocking for the affected farm – it only takes a few SBV deformed calvings and caesareans to spoil a calving season and the temptation to vaccinate when an epidemic is occurring, or when one is expected, is quite sensible – an inactive vaccine is commercially available; a primary course of two injections needs to be completed before breeding to provide sufficient protection. Other control measures include the use of midge repellents or insecticides, or reducing exposure to midge infested grazing. One measure that could make a big difference is changing the breeding period so that cows are not at the critical stage of pregnancy during the midge season, the *vector period* as it is called, although in the authors' experience SBV infected calves have been born in June and July suggesting the dam was infected with SBV in mid-winter. In England it may be that a vector free period does not exist some years, or maybe even in any years – it is not unusual to see a plume of midges on a sunny afternoon in mid-winter in the UK. Countries that experience much harsher winters than the UK may indeed have a vector free period.

MUSCULOSKELETAL DISEASE

Fractures

Fractures in calves are common and usually involve the bones of the limbs below the hock or knee. There is little protective soft tissue coverage in these regions, there is extra leverage at the end of a limb and the bones are thinner than higher up the limb. The fractures are usually caused either by excessive traction with a calving aid or from being stood on by the dam.

Fractures are often readily diagnosed as the limb is bent or pointing in the wrong direction. Where the bone is fractured but the two opposing bones have not moved apart, the site of the fracture may not be obvious, but the calf will be extremely lame. Often the location of one of these so called non-displaced fractures can be identified by palpation of the limb – a painful swelling may be detected – but radiography may be required to confirm a diagnosis. Misdiagnosis of a fracture is possible if it is located adjacent to a joint and the initial presentation may be similar to that of joint ill.

Open fracture versus closed fracture

The skin should be closely examined for any wound associated with the fracture site, if there is a wound this is called an open fracture (Figure 11.7) and requires more intensive management than a closed fracture – the situation carries a poor prognosis (Anderson et al., 2008). The prognosis for an open fracture depends on the degree of infection, the amount of damage to the exposed bone and the amount of damage to the surrounding tissues and blood supply (Anderson et al. 2008). In many cases an open fracture warrants euthanasia but in the case of a particularly valuable animal surgery may be attempted to remove bacterial contamination and damaged bone from the site followed by appropriate dressing, possible wound closure, a prolonged course of antibiotics and pain relief and

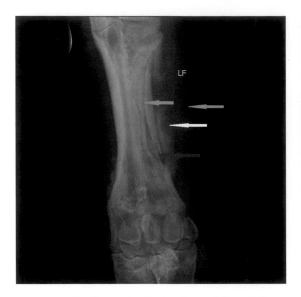

FIGURE 11.7 Radiograph of a fracture of the left fore cannon bone of a young bull (the green arrow indicates the skin, the white arrow indicates air in the wound from an open fracture site, the blue and red arrows indicate fragments of bone from the fracture)

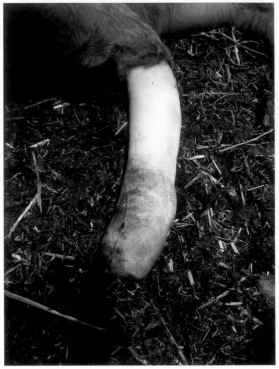

FIGURE 11.8 Cast applied to the front right leg of a 3 week old calf. The site of the fracture was just above the fetlock

of course stabilisation of the fracture site using a cast which, because of the wound, may need changing at intervals during the healing period (Mulon, 2013).

Closed fractures can often be treated by the correct application of a cast, Figure 11.8. Plaster of Paris has been largely superseded by modern synthetic casting materials that are lighter, stronger, faster setting, but also more expensive.

- The leg should be fixed in a slightly flexed position.
- The joints above and below the fracture must be stabilised by the cast or the fracture will still move, and healing will not result.
- There should be a 50% overlap of cast material.
- A calf weighing (less than 150 kg) necessitates 6–8 layers of cast material.
- The foot should be incorporated into the cast (Anderson et al., 2008).
- The animal needs to be confined.
- The cast should be removed and reapplied if required after 3 weeks in the growing calf

(Anderson et al., 2008). In adult animals, the cast is often left in situ for 6 weeks.

- During this time the calf should be monitored for signs of discomfort, rubbing, heat through the cast, and a bad smell which would signify infection or gangrenous necrosis. Any of these developments require the removal of the cast for inspection – euthanasia may be necessary.

Fractures caused by excessive traction with a calving aid can be managed as above although consideration needs to be given to damage to the blood supply and surrounding skin and tissues. It is reasonably common, if the blood supply has been damaged, that the fracture is unable to heal, and this may not become evident until the cast is removed; euthanasia may be required at this point. Calves that are cast soon after birth may be unable to rise and suck their dam so additional colostrum supplementation may be required (Mulon, 2013).

When fractures occur further up the limb above the hock and knee, casting is not possible as the joint above the fracture cannot be stabilised. In these cases, splints have been designed to help immobilise the leg, but they enjoy very limited success. In valuable animals, surgical insertion of orthopaedic implants may be an option.

Fractures are extremely painful and pain relief usually in the form of NSAIDs is essential until the fracture is stabilised.

Joint dislocations

Joints are the sites where two bones meet, where they articulate. The joint needs to be able to move but it needs to retain its structural integrity at the same time. Ligaments, tendons, muscles and joint capsules, and the shape of the articulation itself, help keep the joint in line, in other words, keep it *located*. When a joint dislocates, the ligaments, tendons, muscles and joint capsule may have ruptured or stretched so the two joining bones are no longer held in the right position to work as a functional joint. Where there is dislocation of a joint in the lower limb, then it is possible to apply a cast to immobilise the joint which should then allow the soft tissue structures to repair, tighten up and re-stabilise the articulation. Unfortunately, this is a slow process, slower for example than the healing of a fractured bone. If things go to plan the soft tissues will repair with scar tissue. The joint may go on to work reasonably well but it will tend to be thickened and stiff thereafter. It may be, especially if the bone of the joint was damaged, that the bones either side of the joint fuse together in a bony repair. This fusion of the bone, known as ankylosis, may be sufficiently functional but the fusion will result in mechanical lameness and the fused joint will be very vulnerable to subsequent fracture. If things do not go to plan the joint will fail to re-stabilise, the articulation will fail, the animal will be painfully and mechanically lame, extreme arthritis will develop rapidly in the joint and euthanasia will almost certainly become necessary.

Joint ill (septic arthritis)

Joint ill is a bacterial infection of one joint (septic arthritis) or more than one joint (septic polyarthritis). Bacteria enter a joint either through a penetrating wound straight into the joint or, as is the usual case in neonatal joint ill, from the bloodstream, having entered the body through some port or other, a common one being the umbilicus. Joint ill can also be secondary to a bacterial pneumonia or diarrhoea (enteritis). Whatever the cause it often follows on from a failure of passive transfer of immunity to the calf, often a result of poor colostrum management.

Most commonly infected joints, in descending order, are: the carpus of the front leg (the knee), the stifle (the true knee of the back leg), the hock and the fetlock. Septic arthritis can occur in almost any joint of the body including the articulation between the vertebrae of the spine. The infection is, by name, located within the joint but it can also spread into the adjacent bone, this then being called *osteomyelitis* (infection of the bone), or, where a growth plate is infected, *physitis*.

Once a joint is infected the bacteria attach to the lining of the joint capsule; they may penetrate into the cartilage; they invariably multiply within the fluid in the joint. As with most infections a fight breaks out between the immune system and the bacteria. The toxins, the enzymes and the white blood cells involved in this battle cause collateral damage to not only the offending bacteria but to the structures of the joint itself, most notably the lining of the joint and the cartilage. The cartilage weakens and becomes fragile. The fluid in the joint becomes watery rather than lubricating. The fluid then becomes thick and tacky as the body produces fibrin, in an effort to stabilise the situation. Fibrin ultimately coats the cartilage and joint capsule so limiting its mobility and, of therapeutic consideration, limiting the penetration of antibiotics.

Calves with joint ill are lame, often non-weight bearing on the affected limb or limbs. The affected joints are hot, swollen and painful, and will have reduced movement. The calf will often have a fever and will be off its milk.

Ideally a sample of the fluid from an infected joint should be obtained and sent away to find out which bacteria are involved so as to better understand the problem and to aid in the choice of antibiotic. For example, *Salmonella* and *Mycoplasma* infection can both cause joint ill (along with many other clinical signs and manifestations) and culture of the joint fluid can detect these bacteria which, compared to, say, streptococci or staphylococci (both common causes) require specific treatment and a whole herd control plan.

In the field situation it is often not practical to carry out a joint tap to obtain the sample; the conditions are too dirty, and the sample will be contaminated; a joint tap is a sterile procedure. Furthermore, the calf requires prompt treatment with antibiotics if there is to be any chance of a successful outcome; there is not time to wait for bacteriological culture results. That being the case the field situation usually dictates the immediate use of broad-spectrum antibiotics. In the valuable animal joint lavage may be employed to flush bacteria and inflammatory debris from the joint. Certain antibiotics may be injected directly into the joint in specific cases (this is an off-license treatment). Regardless of method, it is essential that the duration of antibiosis is sufficient. This duration will depend on the severity of infection, the stage of the infection, the nature of the infection, and on the response to treatment, but as a general rule antibiosis should last for a minimum of 7 days after the calf starts to show an improvement.

Often there are irreversible changes to the cartilage – more likely when there has been a delay in the treatment. Certain antibiotics can themselves damage the cartilage as a side effect to killing the bacteria. Either way the calf remains lame due to chronic arthritis, similar to osteoarthritis. If sufficiently painful this will be a welfare concern and euthanasia may be appropriate.

Septic arthritis and chronic arthritis are painful conditions with an inflammatory component so in almost every case anti-inflammatory drugs will be prescribed alongside the antibiotics. Given the pressure to reduce inappropriate antibiotic use it will become more common to admit defeat with severe cases of septic arthritis and replace antibiosis with euthanasia, knowing the outcome will probably be futile, with or without the antibiotics.

SKIN DISEASE

Bovine erythropoietic protoporphyria

Bovine erythropoietic protoporphyria (BEPP) is a hereditary condition affecting only Limousin or Limousin-cross calves (Armstrong et al., 2002). Affected calves show signs from 3 weeks of age – they are subdued, demonstrate hair loss and crusting of the skin around the ears and muzzle, along the back and on the rear end. The condition is caused by a defect in the production of an enzyme, protoporphyrin oxidase, the failure of which results in an elevated concentration of protoporphyrin in the red blood cells and tissue. Protoporphyrin is, ordinarily, a precursor of the all important oxygen carrying pigments, haemoglobin and myoglobin. Failure of this process jeopardises levels of these important pigments but more immediately critical is the build-up of protoporphyrin that is potentially toxic mainly due to its sensitivity to light. When exposed to intense light in superficial blood vessels of the body, especially areas of hairless skin, the surrounding tissues become damaged. The condition can be diagnosed from a blood sample using a technique called fluorescence emission spectrometry. There is no treatment other than to keep affected calves in a darkened environment for fattening. Where that is not practicable euthanasia is required. Genomic testing can now be used to detect the gene in Limousin cattle; as an autosomal recessive gene, only double carriers (homozygotes) exhibit signs of the disease but heterozygotes are carriers. The North American Limousin Foundation, the Canadian Limousin Association and the Australian Breeders Association have promoted a genomic testing programme to reduce the incidence of disease. At the time of writing, this is not currently the case in the UK.

Bovine papular stomatitis

Bovine papular stomatitis (BPS) is a contagious viral disease of young calves caused by a *Parapoxvirus* (Andrews et al., 2004). The virus is transmitted in the saliva and nasal secretions and spreads rapidly in artificially reared calves sharing teats. The gums and muzzle are usually affected with small lesions resembling small red papules, often with yellow/brown centres. They can be up to 1 cm in diameter but usually only 2–3 mm. The calf is usually fit and well and continues to suck. No treatment is required; the calf generates an immune response and lesions subside within 10–14 days.

UMBILICAL DISEASE

The umbilicus, at birth, normally stretches, narrows, tears and seals. Occasionally after rapid expulsion or traction or after delivery by caesarean section the umbilicus may snap relatively abruptly and haemorrhage results. Surgical clamps should be applied to the umbilicus and it should be ligated by a vet. If a vet is not present, then quick action is required by the stockperson – a clamp may have to be improvised to stop the bleeding until the vet arrives or a homemade ligature applied with string or similar. Any procedure involving the umbilicus should be carried out as hygienically as possible as it is a direct portal of entry for bacteria into the calf's body and circulatory system. Any homemade improvisations should be followed up with veterinary consultation.

Umbilical hernia

A hernia is an abnormal enlargement of an opening into a body cavity, in this case the opening that conducts the umbilical cord through the body wall. Body contents can pass through a hernia to varying extents.

Umbilical hernias in the period immediately after birth

On occasion, calves are born with intestines outside the abdominal cavity. They can be either contained within a translucent sac, an out-pouching of peritoneum, or be out with the sac and exposed to the outside world. Veterinary attention is required to replace the intestines to the abdomen. Where the intestines are not encased within the sac there is a poor chance of survival as damage to the intestines is likely, as is a high level of bacterial contamination. Returning the intestines to the abdomen is usually surprisingly difficult as the hernia is often small and the intestines swollen. The vet will usually sedate the calf, inject local anaesthetic into the body wall and temporarily extend the hernia surgically, clean, repair and replace the intestines and finally close the enlarged hernial opening with surgical sutures. This is definitely one for the vet!

Umbilical hernias in the first few weeks of life

Hernias can also occur and are often noticed a few days to weeks after birth as a bulging of the haired skin at the navel. This needs to be differentiated from a navel abscess or infection (navel ill) which is readily done by careful palpation for a hernial opening and of the structures within the swelling. An ultrasound examination can be used to aid diagnosis. The severity of the hernia is dictated by the size of the hernial opening or hernial ring that the abdominal contents are protruding through. In most cases the hole in the body wall can easily be identified and the contents of the sac pushed back up into the abdomen. This is referred to as a reducible hernia. There are various treatment options. The sac of the hernia can be squeezed upwards to empty it and ligating elastic rings then applied to the sac to nip it shut and prevent re-filling. Inflammation caused by the ligation seals the hernial ring in the longer term and the shrivelled up sac below the ring eventually drops off leaving a closed scarred wound where the ring was. This technique can be successful in small hernias. In larger hernias, surgery can be performed under general anaesthesia to return the contents of the hernia to the abdominal cavity and close the hole in the body wall. There is a genetic predisposition to umbilical hernias and females should not retained as breeding animals and male animals should be castrated (Edwards, 1992).

Umbilical infections

Often umbilical infections are confined to the tissues outside the body cavity under the skin – this infection may present as tissue swelling or as an actual abscess (collection of pus). The navel is usually swollen, wet, smelly and painful when touched. Often calves are slightly depressed as is the case in systemic navel ill. Umbilical infections are more common in the following scenarios:

- calves born inside
- failure of passive transfer of immunoglobulins through the colostrum
- bull calves experiencing urine scalding
- dystocia or other causes of the calf lying on warm, damp, contaminated bedding material for longer than normal.

The umbilicus contains two umbilical arteries, an umbilical vein that leads back to the liver, and a structure called the urachus, which carries urine from the calf's bladder to the placenta when the calf is in utero (Chapter 4, Figure 4.9) (Edwards, 1992). These structures recoil and seal after birth but sometimes the seal is incomplete and/or they can become infected and allow bacteria to track up into the body, most notably along the length of the cord (umbilical abscesses) or as far as the

liver and sometimes beyond. Internal abscesses may not be apparent but often the navel is damp and smelly, and the calf is unwell. On palpation a painful thickening of the cord at the navel is often evident. Liver abscessation is not evident but the calf will be ill; it is common after a long-standing navel infection.

Umbilical infections or navel ill, whether affecting the internal or external structures, require treatment with a broad-spectrum antibiotic and an NSAID. In advanced cases, and, where it can be economically justified, surgical intervention may be warranted to remove infected tissue, or in the case of abscesses, to drain them.

Bacteria can, and do, gain entry into the calf's bloodstream via the umbilicus. This is called bacteraemia (bacteria in the bloodstream). The presence of both bacteria and associated toxin in the bloodstream is called septicaemia (blood poisoning). Septicaemia without prompt treatment results in an extreme shock like state known as sepsis – this is usually fatal.

Calves born to cows rather than heifers have a higher incidence of umbilical infections. This is assumed to be due to natural licking behaviour which is known to be more pronounced in the experienced cow than it is in the relatively inexperienced and distracted heifer. The natural behaviour to lick the calf after birth is evolutionary and instinctive and is useful for drying, warming and stimulating the calf but in the case of the navel it can cause extra wetting, contamination and trauma so predisposing it to infection.

A calf is more likely to develop an umbilical infection when the remaining cord is very short from having ruptured closer to the navel than is normal. The assumption is that bacteria can more easily get up a short cord than a longer one before the cord has time to shrivel up.

The risk of navel infections increases with the birth weight of the calf. This is likely to be because heavier calves spend more time lying down and consequently more time in contact with contaminated bedding.

GASTROINTESTINAL DISEASE

Diarrhoea ('calf scour')

Diarrhoea or calf scour is the passage of abnormally soft or liquid faeces. It is a very common condition of neonatal calves and is preventable to a degree, bearing in mind the concept of immunity versus challenge – among other factors good colostrum boosts immunity, good hygiene reduces challenge. Nutritional scour, however, which is not infectious, occurs in pre-weaned calves exposed to fluctuating quantities of milk either from the cow or from artificial feeding systems. In the case of an artificially reared calf a change in milk composition and/or temperature can also induce nutritional scour (Bazeley, 2003). In this situation the content of the intestines is too plentiful and too concentrated – this creates an osmotic pull of fluid into the lumen of the intestine and consequently diarrhoea.

Diarrhoea is a result of too much water in the intestine, either caused by osmosis as described above, or by the intestines of the calf being unable to absorb the water from the faeces before being excreted (malabsorption) or by the cells within the intestinal wall excreting excessively large volumes of fluid into the gut lumen (hypersecretory). If the faecal fluid losses from the body exceed the volume of water the calf is able to drink then the calf becomes dehydrated. Whether osmotic, malabsorptive or hypersecretory the causes are nutritional or infectious. Infectious causes include bacteria, viral and protozoan parasites.

The viruses that can be involved are rotavirus and coronavirus. The bacteria that can be involved are enterotoxigenic *E. coli* (ETEC) and *Salmonella* (typically *S. dublin* and *S. typhimurium*), see Chapter 12.

The protozoan parasites, cryptosporidium and coccidia, will be discussed in Chapter 12 as they typically affect older calves.

It is fairly common that mixed infections of bacteria, viruses and protozoa are involved in calf scour outbreaks. UK data suggests rotavirus is the most common cause of neonatal diarrhoea in calves 1–4 weeks old (Mason and Caldow, 2012) with cryptosporidium coming in a close second.

Salmonellosis and cryptosporidiosis can infect humans; they are zoonotic infections – infections that can spread from animals to people, so personal hygiene is important during outbreaks as is the serious consideration of risk on open farms, especially those visited by children.

All the bacterial, viral and protozoan causes of diarrhoea are ubiquitous, that is, everywhere, in the environment; any environment that contains cattle faeces. Older cattle carry these bugs having long since established immunity and harmony with them. When a young, non-immune calf ingests such faeces directly or through contamination then infection results and disease may or may not follow depending on the balance between immunity, be it specific or non-specific, and the scale of the challenge. To reduce the infectious challenge, hygiene is critical in the control of these diseases – a strong calf that has had an easy calving, plenty of colostrum and is not immunosuppressed by some other infection or nutritional deficiency can ingest a small amount of rotavirus and cope; it will not succumb to disease. The calf's environment also plays a part; warm calves in a cosy well-bedded shed free from draughts and kept dry are non-specifically more immune. Vaccines for rotavirus, ETEC and coronavirus are available. Interestingly they are not administered to the calves but instead to the cows between 12 and 3 weeks pre-calving. The idea is that the cow's immune system produces antibodies in response to the vaccination. These antibodies naturally find themselves in her colostrum which are then transferred to the calf via the all important first meal. This specific immunity adds to the non-specific immune measures the calf is able to deploy providing all else is well. The effectiveness of calf scour vaccination relies, most importantly, on the calf ingesting a sufficient quantity of the vaccinated cow's colostrum. It also relies on the cow herself being well and being vaccinated at the correct time and in the correct manner with a properly prepared and stored vaccine. Salmonella vaccination is also available and works on the same principle – this will be discussed in Chapter 12.

The incidence of calf scour in a herd often increases towards the end of the calving period, especially in cattle that are calving indoors. This is largely attributable to the build-up, over time, of bugs in the environment until levels eventually exceed a threshold at which the challenge overwhelms immunity, be it innate or specific. If cows can be kept outside for calving this usually reduces this effect thanks to outdoor dilution of the bugs. The environment still needs to be reasonably clean and dry though; this is not the case if the land is waterlogged and the cattle are cold, wet and dirty. Where indoors becomes the answer then it clearly needs to be clean, dry, and preferably newly moved into in time for the calving season – a big ask on most farms!

A compact calving period helps maintain hygiene as efforts can be focused. This also reduces the age spread of calves so preventing older calves passing their multiplied pathogens to their younger mates. Compact calving periods also help where a vaccination plan is implemented as cows ideally need to calve within 12 weeks of vaccine administration; where the period extends the late calvers either require a second top up vaccine or the cows have to be vaccinated in two separate groups; late and early.

The faeces from an affected calf can be tested immediately for the presence of rotavirus, coronavirus and ETEC and, with a delay of a day or two, cultured for salmonella. While the presence of a bug does not necessarily prove disease causation it does raise some suspicion when designing a vaccination programme – the problem is that these pathogens can be found in healthy animals so it is difficult to know whether the bug detected in the faeces is actually causing the clinical signs or not. If treatment fails and a calf dies, a post-mortem examination is a valuable tool in obtaining a more accurate diagnosis. Although there is little difference to be seen on gross examination – one scoured, dehydrated calf looks pretty much like any other – but if the carcase is fresh (less than 6 hours since

death) then pieces of intestine can be sampled and processed for examination under the microscope. This process, called histopathology, is very accurate in these cases. The samples are examined by highly trained individuals, histopathologists, who can distinguish the different effects that different viruses and bacteria have on the gut lining. The histopathologist can therefore ultimately diagnose the cause of the scour based on visual evidence rather than guesses and assumptions!

Other than vaccination, the control measures for calf scour are the same irrespective of the pathogen causing the disease. Aside from the environment, compact calving, colostrum, and nutrition, the immunosuppressive effects of BVD virus should always be considered.

In terms of the colostrum factor, when investigating a scour outbreak in calves less than 7 days old, blood sampling the calves to check there has been sufficient passive transfer is recommended (Figure 11.9).

Effective passive transfer in a calf less than 7 days is considered to have been achieved when the blood total protein level exceeds 50 g/l.

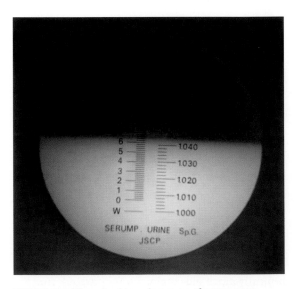

FIGURE 11.9 View looking down a refractometer measuring the level of protein within a calf's blood to assess the level of antibody passive transfer. In this case the result is 62 g/l and is adequate

The main calf scour syndromes

Enterotoxigenic *E. coli*

ETEC affects calves in the first 4 days of life; it rarely affects older cattle (Foster and Smith, 2009). ETEC is a type of *E. coli*; there are many non-pathogenic species and varieties of *E. coli* that live ubiquitously in the environment. ETEC causes disease by the presence of two so called *virulence factors*, special hairs on the bug called K99 fimbria and a particularly nasty heat stable toxin. The special hairs, also known as F5 or K99 antigens, attach the ETEC to the gut wall so it does not just pass straight through the intestinal tract with the milk. The K99 adhere mainly in the ileum where the pH is 6.5 or above, further up the small intestine and into the stomachs the acidity is too high. Once the ETEC attach they multiply, and infection takes hold in the small intestine. Once established the ETEC produces the aforementioned heat stable toxin. This toxin has the effect of switching on fluid secretion in the intestine causing the undesirable phenomenon of hypersecretory diarrhoea – the production of fluid by the intestine at a rate that exceeds its ability to reabsorb the fluid further down the gut (Foster and Smith, 2009). ETEC causes the hypersecretory effect by inhibiting the ability of the gut cells to absorb sodium and chloride (normal salt) but increasing their excretion of chloride into the gut lumen (Grove-White, 2007).

As ETEC is a bacterium, the treatment includes the use of appropriate antibiotics to clear the bacteria from the gut. Rehydration therapy is also needed but care needs to be taken not to use products that contain high concentrations of bicarbonate at risk of alkalinisation of the small intestine and abomasum, an environment which favours ETEC survival.

There are other pathogenic types of *E. coli*, categorised as attaching or effacing. They differ from ETEC as, while they do attach to the gut lining, they do not produce toxins, so they are referred to as enteropathogenic (EPEC) rather than enterotoxigenic (ETEC). The significance of EPEC is unclear as it can be detected in both normal and sick calves.

EPEC causes a malabsorptive type of diarrhoea rather than hypersecretory. These bugs also disrupt the junctions between the gut cells (enterocytes) causing further gut damage. Enterohaemorrhagic *E. coli* (EHEC) also exists which again is of questionable importance in calves but, knowing it affects people, there is a public health concern to consider (Foster and Smith, 2009).

Rotavirus

Rotavirus is, no surprise, a virus; it is very stable in the environment. Rotavirus infects calves through being ingested whereupon it attacks and destroys the cells in the gut lining, especially the villi. Villi are the small finger-like projections that line the gut wall, their job being to increase the surface area for absorption of water, electrolytes and nutrients, and of course colostral immunoglobulins (Figure 11.10). Rotavirus causes diarrhoea by the malabsorptive model (Grove-White, 2007). The gut is left unable to absorb nutrients, water or electrolytes. This alone is bad enough but furthermore the undigested food particles pass to the hind gut and ferment causing the production of the metabolite D-lactate which contributes to a drop in blood pH in the gut and consequently the blood – a state known as acidaemia or, more commonly, acidosis. Rotavirus induced illness is typically seen in calves

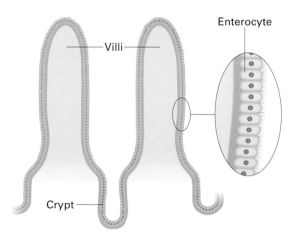

FIGURE 11.10 Schematic diagram of the lining of the small intestine

between 6 days and 3 weeks of life. It has an incubation period of 24 hours (Foster and Smith, 2009).

As stated, the virus targets, invades and kills the mature cells (enterocytes) on the villi rather than those at the base of the villi, in the 'crypts'. This is fortunate as it is in the crypts where new cells are produced and these new cells in turn slide up the villi to replace the lost cells whether lost through natural wear and tear, or, in this context from viral attack. In nature, pathogens often protect the source of their habitat – this is a good example; rotavirus needs enterocytes.

There are no specific medicines to kill the virus and treatment relies on restoring and maintaining hydration status and correcting electrolyte and acid imbalances until the animal's immune measures shed the virus. Plentiful, appropriate fluid therapy achieves this but not all cases survive.

Rotavirus diarrhoea is reported in other species including humans and sheep, but each strain of the virus is species specific; it is not a zoonotic pathogen.

Coronavirus

Bovine coronavirus infection is a cause of enteric disease unlike the well known human coronavirus that causes respiratory disease. Bovine coronavirus is similar to rotavirus and again causes a malabsorptive diarrhoea at 6 days to 3 weeks of age. The clinical signs often last longer than with rotavirus as this virus infects the enterocytes on the villi as well as in the crypts where the new cells are made. This double hit makes the situation worse. Treatment again is through rehydration therapy and even more cases will die.

The scour pathogens themselves do not kill a calf, it is the resulting dehydration, electrolyte loss and drop in blood pH (acidosis) that causes death if not corrected. The acidosis element of the complex is not, however, a feature of hypersecretory diarrhoea, such as is seen with ETEC in the younger calf. This explains the findings of studies that observe acidosis to be more a problem of the slightly older diarrhoeic calf, 6 days old or more that is.

How do we know if a calf is dehydrated?

A calf will not show any outwards signs of being dehydrated until it has exceeded 5–6% dehydration – by that we mean the calf has lost 5–6% of its body weight in water alone. Yes, loss of body fat and other tissue will follow but dehydration hits quickly and can be the sole cause of weight reduction. Death occurs at 14% dehydration. Skin tent, as it is called, is a good indication of dehydration; when the skin of the neck of a calf is lifted and pinched between the thumb and forefinger and then released it should fall flat again within 2 seconds. If it takes between 2 and 6 seconds the calf is 8% dehydrated. Another good place to test skin tent is the eyelid. If the gums are dry to the touch, or pale, this also indicates dehydration. Dehydrated calves have sunken eyes as the fat pad behind the eye shrinks (through water loss and fat burn) and the eye moves further back within the eye socket – this indicates severe dehydration, exceeding 10% (Figure 11.11), which has persisted long enough for fat stores to begin depleting (Grove-White, 2007). In advanced stages of disease, the calf becomes recumbent and unable to stand and the suck reflex and gut motility are lost. The circulatory system then starts to fail, there is reduced blood volume, and blood no longer flows to key organs such as the kidneys; the calf's extremities are cold to the touch, core body temperature drops and then death occurs.

Oral fluid therapy

Oral rehydration therapy (ORT) is a quick and easy technique that farmers can use to treat mild to moderate dehydration without seeking veterinary intervention. ORT is very frequently employed for calves dehydrated by diarrhoea. Oral rehydration is effective while the calf still has a suck reflex. If the calf does not have a suck reflex then it is likely to be so ill that its gastrointestinal tract is no longer functioning properly and the fluids administered

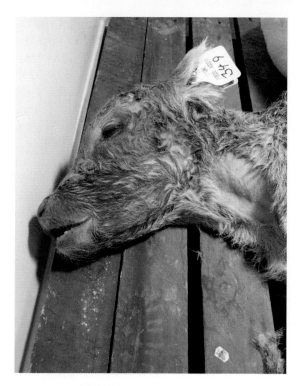

FIGURE 11.11 Calf with sunken eyes suggesting dehydration greater than 10%

will simply sit within the abomasum, they will not move through the gut and they will not be absorbed into the bloodstream. Where this is the case, intravenous fluid therapy is required; this is severe dehydration requiring maximum intervention, here the vet will be needed.

Oral rehydration products need to be formulated with the following in mind (Constable, 2003).

- They need to contain electrolytes (salts), especially sodium, to restore the electrolyte deficit in the calf's body cells.
- They need to contain ingredients that help the damaged gut to absorb sodium and water.
- They need to be alkalinising as neonatal diarrhoea results in the calves becoming acidotic (be careful in cases of ETEC as described previously).
- They should not interfere with milk clotting; unclotted milk passing through the gut can

cause an osmotic diarrhoea that compounds the existing problem.
- They need to provide some form of nutrition, especially energy, for the sick calf. Ongoing milk feeding achieves this but extra energy/amino acids in the rehydration product usefully add to this effect.
- They need to help the gut repair.

A successful formulation contains: sodium, potassium, chloride, acetate or propionate, and glucose. Glutamine is advertised as promoting gut repair but there is limited research to support this (Constable, 2003).

Calves less than a week old have the capacity to hold 3–4 l of fluid in the abomasum at any one time but in the case of a sick scoured calf 2 l of oral fluids is recommended and should be fed every 2 hours initially. The calf still requires its daily intake of milk as well as the water and electrolyte solution to restore dehydration and compensate for ongoing losses. A solution to this may be to alternate 2 l feeds of milk/ORT and water/ORT every 4 hours over a 24 hour period or until the calf is able to suck sufficient quantities itself. Oral fluids can be administered quickly via an oesophageal feeder; the solution will, however, enter the rumen instead of the abomasum. This is not a problem in calves less than 1 week of age but, in older calves, milk fed with an oesophageal feeder will ferment in the rumen and cause a dietary upset. Fresh water should always be available to the sick calf, so it has the choice to drink should it wish to do so.

Intravenous fluid therapy

Intravenous fluid therapy (IVFT), can be administered directly into the bloodstream of a calf via the jugular vein – the large veins on each side of the neck that drain blood from the head back to the heart. An intravenous cannula is inserted into the vein and stitched to the neck; it can remain in place as long as needed, within reason, while fluids are administered (Figure 11.12). This requires

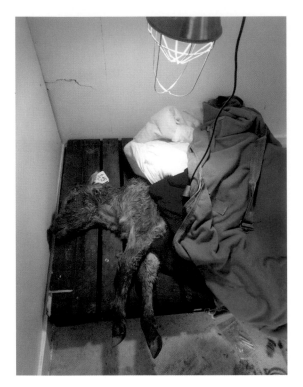

FIGURE 11.12 Calf receiving IVFT while being warmed by a heat lamp and warm air blown from a convection heater underneath a slatted bed

careful supervision as the calf can dislodge the cannula if it is well enough to move about! When vets refer to a percentage value for dehydration, the percentage represents the percentage of the calf's total body weight lacking in the form of fluid, be it blood, or other bodily fluid. For example, a calf that is 10% dehydrated and weighs 50 kg requires 5 l of fluid to restore its hydration status. This does not account for ongoing losses, be they the normal inevitable fluid losses from breathing and urination, or abnormal fluid losses from scour. Consequently, a calf may require up to 15 l of intravenous fluid in a 24-hour period. Initially this can be administered quickly, up to 4 l in the first hour, then at a slower rate thereafter – 1 l per hour. The initial high rate of fluid will restore the volume of blood circulating and help the kidneys to function effectively. The addition of bicarbonate to intravenous fluids has been advocated to neutralise the acid pH of the blood. This has to be

carried out carefully as without advanced laboratory equipment it is impossible to know just how much bicarbonate to administer; too much or too little will not help! It has been suggested by some researchers that as long as standard IV fluids are administered in sufficient quantities to restore kidney function then the kidneys themselves are capable of effectively restoring the pH of the blood, in which case bicarbonate would not need to be added to the fluid. Others prefer the rapid benefit of direct administration of the bicarbonate rather than waiting for kidney function to kick in.

Diarrhoea from calves is potentially infectious to others so affected calves should be moved out of the main calf house for treatment; in the case of the suckled calf the dam will also have to be moved with the calf. If possible, any area they have come into contact with should be cleansed and disinfected. Sick calves are often hypothermic and warming them up, and keeping them warm, is essential for their survival. Heat lamps were traditionally used but they can further dehydrate calves and are a burning, electrical or fire hazard. A heat box is more effective, these are wooden boxes raised off the ground with a slatted floor. An electric convection heater can be placed below the calf – and the warm air rises up through the slats so warming the calf up. Calf coats are also useful in the case of sick calves, but they are only useful for retaining the heat of an already warm calf and will not effectively warm up a cold calf.

SEPTICAEMIA AND SEPSIS

Septicaemia is the state in which an animal has both bacteria and toxins in the bloodstream. Sepsis, the term currently in favour in human medicine, is the inflammatory response the body elicits in the presence of septicaemia.

The most common bacteria detected from culturing the blood of septicaemic animals is *E. coli* (Lofstedt et al., 1999). *E. coli* gains entry into the bloodstream via dirty needles, the navel, the gut or the respiratory tract. When there is inflammation

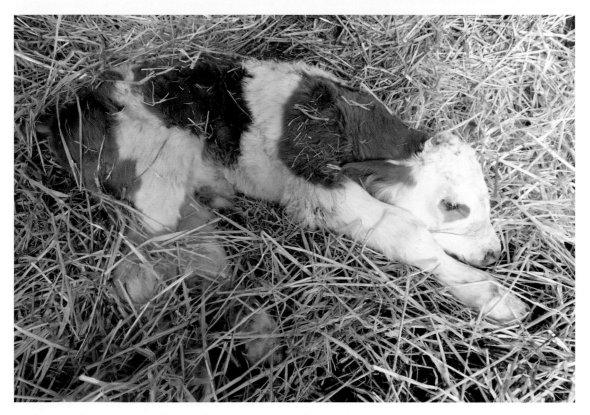

FIGURE 11.13 Septicaemic calf, recumbent, weak and salivating

and damage to the gut lining, as in the case of calf scour, bacteria can cross the wall of the gut and directly enter the bloodstream quite readily; septicaemia and sepsis follow unless the body quickly overwhelms the attack.

Septicaemic calves are weak, have no suck reflex, are recumbent (Figure 11.13) and, initially at least, have a high temperature – above 39.5°C. They often have a wet chin from excessive salivation, they have an elevated respiratory and heart rate, and the normally salmon pink mucous membrane of the eye socket is a darker pink colour, or maybe even brick red.

The bacteria circulating in the bloodstream can infect other tissues such as the brain, the joints and the lungs. The results of this, in order, are meningitis, joint ill and pneumonia. Septicaemia and the subsequent secondary infections are a result of the balance between immunity and challenge, tipping in the favour of the challenge.

A healthy calf has adequate passive transfer of immunity, is well nourished and is living in a clean, dry environment within its thermoneutral zone; this calf has the balance tipped in favour of immunity; it will probably not succumb to septicaemia.

Calves with septicaemia need to be treated promptly with intravenous antibiotics and IVFT and supportive care. The prognosis is poor. Even if the calf survives there may be irreparable organ damage resulting in poor growth rates. Euthanasia is warranted in some cases.

FAILURE OF PASSIVE TRANSFER

Failure of passive transfer is where a calf does not get sufficient immunoglobulins via the colostrum (further information on colostrum management in Chapter 4). When this is further investigated it can be down to three main reasons.

1. The calf did not suck quickly enough – the window of opportunity for immunoglobulin absorption was missed.
2. The calf did not ingest enough colostrum. The 'cow reasons' for this may be the dam not allowing the calf to suck, or her not having milk, maybe due to mastitis. She may not stand; she may not be able to stand. She may kick the calf off, or she may have poor udder conformation or large teats such that the calf cannot suck. 'Calf reasons' for this may be that the calf failed to stand as a result of dystocia. The calf may have trace element deficiencies. The problem may be one of prematurity, or the calf may have been stood on by the cow.
3. The colostrum was of poor quality. It is the stockperson's responsibility to supplement the calf with an alternative source if there are concerns.

It is also the stockperson's role to prevent these reasons arising in the first place!

More research is required into the ability of the calf to absorb colostral immunoglobulins from the gut. There has been research carried out in sheep to suggest that high levels of iodine in the ewe's diet prevents adequate absorption of colostral immunoglobulins in neonatal lambs (Boland et al., 2008). A pilot study has suggested this may also be the case in cows (Moredun, 2019). Further research is required to clarify if this is the case and at what level iodine in a pre-calving ration is no longer safe.

RESPIRATORY DISEASE

While not particularly common, infectious respiratory disease can affect calves at a very young age, depending on the pathogens on the farm, the immune status of the calf and dam and the level of challenge from the pathogen. Bovine respiratory disease is discussed in Chapter 13.

REFERENCES

Anderson, D.E. and St. Jean, G. (2008) Management of Fractures in Field Settings. *Veterinary Clinics of North America: Food Animal Practice* 24, 567–582.

Andrews, A.H. (2004) Other calf problems. In: Andrews, A.H., Blowey, R.W., Boyd, H. and Eddy, R.G. (eds) *Bovine Medicine Diseases and Husbandry of Cattle*, 2nd edn. Blackwell Science, Oxford, 249–264.

Armstrong, S.C. Jonsson, N.N. and Barrett, D.C. (2002) Bovine congenital erythrocytic protoporphyria in a Limousin calf bred in the UK. *Vet Record* 150, 608–610.

Bazeley, K. (2003) Investigation of diarrhoea in the neonatal calf. *In Practice* 25, 152–159.

Boland, T.M., Hayes, L., Sweeney, T., Callan, J.J., Baird, A.W., Keely, S. and Crosby, T.F. (2008) The effects of cobalt and iodine supplementation of the pregnant ewe diet on immunoglobulin G, Vitamin E, T3 and T4 levels in the progeny. *Animal* 2(2), 197–206.

Constable, P. (2003) Fluid and electrolyte therapy in ruminants. *Vet Clinics of North America: Food Animal Practice* 19(3), 557–597.

Davies, I., Vellema, P. and Roger, P. (2012) Schmallenberg virus – an emerging novel pathogen. *In Practice* 34, 598–604.

Edwards, B. (1992) Umbilical hernias and infections in calves. *In Practice* 14, 163–170.

Foster, D.M. and Smith, G.W. (2009) Pathophysiology of diarrhoea inc. *Veterinary Clinics of North America: Food Animal Practice* 25, 13–36.

Grove-White, D. (2000) Resuscitation of the newborn calf. *In Practice* 22, 17–23.

Grove-White, D. (2007) Practical intravenous fluid therapy in the diaroeic calf. *In Practice* 29, 404–408.

Leipold, H.W., Hiraga, T.H. and Dennis, S. M. (1993) Congenital defects of the bovine musculoskeletal system and joints. *Veterinary Clinics of North America: Food Animal Practice* 9(1), 93–104.

Lofstedt, J., Dohoo, I.R. and Glen, G. (1999) Model to predict septicemia in diarrheic calves. *Journal of Veterinary Internal Medicine* 13, 81–88.

Mason, C. and Caldow, G. (2012) Calf diarrhoea. The Moredun Foundation. News sheet 5(14).

Mee, J.F. (1991) Perinatal calf mortality – recent findings. *Irish Veterinary Journal* 44, 80.

Moredun Magazine (2019) Issue 17 Spring/summer, 12–13.

Mulon, P. (2013) Management of ling bone fractures in cattle. *In Practice* 35, 265–271.

Noakes, D.E., Parkinson, T.J. and England, G.C.W. (2009) Dystocia and disorders associated with parturition. In: *Veterinary Reproduction and Obstetrics*, 9th edn. Elsevier, Amsterdam, pp. 270–271.

Otter, A. (1995) Bovine congenital neospora caninum infection. *In Practice* 17, 382.

Patterson, D., Bellows, R. and Burfening, P. (1987) Occurrence of neonatal and post natal mortality in beef range cattle. 1 Calf loss incidence from birth to weaning, backwards and breech presentation and effects of calf loss on subsequent pregnancy rate of dams. *Theriogenology* 28, 557–571.

Penny, C.D., Howie, F., Nettleton, P.F., Sargison, N.D. and Schock, A. (2002) Upper respiratory disease and encephalitis in neonatal beef calves caused by bovine herpesvirus type 1. *Vet Record* July, 89–91.

Perry, V.E.A, Copping, K.J., Miguel-Pacheco, G. and Hernandez-Medrano, J. (2019) The effects of developmental Programming upon Neonatal Mortality. *Veterinary Clinics of North America: Food Animal Practice* 35, 289–302.

Steiner, A., Anderson, D.E. and Desrochers, A. (2014) Diseases of the tendon and tendon sheaths. *Veterinary Clinics of North America: Food Animal Practice* 30, 157–175.

Toombs, R.E., Wikse, S.E. and Kasari, T.R. (1994) The incidence, causes, and financial impact of perinatal mortality in North American beef herds, *Veterinary Clinics of North America: Food Animal Practice* 10, 137–146.

Wernike, K. Holsteg, M., Schirrmeier, H., Hoffmann, B. and Beer, M. (2014) Infection of pregnant cows with Schmallenberg virus – a follow up study. *PLOS ONE* 9(5).

White, P.J. and Windsor, P.A. (2012) Congenital chondrodystrophy of unknown origin in beef herds. *The Veterinary Journal* 193, 336–343.

FURTHER READING

Desrochers, A. and Francoz, D. (2014) Clinical management of septic arthritis in cattle. *Veterinary Clinics of North America: Food Animal Practice* 30, 177–203.

Hartnack, A.K. (2017) Spinal cord and peripheral nerve abnormalities of the ruminant. *Veterinary Clinics of North America: Food Animal Practice* 33, 101–110.

SAC Consulting News (2013) Dwarf calf syndrome, September.

Truyers, I. and Ellis, K. (2013) Case report: bovine congenital erythropoietic protoporphyria in a pedigree Limousin herd. *Livestock* 18(2).

Chapter 12

Disease and production failure in the young calf to weaning

GASTROINTESTINAL DISEASE

Cryptosporidiosis

Cryptosporidium parvum, to give it its full name, is not a bacterium or a virus but is a parasite, a tiny single celled parasite known as a protozoa. There are 65,000 species of protozoa, many are completely harmless and live harmoniously in the environment or in the gastrointestinal tract of many different animals (Taylor, 2000). As with many basic life forms, protozoa have a lifecycle composed of different stages. The protozoa that have adapted to live parasitically have an infectious stage of the lifecycle – this is the encapsulated egg known as the oocyst. The oocyst survives in the environment. After ingestion by the host the oocyst passes through the stomachs. It is while passing through the acidic abomasum that the oocyst hatches and releases the next stage of the lifecycle – four motile sporozoites which have the ability to burrow into the cells of the gut wall, the enterocytes, and indeed do when they reach the ileum in the small intestine (Chapter 11, Figure 11.10). *Cryptosporidium* spp. are actually capable of attaching anywhere in the small or large intestine and not just the ileum, but they do prefer the ileum. The reproductive lifecycle continues in the gut wall; the sporozoites grow up into the next stages which ultimately generate huge numbers of oocysts which burst out of the enterocyte. This stage of the lifecycle is complex but extremely efficient. The faeces of an infected calf can shed up to 100 million oocysts per gram of faeces (Foster, 2009). Infected enterocytes explode and die during the release of the oocysts. So many enterocytes die that the villi (Chapter 11, Figure 11.10) shrink in an attempt to maintain a continuous gut lining with the ever decreasing number of enterocytes left. A malabsorptive diarrhoea results. The recesses, or crypts as they are called, between the villi, do respond by producing new cells as fast as they can to restore the gut lining, but they often fail to keep up with the rate of cell loss. Calves are infected soon after birth and show signs of disease a few days after, typically 7–21 days old. They are subdued and mildly dehydrated with a pasty scour which is usually seen stuck to their tail and back ends. Their coats are dull, and they fail to thrive. In severe cases the calf is severely dehydrated due to a profuse watery scour and is recumbent. Death can result, mainly due to the dehydration.

Transmission is through ingesting oocysts in infected faeces. This can be on the udder and teats, the mother's coat or on the ground or bedding. As with most scour pathogens the number of oocysts in the environment will build up as the calving period progresses, most cases are seen from 3 to 4 weeks into the calving season onwards. Poor hygiene, an extended calving period and high stocking densities are all risk factors for this disease, as it is for some other types of scour. Although infection is most concentrated within buildings, calves can be infected with *Cryptosporidium* spp. while out at grass, particularly if the land is contaminated by natural water courses that contain faeces. This can include human sewage as humans and livestock can share the same species of *Cryptosporidium*; cryptosporidiosis is a zoonosis and can cause severe disease in humans too. This same species of *Cryptosporidium* can also infect lambs and foals too.

Cryptosporidiosis is easily diagnosed by obtaining a faeces sample from an infected calf and examining it under a microscope using a Ziehl–Neilson (ZN) staining technique. This highlights the oocysts. Oocysts are excreted from 6 days after infection and are immediately infective to others; the infectious state lasts a number of weeks (Wyatt, 2010).

Treatment for cryptosporidium should focus on rehydration therapy. Halofuginate is a product licensed in the UK for the prevention and treatment of calf cryptosporidiosis. It is administered prophylactically (as a preventative) to calves orally for 7 days after birth. It is reported to decrease the severity of clinical signs and reduce the number of oocysts shed by infected calves and consequently lessen the environmental contamination (Wyatt et al., 2010). This is only the case while the halofuginate is being administered, after administration stops the calves which are already infected go on to shed high numbers of oocysts and those not already infected are likely to become so (Foster and Smith, 2009). Daily administration of this product is laborious and in the case of protective mothers, dangerous!

An antibiotic – paromomycin – has been used in an attempt to control cryptospordial infection on farm. It is, again, administered every day, orally, to the whole group of calves. As with halofuginate, once treatment stops, infection and shedding resume. The blanket use of antibiotic for prophylaxis is not considered responsible and for this reason alone this is not a viable control option. Decoquinate has also been trialled as a control option for cryptosporidial infection on the basis that it is effective in the control of other protozoal diseases, namely coccidiosis, but studies suggest it to have little or no effect (Foster and Smith, 2009).

With no effective treatment, prevention of cryptosporidiosis is the key. Cryptosporidial oocysts are highly resistant and persist in the environment for long periods of time (Mason and Caldow, 2012). For disinfection of the environment, cleaning is first required. Hot water, 60°C or higher, kills oocysts. Ammonia based disinfectants are most effective against the oocysts but have highly irritant fumes. Other products that are available, that kill oocysts in the environment, are Kenocox™ (an amine), Sorgene 5™ (and other peroxides such as hydrogen peroxide) and peracetic acid-based products (Mason and Caldow, 2012).

Calves and cows do produce antibodies against *C. parvum*, and the antibodies do pass into bovine colostrum. This would suggest that colostral protection is valuable, which is indeed considered to be the case, but also that a dam-administered vaccine could be a potential possibility. Experimentally, cows have been vaccinated with oocysts and their colostrum fed to calves. When the calves were then infected with cryptosporidium oocysts the clinical signs were far less severe and the calves were seen to shed significantly less oocysts subsequently. Unfortunately, the cows required multiple injections to produce a sufficient antibody response and it was deemed not to be practical or cost effective in a commercial scenario (Wyatt et al., 2010). With improved vaccine technology there may still be hope in this area.

Once calves have been infected with *Cryptosporidium* spp. they tend not to suffer from the disease again thanks to residual immunity. Mixed infection of *Cryptosporidium* spp. with an enteric virus (rotavirus or coronavirus) (Chapter 11) or a bacterial infection such as salmonella does occur.

Coccidiosis

Coccidiosis, like cryptosporidiosis, is a protozoal infection, the protozoa in this case being *Eimeria* spp. of which, unlike *Cryptosporidium*, there are many species, some pathogenic (disease causing) and some not. *E. bovis* and *E. zuernii* are the main pathogenic species infecting cattle. Disease associated with *E. alabamensis* has also been reported in calves shortly after turn out (Marshall et al., 1998). Most animals can suffer from coccidiosis – mammals and birds notably, but the *Eimeria* involved are very species specific so different animals do not infect each other – for example cattle do not catch coccidiosis from sheep, or from birds, or vice versa. Mixed infections are the norm with three or four different *Eimeria* spp. routinely being detected in one animal. Co-infections with the likes of salmonella and cryptosporidium are also commonplace.

Infection is through the ingestion of other infected animals' faeces that contain the infectious coccidial oocysts (eggs). The oocysts attack and inhabit the cells in the gut lining of the host. Infections are commonly seen in spring-born calves at grass in early summer, but infection can also occur in housed cattle. Calves are typically between 3 weeks and 6 months when they are infected (Mason and Caldow, 2012). Affected calves present with pasty diarrhoea; red flecks of blood and mucus may be seen. The calves typically strain to pass faeces and appear to have abdominal discomfort. Some coccidial species will attack the small intestine and others the large intestine. Small intestinal infections appear to be less severe – this is largely because the large intestine can compensate by absorbing some nutrients and water. Large intestinal infections are more severe as there is no compensatory mechanism and the turnover of new cells to repair the damage is slower (Taylor, 2000). An infected calf can shed up to 80,000 oocysts per gram of faeces (Bazeley, 2003). As the number of oocysts in the herd's environment increases, more calves become infected but the extent to which they suffer from the disease will vary depending on the species of *Eimeria* they are infected with, the number of oocysts ingested and the immune status of the calf. Subclinical infection is a common finding where the calves are not scoured but have a dull coat and more or less achieve expected weight gains. Up to 95% of coccidial infections are subclinical (Bazeley, 2003). Unfortunately, however,

a coccidial burden does typically decrease feed intakes by up to 60% for up to 28 days so while often subclinical they are nevertheless significant (Daugschies and Najdrowski, 2005).

Coccidial oocysts are easily detected in the faeces of infected animals but this test is limited as animals can show severe clinical signs and die before oocysts are present in the faeces, and also affected animals tend to shed oocysts only intermittently. This simply means a negative coccidial count does not rule out disease. It does, all the same, remain a useful test. The technique to prepare the sample is the same as that used to carry out a worm egg count. Similarly to worm egg counts, a low number is unlikely to be significant and is, in fact, perfectly normal. Different species of coccidia look the same using basic microscopy, Figure 12.1. If a diagnosis of the specific species is required then this requires the expertise of a specialist laboratory who will embryonate the oocysts and then with a skilled eye, speciate the coccidia in the sample. The results are often reported as a percentage of each species within the sample as well

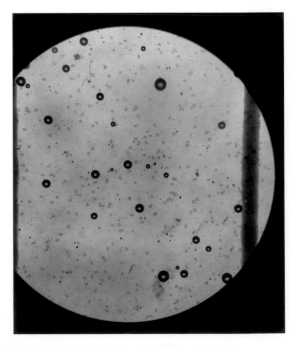

FIGURE 12.1 Coccidial oocysts viewed under a microscope (larger dark circles are air bubbles)

as a total oocyst count per gram. Speciation can take up to 10 days and the calves cannot wait that long before they are treated so a treatment plan is usually instigated before the results come back.

Treatment in severely affected animals involves rehydration therapy and supportive care. Calves should be isolated to minimise environmental contamination. Antimicrobials are sometimes warranted to prevent translocation of bacteria over the damaged gut wall. One class of antibacterial agent, namely the sulphonamides, have activity against coccidia as well as bacteria so they are sometimes prescribed to deliver both desired effects (Taylor, 2000). Decoquinate can be used as a feed additive for the prevention and treatment of coccidial disease but this drug needs to be fed over the entire risk period because it acts only on specific stages of the coccidial life cycle (Daugschies and Najdrowski, 2005). Oral drenches containing diclazuril or toltrazuril are licensed to treat and prevent coccidiosis. The timing of diclazuril or toltrazuril administration should be just before the onset of clinical signs so some immunity is allowed to develop from exposure to a low number of oocysts but before there is growth limiting damage to the gut, and, before there is widespread heavy environmental contamination. Widespread use of anticoccidial treatments in the poultry industry has led to the development of resistance within the coccidial population. It can only be assumed at this stage that the same is possible in bovine Eimeria species. For this reason, control should not rely on anticoccidial treatments alone (Daugschies and Najdrowski, 2005).

Calves enjoy some protection against coccidiosis from maternally derived colostral antibodies; this lasts a few weeks (Taylor, 2000). During this time exposed calves generate a strong immune response and good immunity to coccidial infection, and they go on to be resistant to infection. Low-level exposure, therefore, can be a good thing, the calf becomes immune without suffering from disease. Disease, on the other hand, can occur in older animals if they have not been exposed earlier in life or if they have a weak immune system, or if

the challenge is high. The immunity is not absolute and even healthy adult animals will have a few oocysts in their faeces – this is normal, but it does mean the coccidial lifecycle is perpetuated through ongoing environmental contamination.

Coccidiosis is considered a disease of intensification. The more cattle there are in a given area at a given time the higher becomes the risk of disease. Prevention is through blocking or limiting access by young calves to areas contaminated with oocysts. The oocysts are, unfortunately, ubiquitous in the environment so this preventative approach may prove challenging. For example, the oocysts can survive up to 12 months on pasture in the right conditions and in hay cut from contaminated pastures even after 8 months of storage (Daugschies and Najdrowski, 2005). Hygiene within buildings, namely a clean, dry disinfected environment, can make a difference – oocysts do not like the cool or the dry and certain disinfectants will kill them. Building design should ensure feed and water troughs are not easily contaminated with faeces. Certain pastures that have been grazed by animals shedding oocysts in the past will pose a risk and should be avoided; generally, cows and young calves should not graze the same pastures year on year. Creep feeders should be moved regularly to fresh ground as this is often an area where calves lie, and this inevitably creates a higher challenge from the coccidial oocysts.

Necrotising enteritis

This is a relatively rare sporadic gastrointestinal condition of suckled calves 2–3 months of age. The cause of the disease is, as yet, unknown. Affected calves have diarrhoea associated with ulceration throughout the gastrointestinal tract. Pneumonia and kidney disease are also a feature. Calves usually die from this disease (Caldow and Munro, 1995). The clinical signs are similar to those seen in mucosal disease, the clinical syndrome that eventually befalls cattle that are persistently infected with BVD virus. That being the case the presence of BVD virus should always be ruled out before a diagnosis of necrotising enteritis is assumed (Chapter 15).

Salmonellosis

Salmonellosis is the disease caused by any species of the notable and infamous bacterium that is *Salmonella*. There are many species and subtypes of *Salmonella* – some infect just one species of host, in our case cattle, others infect many host species. *S. Dublin*, for example, is fairly cattle specific whereas *S. typhimurium* affects many different species including cattle, man and others. The most common *Salmonella* species affecting cattle are *S. dublin*, *S. typhimurium*, *S. mbandaka* and *S. newport* (Hateley, 2017). Salmonellosis can, clearly, in some cases at least, be zoonotic (infecting humans) and this is usually a result of direct contact with infected cattle or their faeces or, less usually, through drinking unpasteurised milk or eating unpasteurised dairy products (Henderson and Mason, 2017). It is the second most common reported cause of food poisoning in humans worldwide (Hateley, 2017) Not only can humans contract salmonellosis from cattle, but cattle can from humans, and from other species such as wildlife, and of course from each other. *S. mbandaka* has been isolated from cattle feed containing soya and rape meal, and cattle feed is thought to be the route of introduction of this species into cattle herds (Carrique-Mas et al., 2010). Salmonellosis is a disease seen more commonly in the dairy herd than the beef herd, but infection is still possible and should be considered, especially in more intensive situations.

Salmonellae can be carried, multiplied and shed in the faeces of apparently healthy animals so are easily introduced to a herd inadvertently. These infected healthy animals are referred to as active carriers. Passive carriers also exist, these are the animals that ingest salmonellae, which transiently pass through the gastrointestinal tract and out in the faeces but with no multiplication in the gut. Active carriers are previously infected animals that continue to excrete bacteria in high numbers; 1 million bacteria per gram, and for up to several years if not for life (Jones et al., 2004). They are highly infectious and cause a large amount of environmental contamination. The dose of bacteria required to infect an animal is high compared to other pathogens but the infectious dose that will cause disease is dependent on the health of the animal; again, a balance between challenge and immunity. A calf with adequate colostral antibody, and one that is dry, warm and well nourished, will be less likely to succumb to disease. The acidic pH of the abomasum should be sufficient to kill salmonellae after ingestion but if the animal is not recently fed, or if it happens to before the first feed of colostrum or if the calf is being treated with alkalinising agents such as bicarbonate in an electrolyte formula, the pH will not be sufficiently low to kill the bacteria and they will pass through the abomasum to the small intestine. It is in the small intestine they most commonly cause disease. Salmonellae are able to overcome the natural defences of the intestine and move around in the lumen using a flagella – a small tail like appendage rather like that of a tadpole – to locate an appropriate site where they can penetrate the gut lining and invade the enterocytes, the cells that line the gut. The ileum (the last portion of the small intestine) is the preferred location for salmonellae. Salmonellae stimulate a secretory response by the enterocytes and the gut wall produces large amounts of fluid resulting in diarrhoea. Damaging to the host, this mechanism does assist the bacteria in spreading far and wide and in large numbers in a copious outpouring of watery faecal liquid that helps keep the bug alive while it waits in the environment for its next host.

Salmonellae can, on their own, cause diarrhoea or they can do it in association with other pathogens such as rotavirus as part of a mixed infection. Once within a population, salmonellae travel readily from animal to animal via the ingestion of infected faeces. Hygiene again is therefore of paramount importance in the control of this disease.

In calves up to 6 weeks of age septicaemia associated with salmonellosis is a common presentation; calves are acutely affected, fevered, recumbent, salivating, lacking a suck reflex, dull, depressed, dehydrated and toxic. The bacteria gain entry to the circulation and consequently to other organs, such as the liver and lungs, through the lymph nodes that drain the gastrointestinal tract. Pneumonia, joint ill, sloughing of ear tips and the tail tip and meningitis are occasional manifestations of septicaemic salmonellosis. *Salmonella* spp. has been detected in other organs of the body within 6 hours of infection. Infection of the liver is a classic step by this bug; the bacteria can make home in the gall bladder and be intermittently shed in the bile. This infected bile repeatedly re-infects the gut so resulting in prolonged, chronic, intermittent shedding of the bacteria by the host animal (Jones et al., 2004).

S. dublin infection of adult cows, most frequently dairy cows, has a fairly distinct geographical distribution within the UK finding itself predominantly in the south west and north west of England (Carrique-Mas et al., 2010). This may be an association with the UK's dairy population, the wetter environment or it has been postulated there is a relationship between *S. dublin* and liver fluke infection – fluke infection is traditionally more prevalent in the west where higher rainfall and suitable habitats for the mud snail, a key part of the fluke lifecycle, are commonplace. Adult cows infected with *S. dublin*, with or without liver fluke, present with diarrhoea, a fever and milk drop. Abortion is a common sequel as a result of the fever or bacterial multiplication within the placenta. Abortion can occur before, during or after the cow's apparent illness; sometimes the cow will abort without any signs of illness in herself at all.

The clinical signs and post-mortem changes associated with salmonellosis are not unique to the disease, so further laboratory testing is required to achieve a diagnosis. Salmonellae are readily cultured in a laboratory and as they are excreted in high numbers from affected calves it is usually readily diagnosed. Post-mortem samples can be taken from the liver (particularly the gall bladder), the gut and, for evidence of systemic spread, the lung. If the animal has previously been treated with antibiotics then this can interfere with the diagnosis as the bacteria may have been eliminated. In recent years blood testing for antibodies to salmonellae has been adopted as a diagnostic aid, particularly in dairy herds. This test establishes if there has been exposure of the tested youngstock to salmonellae but does not confirm causal association with any disease observed – this is a matter of judgement. A group of ten calves from each separately managed group are sampled, ideally between 100 and 300 days of age (Henderson and Mason, 2017). As with any antibody surveillance initiative it is a retrospective study; it takes 1–6 weeks for antibodies to be generated to the infection, peaking at 5–6 weeks. Care has to be taken in the interpretation of the results in the case of calves less than 3 months of age; here antibodies in the calf's bloodstream from colostral transfer may still be detectable and provide a false positive result (Henderson and Mason, 2017).

Treatment of salmonellosis requires fluid therapy and, questionably, antibiotic therapy. Interestingly antibiotics are not always used in the treatment of human salmonellosis. They do not shorten the duration of clinical signs and can actually lengthen the period of bacterial shedding post-infection (Jones et al., 2004). Furthermore, inadequate doses of antibiotic worsen the disease by killing only the natural bacterial population of the gut rather than the salmonella itself. The natural bacteria of the gut contribute to the host's defence against infection so removing them helps the salmonellae to colonise the gut. Salmonellae are particularly good at adapting to their environment, the greatest of all survival mechanisms, and their ability to develop resistance to several antibiotics has been a worrying feature of recent times. This is more prevalent with *S. typhimurum* than *S. dublin* (Jones et al., 2004). Despite this backdrop of knowledge in human medicine, antibiotic therapy is still advocated in the treatment of salmonellosis in cattle given the bacteria's ability to spread throughout the body and cause high morbidity and mortality if left untreated. The choice of antibiotic should be dependent on what that particular strain of salmonella is sensitive to; that is only known through laboratory testing.

A vaccine providing protection from S. *dublin* and S. *typhimurium* is commercially available. This vaccine is given to the dam pre-calving. Protection of young calves relies on the colostral transfer of the antibodies produced in response to the vaccination.

Control of salmonellosis within an infected herd is based on the challenge versus immunity concept:

- adequate environment – clean, dry and well ventilated
- isolation of infected animals
- good isolation facility management to prevent infected faeces being transmitted to other unaffected animal on equipment or personnel
- control of concurrent disease such as BVD, liver fluke
- adequate nutrition – including trace element supplementation
- adequate passive transfer and good colostrum management
- sensible stocking density to minimise faecal contamination of the environment
- minimal mixing of animals – group sizes should be small and stable
- biosecurity – purchased/returning animal policies, visitors, equipment, wildlife, vermin and water supplies.

In the case of beef-cross dairy calves, disease control can be improved by removing calves from the calving area and from their mothers as soon as practically possible, a controversial practice known as *snatch calving*. Here the calf, in theory, does not have the chance to become infected from the faeces of actively shedding carrier cows. The pasteurisation of colostrum and the feeding of powdered milk will help further in preventing the infection of youngstock. Calf and heifer housing and workflow on the farm should be designed so that youngstock are not exposed to the faeces of adult cows.

Abomasal ulceration

Abomasal ulceration, areas of loss of the abomasal stomach lining, occurs predominantly in artificially reared calves but is occasionally seen in suckled calves. Affected calves present with abdominal pain, excessive salivation and distention of the abdomen. If the ulcers are haemorrhaging then the faeces may be dark or even black in colour – a result of the presence of tar like semi-digested blood. Affected calves may show no outward clinical signs and the ulcers are only detected on post-mortem examination (PME) as an incidental finding. That is not to say the calves were free of discomfort or experiencing reduced growth rates. These undiagnosed ulcers can be the cause of sudden death if they suddenly result in severe haemorrhage through the erosion of a blood vessel or if they result in acute peritonitis following perforation and the leakage of gut contents and abomasal acid into the abdomen. The exact cause of abomasal ulcers is unknown but it is thought that undigested forage may pass through the rumen to the abomasum and cause physical damage to its lining which is thinner and more fragile than that of the fore-stomachs, which, in their cases are designed for forage. Ulcers are also seen in association with hair balls in the abomasum – again the rough hair may cause physical erosion. Hair balls are formed when calves excessively lick themselves or lick others; this is thought to commonly result from discomfort or stress (Blowey, 2004). In short, abomasal ulceration may be a result of poor calf husbandry.

Ruminal bloat

Ruminal bloat is more common in artificially reared calves but occurs in suckled calves too.

There is an obvious distention of the abdomen predominantly on the left-hand side just behind the ribs. Affected calves are dull, uncomfortable and reluctant to feed. Bloat is an abnormal build-up of gas or froth in the rumen. In the case of gas this is a mix of methane and carbon dioxide produced by the fermentation and respiration activity of the bugs in the rumen. The production of this gas is normal, but three things can go wrong. The first problem that can cause excessive gas accumulation is when the oesophageal groove is functioning incorrectly and ingested milk is entering the rumen instead of the abomasum. Finding itself in the rumen in the presence of yeast enzymes, among others, this milk ferments rapidly and an excessive amount of carbon dioxide is released. This gas blows up the rumen so quickly that it essentially kinks the outlet trapping the gas. The second thing that can cause excessive gas accumulation is when the calf is ingesting too little rough fibre and too much readily digestible carbohydrate, for example in the form of creep feed. The result is an abnormally low pH in the rumen. This acidic liquid is so strong it is capable of damaging the lining of the rumen. This seems to result in paralysis of the rumen and an inability to belch out the gas – the result being bloat. The third thing that can cause excessive gas accumulation is 'choke'. While choke in humans usually refers to a blockage of the windpipe, in cattle we use the term to describe a blockage of the oesophagus. This can be the swallowing of a foreign body like a whole potato or a result of something compressing the oesophagus from the outside, such as an abscess or a tumour. In a state of choke any attempt to belch out gas fails so bloat develops.

Sometimes, although less commonly, the bloat is not the presence of gas but instead a mixture of gas and liquid in the form of a foam – this is known as frothy bloat. The cause is the presence of foaming agents in the diet – typically certain proteinaceous forages like alfalfa, clover, rich leys and kale (Blowey, 2004).

The first course of action is to relieve the calf of the pressure in the rumen which is otherwise painful and potentially enough to compromise the diaphragm and the calf's ability to breath. This should be carried out with an appropriately sized stomach tube. The tube should be passed via the mouth but through a protective casing/tube as it is entirely possible for calves of this age to chew through the stomach tube. When the tube reaches the rumen then gas will be expelled from the rumen; froth is less obliging and may exude slowly or not at all. If frothy bloat is identified, then antifoaming agents should be used – proprietary products including poloxalene or simethicone are available but in their absence linseed oil can be used at a rate of 10 ml per 100 kg bodyweight. All feed should be withdrawn, including milk, for 2 days and electrolyte solution and water alone fed. A standard dose of penicillin can be administered but, on this occasion only, it is to be given orally to kill the population of bacteria (lactobacilli) in the rumen that are causing the excessive fermentation and gas production (Blowey, 2004). This would, ordinarily, be most wrong and ill advised! Feed and milk should be gradually re-introduced into the diet with, importantly, the provision of adequate roughage. If more than one case occurs a systematic review of feeding practices should be carried out.

Necrotic stomatitis (calf diphtheria)

Calf diphtheria is a fairly common condition of the suckled and artificially reared calf between 2 weeks and 3 months of age. It is caused by the bacterium *Fusobacterium necrophorum*, a bug that invades the mucosa, the pink skin like tissue that lines the mouth and covers the tongue. Calves that are affected drool saliva, are reluctant to suck or eat, have smelly breath (halitosis) and sometimes have a swelling or distension of one or both cheeks, the distension resulting from the cheek pouch filling with food. On opening the mouth there is a large area of ulceration and infection. There is usually a white layer covering the affected area – this is necrotic mucosa, hence the name. The infectious agent, *F. necrophorum*, is present in the environment, it usually invades the mucosa secondary to damage from rough creep feed, thistles, very fibrous roughage or straw (Holliman, 2005). The condition is easily treated with penicillin-type antibiotics given by injection for 2–4 days. A dilute iodine solution can also be used as a mouth wash, but care should be taken to avoid ingestion or inhalation of the solution, which could cause toxicity or respiratory damage, respectively. The condition is noticeably infectious with infection passing between calves via teats and water buckets. Affected calves should be isolated, the cause of the abrasions identified and the hygiene of the calf feeding process reviewed.

MUSCULOSKELETAL DISEASE

Hypovitaminosis A (Vitamin A deficiency)

Blindness is the most notable clinical sign of Vitamin A deficiency (Figure 12.2) and can be seen in cattle at any age although growing cattle have a higher demand for Vitamin A making it most prevalent in cattle less than 24 months old. Congenital abnormalities in calves associated with low Vitamin A levels in the dam have been reported; these calves born to deficient dams are not just blind, they have abnormal formation of their eyes and eye sockets, which may be noticable at birth (Mason et al., 2003). Cattle eating green forage or at grass are less at risk than housed cattle on a concentrate or straw ration. Vitamin and mineral supplements added to feed often contain adequate Vitamin A but it deteriorates quickly in stored product, so it is important that the 'best before' date on the packaging is adhered to. The blindness is a result of deterioration of structures and chemicals within the eye and the initial clinical sign is night blindness although this will not be so readily detected. The condition up to this point may be reversible by administering Vitamin A injection (Van Donkersgoed and Clark, 1988).

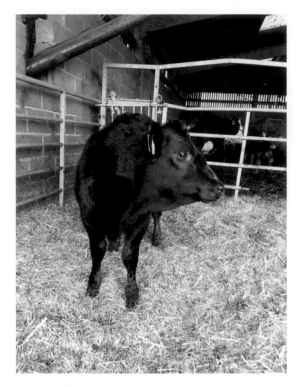

FIGURE 12.2 Suckled calf presenting with blindness that was later diagnosed as having hypovitaminosis A (Vitamin A deficiency)

As the disease progresses there is a narrowing of the bony channel at the back of the eye socket, the channel through which the optic nerve passes. As the optic nerve is necessary for sight the bony compression of the nerve causes irreversible blindness. Supplementation at this stage is futile.

White muscle disease (nutritional muscular dystrophy)

WMD is a nutritional muscular dystrophy associated with a dietary deficiency in Vitamin E and/or selenium. The disease primarily affects well-muscled, young, fast-growing calves. In the early stages of the disease, the calf appears stiff and reluctant to move; muscle tremors may be evident. As time passes the calf can only stand for short periods of time and the skeletal muscle of the rump and shoulder feel firm to the touch; this is symmetrical unlike with some localised soft tissue injuries (Radostits et al., 1994). The disease progresses to recumbency and ultimately death; where the muscles of the heart or breathing are affected (in the case of breathing, the diaphragm and intercostal muscles) then death may follow surprisingly quickly, sometimes within hours, and appearing, at times therefore, as sudden death. Congenital WMD has been reported (Abutarbush and Radostits, 2003) and it is assumed in these cases that the dam was deficient in selenium and Vitamin E so resulting in the calf being born already deficient.

If Vitamin E and selenium levels in the blood are below a required level, cell membranes become damaged; this is particularly evident in highly active muscle cells (Abutarbush and Radostits, 2003). Selenium and Vitamin E have a role in protecting these cell membranes against damage from the inevitable, naturally existing, waste products in the blood known as free radicals. Their main function appears to be an antioxidant effect on the otherwise damaging, oxidising effect these free radicals have on some body chemicals – notably the phospholipids in cell membranes. Once Vitamin E and selenium levels are increased the damage stops and repair begins; the calf returns to normal over a period of a few days. An injectable formulation of Vitamin E, in the form of alpha-tocopheryl acetate, and selenium, in the form of potassium selenate, is available for the treatment and prevention of WMD.

The diagnosis is based on clinical signs, backed up by a biochemical test to detect raised muscle enzymes released into the blood from the damaged muscle cells. The enzyme is not specific to WMD and any muscle damage, for example, from a difficult calving or a traumatic injury, or even from an injection site, will result in raised muscle enzymes. If death has occurred and post-mortem material is available, the changes within the muscle are specific and detectable on microscopic examination of the muscle tissues. Some texts describe grey streaks visible to the naked eye within affected muscle; while suggestive of WMD, this is not always the case.

Vitamin E naturally exists as various tocopherols. Measuring tocopherols in the blood and liver is a good indication of Vitamin E status but this advanced test can only be done by some laboratories. Selenium levels in blood and tissues, such as liver, can also be measured and aid in a diagnosis but again this is a test only done by some laboratories. Liver sampling and testing for Vitamin E and selenium at PME is ultimately very useful in supporting a diagnosis of WMD.

An enzyme called glutathione peroxidase (GSHPx) present within red blood cells is an enzyme that contains selenium and is one of the main anti-oxidant enzymes in the body. GSHPx level in the bloodstream is a good indicator of long-term selenium status and is comparatively cheaper than the more difficult test of measuring blood selenium levels. This is the most frequently performed test in the diagnosis of WMD and in the monitoring of selenium and Vitamin E status. The calves themselves can be tested but also the dams for an earlier pre-emptive warning of deficiencies (Chapter 10).

It is likely that if one animal in a group of animals in the same management system is affected, other calves will be subclinically affected; not showing signs of disease but on the verge of doing so.

WMD can be induced by intense muscular activity resulting from moving or handling the cattle. As soon as muscle cells have to increase their work load the damage due to free radicals increases and disease can ensue.

Blood selenium and Vitamin E content are strongly correlated with the selenium and Vitamin E content of the diet. Ensuring that the diet contains adequate selenium and Vitamin E is therefore essential in the prevention of WMD. For suckled calves this may be through Vitamin E and selenium provision in the diet of the dam; the nutrients are transferred to the calf via the milk. In the artificially reared calf this may be by ensuring that the milk replacer and then the rearing diet contain enough of these ingredients.

RESPIRATORY DISEASE

Laryngeal chondritis

Chondritis means inflammation of cartilage; laryngeal chondritis therefore, is inflammation of the cartilages in the larynx – the voice box and the valve like structure at the opening to the trachea (windpipe). Inflammation, assumed to be caused by infection, of this cartilage narrows the airway of the voice box and a distinctive, highly audible, inspiratory roar is created. In extreme cases where the airway occludes completely the calf will, of course, die. A secondary manifestation of this disease occurs when a piece of infected, dead cartilage is inhaled into the lungs and a secondary pneumonia results. It affects calves anytime between 1 week and 6 months old and appears to be more common in well-muscled, pure- or part-bred, Limousin- or Belgian Blue-bred calves.

The cause and pathway of the disease is uncertain. Bacteria have been found in the inflamed cartilage but what is the sequence of events? Does the bacterial infection cause the inflammation or do the bacteria invade the inflamed cartilage? There would presumably have to be trauma or damage to the lining of the larynx for the bacteria to get into the deeper cartilage? The condition is seen even more commonly in Texel and Beltex sheep where there is a known genetic predisposition (Lane et al., 1987). These sheep have very narrow airways and short necks. It could be that the narrow airway causes increased resistance to the air passing through it with every breath, this eventually inflaming the larynx until secondary bacteria gain entry. It has been suggested there may be a genetic predisposition to the disease in cattle as well (Gustin et al., 1986) and animals should not be retained for breeding (Milne et al., 2000).

The bacteria associated with this condition are *Actinobacillis* and *Fusobacterium necrophorum*. *F. necrophorum* is the causal agent of calf diphtheria and it has been suggested laryngeal chondritis could be part of the same disease complex.

Both bacteria are easily killed with penicillin-type antibiotics, the problem is that the cartilage tissue that is infected has a very poor blood supply so getting a high enough concentration of antibiotics to the site of infection is challenging. It has been reported in the literature that administering intravenous lincospectin for 14 days was used to treat two calves effectively (Milne et al., 2000). Steroids are necessary in the treatment of this condition as they decrease the swelling of the soft tissue in the larynx and make it easier for the calf to breath. The reduction in breathing noise following treatment with steroids is remarkable.

The prognosis is guarded, with a treatment success of just 14% reported in the literature (West, 1997). Post-mortem examination findings are an obvious swelling and redness of the larynx and, on closer inspection, abscessation of the laryngeal cartilages (Figure 12.3).

For cases that do not respond to antibiotics and steroids then surgery is an option (Goulding et al., 2003); a tracheostomy can be performed. A permanent tracheostomy involves making a hole directly into the windpipe halfway down the neck, so the inhaled air bypasses the nose and larynx. The calf will be able to breath unhindered. The down sides of a tracheotomy aside from cost and welfare are the loss of function of the larynx, one of whose jobs is to protect the upper airways from pathogens and dust entering the lungs that would otherwise cause pneumonia. This procedure may not be economically viable and will require significant aftercare and regular inspection of the surgical site.

The incidence of this condition appears to be increasing in the suckled calf population, certainly in the north east of England, and in some herds up to 5% of calves are affected; this has a significant economic and welfare impact with a survival rate of about 50%, negative effects on the growth rates of survivors and the time and cost of treatments. The genetic component of the condition clearly warrants further research.

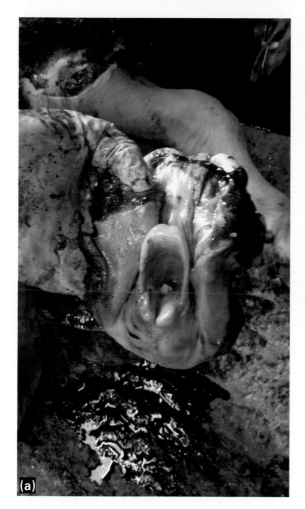 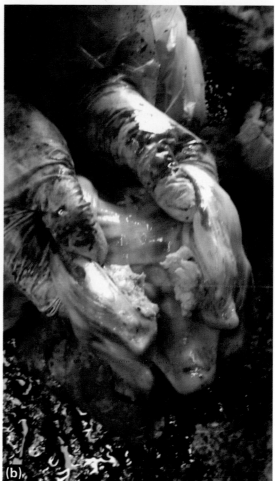

FIGURE 12.3 (a) Photograph of the larynx from a calf at post-mortem examination (a small amount of pus visible); (b) photograph of the same larynx cut open to reveal extensive abscessation

Mycoplasmosis bovis (disease caused by *Mycoplasma bovis*)

Mycoplasma bovis seems to be a relatively new pathogen to contend with in intensively managed beef and dairy cattle. This bug commonly causes unresolving mastitis in dairy cows while in young-stock it is frequently involved in pneumonia outbreaks, septic arthritis (joint ill) and middle ear infections. It was first detected in the UK in the 1970s. Surveillance data suggests that the incidence of *M. bovis* infection is increasing (Ridley and Hateley, 2018).

There are other mycoplasmata that have been

suspected of causing disease in young calves. Their role, however, is not clearly understood; some mycoplasmata are thought to be normal inhabitants of the upper respiratory tract and others are opportunists and only infect an animal after the primary infectious agent has paved the way with the initial damage. Further research is being carried out in this area; *M. bovis*, specifically, is the main focus of mycoplasma research in young calves.

M. bovis is thought to enter herds through clinically unaffected carrier animals that shed the bacteria. The bacteria can be shed in colostrum, milk, respiratory and vaginal secretions. Calves become infected from their dams. In beef-cross dairy systems where calves are removed from their mothers, the disease can be controlled by snatch calving, where the calf is removed immediately at birth from the cow and her environment so reducing the chance of the calf becoming infected. For further control the colostrum can be pasteurised so no bacteria are transmitted by that route to the population in the separate calf houses. Powdered milk is fed from then on, rather than potentially infected milk from the bulk tank. This is clearly not a control method that can be adopted in the suckler herd. Once infection is established in a population of calves it is passed from calf to calf in respiratory secretions.

M. bovis can survive in the environment; up to 3 weeks in straw and 2 weeks on wood and in water. Survival is best achieved in cool humid conditions (Pfutzner and Sachse, 1996). Research suggests that shedding increases when calves are subjected to a drop in ambient temperature from 17°C to 5°C. Another study suggested that calves exposed to a warmer environment were less likely to be infected with *M. bovis* than those exposed to lower environmental temperatures (Maunsell and Donovan, 2009). It follows, therefore, that given the ambient temperatures, and closer proximity of calves at housing, there is an increased rate of diagnosis of *M. bovis* through the winter months (Ridley and Hateley, 2018).

M. bovis is good at evading immune defences and going further to even modulate the host animal's immune response (Maunsell and Donovan, 2009). As with all infectious disease the balance between immunity and challenge is vital. Calves with adequate passive transfer of maternal colostral antibodies and living in a clean dry environment with adequate nutrition are less susceptible to *M. bovis* infection. The exact role of maternal antibodies in the protection of calves from *M. bovis* infection is actually, however, currently unclear.

Mycoplasmata compared to other bacteria are unique in that they do not have a cell wall (Figure 12.4). This means they are classified by some systems as not actually bacteria. It also means that only certain antibiotics can be used to treat infection – penicillin type antibiotics which attack the bacterial cell wall are ineffective on mycoplasmata.

Disease associated with *M. bovis* is usually chronic, debilitating and unresponsive to treatment. *M. bovis* pneumonia typically affects calves from 4 weeks to 24 months of age. *M. bovis* is usually part of a mixed infection with other respiratory viruses or bacteria such as RSV, Pi3, IBR or *Mannheimia haemolytica* (*pasteurella*) (Chapter 13). When the other infectious agents are controlled through vaccination *M. bovis*, although still present, causes less disease, with reduced incidence and mortality. There is no commercially available

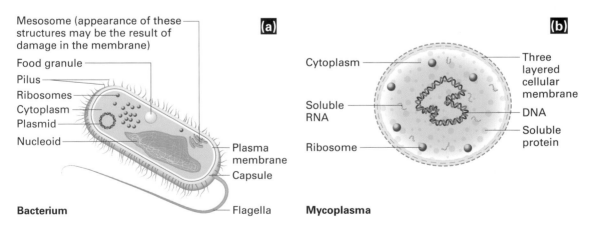

FIGURE 12.4 (a) A normal bacterium compared to a (b) mycoplasma (note the absence of a cell wall in the mycoplasma)

vaccine available for *M. bovis*, although autogenous vaccines have been used with some success. This involves isolating the causal organism from an affected animal (or carcase) and cultivating a safe preparation of the organism to use in a vaccine on that specific herd. There are fairly stringent licensing requirements and safety testing to be carried out with these autogenous vaccines; specialist laboratories are available to provide this service.

It is unclear whether ear infections associated with *M. bovis* are a result of infection ascending from the throat up the small eustachian tube, which connects with the middle ear, or from infection invading the ear canal from the outside world, or from bacteria in the bloodstream. The infection within the ear causes pain, fever, loss of appetite, head shaking and a dropped ear. If the infection progresses and compromises the nerves that run close to the site of infection, then the calf may suffer paralysis of its facial muscles and lose the ability to swallow. In severe cases the infection can pass to the brain causing meningitis, recumbency, staggering, seizures and death.

Calves may suffer from *M. bovis* associated synovitis (joint ill) – this may be with or without the simultaneous presence of respiratory disease. One or more joints may be affected; the calf will be lame and the affected joints hot, swollen and painful. Calves are frequently culled due to poor response to treatment.

Confirming a diagnosis of *M. bovis* can be difficult. *M. bovis* is difficult to grow in a laboratory and requires specialist techniques. It is also relatively slow growing, taking up to 10 days to culture. Despite this, growing the bacteria in the laboratory remains the best means of getting a diagnosis in a disease outbreak where *M. bovis* is suspected. In a live animal swabs can be taken of fluid aspirated from an infected joint or from nasal swabs in the case of pneumonia. It is vital the samples are collected in the acute stages of disease and before the animal is treated with antibiotics. Where a carcase is available for PME, infected tissues can be sampled and attempts made to culture the bug directly from them.

New technologies have recently become available to detect *M. bovis* DNA within an infected tissue. This technique is called polymerase chain reaction (PCR). It is not unique to *M. bovis*; it is also used to find a variety of other bacteria and viruses. It is a very good technique; it has removed some of the frustration associated with trying to culture bacteria with more traditional methods.

As cattle produce antibodies to *M. bovis* it is possible to blood test for the evidence of previous exposure. This method of diagnosis cannot be used during an outbreak of disease as it takes up to 4 weeks for the antibodies to be generated to a detectable level in the blood. In young calves there is uncertainty whether the antibodies detected are the calf's own antibodies produced in response to infection, or whether they are the dam's antibodies transferred to the calf via the colostrum. In summary, blood testing is a useful tool in the diagnosis of *M. bovis* but it must be understood and interpreted with caution.

Treatment of mycoplasmosis needs careful consideration. Beta-lactamase antibiotics work by destroying the bacterial cell wall (Chapter 26), they are therefore completely ineffective in treating *M. bovis* which does not have a cell wall. Oxytetracyclines and macrolides are effective but resistance is increasingly being reported (Maunsell and Donovan, 2009). In practice, synovitis and ear infection are sometimes treated surgically with drainage and lavage of the infected tissues, these techniques are demanding on welfare and cost and they yield variable results.

The lack of treatment options, the difficulty of vaccination options and the severe economic and welfare implications of *M. bovis* make it a serious threat to cattle herds; it is best, therefore, to keep it out of herds in the first place – stringent biosecurity is required to achieve this (Chapter 18). Purchased or returning animals are a high risk but given the environmental survival of the mycoplasma, fomites such as equipment and clothing/footwear are also a significant risk.

TABLE 12.1 Showing the different clostridial diseases and the causal organism

Clostridial disease	Causal *Clostridium species*
Black leg	*C. chauvoei*
Malignant oedema	*C. septicum, C. novyi, C. chauvoei* and *C. sordelli*
Tetanus	*C. tetani*
Black disease (infectious necrotic hepatitis)	*C. novyi* type B
Botulism	*C. botulinum*
Enterotoxaemia	*C. pefringens*
Bacillary haemoglobinuria	*C. novyi* type D
Abomasitis	*C. sordelli*

CLOSTRIDIAL DISEASE

There is a wide range of clostridial diseases that affect domestic livestock in the UK and all over the world. They are caused by bacteria from the *Clostridium* genus. Each of the different pathogenic species of *Clostridium* causes a fairly different and sometimes unique disease picture (Table 12.1).

These bacteria thrive in anaerobic conditions, they are widespread in the environment; in the soil, rotting vegetation, animal matter and in the animals themselves as a normal part of the animal's bacterial flora (Harwood, 2007a). They are not a problem until an event occurs that triggers the bacteria to emerge from their otherwise normal dormant state and start multiplying – this releases their notorious toxins; it is their toxins that do the harm.

Black leg

The sudden death of a young beast, less than 24 months old, at grass, is a common presentation of black leg. It is unusual to see the affected animal alive.

Here an animal ingests the bacteria from the soil contaminated pasture. The bacteria pass into the bloodstream either across the gut wall or through some damage in the gut lining. The bacteria travel in the blood and have a predilection to settle in muscle tissue. There they remain dormant until triggered to multiply whereupon they produce their toxins. The trigger in the case of black leg is usually trauma. This trauma can be from heifers bulling, or escaping through a fence, being caught in a ring feeder; anything that traumatises the muscle. The disease can occur in housed cattle too where the bug has persisted in the housed environment such as in a dark dirty corner. If the animal is seen alive it will be stiff and have a swollen, hot affected muscle. Treatment can be attempted with penicillin-type antibiotics but is usually futile. Where the bacteria target the muscle tissue of the diaphragm, the heart or chest (intercostal muscle), death is instant. Black leg can be diagnosed on PME if the primary lesion can be located within the muscle mass. The lesion appears dark red/black and dry and can extend to a significantly sized area of the muscle. Further testing may be required to confirm a diagnosis; a technique known as fluorescent antibody test (FAT) can be used where an antibody combined with a fluorescent marker attaches specifically to the *C. chauvoei* bacteria which can then be illuminated under a microscope.

Malignant oedema

Malignant oedema is an infection by a combination of up to four different *Clostridia* spp. and is associated with a wound that becomes secondarily infected. As clostridial bacteria prefer to replicate in an environment with little oxygen (anaerobic), a deep puncture wound is a perfect environment for them to set up camp. The bacteria replicate and produce a large quantity of toxins. The tissue around the wound becomes very swollen, quite wet and gelatinous. There is commonly a large amount of gas associated with the wound, so the underlying tissues feel crackly or like bubble wrap. This is a common presentation in cows that have had a traumatic birth or tears to the vulva which become contaminated. Affected animals are seen alive but prompt treatment with penicillin type antibiotics is required if death is to be avoided.

Black disease

The clostridial bacterium responsible for black disease is *C. novyi* type B. This bug chooses to replicate in the liver; preferably in the tracks of damage left behind by migrating fluke. Again, animals are often just found dead and on PME there is a well demarcated dark brown/red/black circular lesion on the surface of the liver extending into the deeper liver tissue. Again, as with black leg, a diagnosis can be confirmed by FAT. The management and control of fluke on the farm needs to be discussed in cases of black disease.

Enterotoxaemia

C. perfringens normally lives in the gut of an animal at a low dormant level. The trigger for its multiplication is usually an abrupt change of diet, such as the move to lush pasture or the introduction of creep feed. It is often the stronger animals in the group that are affected, presumably because they are generally dominant, greedier and manage to eat more of the new food than their contemporaries. In greedy suckled calves there may be overflow of milk from the abomasum to the small intestine; milk is dense in carbohydrate (lactose) and this again triggers *C. perfringens* to replicate. *C. perfringens* like other clostridial species produces toxins that are absorbed into the blood stream. *C. perfringens* is classified into four groups depending on the toxins that the strain produces; in cattle type D is by far the most common.

Animals usually die suddenly so are rarely seen alive but where they are, diarrhoea and neurological abnormalities would be likely clinical signs. Prompt treatment with fluid therapy and penicillin-type antibiotics is required.

The diagnosis of *C. perfringens* type D from a carcase is not particularly easy. There is a misconception that the observation of soft, mushy kidney tissue at PME is diagnostic but this is seen in all animals within a few hours of death; the kidneys 'go off' (autolyse) quickly after death as they are located adjacent to the large fermenting vat of the rumen that remains warm for a number of hours after death. If, however, a PME is carried out soon after death and the kidneys are autolysed then this is indeed suggestive of pulpy kidney. Other clues include glucose in the urine; a dip stick test can be used; in a healthy animal there is no glucose in the urine. There is no point in trying to detect *C. perfringens* in the gut, it will be present in a normal healthy animal and proliferates after death. Looking for high levels of its toxin in the gut contents, can, however, be beneficial but not necessarily diagnostic in its own right. Another way of obtaining an answer is to remove the brain at PME and request a microscopic examination. The *C. perfringens* type D toxin is associated with a characteristic microscopic change in the brain that is diagnostic and also explains the neurological signs seen in the live animal before death.

Abomasal ulcers

C. sordelli has been found to be present in gangrenous abomasal ulcers in 3 week to 3 month old calves. It remains unclear whether *C. sordelli* is the primary cause of the ulcer or whether it invades existing damaged tissue in the abomasal wall and makes the situation worse (Harwood, 2007b). Affected calves present with abdominal pain, a distended abdomen and salivation, followed soon after by death. Treatment is with painkillers, penicillin antibiotics and supportive care but, all too often, is unsuccessful.

Bacillary haemoglobinuria

C. novyi type D (previously *C. haemolyticum*) causes a rare form of clostridial disease known classically as bacillary haemoglobinuria characterised by distinctive jaundice of the carcase and the presence of red urine. The disease is acutely fatal unlike the similar but less acutely fatal conditions of copper toxicity, blue green algae poisoning and non-specific liver disease. Similar to black disease this clostridial infection is linked to fluke infection; the grazing of wet marshy flukey ground is therefore considered a risk factor.

Tetanus

Tetanus, an infamous disease known in the past as lock-jaw, can affect all ages of animal. The clostridium in question is *C. tetani*. The clinical signs are very specific:

- walking very stiffly in a 'wooden' fashion
- recumbency
- raised tail
- stiff jaw
- protrusion of the third eye lid
- drooling
- tremors
- convulsions.

Tetanus is usually diagnosed on clinical signs alone as there are no specific laboratory tests, and culturing the bacterium is very difficult.

Treatment can be attempted in the early stages with penicillin-type antibiotics and tetanus antitoxin. Large amounts of antitoxin are required, and this is prohibitively expensive for commercial cattle especially considering the prognosis is still poor despite this type of treatment. Euthanasia is usually the best course of action.

C. tetani is widespread in the environment but some farms appear to have a higher burden than others. Where there has been groundwork, such as drainage, and the soil has been disturbed, spores can be unearthed; this is a recognised risk factor. Spores infect open wounds, open navels, castration wounds and the like. Following infection, the bacteria may proliferate immediately or, occasionally lie dormant for some time before multiplication and the release of the inevitable toxin in common with other clostridial disease. Sometimes there is no obvious port of entry and *C. tetani* is assumed to have gained entry into the bloodstream via damage to the gastrointestinal tract perhaps following dietary acidosis or parasitic damage to the gut lining.

Botulism

C. botulinum produces the notorious botulinum toxin. If cattle ingest this toxin, or the bug producing the toxin, clinical signs can appear suddenly within 24 hours or in a delayed fashion; up to 17 days after the toxin is ingested. The disease has an acute form where cattle are found dead and a subacute to chronic form displaying the following clinical signs:

- not wanting to drink or eat
- flaccidity (floppiness, lack of muscle tone), weakness, knuckling
- dilated pupils
- flaccid tail, eyelids and jaw
- drooling
- difficulty swallowing
- recumbency.

Mortality is very high at around 90%.

Access to poultry litter is a common cause as it may be contaminated with the carcases of birds which happen to be frequent carriers of dormant *C. botulinum*, which starts to multiply in the dead bird. Housed cattle may be infected if fed forage crops sourced from where poultry litter has been spread. Dead rodent or rabbit carcases in conserved forage are also a potential source as are water courses contaminated with bird and animal carcases. There is a direct correlation between the amount of toxin present on the pasture or within the contaminated feed and the severity of the outbreak. There are no specific signs indicative of botulism on PME; detecting the toxin in a carcase or feed stuff is required to make a diagnosis. Where disease is suspected it should be reported to the relevant authorities as it is a food safety concern; there is some evidence that botulinum toxin can be transferred to humans in meat or milk.

Prevention of clostridial disease

Clostridial bugs are ubiquitous (widespread) in the environment. Animals affected with clostridial disease are rarely seen alive and even when they are treatment is rarely successful and death soon follows. Fortunately, however, affordable, effective vaccines are available for all clostridial diseases (apart from botulism). Clostridial vaccines are all based on the toxin rather than the bacterium itself. The toxin is heat treated to form a safe but similar toxoid that generates antibodies that are capable of attaching to and blocking the effects of the toxin in the vaccinated animal. These vaccines are very effective but usually multiple doses, certainly at

least two, are required to elicit a strong antibody response. Clostridial disease is, therefore, largely preventable. Some vaccines provide protection for only one disease, for example, pulpy kidney, black leg or tetanus. Other vaccines are so called multivalent products, they cover up to ten different clostridial diseases, Table 12.2. Within each vaccine the protection varies depending on the specific bacterial toxin. It is possible to protect very young calves from disease by vaccinating the dam and, in doing so, generating colostral antibodies. This technique is effective providing colostrum is ingested in sufficient quantities, but it also needs recognising that the antibodies produced against each clostridial toxin wain at different times, the longest lasting 12 weeks after birth, the rest, sadly, shorter. It also needs remembering that maternally derived antibody (MDA) (antibodies absorbed from the colostrum) will interfere with the calf's ability to generate its own immune response to a vaccine, so it is recommended that calves do not receive their first dose of clostridial vaccine until 8–12 weeks of age, that being if they are from a vaccinated dam. If calves are not born to or have not sucked a vaccinated dam, they can be vaccinated from as early as 2 weeks of age. A primary course of two injections, 4–6 weeks apart, is required to achieve full protection and this protection relies on annual boosters. Even with this heavy approach some components of the vaccine will not provide immunity for the full 12 months. Where this is the case it will be stated in the data sheet; if these

TABLE 12.2 Some commercially available clostridial vaccines and variation in diseases covered

Vaccine	*C. perfringens* Type A	*C. perfringens* Type B & C	*C. perfringens* D	*C. novyi* Type D	*C. Chauvoei*	*C. novyi* Type B	*C. septicum*	*C. Tetani*	*C. sordellii*
Product C8		X	X	X	X	X	X	X	
Product C10	X	X	X	X	X	X	X	X	X
Product B	X	X	X	X	X	X	X	X	X
Product T				X	X	X	X	X	

diseases are of concern then 6 monthly boosters are required. If cows are expected to transfer antibodies to their calves via the colostrum, they will require a booster between 2 and 8 weeks prior to calving. There is a slight variation in the timing of vaccine depending on the brand; the data sheet should always be consulted before using any product.

Anthrax

It is often assumed that any sudden death in livestock is likely to be related to clostridial infection. However, any sudden or unaccountable death in farm stock should always raise suspicion of anthrax unless an alternative diagnosis is obvious (APHA, UK, 2019).

Anthrax is caused by infection with the bacterium *Bacillus anthracis*. Anthrax infection results from ingesting or inhaling the bacterial spores which may have been dormant in the environment for many years, even decades. The bacteria multiply and release toxins, infection is nearly always fatal. Anthrax is a zoonosis, personnel working with soil contaminated fleeces are particularly at risk hence its old name 'wool sorters disease'. The disease in humans tends to be less serious, mainly skin based.

When the farmer initially informs their private local vet of a sudden bovine death, the vet needs to establish if anthrax can be reasonably ruled out. The questions in Box 12.1 can be used to help decide if anthrax remains a possible diagnosis. If there is any doubt that anthrax cannot be ruled out there is an obligation for the vet to notify the relevant authority. In the UK this would be the duty vet at the Animal Health and Veterinary Laboratories Agency (AHVLA) regional office under Article 4 of The Anthrax Order (1991).

Other findings that may be suggestive of anthrax are a history of anthrax on the premises, recent ditching or soil exposure, or multiple unexplained deaths. Unopened anthrax infected carcases are described as swollen with blood oozing

> **Box 12.1** Questions suggested by APHA, UK, to conclude on the likelihood of anthrax as the cause of death (APHA, UK 2019)
>
> - Age of the animal – is the animal young and therefore more likely to have died from other causes?
> - Has the animal been ill in the last few days or has it been losing condition and weight over a long period, suggesting an acute (but not peracute) or chronic illness?
> - Has the animal been visibly bloated over the last few hours – suggestive of bloat?
> - Is there evidence of convulsions, during a period of grazing on lush pasture – suggestive of hypomagnesaemia?
> - Is there evidence the animal has been in parturition, that is, a dead foetus is partly visible – suggestive of dystocia?
> - Is there evidence suggestive of poisoning as the likely cause, for example, evidence suggesting the likely ingestion of yew or water dropwort?
> - Are there other animals recumbent with flaccid paralysis, others that may have died and a recent history of spreading of poultry litter – suggestive of botulism?
> - Was the body found directly under a tree that has signs of being struck by lightning, or beside a metal fence or object, or are there are scorch marks visible on the carcase – suggestive of lightning strike?
> - Have milking cows died suddenly in a parlour – suggestive of electrocution?

from the nostrils or other natural openings of the body. This is not always the case and these signs are not specific to anthrax so not necessarily helpful in deciding if anthrax may be involved or not.

If an anthrax enquiry is initiated the keeper of the animal should be advised to keep other livestock away from the carcase or any area contaminated by discharges from the carcase. Drains in the vicinity of the carcase should be blocked and the carcase not moved from its location or the premises. Disinfection of the area affected and any equipment or personnel should be carried out as a precaution pending diagnosis. Carcases suspected of or known to be infected with anthrax must not be opened as this is likely to result in an increase in the production of, and contamination from, the bacterium.

REFERENCES

Abutarbush, S.M. and Radostits, O.M. (2003) Congenital nutritional muscular dystrophy in a beef calf. *Canadian Veterinary Journal* 44(9), 738–739.

APHA (n.d.) http://apha.defra.gov.uk/External_ OV_Instructions/Anthrax/index.htm (accessed 27 January 2019).

Bazeley, K. (2003) Investigation of diarrhoea in the neonatal calf. *In Practice* 25, 152–159.

Blowey, R.W. (2004) Digestive disorders of calves. In: Andrews, A.H., Blowey, R.W., Boyd, H. and Eddy, R.G. (eds) *Bovine Medicine. Diseases and Husbandry of Cattle*, 2nd edn. Blackwell Science, Oxford, pp. 231–248.

Caldow, G.L. and Munro, R. (1995) Necrotising enteritis in suckled calves. *Vet Record* 137, 307–311.

Carrique-Mas, J.J, Willmington, J.A., Papadopoulou, C., Watson, E.N. and Davies, R.H. (2010) Salmonella infection in cattle in Great Britain, 2003 to 2008. *Vet Record* 167, 560–565.

Daugschies, A. and Najdrowski, M. (2005) Eimeriosis in cattle: current understanding. *Journal of Veterinary Medicine Series B* 52, 417–427.

Foster, D.M. and Smith, G.W. (2009) Pathophysiology of diarrhoea in calves. *Veterinary Clinics of North America: Food Animal Practice* 25, 13–36.

Goulding, R., Schumacher, J., Barrett, D.C. and Fitzpatrick, J.L. (2003) Use of a permanent tracheostomy to treat laryngeal chondritis and stenosis in a heifer. *Vet Record* 152, 809–811.

Gustin, P., Bakima, J., Lekeux, P. and Lomba, F. (1986) Relationship between ventilation mechanisms of the larynx and laryngeal disorders in double muscles Belgian Blue calves. *Proceedings of the 14th World Congress on Diseases of Cattle*, Dublin, Ireland, 26–29 August, Vol. 1, 697–702.

Harwood, D. (2007a) Clostridial diseases in cattle: Part 1. *UK Vet Livestock* 11(7), 31–33.

Harwood, D. (2007b) Clostridial diseases in cattle: Part 2. *UK Vet Livestock* 12(2), 21–24.

Hateley, G. (2017) Salmonella investigations in ruminants. *Veterinary Record* 181, 366–367.

Henderson, K. and Mason, C. (2017) Diagnosis and control of *Salmonella dublin* in dairy herds. *In Practice* 39, 158–168.

Holliman, A. (2005) Differential diagnosis of disease-causing oral lesions in cattle. *In Practice* 27, 2–13.

Jones, P.W., Watson, P.R. and Wallis, T.S. (2004) Salmonellosis. In: Andrews, A.H., Blowey, R.W., Boyd, H. and Eddy, R.G. (eds) *Bovine Medicine Diseases and husbandry of cattle,* 2nd edn. Blackwell Science, Oxford, pp. 215–230.

Lane, J.G., Brown, P.J., Lancaster, M.L. and Todd, J.N. (1987) Laryngeal chondritis in Texel sheep. *Vet Record* 121, 81–84.

Marshall, R.N., Catchpole, J., Green, J.A. and Webster, K.A. (1998) Bovine coccidiosis in calves following turn out. *Vet Record* 143, 366–367.

Mason, C. and Caldow, G. (2012) Calf diarrhoea. The Moredun Foundation. News sheet Vol. 5 No. 14.

Mason, C.S., Buxton, D. and Gartside, J.F. (2003) Congenital ocular abnormalities in calves associated with maternal hypovitaminosis A. *Vet Record* 153, 213–214.

Maunsell, F.P. and Donovan, G.A. (2009) Mycoplasma bovis Infections in young calves. *Veterinary Clinics of North America: Food Animal Practice* 25, 139–177.

Milne, M.H., Barrett, D.C., Sullivan, M. and Fitzpatrick, J.L. (2000) Successful medical treatment of laryngeal chondritis in cattle. *Vet Record* 147, 305–306.

Pfutzner, H. and Sachse, K. (1996) Mycoplasma bovis as an agent of mastitis, pneumonia, arthritis and genital disorders in cattle. *Revue scientifique et technique* 15, 1477–1494.

Radostits, O.M., Blood, D.C. and Gay, C.C. (1994) Diseases caused by deficiencies in mineral nutrients. In: *Veterinary Medicine*, 8th edn. Tindall Publishing, Philadelphia, PA, pp. 1408–1418.

Ridley, A. and Hateley, G. (2018) Surveillance focus Mycoplasma bovis investigations in cattle. *Vet Record* 183(8), 256–258.

Taylor, M. (2000) Protozoal disease in cattle and sheep. *In Practice* 22, 604–617.

Van Donkersgoed, J. and Clark, E.G. (1988) Blindness caused by Hypovitaminosis A in feedlot cattle. *Canadian Veterinary Journal* 29, 925–927.

West, H.J. (1997) Tracheolaryngostomy as a treatment for laryngeal obstruction in cattle. *Veterinary Journal* 153, 81–86.

Wyatt, C.R., Riggs, M.W. and Fayer, R. (2010) Cryptosporidiosis in neonatal calves. *Veterinary Clinics of North America: Food Animal Practice* 26, 89–103.

Chapter 13

Disease and production failure in growing cattle

HEAT STRESS AND HEAT STROKE

Cattle are poor at dissipating heat in hot conditions. They have a high volume to surface area ratio; that means a lot of body to produce heat and not much surface from which to lose the heat. Furthermore, their large body also contains a huge heat producing fermentation vat – the rumen. Black cattle are more affected by solar gain than lighter coloured cattle and overweight cattle will also suffer more given the higher levels of insulating fat tissue. What is worse is that cattle do not sweat very much – they are rather deficient in sweat glands and the few they have are not particularly functional. The worst scenario arises when there is high humidity and low wind speeds both of which further reduce heat dissipation from the body surface just as it does with us.

Cattle will naturally seek shade and water in hot weather if it is available to them. Trees, even hedgerows, can provide some protection from the sun. They love to paddle in natural water courses although in prolonged periods of hot weather these may have dried up. During hot weather cattle will accumulate heat in the day and then lose heat at night. It takes up to 6 hours for the animal's temperature to return to normal after a very hot day.

Cattle showing signs of heat stress (over heating) salivate profusely, seek shade, drink large volumes of water, appear agitated, pant and, rather paradoxically, cluster together – either for primitive protection reasons or maybe to offer shade to one another. If their body temperature continues to rise, they will suffer from heat stroke; they become recumbent, unresponsive and unable to move, finally terminating in convulsions before death. Although the signs appear similar to a straightforward case of milk fever it is far more serious; prompt treatment is required, this involving cooling the animal down and maybe intravenous fluids. The cooling of an animal is an interesting subject – most research coming from human and racehorse medicine. Racehorses are vaguely similar in size and shape to cattle so what can we learn from the race-track vets? Constant cold hosing is counterproductive – convincing racehorse trainers of this, to them a surprising fact, is difficult! The problem is that over cooling of the skin triggers off vasoconstriction of the cutaneous circulation so the overly warm blood stays in the body's core circulation, it stays overly warm and continues to overheat the brain leading to heat stroke. Instead, the animal should simply be soaked once, briefly and not necessarily with particularly cold water. This way vasoconstriction is not triggered and the hot blood flows through the cutaneous circulation as per nature's way, so releasing heat through the surface of the body. Furthermore, the water on the skin evaporates and knowledge of physics reminds us that this removes energy from the body in the form of the *heat of vaporisation* – that is the principle of sweating.

The feed intakes of heat stressed animals will be reduced and subsequently milk supply and growth rates are affected. Conception rates will be affected if cows are served during this time and the fertility of bulls will also be compromised for several weeks after the testicular temperature has been raised, which this impairs sperm production.

PHOTOSENSITISATION

Photosensitisation put very crudely is sunburn but there's really quite a lot more to it than the simple sunburn we, as humans, are familiar with. It is usually seen in light coloured cattle at pasture in the summer months. It does not have to be particularly hot; it is all about high ultraviolet (UV) light exposure. The condition presents with the light-coloured areas of skin over the animal's back becoming initially swollen, then firm and then hard and raised, almost like large hair covered scabs. The hair covered scabs then 'lift' off and after a number of weeks the affected skin detaches completely leaving new pink skin and new hair shafts behind. The animal can be irritated by the scabs and become itchy during this time. The condition is caused not by simple sunburn but by photo-active substances accumulating under the skin. This can happen in one of three ways.

1. Chlorophyll is the chemical in grass that gives it its green appearance. This pigment captures light energy for the plant to conduct the photosynthesis of sugar. If cattle are grazing lush green pasture, they are ingesting large quantities of chlorophyll and they may become unable to keep up with the metabolism of this pigment and its metabolites. One such metabolite, a chemical called phylloerythrin, is particularly problematic. When it passes through the circulation of the light-coloured skin it is exposed to the UV rays and reacts to produce damaging waste products that harm the skin. Why light coloured skin? It seems that the melanin pigment in dark coloured skin absorbs UV

light and circulating chemicals are, therefore, less exposed.

2. Some plants carry certain photo-active substances that are already photo-active. St John's Wort and buck weed are two such plants found in the UK. Again, the chemicals react to UV when exposed in pale coloured skin and damage results.

3. Photosensitisation can be secondary to liver disease. The metabolites of chlorophyll, such as phylloerythrin, are usually excreted from the liver via the bile duct. If the bile duct is blocked as a result of liver disease, then the metabolites and phylloerythrin accumulate in the circulation and photosensitisation is made more likely. There may be other clinical signs associated with liver disease such as diarrhoea, abdominal pain, weight loss, oedema of the throat (bottle jaw) or brisket, loss of appetite and a yellow tinge to the gums and the whites of the eyes (jaundice).

To treat the condition effectively, it is obviously necessary to accept that UV light is part of the problem but it is useful to have an idea of the rest of the causation. Often the grazing history provides some answers and blood tests can establish if the liver is functioning correctly.

The affected cattle should be housed with as little exposure to sunlight as possible. They should be treated with anti-inflammatory, unless the cause is liver failure in which case the vet may decide to withhold anti-inflammatories, some of which can exacerbate liver damage. Emollient cream should be applied to the lesions to reduce moisture loss and to provide a moist healing environment for the skin and undoubtedly some comfort. If photosensitisation is secondary to liver disease, then the cause of the liver disease needs addressing.

BESNOITIOSIS

Bovine besnoitiosis is a condition seen in mainland Europe but is yet to be reported in the UK although a case was reported in an Irish dairy herd, which was also unusual as the cases in Europe have predominantly involved beef cattle (Ryan et al., 2016). The disease is caused by a protozoan parasite, *Besnoitia besnoiti*. This parasite's lifecycle is poorly understood; it may have an indirect lifecycle involving wildlife and/or biting flies. Once cattle are infected, they remain carriers for life. The disease initially presents in the acute form as fever, swelling of the skin around the head and neck, enlarged superficial lymph nodes, pain on movement due to swelling within the joints, swollen and painful testicles in the case of male animals, discharge from the eyes and nose, and, difficulty breathing. After 3 weeks the disease progresses to a chronic form with hard thick skin folds on the head and neck with skin thickening and hair loss elsewhere on the body; bulls become infertile due to irreversible changes within the scrotum. A fairly specific clinical sign is the appearance of cysts (fluid-filled vesicles) on the eyeball and, in females, on the vulva (Ryan et al., 2016).

There is no statutory testing for this disease and there is concern that carrier animals may be imported to the UK. The disease is not notifiable in the UK. The clinical signs are similar to photosensitisation or pneumonia until tissue cysts appear. An antibody test is available to confirm exposure to the disease and biopsies of the skin from the rump are also diagnostic.

COPPER DEFICIENCY

Copper plays a part in many physiological processes in the body. A lack of copper causes infertility, impaired immune function, poor growth rates and weak connective tissues including those of the skin. Outwardly cattle may show depigmentation of the hair surrounding the eyes, brown tinged coats, and abnormal development of tendons and bones. These are often referred to as copper responsive disorders rather than copper deficiency (Laven and Livesey, 2005) for the following reasons.

Copper deficiency can be due to a lack of copper in the diet, a primary deficiency or, in the case of secondary deficiency, there is adequate copper in the diet but there are high levels of antagonists disturbing the absorption of the dietary copper from the digestive tract. Antagonistic disruptors of copper absorption from the gastrointestinal tract include sulphur, molybdenum, iron, zinc and, perhaps indirectly, calcium carbonate. This is based on certain chemical reactions that occur in the rumen; a relevant one being when sulphur and molybdenum combine to form complexes called thiomolybdates. These thiomolybdates bind with soluble copper in the rumen and prevent it from being absorbed. One method of overcoming this reaction is to feed enough soluble copper to bind all the thiomolybdate leaving enough remaining soluble copper to be absorbed. Some researchers have suggested that thiomolybdate that is not bound to copper is absorbed into the circulation and the clinical signs we traditionally associate with copper deficiency are actually thiomolybdate toxicity rather than primary copper deficiency – in other words a secondary copper deficiency as there simply is not enough copper to overcome the thiomolybdate. To challenge this theory, it has been suggested that cattle are actually unable to absorb enough thiomolybdate from a normal diet to reach toxic levels; toxic levels have only ever been demonstrated in trial conditions (Laven and Livesey, 2005). There are strong opposing views between researchers on primary copper deficiency versus thiomolybdate toxicity (or what could be described as secondary copper deficiency).

Measuring the copper status of an animal is difficult. Copper is stored in the liver and the blood copper levels are, through some poorly understood mechanism, topped up as required by the body. The most accurate measure of an animal's overall copper status is, therefore, to measure the amount of copper stored within the liver. Although there have been techniques described within dairy cows for vets to perform liver biopsies in the live standing animal this is not widely practised and certainly not in suckler cows. The procedure is invasive and there is a risk of infection and haemorrhage. It is also poorly understood how painful the procedure is for the cow. An alternative approach is to test livers from cull cows that have either died on farm or been slaughtered – either way the liver can be harvested/sampled and sent for testing. A reasonable number of cows should be assessed for a meaningful interpretation of overall herd copper status – there could be individual variations in copper status that, viewed in isolation, could be misleading.

Copper blood levels are a second-best method of assessing herd status; they only tell us what is in the blood, not what is in the body overall and only on that day, bearing in mind copper in the blood fluctuates more than it does in the liver. As the blood is topped up from the liver, blood levels may measure in the acceptable range despite the animal being low in the liver and being fed a deficient diet. The blood levels may not fall below acceptable levels until the liver is emptied of copper and given that copper levels will fluctuate over time anyway, one sample will give no indication as to whether the levels are in the process of rising or falling. As with liver sampling, blood testing just one individual animal is not useful in assessing herd levels as copper absorption can be affected by other things such as gut parasites, fluke or Johne's disease. Ten animals from a group that have had the same nutritional management should be sampled and the results averaged to iron out variations. Testing ten animals at regular intervals, every 6 months for example, allows a trend to be identified and helps to make informed decisions on copper supplementation for the whole herd.

COPPER TOXICITY

Copper toxicity can be acute or chronic depending on the level of copper exposure and by what route it is entering the body. Acute copper toxicity is usually a result of an overdose of an injectable or oral copper preparation. Chronic toxicity could be from an accumulation of copper from a number of sources, for example, powdered mineral, copper-enriched concentrate feed, boluses, injections or naturally high levels in the water or forage. Acute toxicity is dramatic with the sudden appearance of one or more very sick or dead animals; chronic toxicity tends to be less obvious. Copper accumulates in liver cells and eventually reaches toxic levels where it causes damage; the liver cells (hepatocytes) practically 'burst' and there is a mass degeneration of the liver releasing large amounts of this accumulated copper into the circulation. Large amounts of copper released into the blood at any one time can cause destruction of the red blood cells resulting in the clinical signs of anaemia and jaundice. Typically, the acutely poisoned animal is pale, with an increased respiratory rate, lethargic, it has dark red urine and yellow tinged mucous membranes (jaundice). There are other diseases which will cause this clinical presentation such as babesiosis, blue green algae poisoning, leptospirosis, brassica poisoning and *Clostridium noyi* type D disease. Further investigation of suspect cases is required to achieve a diagnosis.

As damage occurs to the hepatocytes, they release liver enzymes into the blood. These enzymes are detectable on a blood test but are not specific to copper toxicity; elevated liver enzymes indicate liver damage, which could be caused by a number of different disease processes. A diagnosis of acute copper toxicity in the live animal would require liver enzymes to be elevated *and* blood copper levels to be extremely high (>50 umol/l) (Livesey et al., 2002). On PME copper levels within the kidney will be high and microscopic examination of the liver will show degenerating or 'burst' liver cells. Liver copper levels in this scenario cannot be relied upon: First, because the liver can store potentially large amounts of copper without illness. Second, as once the liver cells have burst the copper is released into the circulation so, for this reason, liver levels might not be as high as expected (Laven and Livesey, 2004).

Chronic toxicity can be less obvious or may even be subclinical; a cost to production without any obvious outward signs of disease.

Careful consideration is needed when interpreting blood copper levels as the copper in blood is bound to a protein associated with inflammation; falsely high copper levels can be due to inflammation rather than the release of copper into the blood – the rising protein levels seem to grab copper from somewhere, presumably the liver. Studies suggest, however, that elevated copper levels due to unrelated inflammation would not usually exceed 30 umol/l so levels higher than this are likely to be genuine toxicity (Laven and Livesey, 2004).

Analysing the inclusion rate of copper in the diet can be a valuable tool but does not always indicate if the diet is over supplemented or deficient. What is fed in the diet is not correlated directly to what the cow absorbs from the diet. Copper absorption from the gastrointestinal tract is influenced by many factors as stated above. For example, cattle grazing pasture have a high iron content in their diet simply from the soil they ingest. This may also be the case in grass silage-based rations. The mineral content of the water also needs to be taken into account especially when natural waterways or bore-hole water is utilised.

Copper deficiency and toxicity is complicated! Copper toxicity is also a food safety risk as high levels in meat and milk are a risk to human health - where suspected or confirmed the responsible authorities need notifying.

SELENIUM TOXICITY (SELENOSIS)

In the UK selenium toxicity (selenosis) is only ever caused by over supplementation of selenium either in the diet, through an oral drench, by bolus or by injection. In other countries, however, for example the US, natural toxicity can occur – some plant species contain high levels of selenium and cattle can ingest high levels of selenium over a long period of time so leading to accumulation and chronic toxicity. Selenium toxicity is relatively rare, approximately 50% of selenium ingested is excreted in the faeces (Aitken, 2001). A safe dietary level is considered to be up to 0.3 mg/kg

DM (Aitken, 2001). Toxicity can be induced with >0.5 mg/kg body weight of selenium by injection.

Selenium has a vital role in the body as an antioxidant protecting cells from damage by free radicals (chemicals that naturally occur in the blood and damage cell membranes). There is, however, a delicate balance; too much selenium actually causes cell damage. Selenium also displaces sulphur within keratin and disrupts hoof and horn growth.

Selenosis can be classified into acute and chronic (Watts, 1994).

- **Acute selenosis**. The clinical signs include depression, salivation, blindness, partial paralysis, difficulty in breathing, sometimes abdominal pain, diarrhoea and death
- **Chronic selenosis**. Here the clinical signs are weight loss, hair loss, rough coat, hoof deformities starting at the coronary band, sloughing of the hooves, lesions at the base of the horn, infertility, diarrhoea and ultimately death.

Selenium, like copper, is present in both meat and milk and, in toxicity cases, should be considered a food safety risk – the responsible authorities need notifying of potentially high levels in food to ensure that human health is not at risk.

As discussed in Chapter 10, glutathione peroxidase (GSHPx) is used as an indirect measure of body selenium levels in order to diagnose deficiency, but GSHPx levels are not raised in selenium toxicity – the body does not produce any more of the enzyme than it needs to. A diagnosis of toxicity can only be obtained by directly measuring selenium levels in the blood. This is useful particularly in cases of acute toxicity but blood levels drop almost immediately the exposure levels drop so blood selenium is not a reliable indicator of chronic toxicity. Hair and horn selenium levels are, conversely, useful in the diagnosis of chronic selenosis as the levels incorporated in these stable tissues are non-fluctuating (Watts, 1994). Post-mortem liver and kidney samples are also a reliable indicator of an animal's selenium status, in both the short and long terms.

There is no specific treatment for selenosis, but the source of the selenium should be removed, if possible, and the animal fed a low selenium diet. It has been reported that the excretion of selenium in the bile can be increased by feeding arsanilic acid to the feed (Aitken, 2001), whether this is a practical solution or not is a different matter!

LEAD POISONING

The source of lead in a poisoning case is usually identified as a battery, bonfire ashes, old flaking lead paint, lead flashing, sump oil, old lead shot or old lead based clays from clay pigeon shoots. Batteries remain the most common source as reported by the then Veterinary Laboratories Agency UK (VLA) now part of APHA (Payne and Livesey, 2010). The source of lead can sometimes be introduced by 'fly tipping' and remain unknown to the farmer until the boundaries of the field are closely inspected. Lead contamination of feedstuffs is also a consideration. Lead is present naturally in the earth and background levels of lead in the diet are usually normal and safe. In lead mining areas, however, the environmental levels in the soil are usually naturally high – this may not be consistent across an area or even a field but in small pockets of mineral deposition. It is therefore difficult to get a representative sample of soil for estimating the local risk. Areas where spoil from lead mines was disposed of tend to be highly contaminated over and above the natural level that may be high to start with. If flooding or erosion mobilises these deposits toxicity can occur miles away from the original source. This can happen on flood planes or downstream. Very little lead is absorbed from the soil into the leafy parts of the plant so soil ingestion poses the highest risk, not forage itself. This is a problem on occasions of poor grass cover, mole hills, feeding from troughs or heavy poaching.

Lead is more readily absorbed by pre-ruminants than ruminants, the reason being that the mature rumen contains compounds that bind to soluble lead and make it insoluble in the rumen liquor and unabsorbable for the body. Young animals are also the most inquisitive with their characteristic licking of abnormal objects or painted surfaces being a common behaviour.

Acute lead poisoning, likewise, seen more commonly in the young pre-ruminant animal, can present as sudden death. If found alive, neurological signs are the predominant clinical feature. Tremors, muscle twitching, rolling eyes, snapping of the jaw, grinding of the teeth (bruxism), salivation, convulsions, staggering and frenzied behaviour are all to be expected.

Subacute toxicity, the more likely presentation in older animals, where animals live for a number of days before death, typically presents with a loss of appetite, grinding of the teeth (bruxism), blindness, incoordination, circling, abdominal pain and diarrhoea. In the authors' experience affected animals develop an unusual smell.

Both acute and subacute clinical signs are similar to cerebrocortical necrosis (CCN) (Chapter 14), Vitamin A deficiency (Chapter 12), ketosis (Chapter 17) and meningitis (Chapter 11).

The presentation of chronic disease, caused by exposure to environmental lead in the soil, can cause osteoporosis and weak bones. This is because lead can displace calcium in bone and weaken it as a result; an increased number of fractures are likely. Contracted tendons and gait abnormalities are, for the same reasons, a frequently observed clinical feature. Anaemia and kidney disease can also develop.

When diagnosing lead toxicity, blood levels are a good indicator. Lead is incorporated into the red blood cell so whole blood is required for analysis rather than serum or plasma from a separated sample. Kidney and liver levels are useful tissues for testing post-mortem; bone lead is a measure of long-term exposure. As lead toxicity causes anaemia, then haematology (a count of the number of red and white blood cells) can be used to support a diagnosis.

Treatment for lead toxicity includes what is known as *chelation therapy*. Chelation involves using a drug to bind the toxic substance rendering it safe or rendering it fit for excretion from the body. For lead, sodium calcium edetate is commonly used and can be administered intravenously by a vet. Thiamine hydrochloride administered by intramuscular injection (readily available and used to treat CCN in ruminants) is also a specific treatment as it reduces the amount of lead deposited in tissues (Reis et al., 2010). Other therapy is merely supportive, for example, sedatives to control convulsions, fluids to help kidney function and supportive nursing to aid recovery.

Lead poisoning in food producing animals is a food safety risk and advice from the authorities is required to protect human health. There is often a withdrawal period to observe before the animal or others from the group can enter the food chain; blood testing may be needed to clarify the position. If exposure is from environmental lead, animals should be removed from high-risk pastures for at least 16 weeks before slaughter (Payne and Livesey, 2010).

POISONOUS PLANTS

When cattle are out at pasture, plant poisonings should never be discounted as a possible cause of disease. Certain situations make plant poisoning more likely; for example, if cattle have not grazed a particular pasture before or if there has been stormy weather and otherwise inaccessible branches have fallen into the field. If there is a lack of grass to graze then cattle may reach to hedge rows and eat plants they would not usually entertain but do so when hungry enough – there are few poisonous plants that an animal would choose to eat over lush grass. Along the same lines, if cattle are outwintered and there has been heavy snow fall, cattle may look for alternative forage. There is always a risk that garden cuttings may be dumped over field boundaries and unbeknown to the perpetrator cattle consume the foliage, which may turn out to be poisonous. Cattle that have escaped from a field may have ingested plants on their exploits that may be toxic. Housed cattle are also

at risk; conserved forage may contain poisonous plants that grew undetected in among the forage crop – that said, many plants lose their toxicity when cut and dried but that is certainly not always the case. In addition, poisonous plants and trees can grow through the walls of sheds and provide nibblings for the cattle housed within.

Many toxic plants cause death within a few hours and a diagnosis is obtained from finding partially digested leaves within the rumen that, by the trained or experienced eye, can be identified.

Rhododendron poisoning

Rhododendrons are abundant especially in the estates of grand houses in the UK and especially in slightly acidic soils (Figure 13.1). Cattle show clinical signs within 3 hours of ingestion of the plant and present with incoordination, and abnormal rumen function resulting in ruminal fluid spilling from the nose and mouth (incorrectly often referred to as vomiting), and, abdominal pain. This is often followed by recumbency, convulsions and death after 48–72 hours. Oral administration of cold tea was always advocated in the past but there is little evidence for its effectiveness. With supportive care some animals will recover.

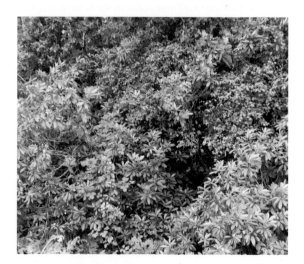

FIGURE 13.1 Rhododendrons just at the end of their flowering period in mid-summer

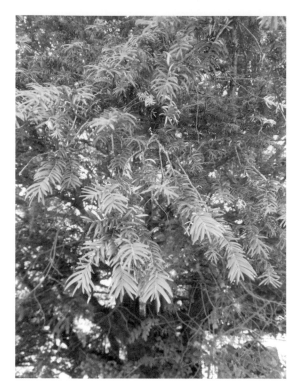

FIGURE 13.2 Yew tree in a church yard

Yew poisoning

Yew is the deadliest of all plants; sudden death very soon after ingestion is the norm, sometimes the animal dies with the plant in its mouth (Figure 13.2). Yew is abundant in the countryside and is often found in or near church yards. Yew contains *taxine*, which has a fatally depressive effect on the heart and respiration.

Nitrate poisoning

This is more of a problem for cattle grazing clover, or, brassica crops such as kale, swedes, turnip, forage rape or fodder beet. Nitrates are taken up by the roots of a plant and, as the next step on from photosynthesis, converted into protein. In drought conditions nitrates remain in the soil and are taken up by the plant in large amounts when it next rains. In overcast conditions the nitrate remains in the

leaves rather than being converted into protein. This makes the plant a potential cause of nitrate poisoning to the herbivore that eats it. The roots of a plant usually contain more nitrate than the leaves (Sargison, 2008b) so aggressive or hungry grazing makes matters worse.

Nitrates are normally converted into nitrites in the rumen and these nitrites are then converted into ammonia. The final conversion to ammonia requires carbohydrate. If there is insufficient carbohydrate in the diet for this to happen, nitrite accumulates and binds with haemoglobin in the red blood cells in significant amounts. The haemoglobin in red blood cells is responsible for transporting oxygen around the body. This nitrite effect renders the haemoglobin dysfunctional by converting it to the ineffective *methaemoglobin*; the tissues of the body are starved of oxygen. The affected animal gasps for air, the heart rate is increased, the muscles tremor and the mucous membranes (gums, pinks of the eye and the lining of the vulva) turn brown. Death ensues and a PME along with the history is usually sufficient to obtain a diagnosis. The carcase and a blood sample from the carcase is characteristically brown in colour. In an outbreak situation there are usually one or two affected animals but the rest of the group grazing the field are at risk and should be promptly removed and fed a high carbohydrate diet. Treatment of ill animals may be attempted and involves the unlicensed use of intravenous methylene blue administered by a vet. The methylene blue supposedly helps reconvert methaemoglobin back to haemoglobin.

Bracken poisoning

Bracken poisoning is a chronic state that results from prolonged ingestion (over a number of weeks) of fresh (Figure 13.3) or conserved bracken plants. Affected animals have evidence of otherwise unexplained bleeding and anaemia. Blood in the urine is a common finding and can be confused with babesiosis. Bracken affects the bone marrow, which is responsible for the production of new red blood

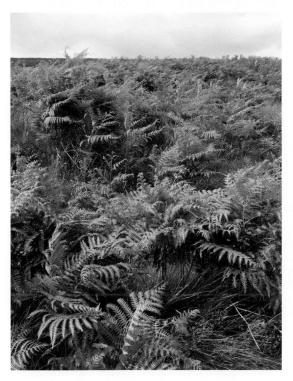

FIGURE 13.3 Bracken on upland in North East England

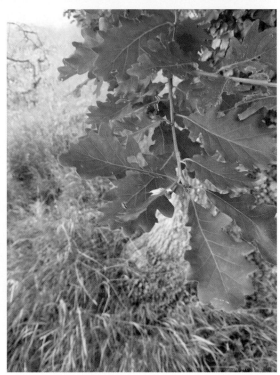

FIGURE 13.4 Oak leaves

cells and platelets (platelets help with blood clotting). Anaemia leaves the animal lethargic, weak and reluctant to move when required. There is also a depletion of white blood cells, so cattle are more susceptible to infection. Death can occur and at post-mortem there may be multiple small haemorrhages within organs such as the liver or kidney or a large, fatal bleed into the abdominal or thoracic cavity. Bracken is also carcinogenic and tumours in the reproductive tract can result from prolonged ingestion of bracken, and similarly for the jawbone tumours in sheep. Bracken poisoning is a potential food safety concern and cattle must have been free from exposure to the plant for 15 days prior to entering the food chain.

Oak poisoning

Although oak trees are commonly situated in cattle pastures, cases of oak poisoning are rare.

Oak leaves (Figure 13.4) and acorns contain tannins, which are hydrolysed in the rumen to gallic acid, pyrogallol and other compounds. These tannins can be poisonous if ingested in sufficient quantities. Young immature leaves and acorns are known to contain more tannin. Normally the rumen microbes sufficiently detoxify these compounds but when overwhelmed the break down products of the tannins survive and this causes cell damage (Dunn, 2006). Overwhelming ingestion may follow a storm when extra leaves and acorns fall and get eaten by animals sheltering under the tree. Kidney failure results and the affected cattle present with abdominal pain, poor rumen function, abdominal distention and constipation. Depending on the degree of kidney damage the animals can die within a few hours or survive a number of days. There is no specific treatment; cattle should be removed from high-risk pastures and fed normal safe forage. Fluid therapy, perhaps intraruminal fluids, but only in the absence of rumen stasis and distension, will help to support the damaged kidneys. Otherwise, intravenous fluids could be attempted but this is expensive in the face of a prognosis that is poor – renal failure is usually irreversible. Adding 10% calcium hydroxide (hydrated lime) to the drinking water prior to cattle grazing high-risk fields has been suggested as effective (Dunn, 2006) but this is rarely practicable. Fencing off oak trees within grazed pastures seems a more sensible option.

Foxglove poisoning

Foxgloves are not usually eaten by cattle, but they can sometimes seemingly develop a taste for them (Figure 13.5). Foxgloves contain the infamous digoxin that is pharmacologically classified as a cardiac glycoside, a class of drug which increases the contractions of the heart muscle. Used carefully it is a useful drug, but excessive amounts cause

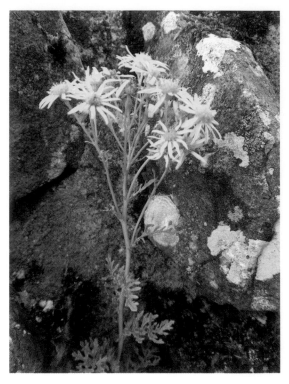

FIGURE 13.6 Ragwort in flower

fatal heart failure usually seen as sudden death (Payne and Murphy, 2010). Foxgloves usually grow in small clusters and their large pink flowers mean they are readily identified and are easily pulled from the ground by the diligent farmer.

Ragwort poisoning

Dried mature plants are more palatable and appealing to livestock than fresh plants (Figure 13.6), especially when bundled up with hay. Ragwort contains pyrrolizidine alkaloids which, once metabolised, are toxic to the liver. Accumulation over time causes the symptoms of liver disease namely: ill thrift, diarrhoea, jaundice, and abdominal pain. Horse owners are, justifiably, hugely concerned about ragwort as the plant is much more toxic to horses than it is to cattle and sheep.

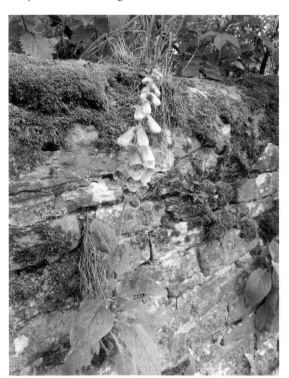

FIGURE 13.5 Foxgloves

Hemlock poisoning

The whole plant is toxic, that is the leaves, stem, roots and flowers but toxicity is reduced by drying, as it is when bundled in conserved forage. The toxin is an alkaloid that causes regurgitation, salivation and a slow heart rate followed by a rapid heart rate, rapid respiration, then decreased rumen motility, dilated pupils and a staggering gate. The prognosis is poor, but treatment can be attempted by administering tannic acid, such as very strong cold tea, to neutralise the alkaloid (Sargison, 2008b).

Laburnum poisoning

Laburnum poisoning is similar to hemlock as it is caused by a similar alkaloid, in this instance, cytisine. Animals present with abdominal distention, diarrhoea, muscular spasms, incoordination and regurgitation (Sargison, 2008b).

Other poisonous plants

- bog asphodel
- buttercups
- crowfoot
- laurel
- deadly nightshade
- privet
- laurel, for example, cherry laurel
- fat hen
- dog's mercury
- bluebell
- lilly of the valley (Payne and Murphy, 2010)

GASTROINTESTINAL DISEASE

Parasitic gastroenteritis (gut worms)

Gut worm infections are acquired by cattle through ingesting the infectious parasitic larvae on the pasture. The larvae have hatched from eggs that were shed in the faeces of another animal and were produced from the adult worms that live within the gastrointestinal tract. The larvae in the faeces are first-stage larvae that then develop on the pasture to second stage and then third stage whereupon they become infective. There are two species of worms that are of particular concern to cattle in the UK, *Ostertagia ostertagi* and *Cooperia onchophora*. The adult worms live in two different sites in the gastrointestinal tract; *C. onchophora* lives in the small intestine, *O. ostertagi* in the abomasum. Once the third-stage larvae reach their target site, they develop to fourth stage larvae and then into adults – this takes about three weeks. Male and female worms are required for reproduction and therefore to produce more eggs. The larvae and adult worms cause disease; a moderate burden of adult worms may not cause any outward disease but can affect growth rates by up to 30% in young cattle. Heavy burdens can cause obvious disease; diarrhoea, emaciation and sometimes death. This is typically seen later in the season when larval pasture contamination is at its highest.

The worm larvae are host specific so cattle larvae can be eaten by sheep but will not develop into adult worms and, likewise, cattle can ingest sheep larvae but, again, they do not develop into adults. The one exception to this is *Nematodirus*, a common parasite of sheep but occasionally young calves also; both species are affected, usually in the spring after turn out and both presenting with a profuse scour (McCoy et al., 2004). In one particular report the pasture had not been grazed by sheep in previous years but young artificially reared calves had been grazing there in previous successive springs. This suggests that calves alone can sustain the *Nematodirus* life cycle from season to season without the involvement of sheep. Despite this knowledge, *Nematodirus* is not routinely considered in parasite control on cattle farms but maybe should be; it should certainly be considered in any outbreak of profuse scour in young calves at spring grazing.

The hatching of the eggs and the development of the infective larvae that cause parasitic gastroenteritis (PGE) depends on the moisture in the faecal pat and the ambient temperature. It can be as little as a week in a warm, wet summer where temperatures are between 15–23°C, but it can take up to 3 weeks when temperatures are 10°C (COWS, 2014a). The larvae are not particularly motile, they can only move a few centimetres, but they do need to move away from the pat and onto the herbage to stand a reasonable chance of being ingested by grazing cattle. This is facilitated by moisture; rain will disperse a faecal pat and help the larvae to move. If the weather is too dry the eggs and larvae desiccate and die.

Knowing the likelihood of larvae surviving and how long it will take them to develop is useful in PGE control. Knowing the pre-patent period for each species of worm is also useful, especially when monitoring for disease and monitoring the effectiveness of anthelmintic treatments. The prepatent period is defined as the time it takes from a larva being eaten by the host, developing into a mature adult worm and finally it laying eggs and them appearing in the animal's faeces. This is not always as quick or straightforward as might be expected; *O. ostertagi* has a unique strategy to survive the winter months. This parasite has the ability to stop its life cycle in early winter at the larval stage while taking refuge in the gastric gland of the host's abomasum. Towards the end of the winter period the larva resumes its lifecycle and there is a synchronised emergence of larvae which causes damage to the lining of the abomasum causing clinical signs such as abdominal pain, inappetence, diarrhoea and even death. This is known as *type 2 ostertagiosis* and is seen in late winter or early spring. Even though many animals in a group may be affected only a few may show clinical signs of this disease.

Most cattle at grass will be infected with both *O. ostertagi* and *C. onchophora* worms; the effects of being infected with both worms is worse than being infected by just one species alone. The impaired protein digestion in the abomasum that results from ostertagiosis is bad enough but the damage to the small intestine as result of a *C. onchophora* infection ensures a significant effect

– a subclinical reduction in performance or full blown disease (COWS, 2014a).

Young cattle develop immunity to the larvae and once achieved can prevent an adult population becoming established in their gut; this means no reproduction by the worms and no further contamination of the pasture with eggs. Adult cows (and sheep) act like vacuum cleaners ('hoovers') and keep the burden on pastures low (Figure 13.7.) The development of immunity takes a whole grazing season for *C. onchophora* and two seasons for *O. ostertagi* (COWS, 2014a). Unfortunately, this is not absolute and some older cattle will still harbour adult worms and still pass a few eggs although with no outward signs of disease and probably no subclinical reduction of performance either. If cattle have not been allowed to graze pasture as young animals and have therefore had no exposure to worms then they are unlikely to have developed immunity.

Knowing the life cycle of the two main worms allows us to have an idea of the factors resulting in high-risk pasture as opposed to low risk.

- **Example Pasture 1**. A pasture grazed late in the autumn will be heavily contaminated with eggs and over wintered larvae. The following spring and summer the cattle grazing this pasture will ingest these infective larvae. If the cattle are naïve, that is they have not seen parasites before, they will become infected and shed a large number of eggs onto the pasture. If these cattle are not grazed with their mothers, for example artificially reared calves in their first grazing season, pasture contamination will be even higher and there will be no hoovering effect to help reduce the challenge. This is high-risk pasture.
- **Example Pasture 2**. A pasture that has not been grazed that season but closed off for silage or hay making. Few larvae will have survived from the previous autumn and by late summer when the pasture is released for grazing the larval levels will be very low. This is low risk pasture.

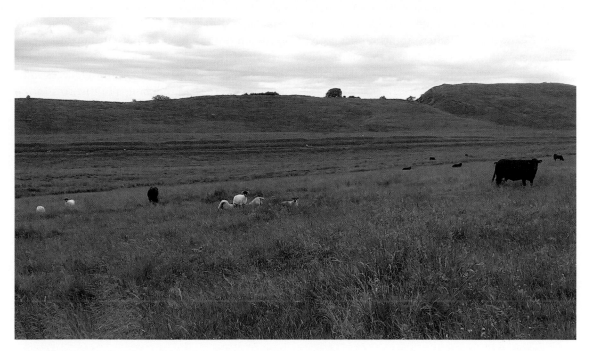

FIGURE 13.7 Mixed grazing with cattle and sheep can reduce the worm burden on the pasture for both species

- **Example Pasture 3**. A colder winter is conducive to larval survival as it encourages the larvae to hibernate and survive with a very low metabolic rate. Snow cover, ice and cold moisture also reduce the chance of larval desiccation (a typical UK winter!). So, after a cold winter the pasture is high risk (COWS, 2014a).
- **Example Pasture 4**. In a warm winter the metabolic rate of the non-hibernating larvae is relatively high and they may well die off before the spring when the cattle are turned back out to graze. Pasture after a warm winter is low risk (COWS, 2014a).

At turn out, if non-immune cattle are grazing fields that were grazed by cattle in the previous autumn they will be ingesting overwintered larvae. Anthelmintic drugs can be used to kill the worms in the gut before they fully mature and start shedding eggs – otherwise it is obviously this cycle which perpetuates and contaminates the pasture further. As the pre-patent period (the time taken for a worm to develop to the stage of laying eggs) is 3 weeks then this treatment needs to be approximately three weeks post turn out. This can then be repeated at regular intervals through the summer months, assuming, that is, the cattle continue to graze the same pasture. Alternatively, young cattle can be closely observed and anthelmintic only used when there is a perceived effect on production. The downside to this is that gut damage will have taken place, this gut damage may be irreparable, the cattle may be unable to compensate for the reduced production, and, finally, further levels of pasture parasitic contamination will have occurred. This technique exists nevertheless and has been adapted and developed and is now referred to as targeted selective treatment (TST).

Targeted selective treatment (TST)

PGE is observed to be the most common growth limiting factor in cattle production. With TST, growth rates are monitored and any animals not achieving expected target weights, targets based on well researched algorithms, receive an anthelmintic treatment. TST allow anthelmintics to be administered in good time, before there are irreversible effects on production. TST also decreases the number of anthelmintic treatments administered as animals are only treated if there is a need. Fewer treatments lessens the resistance pressure on the worm population.

At the end of the grazing season it is still a frequent recommendation that cattle are treated at or just before housing (if products with persistent activity are used then the product could be given in advance of housing, knowing it will still be working come the actual point of housing). Why administer a housing dose of anthelmintic?

- The cattle will be spared a worm burden over the winter months, which would otherwise cause likely production losses.
- The risk of type 2 ostertagiosis developing in springtime is reduced providing the drug is capable of killing the dormant worms in the gut lining. ML are highly effective, benzimidazoles have variable activity and levamisole is ineffective at killing dormant worms in the gut lining. Anthelmintic classification is covered in more detail in Chapter 26.
- Cattle cleared of worms over winter will not shed eggs on to the pasture at turn out so preventing unnecessary pasture contamination very early in the grazing season, which would otherwise be a problem to young naïve co-grazers.

Measuring worm burdens, faecal worm egg counts

Faecal worm egg counts (FWEC) are used to measure the number of eggs shed in the faeces of an animal at one point in time. The results are quoted as the number of eggs per gram of faeces. A representative sample should be taken from 10–15 cattle. The cattle will be selected, ordinarily, as not having been wormed so the truest picture can be

established. To calculate the animal's total daily excretion this needs to be multiplied up by an estimation of the amount of faeces that that animal will produce in 24 hours. Eggs in the faeces indicates there are egg producing adult worms in the gut. If there are no eggs in the faeces this does not, however, rule out infection as the worms may be in the prepatent period or the worms may be hibernating in their larval stage as is the case in overwintered *O. ostertagi*. The actual number of eggs in the faeces is not well correlated to the number of adult worms in the animal's gut nor is it well correlated to the weight gain or weight loss of the animal. They are useful nonetheless at giving an indication of infection and of the level of pasture contamination that may ensue over the next few weeks. In summary, faecal egg counts are worthwhile but their limitations need to be borne in mind.

The technique used to count the number of eggs per gram of faeces is called the McMaster technique. When samples are collected from the ground in the field it is important that faeces are collected from multiple areas in the cow pat so the sample is representative of overall gut output. The McMaster method involves mixing a certain weight of faeces, typically 3 grams, with a saturated salt solution. The mixture is then passed through a sieve to remove the fibrous faecal material and the solution that remains is then syringed into a special recessed microscope slide that is overlaid by a grid (Figures 13.8 and 13.9). The number of eggs in the grid are counted and the number of eggs per gram of faeces tested can then be calculated. Each egg seen typically represents 50 eggs per gram. Eggs from *Ostertagia* and *Cooperia* species cannot be differentiated by this method – put bluntly, they both look the same!

Faecal worm egg counts can also be used to see if an anthelmintic treatment has been effective or not. Here, the animals sampled *have* been wormed. At a certain interval post treatment, depending on the type of product, a post treatment faecal sample can be examined for the presence or absence of eggs. This is called a *drench check* or an

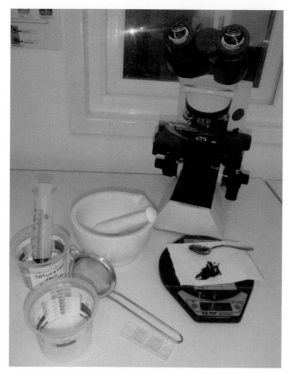

FIGURE 13.8 Equipment required for a faecal worm egg count

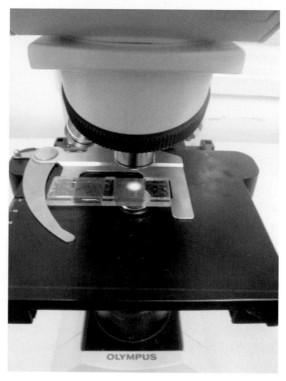

FIGURE 13.9 McMaster slide on a microscope stage

anthelmintic efficacy check or a faecal egg count reduction test (FECRT).

Pre-dosing sample results need to have been done first to ensure there was actually a worm burden there to start with! These pre-dosing samples will have been performed in the usual manner, that is, individual faeces samples collected from 10–15 identified young animals in their first grazing season. The FWEC should exceed 200 epg (eggs per gram) to ensure the anthelmintic treatment has something to work on.

The cattle are then weighed and treated with the required amount of anthelmintic, administered correctly, all in accordance with the data sheet.

The second faecal samples should be collected at fixed times – 14 to 17 days after a treatment with a benzimidazole (white wormer) or macrocyclic lactone (clear wormer) or 7 to 10 days after a levamisole (yellow wormer) treatment.

Anthelmintic resistance is said to exist if more than 5% of worms survive treatment. The results

are expressed as a % reduction in the egg count and this is assumed to roughly equate to the percentage reduction in the adult worm population count.

For example: for a pre-worming egg count of 550 epg, and a post worming egg count of 50 epg, the reduction percentage is as follows:

$$\text{Absolute reduction: } 550-50 = 500$$

$$\text{Percentage reduction: } 500/550 \times 100 = 90\%$$

In this case the egg count has reduced by 90%, which sounds quite good but it means an estimated 10% of adult worms have survived the treatment; resistance is over 5% so should be considered a problem. When using a conventional McMaster technique each egg seen represents 50 epg of faeces. Using a more sensitive dilution ratio, for example, where one egg represents 10 eggs per gram, it is important to factor this into the calculations to avoid the misclassification of resistance.

The responsible use of anthelmintics and anthelmintic resistance is discussed further in Chapter 26.

Blood testing for gut worms

Pepsinogen is a chemical, a pro-enzyme, that is secreted by the glands in the abomasal wall and converted to the enzyme, pepsin, when it encounters the gastric acid of the stomach. Pepsin is the enzyme involved in protein digestion, it breaks proteins down into their component amino acids, which can then be absorbed by the body for subsequent rebuilding into bodily proteins as required by the animal. When the abomasal glands are damaged, most typically by infestation with *Ostertagia* larvae, the glands spill out the pepsinogen which is detectable in the blood. Some pepsinogen in blood is normal, but high levels suggest parasitism, but, quite specifically, *Ostertagia*; pepsinogen levels do not give any indication of the involvement of *Cooperia*.

Post-mortem diagnosis of PGE

Ostertagia are clearly visible on the abomasal wall. Where there has been significant gastric gland inhabitation by hibernating *Ostertagia* larvae, the abomasal wall will have a cobbled appearance. *Cooperia* are harder to detect with the naked eye.

PERI-WEANING SCOUR SYNDROME

Peri-weaning scour syndrome (PWSS) is a chronic scour and wasting syndrome of artificially reared dairy calves commencing at 5–10 weeks of age and typically coinciding with weaning. The calves continue to eat with no reduction in appetite but can scour for up to 6 months. The condition has a 10% mortality rate (Mason, 2004). The calves appear ill thriven, pot bellied and dull coated. The exact cause of the condition remains unknown but is thought to be multifactorial. From pre-weaning

through to becoming a fully developed ruminant the gastrointestinal tract has to change dramatically and at this young age calves are exposed to a variety of pathogens such as *Cryptosporidium* spp. and Coccidia, which damage the intestinal tract. A combination of infectious diseases, dietary mismanagement and non-specific stress is likely to contribute to PWSS. As part of an investigation into PWSS a full evaluation of pre and post-weaning practices is required (Mason, 2004). In terms of treatment, badly affected calves should be returned to a whole milk diet and the weaning procedure started again after 3–4 weeks. The calves should be tested for BVD virus; either persistent or transient infection would be of interest. Salmonella and coccidial infection should also be ruled out through faecal testing.

MALIGNANT CATARRHAL FEVER

Malignant catarrhal fever (MCF) is a viral disease with a high mortality rate. Ovine herpes virus 2 (OHV2) is responsible for causing the disease; a virus that exists in most sheep populations without causing disease in the sheep (Russell, 2009). As is typical of most herpes viruses, sheep only shed the virus when under stress and for very short periods of time. The virus is shed in the sheep's nasal secretions. Lambs are infected at a young age by adult sheep; the lambs then shed virus for a number of weeks until they develop immunity after which shedding only occurs intermittently.

Cattle infected with OHV2 exhibit a combination of the following clinical signs: a fever, salivation, watery eyes and nose, whitening of the eyes, crusty scabs on the nose, ulcers in the mouth and diarrhoea. Affected cattle do not multiply or shed the virus so are not infectious to others. Cases are therefore often sporadic, but outbreaks can occur when a number of susceptible cattle are exposed to sheep that happen to be stressed and are shedding the virus.

There is no treatment for the disease and most

infected animals die, this can be fairly acute or take a week or more.

The clinical appearance of MCF is not dissimilar to a number of other viral diseases affecting cattle, diseases such as foot and mouth disease and BVD. MCF can be diagnosed through testing the blood of an infected animal. Based on a positive diagnosis the animal should be euthanased to prevent unnecessary suffering as recovery is highly unlikely although not impossible.

There is no commercially available vaccine for MCF; the main control measure is to minimise contact between cattle and sheep. There is a higher risk of transmission at housing or when cattle and sheep are sharing water and feed troughs. There is less risk when co-grazing outside although the risk is not entirely eliminated.

RINGWORM (DERMATOPHYTOSIS)

Ringworm is a fungal infection of youngstock that typically appears as grey, slightly raised circular lesions, predominantly on the head and neck. There are many strains of ringworm but the most common is *Trichophyton verrucosum*, closely followed by *T. mentagrophytes* (Scott, 2017). The lesions are hairless and are non-itchy unless they become secondarily infected. The lesions can spread and cause quite dramatic large areas of hair loss. Debilitated calves with poor immune function are more likely to succumb to infection. Ringworm is contagious, and spores live in the environment for long periods of time (the spores can survive for up to 4 years in typical conditions). Calves can be infected from spores in the environment or from direct contact with one another – the disease is more prevalent in the winter months for this reason. The incubation period is 1–4 weeks. The disease is usually self-limiting as calves produce an immune response over time but topical preparation, in the form of enilconazole washes, can be used to kill off the fungus and stop further spread to others in the group or further

spread on the affected animal itself. Vaccination is an option for the prevention of infection, it is a live vaccine of *T. verrucosum*. Two injections are required 10–14 days apart well in advance of the risk period. Vaccination is also advocated in the treatment of disease at twice the preventative dose rate, again two injections 10–14 days apart. Onset of immunity is 3 weeks after completion of the primary course.

The lesions, although quite distinctive, can be confused with viral papillomatosis (warts) or dermatophilosis (rain scald). Ringworm can be diagnosed through examining hairs plucked from the affected region. The hair can be examined immediately using potassium hydroxide and a microscope to see if there are spores on the hair shaft or they can be cultured in a special culture medium which changes colour with a positive result. *T. verrucosum* is a particularly slow-growing fungus and it will take a few weeks until a diagnosis is reached.

Historically ringworm had an impact on the quality of hide for leather production. Now the main economic impact comes from the unsightly appearance of cases and the consequential restriction of trade that infected cattle experience; affected cattle are infectious to others and contaminate the environment as they go, so they should not be moved or mixed with others. This includes auction marts. This poses a problem if cattle are infected just before the sales period as it may take a number of months for lesions to disappear. In this scenario, once treated the lesions are not likely to be infectious but given that the lesions are still visible there will be understandable concerns raised as it is not easy to tell whether the lesions are in fact infectious or not and the movement or sale of the animal is likely to be restricted simply to err on the side of caution.

Ringworm is also a zoonosis and personal protective equipment should be worn to eliminate contact between human skin and infected cattle. This would include wearing disposable gloves.

ECTO-PARASITIC DISEASE

Louse infestation (pediculosis)

Lice are parasitic insects that cannot survive off the host for any period of time and require direct contact between hosts during yarding, handling or housing for transmission to take place (Urquhart et al., 1987). The life cycle lasts 4–5 weeks and adult females lay 2–3 eggs every 5 days. The eggs attach to the hair shafts, so they do not fall off the host; in human infections the eggs are called nits! In ideal conditions the eggs hatch and turn into nymphs within 30 days but many fail to hatch, and some nymphs do not develop into adults. Lice do not like high moisture or high temperatures which is why infestations are more common in housed cattle during the winter months. The thicker coats grown in the winter are also an ideal habitat for multiplication and survival; the shedding of the winter coat and warmer temperatures seem detrimental to their survival. Infestations are more common in malnourished, immunocompromised animals (Otter et al., 2003); yet another example of the challenge versus immunity balance.

There are two types of louse – they differ mainly in their mouth parts and how they feed – sucking lice and biting lice.

Sucking lice include *Linognathus vituli* (the long nosed louse), *Haematopinus eurysternus* (the short nosed louse) and *Solenopotes capillatus*. Sucking lice have piercing mouth parts and feed on blood, they can cause irritation and anaemia when infesting in high numbers.

Biting lice, sometimes referred to as chewing lice, include *Bovicola bovis*. These lice feed on skin and hair and cause more extensive hair loss than sucking lice. They are also a source of irritation.

Adult lice can be seen with the naked eye and are often an incidental finding when handling or examining the animal for another purpose. Clinical signs include itching, rubbing and excessive licking and hair loss. Both forms of louse infestation have been reported to affect growth rates, and heavy infestations of *L. vituli* have been

reported to cause deaths of young calves (Otter et al., 2003).

Treatment is relatively easy with the use of pour-on preparations containing synthetic pyrethroids (deltamethrin, permethrin, alpha-cypermethrin) all of which are effective against both sucking and biting/chewing lice. It takes 4–5 weeks after treatment for all lice to be killed as it takes this long for them all to hatch from the relative and temporary safety of the egg. In a small number of cases a few lice may evade treatment and survive. Resistance is a growing problem and has been reported in the UK. The application of tea tree oil to the skin at 2 week intervals has been demonstrated to be effective in horses and could be used as an alternative in organically reared cattle or where resistance is suspected (COWS, 2014b). Some human preparations supposedly make the hair too slippery for the lice or eggs to grip although this is not thought to be the mechanism with tea tree oil. Some preparations are thought to suffocate the lice – this may be the mechanism with oils.

Macrocyclic lactones (ML) (moxidectin, ivermectin, eprinomectin, and doromectin) in pour-on or injectable formulations are variably effective. The ML injectable forms are more effective against sucking lice than chewing lice whereas the ML pour-ons are effective against both biting/chewing and sucking lice. Depending on the time of year, the age of the cattle and the grazing management, the use of MLs may not be appropriate in respect of their anthelmintic properties, that is, where their inappropriate use on lice could inadvertently contribute to anthelmintic resistance.

Flies

There are many species of flies that have some relevance to cattle. Some purely create a nuisance such as the face fly (*Musca autumnalis*) and head fly (*Hydrotaea irritans*). Others actually bite, these flies include the horn fly and cattle biting fly (*Haematobia* spp.*) and the stable fly (*Stomoxys calcitrans*). Blowfly, as they are called, such as

Lucilia spp. lay eggs in living tissue that hatch into flesh-eating larvae, commonly known as maggots. These are a bigger problem in sheep and rabbits.

Flies move from animal to animal and farm to farm carrying bacteria, laying eggs and creating a nuisance wherever they go. They are responsible for the transmission of diseases such as summer mastitis (Chapter 15) and New Forest Eye (Chapter 16).

Fly strike

Blow flies are attracted to warm, moist, damp dirty coats and open wounds such as navels, dehorning sites, castration sites and ear tag injuries. Their lifecycle is independent of a host other than being a site to lay eggs which then develop into maggots within 24 hours – this could equally be a piece of dead flesh rather than a live host. The maggots burrow into the skin and release enzymes digesting tissues as they go. This allows secondary bacterial infection to develop and the process attracts more flies. Toxins are released by the affected tissue and ammonia is secreted by the maggot; both are absorbed into the animal's circulation causing them to become ill. After about 4 days maggots pupate and fall off the host, and within 3–7 days, they hatch into young, adult flies. The pupae can survive over winter and emerge as the weather warms up in the spring. Fly populations are worst in the warm, humid summer months; sheltered pastures near trees and water pose high risk for the cattle (Sargison, 2008a).

When an animal is infested with maggots it is said to be 'struck'. This requires prompt treatment. The area should be clipped and cleaned, all maggots removed, and a cypermethrin product applied to the area. Topical antibiotic spray may be prescribed.

A pour-on or spot-on synthetic pyrethroid (deltamethrin, cypermethrin, alpha-cypermethrin, or permethrin) is required for prevention and can be used safely from a young age. Repeat application is needed every 3–4 weeks through the summer months or as directed by the data sheet. Ear tags impregnated with cypermethrin

are available and are inserted into the ear flap at the beginning of the grazing season and removed pre-housing. Some ML pour-on and injectable preparations have activity against horn flies (Urquhart et al., 1987).

It is impossible to eradicate flies from a farm, but measures can be taken to minimise how attractive an animal or field can appear to flies; dead carcases should be disposed of promptly, management tasks such as castration and dehorning should be avoided during the summer months, body parts should be cleared up and disposed of, animals with wounds or infected feet should be kept under close observation or better still, housed. Good standards of hygiene help to reduce fly populations.

Warble fly (*Hypoderma bovis* and *H. lineatum*)

Hypoderma bovis has been eradicated from the UK and is a notifiable disease – suspected cases should be reported to the duty vet at the local animal health office. The eradication campaign started in 1978 when there was estimated to be 4 million cases of warble fly each year. Voluntary seasonal treatments and compulsory treatments of affected animals as well as a publicity campaign resulted in a dramatic reduction to just 500 cases per year by 1983 with complete eradication by 1990 (Defra Fact Sheets, 2019).

The adult flies lay their eggs in spring and attach them to a hair shaft. After 3–7 days the eggs hatch and the larvae crawl down the hair shaft, penetrate the skin and start to migrate through the connective tissue layers of the subcutis throughout the ensuing months; the direction of migration is upwards towards the animal's back. During the following winter the larvae end up clustered under the skin overlying the backbone. In the following spring the larvae emerge from the back by making themselves a hole to crawl out from; the larvae fall to the floor. Over the next 1–3 months the larvae develop into adult flies and the process starts again.

The cattle fear this large fly and run to escape it, this is referred to as *gadding*; warble flies are, consequently, occasionally referred to as *gad flies*. The emergence of the large larvae through holes in the back of the animal causes damage to cattle hides and was once a significant industry problem especially in the manufacture of water pouches for American cowboys! Warble larvae are killed by MLs but if they are therapeutically killed in a space too close to the spinal column then paralysis may result from inflammation impinging on the spinal cord (Catts and Mullen, 2002).

Chorioptic mange

Mange is the term used to describe the infestation of the skin by microscopic mites. Chorioptic mange is the commonest form of cattle mange seen in the UK. The mites responsible are *Chorioptes bovis* and *C. texanus* (COWS, 2014b). Many cattle will carry a small mite population with little or no clinical signs. Mites multiply in the skin during the winter months with an associated itchy, scaling and crusting on the legs, the base of the tail and the udder. Pour-on MLs are the most effective treatment; injectable MLs are less effective and permethrin is the only pyrethroid with an activity claim. It is thought that mites can survive off the host for up to 3 weeks so treated cattle should be moved immediately to a 'clean' area to prevent reinfection and the area from which they came vacated for the same crucial 3 weeks.

Sarcoptic mange

Sarcoptic mange, caused by *Sarcoptes scabei*, is less common than chorioptic mange. It is more common in dogs, people, goats and pigs; cross infection can occur. Again, clinical signs can range from unobservable to severe and include loss of hair and scaling of the skin, especially on the neck, face and tail head. Treatment with pour-on or an injectable ML preparation is recommended (COWS, 2014b).

Psoroptic mange

Psoroptic mange is caused by a mite that appears very similar to the sheep scab mite but there is no evidence of cross infection between cattle and sheep. There had been no reported cases of psoroptic mange in cattle since the 1980s, however, in 2007 a case was reported in Wales and there have been a handful of cases since. This mite infestation appears as a scabby skin disease, which is intensely itchy. Skin lesions are seen predominantly along the back, neck and shoulders of the animal. The mite lives off the host for up to 12 days (Lonneux and Losson, 1996) so although the main route of introduction to a herd is through purchased cattle, markets, shared handling facilities and vehicles are all possible sources of initial infection. The mites are less active in the summer months so infected cattle may show few clinical signs until housing. The mites cannot be seen with the naked eye but skin scrapings from the edge of the lesions often contain mites that can be viewed under the microscope so enabling a confirmation of the diagnosis. As yet there is no commercially available blood test for psorptes in cattle; there is an antibody blood test for sheep.

MLs are licensed for the treatment of psoroptic mange but the efficacy of a single such treatment is being challenged (Mitchell and Damaso Peksa, 2018). It has been suggested that two injections of ivermectin, 10 days apart, are required (similar to the treatment of sheep scab). Alternatively, frequent applications of permethrin pour-on have been shown to be effective. The affected cattle and any in-contact animals should be treated. Animals with scabs and sores need to be clipped and washed with antiseptic shampoo to remove any secondary infection. The scabs should be disposed of appropriately as they are highly infectious.

Psoroptic mange is common in certain parts of Europe and there is a concern that the mite could be brought into the UK through imported cattle. Pre-import requirements stipulate the need for a ML injection but this has not been sufficient to prevent some of the more recent reported cases.

Tick infestation

Ixodes ricinus is the most common UK tick affecting cattle but also sheep, game birds, rabbits and dogs. Ticks are a problem in certain geographical areas in the UK, typically rough hill ground. Ticks prefer humid climates and an average daily temperature above 7°C (Sargison, 2008a) so they are traditionally associated as a spring/summer disease but with warmer winters this seems no longer the case and ticks can be found on animals throughout the year. Ticks, when they bite may, in high numbers, cause anaemia in the young animal, but they are most famous as vectors for other diseases such as TBF, louping ill, babesiosis and non-specific septicaemia (tick pyaemia).

The tick life cycle is interesting; they go through phases of development called *moults*, they spend most of their time away from their host in vegetation, but they require one huge 7 day blood feed from a host every year; they do this prior to a moult. It takes 3 years and three different hosts for a tick to go through all its moults and become an adult. This multi-host feeding pattern make them a great mode of transmission for disease!

Louping ill and TBF are the biggest risks from tick bites in young cattle.

Louping ill

This is an acute viral disease transmitted by ticks. Ticks themselves become infected with the virus from feeding on a host that is infected with the virus. The tick then transmits the virus to the next host it feeds off. In affected hosts the virus attacks the central nervous system (the brain and spinal cord). Sheep and game birds are affected more than cattle.

When a tick, inadvertently with its mouthparts, injects the virus into the host, the amount of virus in the blood (viraemia) is at a high level for only a few days. Other feeding ticks become infected with the virus during this time and can then pass it on at their next blood meal. A variable number of infected animals develop clinical signs; in some

heavily infected areas many animals develop only mild signs, with only a few progressing to those neurological. After infection, providing not fatal, the host's antibody response eliminates the virus and provides strong life-long immunity. Protection is passed to newborn calves from their dams via antibodies in the colostrum but this protection lasts only 3–4 months, after which the calf has no protection against this disease. Disease is most prevalent when infected cattle are purchased and introduced to an area where there are ticks but no louping ill – these populations have no immunity against the virus.

Clinical signs of louping ill:

- signs develop 6–18 days after infection
- initial fever, depression and lack of appetite
- subsequent muscle tremors often develop
- unsteady or characteristic high stepping gait
- seizures and paralysis may occur
- coma and death (5–60% of cases)
- clinical disease only seen in some of the population and, in sheep, is associated with exercise and/or stress of some sort.

The existence, current or previous, of louping ill virus in a population can be demonstrated by an antibody blood test. The antibodies are not detectable immediately upon infection; it takes a few weeks for the immune system to release antibodies into the blood. In severe cases an animal may die from louping ill or have to be euthanased due to the severity of the neurological signs. On PME there are no visible signs specific to louping ill but if the brain is removed and examined microscopically there are specific cellular changes that are diagnostic of the condition.

A vaccine is available for sheep but it has no license for its use in cattle.

Tickborne fever

TBF is a blood based parasitic disease caused by a rickettsia. Rickettsias are like bacteria but are actually classified as parasites. *Anaplasma phagocytophilum* is the parasite in question, it is carried by the tick and transmitted to the host during a blood feed. It subsequently infects white blood cells and ultimately destroys them in the process. The infection initially, and within just 24 hours, causes a persistent high temperature, anorexia and depression. Cattle of all ages can be affected. Colostrum provides no protection for young calves. The infection, presumably through its effect on white blood cells, suppresses the immune system and calves especially are more susceptible to other infectious diseases such as bacterial pneumonia. Pregnant cows exposed to TBF for the first time are likely to abort and naïve bulls that become infected may be infertile for up to 2 months after infection. Although cows exhibit signs of clinical disease, overt signs are more commonly seen in sheep. Cattle can be unaffected carriers of the parasite and act as a reservoir of infection for ticks to pick up and spread.

TBF can be diagnosed by detecting the pathogen within a blood sample. Although there are no specific findings at PME the spleen can be enlarged and again the pathogen can be detected within this tissue and in lymph nodes. There is no commercially available vaccine, so prevention of the disease is through tick control.

Redwater fever (babesiosis)

Babesia is another blood-based parasite, a single celled protozoon related to amoeba whose full name is *Babesia divergens*. Babesia is transmitted between cattle by ticks. The parasite, once injected into a bovine host by a feeding tick, infects red blood cells, destroying them in the process and causing a type of anaemia known as a haemolytic anaemia (Taylor, 2000). Haemoglobin (the oxygen carrying pigment) is spilt from the damaged red blood cells in such quantities that the body cannot metabolise it. The surplus pigment finds itself in the urine giving it a red brown appearance, hence the name redwater. Cattle present, 2 weeks after initial infection, with not only dark coloured urine,

but with fever, lethargy and a raised heart rate due to the anaemia. Some cattle develop diarrhoea in the early stages of the disease. Death can result if untreated. Cattle less than 9 months old, oddly, do not develop clinical disease but manage to produce an effective long lasting immunity. A herd with a long history of infection will, consequently, rarely experience disease problems. A diagnosis is obtained by examining blood smears under a microscope where at certain stages of the disease the parasite can be seen within the red blood cells. Babesiosis can be prevented and treated by administering imidocarb. Imidocarb can be used as soon as one or two animals in a group are affected, it should be used to treat the affected animals and all others in the group. An alternative strategy would be to treat susceptible cattle immediately they are introduced to tick inhabited pastures. Imidocarb provides lasting protection for up to 4 weeks. During this time if the cattle are exposed to Babesia they will become immune and not develop clinical signs. The treatment may be toxic so must be administered by a veterinary surgeon; it has a very long meat withdrawal period which absolutely must be observed. Supportive treatment may be required for the anaemia – in mild cases this may take the form of multi-vitamin injections or in severe cases a blood transfusion. Those that recover from infection have a long lasting immunity to further infection.

There are no licensed preparations for cattle in the UK for the prevention of tick bites although it has been suggested synthetic pyrethroids can be applied to young animals before turn out on to high-risk pastures. This may need to be repeated through high-risk periods.

BACTERIAL SKIN DISEASE

Bacteria exist on healthy bovine skin without causing disease but if the skin is damaged in any way or if the animal's immune system is compromised, these superficial bacteria can invade and an infection can become established. Skin infections are common around ear tags especially in the summer months when they have been irritated by flies. Bacteria frequently involved include *Dermatophilus* spp., *Staphylococcus aureus*, *Trueperella pyogenes* and *Actinobacillus* spp. Treatment of superficial skin infections involves clipping and cleaning of the affected area with an antibacterial solution such as chlorhexidine. If there is abscessation then surgical drainage and lavage is required. Injectable antibiotics may be prescribed in severe infections where the deeper layers of the skin are affected and there is local swelling, or if the animal is unwell.

BOVINE RESPIRATORY DISEASE

BRD, also loosely and commonly referred to as *pneumonia*, or, in a veterinary context, as *enzootic calf pneumonia*, is not a disease caused by a single pathogen but is a multi-pathogen and, furthermore, a multifactorial disease involving more than one pathogen and multiple management and environmental stressors. The managemental and environmental prevention and control of BRD is covered in Chapter 6; this chapter will focus on the specific infectious agents and the treatment of BRD. It should also be acknowledged that the term bovine respiratory disease does, technically, pertain to any part of the respiratory system, be it from the nostrils all the way down to the lower reaches of the lungs and the surrounding pleural cavities. The term pneumonia, however, pertains only to the lungs and is actually defined as infection, congestion and consolidation of the lungs as opposed to simple inflammation of the lungs which is called pneumonitis.

The clinical signs of BRD are often similar irrespective of the causal agent. They do, however, vary in severity depending on the immune status of the calf and the stage of the disease. Some cases of BRD will present as a sudden, unexplained death, others will grumble on for weeks or even months. The initial sign of disease is often a fever followed by a nasal and ocular discharge (Figure 13.10),

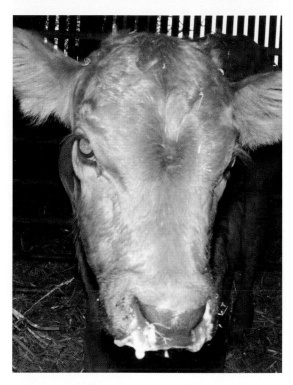

FIGURE 13.10 Calf showing signs of an advanced case of pneumonia with purulent nasal discharge

inappetence and an increased respiratory rate. As the disease advances the calf finds it difficult to breath and can become very distressed before death occurs. At PME there are obvious findings within the trachea, chest cavity and lung. The trachea can have a red inflamed lining and contain a large amount of froth. The chest/pleural cavity may contain pus, free fluid or deposits of sticky, jelly like inflammatory material known as fibrin. With this degree of fibrinous inflammation, the lung often sticks to the chest wall. The lungs themselves have areas of consolidation which appear dark in colour and are firm to touch. In these areas of consolidation, the air sacs of the lung that were once filled with air are now filled with inflammatory tissue and are no longer functional. As more of the lung becomes affected the calf is unable to breath and death occurs. Abscesses within the lungs are also a common finding and they vary in size from a few millimetres to a few centimetres in diameter.

The primary infectious causes of BRD include viruses, bacteria, bacteria like pathogens called mycoplasma and, rarely, fungi.

Viral BRD

Of the viruses that cause BRD, RSV is of major importance, as is bovine herpes virus Type 1 which causes infectious bovine rhino tracheitis (IBR). Other viruses include parainfluenza 3 (PI3), adenovirus and coronavirus all of which have clinical significance. While not a direct cause of BRD, the immunosuppressive effects of bovine viral diarrhoea virus (BVDV) should not be underestimated and may underpin a multifactorial BRD outbreak.

RSV is considered to be one of the major pathogens in the BRD complex. It causes primary damage allowing secondary bacteria to enter damaged lung tissue but, importantly, it can also cause acute deaths on its own. Typically, it affects younger calves from 5 days old upwards but can affect growing cattle up to 6 months of age. Antibodies to RSV are present in bovine colostrum but they do not appear to provide complete protection to the calf. There are effective intranasal and injectable vaccines providing protection against RSV. The intranasal vaccines can be used from a young age as they are unaffected by the maternally derived antibodies.

IBR virus infects the cells in the nasal lining where it replicates very quickly producing large numbers of viral particles which can then go on to infect others (Figure 13.11). Transmission can be over 4 m in *aerosol* and can be carried in nasal secretions on clothing or equipment (Thiry et al., 2002). The virus is unique among other respiratory viruses in that it has an ability to become latent; the animal becoming an intermittent shedder of the virus for the rest of its life while largely unaffected itself. These carriers are a constant source of infection so the mixing of age ranges within a shared air space is a known risk factor for IBR outbreaks. IBR antibodies are passed on in the cow's colostrum offering the calves some protection at a young age.

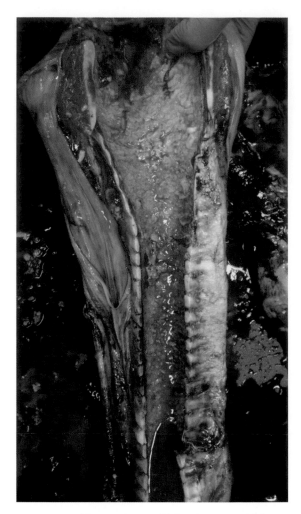

FIGURE 13.11 The trachea at PME of a case of IBR

There is a range of effective IBR vaccines, both live and inactivated, which provide protection to naïve animals but also decrease the shedding of virus in latently infected animals.

Mycoplasma BRD

Mycoplasma bovis, *M. dispar*, *M. bovirhinis* and the closely related *Ureaplasma* spp. have all been associated with pneumonia outbreaks in the UK. *M. bovis* is the most commonly isolated mycoplasma in pneumonia outbreaks and is considered to be the most pathogenic and invasive (Bryson, 2000)

(Chapter 12) and *M. bovis* causes infectious disease of the inner ear and joints of young calves as well as causing pneumonia. The main source of infection is carrier cows who pass the agent on through colostrum and milk. The bacteria can survive for weeks in the environment but do not withstand UV light.

Bacterial BRD

Mannheimia haemolytica serotype A1, *Pasteurella multocida*, *Trueperella pyogenes* and *Histophilus somni* are the bacterial pathogens most commonly involved in BRD (Bryson, 2000). Bacteria such as *M. haemolytica* and *H. somni* can be the primary agents in a case of pneumonia but can equally behave as secondary pathogens hitching a ride on the damage caused by initial viral damage to the lung.

M. haemolytica is an inhabitant of the nasal cavity and tonsils of a normal healthy calf. It is a member of the same family as Pasteurella, a large group of gram-negative bacteria. *M. haemolytica* is divided into different serotypes based on the composition of the outer capsule – there are 12 different serotypes in total. In a normal calf serotype A2 predominates in the nasal cavity but if the natural population of bacteria is disrupted then A1 multiplies and causes disease (Griffin et al., 2010). Serotype A6 is of growing interest, seemingly increasing in prevalence in recent times (Bryson, 2000). There are several commercial vaccines providing protection against various serotypes of *M. haemolytica*.

P. multocida is another member of the Pasteurella group and is also a normal inhabitant of the nasal cavity in up to 60% of normal calves (Griffin et al., 2010). It is seen in younger cattle in particular and is occasionally linked with cases of pneumonia in the UK. It is very commonly found in fatal cases of shipping fever in the USA after transportation, especially after the mixing of large numbers of stressed cattle. There is no vaccine available in the UK for *P. multocida*.

H. somni is again a commensal (normal co-inhabitant) of the upper respiratory tract but it can cause disease when it colonises the lungs. This bacterium is able to gain entry into the bloodstream and following spread and settling out can cause meningitis, joint ill, laryngeal abscesses, and damage to the heart muscle. These infections elsewhere in the body usually occur a few weeks after *H. somni* first infects the lungs (Griffin et al., 2010). There is an effective vaccine in the UK against *H. somni*, a vaccine which also incorporates *M. haemolytica*.

T. pyogenes is a bacterium often isolated from long-standing infections including abscesses. It is considered to be a secondary bacterial invader in cases of pneumonia where the primary agent has long since gone and left behind necrotic (dead) tissue which offers a suitable environment in which *T. pyogenes* can multiply.

Treatment of BRD

There are more antimicrobials on the market licensed for the treatment of BRD than for any other disease of cattle (Potter, 2011). Tetracyclines, florfenicols and macrolides (tulathromycin, tilmicosin, gamithromycin and tildipirosin) are all antimicrobials commonly used to treat BRD. The different formulations and preparations of these active ingredients involve different routes of administration, dose rate, meat withdrawal, duration of action and cost. When a vet prescribes an antibiotic for the treatment of BRD they do not usually have all the required information for the perfect decision. In an ideal world the vet would know the pathogen causing the disease and if indeed it was a bacterium they would then have a sensitivity report detailing which antibiotics the said pathogen is sensitive to. They would also know the exact details of the location of the infection, whether it is walled off in abscesses or not, whether it has got into other tissues or not, exactly how heavy the animal is, how close or not to slaughter it is, what route of administration the stockman prefers, how easily restrained the animal is and so on. Regardless, the animal requires treatment as soon as possible for its own welfare, to minimise the spread of pathogens into the environment and to give the animal the best chance of survival and an ongoing productive life. The vet usually makes a decision based on not only a knowledge of pharmacology but on pattern recognition; the clinical presentation of the animal and previous experiences on that farm and on others. The antimicrobial should have activity against the suspected infectious agent, it should reach the site of infection and it should achieve the right concentration to do its job. The treatment should also be for an appropriate duration, long enough to fully clear the site of infection (Potter, 2011).

In years gone by there was a widespread practice of the prophylactic treatment of groups of animals with antimicrobials, usually via the milk or feed but sometimes by whole group injection. Based on the 'prevention is better than cure' adage, prophylactic treatments are administered in anticipation of disease, rather than after it strikes. For example, it would be routine procedure to inject all calves with antibiotic, pre-housing or in advance of a stressful management procedure, even if they were all fit and well at the time of administration. This results in a lot of animals being exposed to antimicrobial drugs with no certain need. Prophylactic treatments are no longer practised in the UK for the control of BRD.

Metaphylactic treatment is slightly different, this is where antimicrobials are administered to apparently normal animals within a group when some of their cohorts within the group have started to show signs of disease. Again, this results in some animals being exposed to antimicrobials that may have never succumbed to disease, are perfectly healthy, and simply did not need the drug. For these reasons this approach, while occasionally resorted to, is not routinely practised in the UK and it is generally discouraged – the premise being only to use antimicrobials when the need is certain.

The use of NSAIDs alongside antimicrobials is advocated to reduce excessive inflammation

associated with the immune response to the pathogen, to reduce pain and to hopefully reduce lung consolidation (Mahendran et al., 2017). To help the stockperson abide by this advice some antimicrobial injections are combined with an NSAID, usually either meloxicam or flunixin. Otherwise the two drugs can be administered separately – here the withdrawal period of the multiple product treatment would need discussing with a vet.

The early recognition and treatment of calf pneumonia improves treatment success and reduces spread to other animals. The early signs of pneumonia are subtle: the initial fever of infection may appear as malaise, weakness and inappetence; a nasal discharge typically appears 19 hours after the initial fever and a cough 65 hours after the fever develops (Timsit et al., 2011). Tools have been developed to help early recognition of disease; as fever is the initial detectable sign this has been the main focus of early detection systems such as behaviour scoring to detect malaise, reticulorumen boluses to detect inappetence and digital thermography to detect fever (as was used in airports during recent human viral pandemics). These systems have enjoyed very limited use in the field unlike the use of temperature sensor ear tags, one technology which has proven quite popular. The ear tag is inserted into the ear flap (pinna) and a small wire inserted into the ear canal. When the temperature of the ear canal rises above a certain temperature the light on the tag changes colour. The temperature change is assumed to be due to respiratory disease, by far the most likely cause, and the calf can then be treated promptly. If the diagnosis is wrong, then this approach is guilty of breaching the responsible use of antimicrobials codes so the practice will undoubtedly find itself under scrutiny.

In most cases of pneumonia, the treatment does involve an antimicrobial treatment and an NSAID. With the international pressure to decrease antimicrobial usage to only when absolutely necessary there is an interest in testing this assumed need. In a large number of pneumonia cases a viral infection is the primary infection followed by secondary bacterial invasion. Viral infections are not treatable by using antimicrobials. If the disease is caught early enough, in its viral stage, then it has been hypothesised that NSAID alone may be enough to treat pneumonia. Studies have been carried out to test this theory and although 25.7% of calves were successfully treated with NSAID alone, 74.3% of the calves continued to demonstrate a fever and antimicrobial therapy was deemed necessary as a secondary treatment. It was observed, however, that the delay in administering the antimicrobials appeared to have no effect on the outcome of the pneumonia and the future performance of the calf (Mahendran et al., 2017). This study suggests the importance of continually monitoring calves even after treatment. It is well recognised that calves that have suffered from pneumonia once are likely to have repeated bouts of pneumonia, certainly in the next month but often throughout their entire life. Relapses within a month are reasonably blamed on disruption of the lining of the respiratory tract and such calves deserve a second treatment. The repeated treatment of longer term chronic cases with antimicrobial is, however, irresponsible from the antimicrobial usage and welfare perspective. On PME of these chronic cases of pneumonia the damage is extensive with adhesions and advanced abscessation; it becomes very clear why there was only a temporary response to treatment with an antimicrobial. It is then easier to see that euthanasia would have been preferable.

Many vets would argue that pneumonia is caused by a number of infectious agents and the principles of control are the same despite the infectious agent. They have a point but it is good practice to find out exactly the predominant infectious agent – this certainly helps with designing vaccination protocols.

Problems with identifying the infectious agent in BRD

1. The infectious agent isolated from one calf may not be representative of the rest of the group.

A minimum of four calves is, ideally, required as a representative sample although, practically, there may not be four cases available that are suitable for sampling.

2. The agent isolated may be a harmless *commensal* and not part of the disease process.

3. The infectious agent detected may be a secondary pathogen and the primary pathogen may have gone.

4. Infectious agents may vary from year to year especially if the herd is purchasing and mixing cattle. This needs to be taken into consideration when designing vaccination protocols based on previous outbreaks.

5. The key to getting a reliable representative result is to choose the correct animals to sample depending on the testing carried out. For example, there is no point asking a laboratory to culture bacteria from a sample if the calf has been treated with antibiotics, unless, that is, there is a strong suspicion of antibiotic resistance.

BRD infectious agent identification in the live animal

1. **Nasopharyngeal swabbing**. Long nasopharyngeal swabs can be inserted into the nasal cavity – they need to be long as the cavity extending all the way back to the throat. Swabbing needs to be of an acutely sick animal. It is important it is an acutely sick animal with a clear nasal discharge rather than a chronically infected calf with a white nasal discharge. Viruses (RSV, PI3 and IBR) can be picked up and detected by a technique called PCR where the viral DNA material is replicated to a detectable level in a laboratory. Bacteria (*P. multocida*, *M. haemolytica*, *Mycoplasma* spp. and *H. somni*) can be cultured and identified in the lab and an antibiotic sensitivity profile produced. As with viruses they can now increasingly be detected using PCR technology. The swabbing technique is simple but the problem in the case of bacteria

is that many inhabit the nasal cavity in a normal animal so false positive results are common – the results need careful interpretation by a vet.

2. **Bronchoalveolar lavage (BAL)**. This is a technique that involves 'washing' infectious agents from the airways and sacs of the lungs and *harvesting* them in special fluid, all via a tube inserted down the nose. The technique is, with some practice on the part of the vet, relatively simple but causes visible distress to the calf – for this reason there needs to be good cause to commit to the procedure. The technique is, however, preferable to nasopharyngeal swabbing as the washings are from deep in the lung where any isolated infectious agents are likely to be significant, unlike the commensal contaminants that can be sampled from the nose.

3. **Trans-tracheal aspiration**. This procedure is more invasive than BAL as a needle is introduced through the skin at the base of the neck and into the trachea, whereupon a washing is obtained in a similar fashion to a BAL. It bypasses the upper respiratory tract so the infectious agents detected are considered significant but there are no other advantages over a BAL and any bugs lower down the airways could be missed. This technique is no longer commonly practised the UK.

4. **Serology.** As with most other infectious diseases calves produce antibodies to BRD infections, notably RSV, PI3, *M. bovis*, *H. somni*, IBR and BVD. The production of detectable levels of antibody can take up to 4 weeks. A technique called paired serology is recommended. Here, a base or reference blood sample is taken when the animal first shows signs of disease. The animal is treated and identified and 4 weeks later a second blood sample is obtained. The two samples are tested at the laboratory for antibodies to the chosen agents. If there is a significant rise in antibodies between the first and second sample, it suggests the calf has been exposed to that particular infectious agent around the time of the illness in question. It is possible to take just one sample 4 weeks after a pneumonia

outbreak but, without a base line sample, interpretation is more difficult – the antibody level may have already been high and unrelated to the illness. This technique of *single serology* is, to be fair, very useful when used at the end of the housing period where there may have been a number of cases of BRD throughout the winter and diagnostic testing was not carried out at the time. Serology at this stage gives an idea of all the different bugs encountered during the winter but without an indication of exactly when in the winter, or even sooner as could be the case. Serology is generally used on a group of animals, a minimum of six, rather than individuals. More weight is given to the result if more than 50% of the sampled calves show a raised antibody response. Serology is difficult to interpret in young calves that may have obtained antibodies from the colostrum of their dam. It is recommended that if calves are less than 12 weeks of age the number of calves is increased from 6 to 12 and a positive antibody response in 25% of the calves sampled is considered significant (Mason, 2013).

BRD – post-mortem examination

If a carcase is available for PME (Figure 13.12), this can often give the best chance of obtaining a diagnosis. If the animal is in the advanced stages of

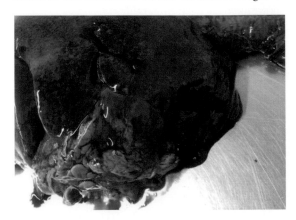

FIGURE 13.12 Bovine lung at PME; the dark red region to the right of the picture is consolidated lung tissue; pneumonia

chronic pneumonia, there is little value in obtaining samples in pursuit of the primary agent as it will no longer be present. Different infectious agents are associated with certain classic changes in the respiratory system at post-mortem but they are not to be considered confirmatory but merely suggestive of the causative agent. For example, IBR typically causes inflammation and sloughing (detaching) of the lining of the trachea. RSV causes large gas filled pockets on the surface of the lung – a change known as emphysema. *M. bovis* causes multiple tiny abscesses throughout a purple, consolidated lung lobe.

At PME samples of lung can be taken and sent, unpreserved, to the lab for culture or PCR. Specific samples can be preserved for examination under the microscope; histopathology. Typically, samples are taken from affected lung, normal lung and the border between affected and unaffected tissue. Under the microscope the cellular changes can be examined and this sometimes gives evidence of whether more than one infectious agent was involved and which one was the primary pathogen.

In summary, BRD is a major problem of the industry but it is preventable through good husbandry, environmental management and, where necessary and appropriate, vaccination. Preventative measures, including vaccination, are discussed in Chapter 6.

REFERENCES

Aitken, P. (2001) Selenium toxicity. *In Practice* 23, 286–289.

Bryson, D.G. (2000) The calf pneumonia complex – current thoughts on aetiology. *Cattle Practice* 8(2), 103–107.

Catts, P.E. and Mullen, G.R. (2002) Myiasis. In: Mullen, G. and Durden, L. (eds) *Medical and Veterinary Entomology.* Academic Press, Bambridge, MA, pp. 317–348.

COWS (2014a) Control of parasitic gastroenteritis in cattle. Control of Worms Sustainably, April.

COWS (2014b) Control of ectoparasites and insect pests of cattle. Control of Worms Sustainably, November.

Defra (2019) Livestock notifiable disease factsheets warble fly. Available at: http://www.adlib.ac.uk/resources/000/110/003/LNDF26.pdf.

Dunn, K. (2006) Oak poisoning in cattle. *UK Vet Livestock* 11(5), 47–50.

Griffin, D., Chengappa, M.M., Kuszak, J. and Scott McVey, D.S. (2010) Bacterial pathogens of the bovine respiratory complex. *Veterinary Clinics: Food Animal Practice* 26: 381–394.

Laven, R.A. and Livesey, C.T. (2004) The diagnosis of copper related disease: do we have the necessary tools? Part 1: prevalence of disease and the diagnosis of copper toxicity. *Cattle Practice* 12, 265–269.

Laven, R.A. and Livesey, C.T. (2005) The diagnosis of copper related disease: Part 2: copper responsive disorders. *Cattle Practice* 13, 55–60.

Livesey, C.T., Bidewell, C.A., Crawshaw, T.R. and David, G.P. (2002) Investigation of copper poisoning in cows by the veterinary laboratory agency. *Cattle Practice* 10, 289–294.

Lonneux, J.F. and Losson, B. (1996) Epidemiology of cattle mange. *Annales de medecine veterinaire* 140, 317–327.

Mahendran, S.A., Booth, R., Burge, M. and Bell., N.J. (2017) Randomised positive control trial of NSAID and antimicrobial treatment for calf fever caused by pneumonia. *Vet Record* 181, 45–50.

Mason, C.S., (2004) Peri-weaning scour syndrome of dairy calves: an update. *Cattle Practice* 12(2), 115–119.

Mason, C. (2013) Practical guide to diagnosis of bovine respiratory disease (BRD).

McCoy, M.A., Kenny, J. and Hill, J. (2004) Outbreak of *Nematodirus battus* infection in calves. *Vet Record* 154, 370–371.

Mitchell, S. and Damaso Peksa, A. (2018) Important ectoparasites of sheep and cattle. *Veterinary Practice.* Available at: https://veterinary-practice.com/article/important-ectoparasites-of-sheep-and-cattle.

Otter, A., Twomey, D.F., Crawshaw, T.R. and Bates, P. (2003) Anaemia and mortality in calves infested with the long-nose suckling louse (*Lingonathis vituli*). *Vet Record* 153, 176–179.

Payne, J. and Livesey, C. (2010) Lead poisoning in cattle and sheep. *In Practice* 32, 64–69.

Payne, J. and Murphy, A. (2010) Plant poisoning in farm animals. *In Practice* 36, 455–465.

Potter, T.J. (2011) Antimicrobial selection for calf pneumonia. *Cattle Practice* 1(2), 120–122.

Reis, L.S., Pardo, P.E., Camargos, A.S. and Oba, E. (2010) Review: mineral element and heavy metal poisoning in animals. *Journal of Medicine and Medical Sciences* 1(12), 560–579.

Russell, G.C. (2009) Malignant catarrhal fever (MCF). The Moredun Foundation. News sheet Vol 5, No 3.

Ryan, E.G. Lee, A., Carty, C., O'Shaughnessy, J., Kelly, P., Cassidy, J.P., Sheehan, M., Johnson, A. and de Wall, T. (2016) Bovine besnoitiosis (Besnoitia besnoiti) in an Irish dairy herd. *Vet Record* 178, 608–615.

Sargison, N. (2008a) Skin and eye diseases. In: *Sheep Flock Health A Planned Approach,* John Wiley and Sons, Hoboken, NJ, pp. 346–431.

Sargison, N. (2008b) Unexpected disease or death. In: *Sheep Flock Health A Planned Approach*, John Wiley and Sons, Hoboken, NJ, pp. 228–274.

Scott, P. (2017) NADIS Fact Sheet. Ringworm (Dermatophytosis). Available at: https://nadis.org.uk/disease-a-z/cattle/calf-management/ringworm/.

Taylor, M. (2000) Protozoal disease in cattle and sheep. *In Practice* 22, 604–617.

Thiry, E., Lemaire, M., Keuser, V. and Schynts, F. (2002) Recent developments in infectious bovine rhinotracheitis. *Cattle Practice* 10(1), 43–49.

Timsit, E, Assie, S., Quiniou, R., Seegers, H. and Barreille, M. (2011) Early detection of bovine respiratory disease in young bulls using reticulorumen temperature boluses. *The Veterinary Journal* 190, 136–142.

Urquhart, G.M., Armour, J., Duncan, J.L., Dunn, A.M. and Jennings, F.W. (1987) Veterinary entomology. In: *Veterinary Parasitology*, 1st edn. Longman, Harlow, pp. 164–168.

Watts, D. (1994) The nutritional relationships of selenium. *Journal of Orthomolecular Medicines* 9(2), 111–117.

Chapter 14

Disease and production failure in fattening cattle

The finishing period is the final stage before slaughter, in which cattle have largely completed the growing of their frames and laid down fat. Historically, it was referred to as the fattening period. However, terms such as fatstock and fattening are, these days, unappealing to consumers, and the term 'finishing' is more often used now.

MUSCULOSKELETAL DISEASE

Musculoskeletal disease usually manifests itself in the form of lameness. Lameness in one limb is classic lameness – a 'limp' or a blatant disinclination to bear weight on that limb. Lameness in more than one limb can be less clear cut but will undoubtedly appear as an abnormal gait of some kind. Lameness can be a result of pain or alternatively it can be due to mechanical impairment in much the same way that Long John Silver limped on his wooden leg – it was not necessarily painful but he limped, nonetheless. In our context a finishing beast with a shortened or deformed leg, from an old fracture say, may well limp but it may not be painful. Sadly, however, lameness usually is pain related; it is a debilitating painful state, and it has a huge economic impact on growth rates, fertility and milk yield. Pain induced lameness has also been demonstrated to cause a heightening of pain responsiveness in general, a phenomenon known as *hyperalgesia*. In hyperalgesia animals are not only suffering chronic unyielding pain from the primary lesion, in this case the limb, but any other painful stimulus appears to be more painful than it normally would – pain 'wind up' as it is sometimes called. Lameness is a major welfare concern and for that reason alone, aside from the devastating production hindrance, we need to be able to identify, diagnose, treat and prevent it.

Pain related lameness can be caused by an injury, infection or other disease within the foot or the leg. Injury induced lameness in fattening cattle can often be due to trauma from bulling behaviour or fighting and other fractious behaviour.

Poor housing design can contribute to lameness; poorly designed surfaces, sharp edges, tight turns, all increase the risk of musculoskeletal injury. In adult cows, 90% of lameness is caused by a condition of the hoof; for younger cattle, however, there is an equal chance that the cause of the lameness is either in the foot or higher up the limb.

On initial presentation the animal needs to be assessed on a flat even surface and walked calmly. There a few questions to be asked.

Is the animal lame on one or more legs and which legs?

Multi-limb lameness cases are hard to detect as affected animals will alter their gate accordingly to keep weight from the *most* painful limb, often disguising the lameness of another slightly lesser painful limb.

The rise and fall of the head should be noted. Often cattle who are lame on a front leg will raise their head when the painful limb bears weight – this is actually the animal attempting to throw its weight upwards when landing on the painful limb and then nodding the head back down when the sound leg bears weight.

The evenness of the stride is an indication of lameness; one back foot should at least reach the level of the imprint left behind by the other back foot.

When a lame animal is left to stand, they will often 'spare' or rest the lame limb.

There may be a swelling or a wound that provides additional information to the site of pain. Such swellings may be subtle, and it can take practice to spot them.

When assessing foot placement, it may give clues as to the site of a foot lesion; the animal will refrain from allowing the painful part of the foot from touching the ground first. For example, a cow with a lesion on the outer claw will try to bear as much weight as possible on the medial claw.

How severe is the lameness?

Mobility scoring is discussed in Chapter 7 and the degree of lameness is graded 0–3, with 0 being normal and 3 being severely impaired mobility. This scale can be used when discussing clinically lame cattle as well. Vets commonly refer to a severely lame animal as non-weight bearing. Even when encouraged to move they still refuse to bear any weight on the limb. This does not provide any information as to the cause of lameness but it does indicate that the animal is in severe pain and requires immediate attention.

Is the lameness due to pain?

A mechanical lameness is not associated with any pain but may be due to a failure of the musculoskeletal system to function – to move and work in the recognised manner, for example, in a case of fixation of the joints – arthrogryposis – a congenital malformation. Another consideration is whether the apparent lameness is actually due to damage of a nerve supplying the leg rather than to the muscles or the bones themselves – the primary components of the musculoskeletal system. Damage to the radial nerve, which supplies the front leg, for example, presents as an animal unable to advance the limb and instead drags its toe or develops the knack of throwing its leg forward. Radial nerve paralysis is a common condition as the radial nerve runs across the bone at the point of the shoulder where there is little protection and is, consequently, commonly traumatised by cattle crushes, gates, feed barriers or head butts while fighting. With rest, the nerve usually regains its function and the animal resumes a normal gait.

Lameness in the foot

The vast proportion of lameness in adult cattle is in the foot although in finishing cattle the proportion is less. Foot lameness can be divided into infectious and non-infectious. Normal anatomy of the foot and preventative hoof care are discussed in Chapter 7.

Non-infectious foot lameness

White line disease

White line disease (WLD) starts from the entry of gravel or dirt into the junction between the hoof wall and the sole. This gravel or dirt is continually pushed deeper until it reaches the corium, the moist sensitive layer, where the inevitable bacteria carried in by the dirt start to replicate. Pus is produced in reaction to the infection and the subsequent pressure build-up causes pain and the animal becomes lame. The pus may track up the hoof wall and burst out at the coronary band or it may track horizontally between the sole and the

Block correctly positioned

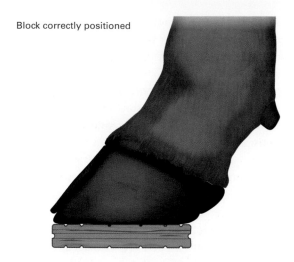

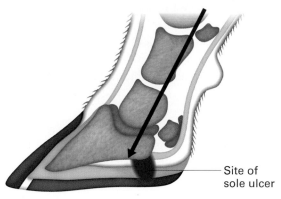

FIGURE 14.2 Site of sole ulceration

Site of
sole ulcer

FIGURE 14.1 Correct positioning of a wooden block

sole corium, causing the sole to separate away from the corium leaving the corium the task of growing a new sole – the so called *false sole*.

Treatment is to remove all *under-run* horn to expose the infected corium beneath and allow the pus to drain. The corium is a sensitive tissue and when exposed to the outside world, with no protection from the horn, it is painful to the touch and therefore should not be expected to weight bear. This can be achieved by elevating the other claw using a wooden or plastic block (Figure 14.1). If there is a poor response to treatment it is usually due to poor drainage and the lesion needs to be re-opened. The lesion may take several attempts to get it right; the inside (axial) wall is particularly slow to repair (Blowey, 1992).

Sole ulcer

Sole ulcers are a result of continual damage to the cells within the sole corium, the cells that are responsible for producing new horn. They are most commonly seen in the back lateral (outside) claw or the front medial (inside) claw where, in each case, there is most weight bearing and specifically there is a spot on the sole two-thirds of the way to the heel, which corresponds to the position of the extensor process (a small protrusion of bone on the bottom of the pedal bone) which has the effect

of nipping the corium at this pinch point (Blowey, 1992) (Figure 14.2).

The compression and damage of these essential delicate cells is made worse by long periods of time standing on concrete. Another factor is horn overgrowth on the sole that essentially forces the sole to bear weight more than it should (the walls are the intended weight-bearing structures of the hoof in most *ungulates*, they being hooved animals). One other risk factor is calving – the ligaments within the foot that hold the pedal bone in place slacken due to hormonal change around calving (the hormones responsible for the relaxation of the pelvic ligaments and birth canal necessary for calving). In the foot the relaxation of the ligaments drops the pedal bone inside the hoof capsule which compresses the sole corium below (Archer et al., 2010).

The sole corium responds to this compression and damage by producing granulation tissue; red, vascular new tissue which, in early cases, presents just as a small haemorrhage on the sole but in advanced cases, a large lesion of bright red haemorrhagic tissue that is particularly vulnerable and painful. These lesions are slow to heal and in severe cases may never fully recover despite repetitive trimming throughout the animal's life. Prompt treatment of sole ulcers is essential. Applying a block to the sound claw allows the lame claw to be relieved of any weight bearing, which will help reduce the pain. Treatment involves reshaping the claw so that the walls resume their weight bearing role, and in addition the granulation tissue protruding through the ulcer needs skilfully removing and the ulcer trimmed back so that the corium has a flat surface across which it can heal the defect.

Foreign body

Nails, screws, sharp stones, and even shed teeth can penetrate the sole of the foot. On occasions the foreign body (FB) is present and can be removed though often there is no sign of the initial foreign body but instead a black lesion, similar to a white line lesion, but on the sole, or indeed the white line for that matter, but when in that location is usually classed as WLD. As with WLD the lesion requires opening up with a hoof knife and then allowed to drain. If the foreign body has dropped out of the foot and the hole has sealed over, an abscess will form which again needs to be identified and opened up with a hoof knife to allow the pus to drain out or squirt out as is sometimes the case! Where a foreign body has not penetrated the sole but just caused severe bruising an animal may be lame for a few days but if housed on a soft bedded area the bruising resolves without paring. Bruising appears as a pink/red discoloration of the sole.

Fracture of the pedal bone

Many cases of acute onset severe lameness without heat, swelling or an identifiable lesion in the foot are diagnosed as a fractured pedal bone. It is not actually possible to diagnose this without radiography but that is often impractical on farm. The hoof capsule provides a good splint and the fracture will heal after 6–8 weeks with a full return to soundness (Blowey, 1992).

Vertical sandcrack

The periople is the white soft tissue that lies on top of the hoof wall adjacent to the coronary band encircling the top of the hoof. It produces a waxy coating that keeps the hoof horn moist and sealed so preserving its condition, especially that of the newly produced horn that grows down from the coronary band. When the periople is damaged or in very dry conditions, the coronary band fails to produce good quality horn and a crack appears somewhere in the wall starting at the top and travelling down. These cracks, often in dry conditions, are sometimes referred to as *sand cracks*. In advanced or severe cases, the crack extends from the coronary band right down to the ground. This does not always cause lameness but the crack can become infected and if there is movement between the two sides of the crack the underlying corium will be painfully nipped and damaged, to which the corium responds with the production of granulation tissue. Both pus, dirt and granulation tissue need to be removed from these lesions. A block can be applied to the sound claw meaning the affected claw is no longer weight bearing so the crack no longer nips with each movement. Cracks that start at the ground and travel upwards but not necessarily all the way to the coronary band may be related to splaying of the hoof wall due to overgrowth rather than problems with the periople function –these *grass cracks* as they are sometimes called can be different. The problem may be a bit of both and the underlying problems would need to be established. Simple overgrowth would of course need standard correct paring with some additional paring out of the crack if necessary.

Horizontal crack

Horizontal cracks in the hoof wall are due to a disruption in horn production at the coronary band some time ago. The disruption is usually due to a change in nutrition, or a response to stress or illness, a bit of both, or calving. The hoof continues to grow down and the lesions will grow out over a period of months. The cracks are seen in more than one foot and lameness results if the corium is reached or if dirt contaminates the crack and an infection establishes. Sometimes they appear just as a dark line (not easily visible in black hoofed cattle) that extends around the hoof, with no visible crack. Horizontal cracks are sometimes referred to as hardship lines.

Heel erosion or slurry heal

The heel is required to provide flexible support and cushioning to the animal and to maintain the correct hoof conformation and angle. When cows stand in wet conditions, especially slurry, for any length of time the heel horn dissolves away and becomes roughened and pitted. This alters hoof conformation – the heel lowers and the foot tips back – this puts stresses on the limb but also increases the probability that the sole corium will be compressed and nipped and that a sole ulcer will result. The tempting amateurish trimming of the heel horn without a balancing of the foot further advances the disease progression. Treatment and prevention include ensuring a clean dry environment for the cattle.

Interdigital hyperplasia

This condition is an overgrowth of normal skin between the digits just below the coronary band. It is thought to originate from constant irritation of the skin from dirt or sods and seems to be more common in heavy breeds of cattle with slightly splayed digits, breeds such as the Hereford or Aberdeen Angus. There may indeed be a genetic predisposition to the condition. The overgrowth of skin is seen as a defined lump and can be surgically amputated, but this may be an overreaction – the preferred treatment initially would be to rebalance the feet with good paring and improve the conditions for the animal.

Laminitis

Laminitis was named after, and thought to be, inflammation of the lamellae of the hoof, although over recent years this theory has been challenged. The lamellae are the vertical folds of tissue that line the inner surface of the hoof wall and support the tiny ligaments that attach to the pedal bone and suspend it within the hoof capsule. Laminitis is well researched and reported in horses, but the cause of the disease cannot be extrapolated to cattle, they seem to be two distinct conditions.

Accepting, however, that laminitis, although poorly understood, is nevertheless a recognised condition in cattle, it needs as full a discussion as possible. Cattle with laminitis are reluctant to move; when they are encouraged to do so, they walk steadily and carefully with short steps. They often appear worse on concrete or gravel than on grass or straw. When standing they may stand with all four feet directly underneath them, like an elephant on a drum! There may be some swelling above the coronary band and the feet are 'hot' to touch. When the feet are trimmed there are haemorrhages within the sole but these can equally be coincidental and represent un-associated bruising.

Laminitis in dairy and beef cattle was thought to be caused by high levels of carbohydrate feeding. It was thought that the laminitis was induced through subclinical ruminal acidosis, a drop in rumen pH, due to poor feeding practices (discussed under ruminal acidosis). This acidosis kills gram-negative bacteria in the rumen causing them to spill out endotoxin which supposedly damages the sensitive laminae within the foot. Modern thinking still considers there to be a nutritional element to laminitis; it cannot be denied that affected cattle are nearly always on a highly energy-dense diet, but there may also be environmental factors involved such as floor design, standing times and stressful events. Why would stressful events lead to laminitis? Stress causes the release of a number of chemical messengers (hormones and neurotransmitters) that trigger specific events to occur within the hoof capsule. These biological messengers, their exact role and the precise trigger factors are yet to be fully elucidated and this is an area of advancing research. What is known to date is that the pedal bone suspended in the hoof capsule ultimately rotates and sinks within the hoof and the subsequent production of horn is disrupted (Greenough, 2015).

The rotation or sinking of the pedal bone is permitted by the stretching of the ligaments that exist between the pedal bone and the laminae. As the pedal bone sinks it squashes the sensitive corium of the sole, causes pain and predisposes the animal to sole ulcers where the extensor process of the pedal bone is particularly insulting to the corium.

Normal horn production is affected during laminitis by a compromise of the blood supply to the foot and a consequent reduction in oxygen availability. In young animals new blood vessels form and the blood supply is restored and recovery is possible. With age and with every subsequent bout of laminitis more scar tissue forms and there is a less successful healing of the situation each time (Greenough, 2015).

As the exact cause and pathway of the disease is poorly understood there is little in the way of treatment or preventative advice. Historically, treatment involved housing cattle on a deep straw bed, administering anti-inflammatory drugs and feeding a forage only diet. Resolution of clinical signs happens over a period of 2–6 weeks. In terms of prevention, it still seems to stand that a review of feeding management and rumen health is appropriate.

Infectious causes of lameness in the foot

Digital dermatitis

Digital dermatitis is caused by an infectious agent called *Treponema* of which there are many different species all belonging to the family of Spirochaetes (spiral shaped bacteria) that includes other famous bugs such as *Leptospira*, *Borrelia* (Lyme's disease) and syphilis. Following apparent import from Italy in the 1990s it is now the leading cause of lameness in dairy cows and has gradually been introduced into suckler herds. It is a surprisingly painful condition and difficult to control due to its ability to survive in the environment. The lesions affect the haired skin just above the coronary band usually at the back of the foot and may affect one or more feet

at any one time. There is a raised area of matted hair, with a yellow brown discolouration which elicits a pain response when touched. Treponema will also infect existing lesions such as cracks and slurry heel. An existing lesion that is already difficult to treat becomes almost impossible. Any invasion of the cells at the coronary band disrupts horn growth and can result in permanent horn deformation – this is less troublesome at the heel but when the coronary band of the walls or toes are affected the disruption of new horn production results in a devastating void or wide crack that extends downwards with time, a big problem.

Treatment of early cases involves, first, cleaning and drying the lesions on the coronary band and then applying topical antibiotics for three consecutive days (Archer et al., 2010). In the case of beef animals where handling may be difficult, applying antibiotics and covering the medicated lesion with a bandage dressing may suffice to increase the contact time. The bandage must be removed after 3 days. Prevention is always better than cure. Providing a dry environment is the key starting point. As with any infectious disease, limiting spread is important; identifying and isolating affected animals, prompt treatment, regular foot bathing, dry clean conditions and stringent biosecurity.

Foul of the foot (interdigital necrobacillosis)

An ancient condition with an ancient name – *foul*! This is a bacterial infection involving *Fusobacterium necrophorum*. There must be initial damage to the skin to allow penetration of this bacterium; this may just be from long grass, thistles, stones or just wetting damage to the skin from continually standing in wet, muddy conditions (Figure 14.3). Between the digits a split in the interdigital skin develops; this starts red, smelly and sore and becomes grey and necrotic as the tissue dies. The bacteria cause secondary swelling and heat in the tissues between the digits and around the coronary band which can extend up to the leg – a distinctly swollen foot in other words and

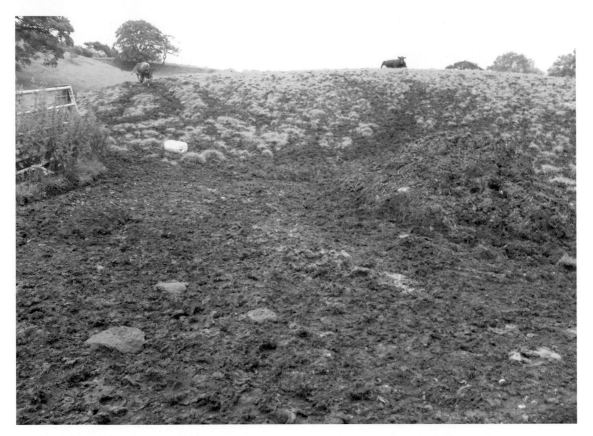

FIGURE 14.3 Poached land will predispose cattle to foul of the foot and other foot injuries due to constant wetting and trauma to the sole and interdigital space

one very characteristic of this classic condition. If untreated the infection may spread into the coffin joint – this has a poor prognosis. Prompt treatment with injectable antibiotics is successful; oxytetracycline or basic penicillin is the antibiotic of choice as the bug is easily killed.

Toe tip necrosis syndrome

This condition is most reported in the USA as a presentation of lameness in calves soon after moving to feedlots. There are a few reports of the condition in the UK (Penny et al., 2017). There appears to be a link with a close succession of numerous handlings; scrabbling on chequer plate aluminium flooring in cattle crushes is thought to be a possible cause as is standing and scrabbling in concrete holding pens while awaiting handling.

The sole horn at the tip of the toe becomes eroded and allows entry of bacteria into the hoof capsule which can then infect the tip of the pedal bone itself or track up through the foot resulting in swelling of the coronary band and sometimes extending further up the leg. Hind limbs are more commonly affected than the front and with group handlings and husbandry tasks it is usual to see more than one animal affected at any one time.

Diagnosis of foot based lameness

It is absolutely imperative that the foot of a lame leg be searched for a cause of lameness before *assuming* a diagnosis or before attempting what would be a blind treatment. No amount of injections will remove an FB from an animal's foot. To not lift the foot and look properly is neglectful. Admittedly if a diagnosis of limb based lameness can be made then it would then become inappropriate to lift the foot but unless absolutely sure of a diagnosis then every lame foot should be inspected by a suitably trained stock person, foot trimmer or vet.

Treatment of lameness

Appropriate corrective paring and the use of foot blocks are nearly always an integral part of the treatment of most foot based lameness but not all – the basic hoof balance in some cattle with digital dermatitis or foul of the foot may actually be fine. That said, the act of lifting the foot for careful inspection creates the opportunity for a routine pare, however minor, even if it is to simply scratch the dirt off the sole to check for additional sole lesions.

Non-steroidal anti-inflammatory drugs

NSAIDs have anti-inflammatory and analgesic (painkilling) properties and can alleviate some of the pain and discomfort experienced by lame animals. Studies in dairy cows have demonstrated that the lameness cure rate is maximised when NSAIDs are used in conjunction with other standard therapies in the treatment of claw horn lesions, such as sole ulcers and WLD (Thomas et al., 2015). Furthermore, ketoprofen, a widely used NSAID, has been demonstrated to decrease the level of hyperalgesia suffered by lame cows (Whay et al., 2005). Consideration should be given to the administration of NSAIDs to all lame animals and where necessary, repeatedly until the acute stage is resolved (the dosing interval is variable depending on the choice of NSAID, typically from 12 to 72 hours). It is essential that NSAIDs are not solely relied upon, however. Other standard therapies must be used. These may include appropriate corrective paring, antibiotics where indicated, foot blocks or even surgery.

Digit amputation

In severe, unresolving cases of lameness affecting only one claw of one foot, a digit amputation can be performed by a vet. Cows manage well on one digit on one foot for a short period of time, long enough to manage a cow through a single lactation or pregnancy or to attain salvage value through a return to soundness, fattening and tolerable transportation to an abattoir. The remaining digit of the foot needs to be in good health as it will be bearing the weight of both digits. Cows should be kept outside or in straw yards after amputation rather than on slats or in cubicle housing. Amputation is an act of veterinary surgery and should be performed only by a vet. The hoof is raised into an accessible position and the sound claw examined for good health and the hoof and interdigital space cleaned and prepared for surgery. A tourniquet is applied to the leg and local anaesthetic is injected into the vein of the leg. The local anaesthetic spreads through the blood vessels of the foot and diffuses out of the blood into the tissue of the foot thereby rendering it numb. The digit is removed above the coronary band at an oblique angle. There is a high risk of haemorrhage, so a pressure bandage is applied before the tourniquet is removed. The bandage should be removed and replaced, if necessary, after 2–3 days. A 3 day course of injectable penicillin antibiotics is advisable to prevent infection of the stump.

Non-foot based lameness in finishing cattle

Osteochondrosis

Osteochondrosis is a disease of the cartilage of the joint where the cartilage is growing so fast it outgrows its blood supply and the cartilage starts to fall apart and develops 'pitting' and flaps. Sometimes the flaps break off and calcify forming so called 'joint mice'. Young fast-growing animals are most commonly affected and present with lameness in one of more limbs, each with swollen, distended joints. The exact cause of the condition has not been established but there is thought to be a causal relationship with gender (male), lack of exercise, growth rate (rapid) and a genetic predisposition (Davies et al., 1996).

Rickets

Rickets is caused by a deficiency of Vitamin D in the diet. Young, growing cattle present with lameness of one or multiple limbs and hard swellings towards the end of the affected bones. The firm swellings are painful to the touch. Rickets responds rapidly to increasing the level of Vitamin D fed in the diet and is helped along by sunlight which catalyses the animal's own manufacture of Vitamin D in the skin.

Osteomalacia

Osteomalacia is the softening of bone because of inadequate bone mineralisation due to a deficiency of phosphorus/phosphate in the diet. A deficiency of Vitamin D can contribute to osteomalacia in adults. Phosphorus/phosphate deficiency presents as weight loss, stiffness, lameness, recumbency and sporadic fractures (Weaver, 2004). Cattle also seek to eat unusual materials that are not readily digestible such as soil, rocks, and other foreign items. A diagnosis can be reached through measuring blood levels of phosphate supported by a mineral analysis of the ration. Treatment is with an injectable phosphorus preparation and an appropriate balancing and supplementation of the ration.

Calcium deficiency

Sporadic fractures and nondescript lameness cases have been reported and linked to insufficient dietary calcium (or excessive phosphorus/phosphate). Fattening cattle fed a high cereal diet are at risk of this and mineral and vitamin balancing and supplementation is required.

GASTROINTESTINAL DISEASE

Wooden tongue (actinobacillosis)

Wooden tongue is a bacterial infection of the tongue muscle and it presents very much as it sounds with an abnormally hard or lumpy tongue. On many occasions the initial clinical sign is weight loss and this presentation should always involve an examination of the mouth. All too often there is an FB, such as string, wrapped round the tongue or a sharp object stuck somewhere in the mouth so this needs ruling in or out, before a diagnosis of wooden tongue is made; wooden tongue is actually quite rare. When it does occur, the affected tongue becomes largely inflexible, so the animal is unable to prehend food or swallow properly. The animal may, consequently, drool saliva and also drop food. The bacterium responsible for wooden tongue is called *Actinobacillus lignieresi* and is found *normally* in the mouth and tonsils of cattle; infection occurs when there is damage within the mouth from rough forage, thistles or a foreign object that allows the bacteria entry into the soft tissues of the tongue. The bacteria form multiple small abscesses in the tongue, below the surface so they are not obvious on examination. *A. lignieresi* can also infect further down the oesophagus and into the rumen. This infection further down the alimentary tract is not as easy to diagnose but should be considered in cases of bloat and vagal indigestion.

Prompt treatment with a streptomycin containing antibiotic for 10 days is usually successful. If cases are left for longer than 2 weeks without treatment the prognosis is poor (Eddy, 2004). Potassium iodide is sometimes administered orally as part of the treatment; it helps the antibiotic to penetrate the abscesses and improves the treatment success rate, but, iodine toxicity is a risk and the treatment is unlicensed in most countries.

Choke

The use of the word choke in veterinary medicine differs from its use in human medicine – it is not blockage of the windpipe with acute death but rather a less imminently fatal blockage of the food pipe, the oesophagus. In the case of cattle this is often due to potatoes, root vegetables or apples that have been swallowed whole without chewing and become stuck some way down the oesophagus. Occasionally it may happen with anthelmintic boluses that have been administered to the wrong size of patient. The animal presents agitated with excessive salivation and bloat. The obstruction may be visible in the neck, but obstructions are more common at the back of the throat or at the thoracic inlet so are more difficult to appreciate by sight or palpation. The thoracic inlet is where the oesophagus passes from the neck through the entrance to the chest, it then continues past the heart, another sticking point for FBs, and finally through the diaphragm into the reticulorumen – this entrance being the final common sticking point.

If the animal appears very bloated, then the bloat should be relieved by inserting a large needle or trochar/cannula into the left sublumbar fossa (flank). Then, at relative leisure, the obstruction needs to be removed; if the obstruction is in the throat, very carefully and by using a mouth gag to prevent the operator losing fingers, it may be possible to remove it by hand, usually with the animal sedated so therefore best done by a vet. If the obstruction is further down the oesophagus but still in reach of the vet then a deeper sedative or anaesthetic can be administered and an attempt made to remove the item, usually a potato, with a narrow corkscrew (this is difficult and dangerous to the patient). Alternatively, a 'pro-bang' or stomach tube can be passed and a gentle attempt made to dislodge the obstruction. Water can be pumped down the stomach tube but care needs to be taken that water does not pass into the trachea – to prevent this from happening the animal needs to have its throat elevated with a wad of straw so its mouth is below the throat. This can be a frustrating and time-consuming task. If the obstruction will not move then, as long as there is a rumen cannula in place to deal with the bloat, the animal can be left without feed and water for 4 hours and then another attempt made to remove the item, which, by this stage, may have softened. Certain medications can be used to relax the smooth muscle of the oesophagus and this may aid removal (it may even allow the blockage to move on without further intervention). Anti-inflammatory drugs, perhaps even steroids, are also beneficial as there will be bruising and swelling of the oesophagus as a result of the blockage and the interventions.

Ruminal acidosis

Ruminal acidosis describes an increase in acidity, in other words a fall in rumen pH, to out with the normal physiological levels. Normal rumen pH is 6.2–7.0 (Gordon, 2004). Acidosis is usually a result of consuming excessive amounts of cereal based carbohydrates of the types that are rapidly fermented in the rumen by certain bacteria, namely lactobacilli and streptococci (normal inhabitants of the rumen bacterial population), this leading to excessive lactic acid production. Lactic acid draws water from the circulation into the rumen causing acute dehydration. The rumen pH can drop as low as 4.5 killing all the 'good bugs' of fermentation. The lactic acid is converted into sodium lactate, which enters the small intestine, again drawing water into the lumen of the gut causing further dehydration and diarrhoea. The sodium lactate is then absorbed into the blood and causes the blood pH to drop, making the animal even more ill. The acidic pH of the rumen causes damage to the rumen wall allowing bacteria to pass into the circulation but also the toxins from the mass death of rumen microbes causes the animal to become toxic (Eddy, 2004).

The gorging of carbohydrate can occur when cattle have had accidental access to feed, such as breaking into a grain store, or sometimes it is seen when cattle are first introduced to cereals/

concentrates or when they have been left without feed and then gorge themselves when the feed is re-introduced. The type of feed is significant; the risk of acidosis is higher when feeding wheat, barley, oats and maize in descending order (Gordon, 2004).

Cattle present with clinical signs from 12 to 36 hours after engorgement (Eddy, 2004). The disease varies in severity depending on how much and what type of concentrate/cereal has been ingested. Initially the animal presents as being 'drunk', weak, wobbly, incoordinate, and dehydrated with tenting skin and sunken eyes. There is little urine production. The animal may be bloated and be in severe abdominal pain, kicking at the abdomen and grinding its teeth. The animal may present with diarrhoea and the faeces often contain a large amount of grain that has passed through undigested. In severe cases recumbency and death follow.

The diagnosis of acidosis is usually apparent on the history and clinical signs alone. On PME the rumen contents are rich in cereal/concentrate (Figure 14.4). Measuring the pH of the rumen fluid with a pH meter may support a diagnosis. In cases of acute acidosis, the pH will be less than 5.2 (Gordon, 2004). This is only a valid test in a recently dead animal – the pH of the rumen rises after death due to the opposing actions of the post-mortem rumen microbes.

Treatment depends on the severity of disease.

When the animal is recumbent surgical emptying of the rumen may be appropriate. This procedure is called a rumenotomy and involves accessing the rumen via the left flank and emptying the rumen content onto the floor and lavaging

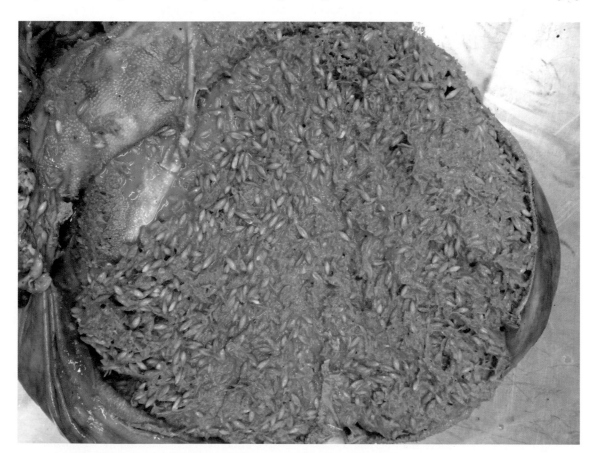

FIGURE 14.4 Rumen content at PME; a large amount of grain visible

the rumen with clean water. Every effort should be made to avoid rumen contents leaking into the abdomen as this would cause peritonitis which is difficult to treat in its own right.

If the animal is still standing, the oral administration of magnesium oxide, magnesium hydroxide, aluminium hydroxide, magnesium carbonate or magnesium trisilicate mixed with 10–20 l of water may provide sufficient neutralisation and rehydration without the need for surgery. Other treatments include intravenous B vitamins, calcium, dextrose, NSAIDs and bicarbonate and additional fluids administered intravenously (Eddy, 2004). Antibiotics are used by some clinicians to reduce secondary bacterial infections elsewhere in the body following bacterial penetration through the damaged rumen wall into the circulation. For this to be effective the duration of the course of antibiotics needs to exceed the time it takes for the rumen wall to repair. A forage-based diet should be fed for 7 days with a gradual re-introduction back to concentrate feeds. A probiotic supplement will help the rumen to restore the normal flora. A full feed review needs to be conducted looking at the feed constituents and how the ration is fed. There are a number of proprietary additives that are mixed with finishing diets that claim to reduce the risk of acidosis, an evidence-based review is required to ensure they 'do what they say on the tin'! Vitamin B injections have been popularly used over the years – while this can only help, quite how much it helps is also lacking evidence!

Liver abscesses

Liver abscesses occur in all ages of cattle but where they cause most economic loss is in finishing cattle where condemnation of the liver at slaughter is a problem. Liver abscesses are clearly visible at PME or at slaughter as encapsulated white pus-filled pockets. Sometimes they are only visible when cutting into the liver, there may be one abscess or they may be multiple and they vary in size typically from 2 to 15 cm although monstrously huge ones are occasionally seen. They often do not cause any clinical signs in fattening animals, however, if they reach such a size to cause disruption of liver function then signs of liver disease will be evident; abdominal pain, weight loss, scour, and jaundice. As the liver is a very vascular structure it is not uncommon for bacteria to seed off from a liver abscess and migrate around the body in the circulation, setting up infections at additional sites such as the lung or within the valves of the heart. On very rare occasions an abscess may rupture and release pus into the abdomen, causing peritonitis – a life-threatening condition if not diagnosed and treated promptly. Depending on the location of the abscess in the liver it may erode blood vessels. This can have catastrophic results in one of two directions: the pus can burst from the abscess into the circulation, sending a fatal bolus of toxic pus into the circulation or alternatively blood can haemorrhage out of the blood vessel through the erosion, causing fatal shock.

Liver abscesses can be detected by ultrasound examination placing the probe on the left-hand side just behind the ribs or in between the ribs. However, not all of the liver can be examined by ultrasonography as it hides behind a lung lobe (Nagaraja and Lechtenberg, 2007). Blood testing and analysing liver enzymes in the blood can indicate there is liver disease of some sort, but it is no more specific than that.

Liver abscessation is classically preceded by a low rumen pH (acidosis), which allows bacteria that are normal inhabitants of the rumen to cross the inflamed rumen wall (rumenitis) into the bloodstream. The variation in incidence on farm varies as is it dependant on feeding practices and is therefore largely preventable. Alternatively, the rumen wall may be damaged or penetrated from foreign material such as a wire or rough feedstuffs, again allowing entry of bacteria into the bloodstream and liver.

The two main bacteria associated with liver abscessation are *Fusobacterium necrophorum* and *Trueperella pyogenes*.

F. necrophorum is a natural inhabitant of the environment, the soil and the rumen where it lives in the microenvironment of the rumen wall. Its optimal pH is 7.4, near neutral, but when the pH is lowered the resulting damage permits entry of *F. necrophorum* into the circulation. The first port of call from the gastrointestinal tract via the bloodstream is the liver via the hepatic portal vein. *F. necrophorum* does not replicate at this low pH but the population in the rumen increases 10-fold when the diet is first changed from roughage to a grain diet, a predisposing factor for acidosis (Nagaraja and Lechtenberg, 2007).

T. pyogenes is again a normal inhabitant of the rumen wall and is also found within the upper digestive tract generally and the respiratory tract. It is commonly found in abscesses of other organs such as the skin, udder and foot.

Rumen acidosis is associated with lack of forage within the diet or what is more commonly referred to as a poor concentrate : forage ratio. Processed grains (crushed/rolled) present, through a larger surface area and through a breaking of the grain, more readily digestible starch that ferment quicker and cause a larger drop in the rumen pH, so much so the rumen is unable to buffer the fluctuation. Irregular feeding times and leaving cattle without feed intermittently can cause these larger fluctuations in rumen pH.

Liver abscesses are more commonly seen in the last 60 days of the finishing period as the cattle are fed an even higher energy-dense diet with a high cereal or concentrate inclusion rate and they are exposed to an acidogenic diet for a longer if not continual period. There will, however, be variation in dietary intakes in some cattle who will take more than others and be more predisposed to acidosis (Nagaraja and Lechtenberg, 2007).

Maintaining rumen health through dietary management is the main method of prevention of liver abscessation and is discussed in full in Chapter 7.

Bloat

Bloat is a gaseous distention of the rumen. The abdomen appears enlarged, there is a distinct massive bulge on the left-hand side behind the ribs below the transverse processes of the spine (the upper left flank referred to as the left sublumbar fossa). On tapping this area, it sounds like a drum. At a very basic level there is either excessive gas production within the rumen or for whatever reason gas is unable to escape from the rumen. As the rumen gets larger it inhibits the function of the diaphragm and the animal is no longer able to breath. The rumen also compresses the large vein, called the vena cava, that is responsible for returning blood back to the heart, the animal's circulation is duly compromised. Both scenarios contribute to the animal's death. Acute bloat is considered a veterinary emergency – the pressure must be relieved.

There are two types of bloat.

1. **Free gas bloat**. This occurs when the top portion of the rumen is filled with a large amount of gas and can be caused by the following.
   a) An oesophageal obstruction such as an abscess or infection (wooden tongue), or a foreign object such as a potato. This can sometimes be palpable in the neck where the blockage is high enough and is usually accompanied by large amounts of salivation.
   b) External pressure on the oesophagus from an enlarged structure out with the oesophagus, for example, a large lymph node or abscess in the throat, neck or chest.
   c) A downer animal where the roughage/fibre mat and/or liquid portion of the rumen contents are overlaying the entrance to the rumen rather than the gas cap so the gas cannot get belched out. The animal may be recumbent for a number of reasons; bloat is commonly seen in cases of hypocalcaemia (milk fever) and, more unusually, tetanus where paralysis of rumen motility further compounds the problem.

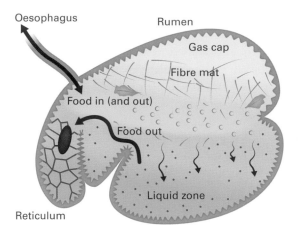

FIGURE 14.5 Normal composition of the rumen contents (courtesy of The Vet Group)

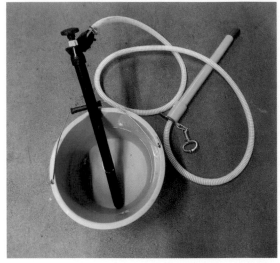

FIGURE 14.6 Modified stomach tube with mouth guard to prevent damage to the tubing. Pictured with pump attached

d) Excessive cereal consumption resulting in overly rapid fermentation and excessive gas production which overwhelms the animal's ability to eructate (belch) and with the distension of the rumen eventually kinking and distorting the entrance to the oesophagus to the point that eructation becomes physically impossible.

2. **Frothy bloat**. Occurs when the composition of the rumen is altered; instead of a liquid zone, fibre mat and a gas cap, the gas cap is made up not of free gas but of froth (Figure 14.5). The particles in the froth interfere with the receptors and the signalling system responsible for eructation and therefore there is further accumulation of gas within the froth. Frothy bloat is caused by lush spring high protein pastures, typically clover, or by feeding finely milled grain.

There are heroic stories of farmers needing to puncture the side of cattle at the sublumbar fossa to relieve the gas and save the animal. This may be warranted if the animal is found in severe distress on the point of death, but often passing a stomach tube, if there is time to do so, is a much more humane, constructive and successful method of relieving the gas; fatal peritonitis often follows poor-quality stabbing of the rumen.

Passing a stomach tube is also the useful first step in assessing the cause of a case of bloat (Figure 14.6). In cattle a stomach tube is passed through the mouth although vets will occasionally use the nasal passage. Care needs to be taken that the tube is protected and not chewed in half by the patient. A piece of alkathene piping held in the mouth for the stomach tube to pass through will prevent this happening but there are now specifically designed stomach tubes with built-in mouth guards and nose clips to make this job easier and more manageable for a single operator.

On passing the stomach tube it is important to pass the tube over the back of the tongue as far as the throat and then wait for the animal to swallow. The tube is then passed into the oesophagus (food pipe). If too much force is used it may cause damage to the throat or the tube may be forced into the windpipe rather than the oesophagus or it may bend or kink. When the stomach tube is in the oesophagus it may be seen through the skin of the neck as it is advanced towards the rumen – this can be a reassuring sight! In cases of bloat where the stomach tube will not advance then there may indeed be an obstruction in the oesophagus that needs to be further investigated and removed. Consideration should be given to the fact that the

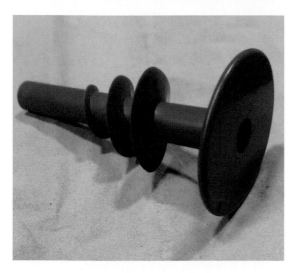

FIGURE 14.7 Red Devil™ rumen trocar

obstruction may not be in the oesophagus but being caused by an adjacent structure such as an enlarged lymph node – this is common in finishing cattle if they have had cases of pneumonia and the local lymph nodes have been repeatedly stimulated and become enlarged as a result. It may be that, on passing the stomach tube, these structures are pushed to one side and, although the obstruction is not detected on examination, the bloat recurs soon after. Recurrent cases warrant the use of a rumen cannula or a permanent rumenostomy or rumen fistula (Figure 14.7 and 14.8); a permanent surgical hole in the flank and rumen wall that allows gas

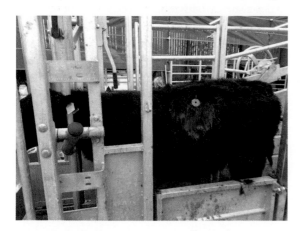

FIGURE 14.8 Red Devil™ in the left flank of a fattening animal

to escape freely. Both these procedures are often sufficient to allow an animal to fatten and get to slaughter but they are not really suitable for long-term management, for example, in a breeding cow or bull; the wounds can become infected and contaminated with overflowing rumen contents and attract flies. That said, it is possible to maintain a valuable animal semi-permanently if deemed really necessary.

If a stomach tube is passed, without resistance, in a case of free gas bloat, gas will be released immediately. If the end of the stomach tube drops into the liquid or fibre mat the tube may block and the tube will need repositioning to allow more gas to leave. Often, *balloting* (bouncing) the left-hand side of the cow facilitates this repositioning and a re-floating of the gas back to the top of the rumen. Once the gas has been relieved, if the cause of the bloat is yet to be identified, the animal should be comprehensively examined to establish the cause. In cases of frothy bloat, the gas does not exit the tube, the tube just blocks with the rather viscous foam. If this is the case an antifoaming agent can be administered down the tube to disperse the froth. These preparations can be purchased in a proprietary format although 500 ml of sunflower, linseed or general vegetable oil is cheaper and nearly as effective. To prevent further cases of frothy bloat the cattle should be removed from the offending pasture (usually clover rich) and fed a basic forage-based diet before being gradually re-introduced to the pasture, starting with just 10 minutes per day.

When cattle are grazing high-risk pastures or fed a finely milled ration then ensure sufficient roughage is fed which will help to prevent cases of bloat. Cattle should be gradually introduced to any change in feed and that includes introduction to pasture. If the pasture is very lush or dense with clover or legume species, then feeding oils for 14 days post turn out may reduce cases. Anecdotally, adding 60 ml per head of liquid paraffin in brewer's grains daily for 14 days is sufficient and beneficial.

Vagal indigestion

Vagal indigestion is a relatively rare condition of well grown and adult cattle. It occurs as a result of damage to the vagus nerve. The vagus nerve leaves the back of the brain and travels out with the spinal column down the neck, through the chest and through the diaphragm to the organs of the abdomen, including the stomachs. The nerve is responsible for stimulating function in the abdominal organs such as getting the rumen to contract, and the movement of digesta from the rumen into the abomasum, and then, from the abomasum into the small intestine. Because the nerve is long and relatively exposed it is prone to damage or compression from a variety of insults: local peritonitis, a wire, post abdominal surgery, abscesses in the chest, an enlarged infected heart/pericardium or enlarged lymph nodes in the chest following repeated bouts of pneumonia. When the vagus nerve fails, the rumen and abomasum also fail and there is an accumulation of feedstuffs in the stomachs. The predominant clinical sign is a distended abdomen. The abdomen has a characteristic appearance; the right side of the abdomen develops a pear shaped swelling low down; this corresponds to the abomasum, which is distended. The left flank is also distended at the left sublumbar fossa but is firm to touch rather than gassy as is the case with bloat. On rectal examination the rumen is 'full' and felt as far back as the pelvis. The vagal nerve also has an influence on heart rate and some cases have a heart rate of as low as 40 beats per minute (Eddy, 2004). A small amount of dry faeces is usually present in the rectum or nothing other than mucus – a sign of nothing having passed through for a while.

Treatment is largely unsuccessful and immediate slaughter is advised. Where treatment is to be attempted, oral fluids should be avoided as they will further distend the stomachs; fluid therapy in which case, if to be attempted, needs to be intravenous. Steroids, typically dexamethasone, can be administered where there is suspicion that chronic pneumonia and enlarged lymph nodes are thought to be interfering with the nerve. In a high value animal, surgery to explore the abdomen and identify the cause of the digestive upset can be attempted. This may involve entering the rumen. Cases of plastic wrap engorgement have a similar presentation; this occurs when plastic sheeting has been eaten from baled silage or sheeted pit silage where the stockperson has failed to remove it all before feeding to the cattle. Once the plastic is removed from the rumen the animal usually makes a full recovery.

Traumatic reticuloperitonitis ('wire disease')

Traumatic reticuloperitonitis (TRP) is caused by the ingestion of a sharp metallic item that becomes lodged in the wall of the reticulum. The reticulum and rumen together form a large conjoined structure referred to as the reticulorumen. Some metallic FBs may stay within the reticulum or rumen for long periods of time and not cause any problem. When they are particularly sharp the strong muscular contractions of the reticulorumen can force the object to penetrate the wall and then cause a localised infection within the abdomen. Depending on the position of penetration and the degree of migration of the metallic FB it may go on to penetrate the diaphragm and then the pericardial sac surrounding the heart.

TRP presents differently depending on the stage of infection and the location of the FB. In the initial stages there may be only signs of mild intermittent discomfort as the FB scratches the reticulorumen wall. If penetration has occurred, an acute peritonitis will result where the animal is off its food, with a fever and abdominal distention. Sometimes, however, peritonitis can be localised and contained with little or no clinical signs at all – here the body successfully fights the infection with an inflammatory response and in chronic long-standing cases the body will attempt to 'wall off' the foreign object with fibrous tissue. If the wire then migrates through the diaphragm, then the pericardial sac may be penetrated causing it to fill with inflammatory fluid and compress the heart. If the wire leaves the reticulum sideways then the liver may be affected or if a large blood vessel is punctured internal haemorrhage and sudden death may result.

TRP can be considered in many disease presentations; there are a few clues to look out for.

- In 50% of cases there is a tucked up, arched back appearance (Orpin and Harwood, 2008).
- When an operative pushes down on the withers the animal resists, dipping its back and showing notable discomfort, often making a grunting noise.
- The animal may have difficulty lying down, getting up and, sometimes, walking around corners.
- The animal may grunt when moving or lying down or rising.
- The animal may display peculiar lying positions in an attempt to find a comfortable position.
- The 'bar test' (Orpin and Harwood, 2008) is a useful crude diagnostic tool. A bar is held by two operatives either side of the patient halfway between its elbow and its udder, if it has one. The bar is raised slowly and dropped quickly; in cases of TRP the cow exhibits signs of discomfort and a ridged stance, and maybe a grunt.
- Where the foreign body has entered the chest cavity a stethoscope may pick up muffled or 'washing machine' heart sounds and/or a heart murmur.

There are two options for treatment: conservative medical treatment and surgical treatment. Where the wire has been recently ingested and still within the reticulum with limited migration it can be effectively removed by surgery. The surgical procedure involves an incision into the left flank and rumen with the surgeon then searching the reticulorumen by feeling forward and down towards the animal's sternum whereupon the wire may be felt and removed. In chronic cases where there is substantial peritonitis and fibrosis it may be impossible to detect or remove the wire; the local infection may also be too advanced to treat with antibiotics and treatment will be unsuccessful. Alternatively, a conservative approach in acute cases would involve administering not only antibiotics but also a magnetic bolus which would attach to any metallic objects in the reticulorumen and prevent them from migrating. If the metallic object has already penetrated the wall and started to migrate this will be ineffective. The magnets are more routinely used for prevention rather than treatment.

Where disease is more advanced, and migration has occurred, medical treatment with NSAIDs and antibiotics may, on rare occasions, have some success. The animals own inflammatory response may be able to 'wall off' and compartmentalise such infections and the metallic FB may be contained within a fibrous capsule with no further clinical signs. Many metallic foreign items are found at slaughter in the reticulorumen or walled off within the abdomen or chest having caused no outward signs of disease or decreased productivity.

The metallic FB may be a fencing wire, a nail, a screw or a wire from a tyre (Figure 14.9) – the disease is sometimes referred to as hardware disease! A Danish study examined 1491 animals at slaughter for the presence of metal objects within the reticulorumen, the existence of TRP and the presence of a magnet. They found a metal object in 16% of the animals examined and of those 10% had evidence of chronic TRP. Of the metal objects identified, 14% were fencing wire, 11% tyre wire, 9% screws, 5% nails and 22% were the remains of antiparasitic boluses, which had not caused any associated damage to the reticulorumen wall. Out of all the foreign bodies tyre wire was considered the most traumatic due to its narrow, sharp structure (Cramers et al., 2005).

The metallic objects enter the ration in a variety of ways; falling off machinery during silage foraging or feeding, metal contaminated silage pastures, or from disintegrated tyres used to compress the silage pit sheeting (Figure 14.10 and 14.11). A large

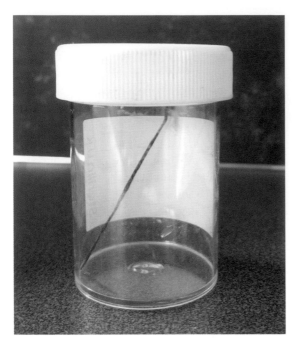

FIGURE 14.9 Tyre wire removed from the pericardium of a cow at PME

number of cases are seen in close succession when metal fragments are fed en masse, for example, a blade in the mixer wagon shatters or a tyre inadvertently gets added to the mixer wagon and gets chopped up and fed with the ration.

Magnets are a useful preventative measure. They can be attached to silage machinery (for the benefit of the machinery as well as the cows!) and magnetic boluses can be administered to adult cattle at risk. Magnetic boluses are administered by the same method as a trace element bolus would be. They are heavy and rarely regurgitated and sit for long periods of time in the reticulum gathering metal particles. There have been cases of TRP in older cows where the magnet has become full, often just with the long-term accumulation of metal filings. Some consideration should be given to administering a follow up magnetic bolus every 3–4 years.

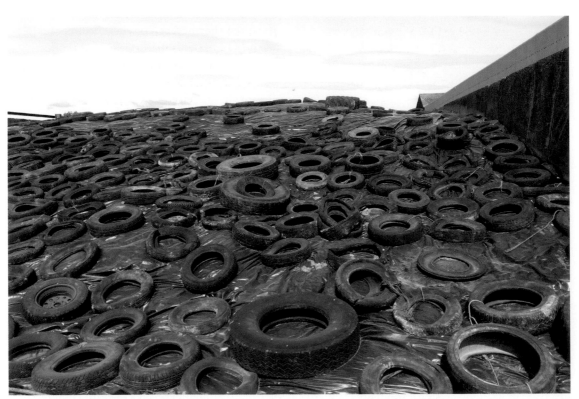

FIGURE 14.10 Silage pit covered in tyres

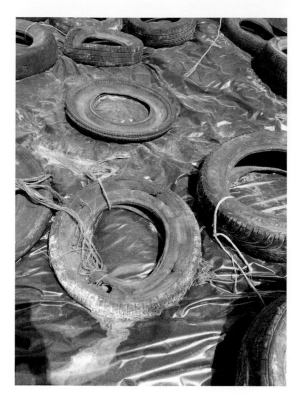

FIGURE 14.11 Close up of a perished tyre with exposed wires

NEUROLOGICAL DISEASE

Cerebrocortical necrosis (polioencephalomalacia)

Cerebrocortical necrosis (CCN) is a disease of the brain in cattle and sheep involving damage to the grey matter. This is associated with altered glucose metabolism as a result of Vitamin B1 deficiency. Glucose is the main energy source for the brain. Vitamin B1 is normally synthesised by the rumen microbes, rather than being fed to an animal in the diet. Consequently, the animal's reserves of Vitamin B1 are entirely dependent on a healthy normal functioning rumen. There are, however, bacteria that naturally occur in the rumen that produce an enzyme called thiaminase, which destroys Vitamin B1. If there is a change in the rumen flora due to a change in diet or a bout of acidosis there may be an overgrowth of these thiaminase producing bacteria; Vitamin B1 deficiency results (Sargison, 2008).

The clinical signs attributed to the resulting brain damage are quite dramatic and usually affect cattle between 6 and 18 months of age. Cattle generally stand away from the group, they are wobbly, uncoordinated, dull and depressed and often go blind. In advanced stages they will be recumbent and lie with their head straight back (opisthotonos). Death occurs within 1–3 days. The clinical signs are not dissimilar to meningitis, lead poisoning, *H. somni* encephalitis, listeriosis, acidosis, salt poisoning (water deprivation) or louping ill.

The diagnosis of CCN in a live animal is based on clinical signs and the response to treatment. Blood thiamine levels have no relation to the clinical presentation and cannot be used as a diagnostic tool. The condition can be diagnosed from microscopic examination (histopathology) of the brain of a dead animal, although processing the tissue for examination can take up to a week so cannot be relied on for a quick diagnosis for the group.

The affected animals respond relatively quickly, within 12 hours, to the intramuscular or intravenous administration of Vitamin B1. Twice daily injections for 3 days are recommended. Supportive care involves housing the animal in a quiet environment and providing easy access to water and food as blindness is often the last clinical sign to resolve.

Sulphur toxicity

Similar brain pathology to CCN results from sulphur toxicity which, in this condition, affects all areas of the brain, not just the grey matter – interestingly the clinical signs are still similar to CCN but without the throwing back of the head. Sulphur toxicity is, perhaps not surprisingly, unresponsive to supplementation with Vitamin B1 (Sargison, 2008). Again, histopathology of the brain is diagnostic, and the sulphur content of the diet needs to be reviewed as the cause is invariably excessive sulphur in the diet.

Listerial meningo-encephalitis

Listerial meningo-encephalitis is caused by infection of the brain with the bacterium *Listeria monocytogenes*. Listeria exist in the environment, in soil and water, and tolerate a wide range of temperatures and pH. They are easily killed by disinfectants and temperatures in excess of 60°C. Cases in cattle are usually a result of ingesting silage contaminated with soil, soil which itself is contaminated with the bacteria and which is offering the ideal conditions for the listeria bacteria to multiply and reach an infective dose. Round bale silage with a high dry matter and low sugar content enjoys less effective fermentation. This means less lactic acid production and a higher pH. If in combination with these conditions there is sufficient oxygen in the bale, which is more likely in less packed high dry matter silages, and in bales with holes in the wrap, then listeria bacteria will proliferate (Sargison, 2008). The same conditions can arise in poorly managed silage pits too. Because of the association between silage feeding and listeriosis, cases are most commonly seen over the winter months (Erdogan et al., 2001). It is also possible for cattle to be infected directly from soil if there is a low sward height and cattle end up eating soil, or, where they are fed soil contaminated root crops.

Listeriosis does not only target the brain, it can cause mastitis, neonatal septicaemia, eye infections, and abortions (Guyot, 2011). Listeriosis is also associated with uveitis of the eye although it is not clear if this is a direct infection of the eye or an immune system reaction to infection elsewhere in the body that manifests indirectly in the eye. The brain form is more common in younger animals that are in the process of erupting teeth; the organism gains entry and travels up the nerve that connects the tooth to the brain (Erdogan et al., 2001); this takes some time; the incubation period is estimated to be 2–3 weeks (Barlow, 1989). It is important to remember this when deciding which feedstuff to blame – the disease was not caused by the feed the animal was eating when it developed clinical signs but rather the feedstuff it was eating 2–3 weeks beforehand.

Listeriosis involves abscesses within the brain and the clinical signs observed are dependent on the location of these abscesses (Sargison, 2008) – different regions of the brain have different jobs. Clinical signs can include any of the following and are usually unilateral (one-sided): drooping of one ear, slight droop of one eyelid, saliva drooling from one side of the mouth and a one-sided droopy lip. The paralysis to the muscles on one side of the face make it difficult for the animal to prehend (bite) food and to drink water. As the infection progresses the animal may start to circle in one direction, this progresses to recumbency and, after 7–10 days, death through starvation.

The diagnosis of listeriosis is based largely on clinical examination and the history of silage feeding. Examination of the silage present at the time of clinical signs is irrelevant but silage making practices in general should be reviewed, particularly to minimise soil contamination but also better packing and wrapping (Chapter 25). A diagnosis can be obtained for a dead animal through bacterial culture of the fluid surrounding the brain or the brain itself. Alternatively, sections of the brain can be prepared for microscopic examination (histopathology) (Guyot, 2011).

Treatment is a long course, at a high dose rate, of penicillin. The response to treatment is slow. In the authors' experience, if the animal is still able to stand when treatment commences, there is a fair to good prognosis. Animals that survive may have a permanent paralysis of half the face or a head tilt.

URINARY DISEASE

Urolithiasis

Urolithiasis is the obstruction of the urinary tract with urinary stones. A urinary stone is called a calculus or urolith. The urinary tract includes the kidneys, the ureters, the bladder and the urethra. The urethra is the tube that connects the bladder to the outside world and is responsible for the passage of urine during urination. The urethra is the most commonly diagnosed site of urolithiasis. If the urethra becomes blocked the animal is unable to urinate and urine backs up, causing bladder distention and ultimately increased pressure in the kidneys. The urinary tract eventually bursts and/ or the kidneys are irreparably damaged, death results. Male ruminants more commonly suffer from urolithiasis than females as they have a narrower and longer urethra. The urethra is narrower in castrated males compared to their entire counterpart. Castrated male calves at around a year old are most commonly affected.

The condition is to be considered of nutritional origin. Ruminants fed high concentrate diets are predisposed. This is usually due to a low calcium: phosphate ratio or a feed containing high levels of magnesium (Divers, 2013). There are many types of uroliths depending on their mineral composition, *struvite* uroliths are the most common in the UK. Normal urine is pH 7 or above. Struvite uroliths form in alkaline urine so this is a physiological predisposition. Inadequate water intake predisposes to urolithiasis and this combination of factors means that it is most commonly seen in housed, concentrate fed young cattle in the winter months, possibly after a period of cold weather where the water supply has been restricted.

In the early stages of the disease the passage of urine may be intermittent, possibly blood stained but it is not until there is a complete obstruction that noticeable clinical signs are apparent. The affected animal is uncomfortable, grinding its teeth, kicking its abdomen, repeatedly straining to urinate and tail swishing. There may be tiny white calculi and/or blood visible on the preputial hair. There may be inappetence and lethargy. A suspected diagnosis can be supported by examining the bladder via the rectum using a gloved hand, in patients large enough for the procedure, or by abdominal palpation in smaller patients. A large distended bladder would support a diagnosis of urolithiasis. Blood tests to assess kidney function and electrolyte balance, ultrasound examination

and testing any urine that is available for calculi (if any) will help confirm a suspected diagnosis.

Initially a small tube (urinary catheter) can be passed up the urethra and flushed with saline solution to see if the urolith can easily be dislodged. Antispasmodic drugs may also help relax the urethral muscle and help the passage of the uroliths and catheter. The anatomy of the bovine penis does not make passing a catheter particularly easy for the same reason that uroliths get stuck! There is an 'S' bend in the penis, called the sigmoid flexure, past which a catheter will not easily pass. Catheterisation is, therefore, only a useful technique if the blockage is towards the end of the penis. There are techniques where local anaesthetic can be applied to deactivate specific nerves and allow the penis to relax which may help to both dislodge the urolith or to pass the catheter.

If the animal is a castrated male or an entire male not intended for breeding then a *urethrostomy* can be performed. A urethrostomy is a surgical opening into the urethra exiting out through the skin, usually at the perineum, just below the anus. The surgery involves dissecting between the tissues and identifying the urethra. The urethra is cut and stitched to the skin of the perineum. The post-surgical male animal is now able to urinate like a female. This procedure is obviously only successful if the obstruction is below the urethrostomy, not if the obstruction is nearer the bladder. Supportive medical treatment such as fluid therapy will be required to flush the kidneys and help restore a physiologically normal electrolyte balance.

If urolithiasis is untreated, the unrelieved pressure causes a rupture of the urinary tract approximately 48 hours after obstruction. There is a temporary improvement in the patient's demeanour as the pressure is released. The bladder itself may rupture releasing urine into the abdomen – this can be seen on ultrasound examination. The fluid within the abdomen can be sampled with a long needle inserted into the lowest part of the abdomen and analysed. Cattle can survive for a surprisingly long time, up to 2 weeks, after the bladder ruptures, their condition progressively worsens, and abdominal distention and discomfort become more apparent. The rupture may occur in the urethra releasing urine into the tissues of the prepuce or perineum. The area becomes swollen, cold to touch and touching the area leaves pitted fingerprints – a sign of tissue *oedema*.

Preventative measures are crucial to prevent further cases. The calcium : phosphorus ratio of the diet should be adjusted to the optimal 2 : 1 (Divers, 2013); there should be free access to water. Acidification of the urine may also prevent the formation of some uroliths; ammonium chloride is commonly used at 50–80 g/head/day for a 240 kg steer (Divers, 2013).

REFERENCES

Archer, S., Bell, N. and Huxley, J. (2010) Lameness in UK dairy cows: a review of current status. *In Practice* 32, 492–504.

Barlow, R.M. (1989) Listerial encephalitis (circling disease) of sheep and cattle. The Moredun Foundation, News sheets 1–30, Volume 1: 91–98.

Blowey, R. (1992) Diseases of the Bovine digit: Part 1 Description of common lesions. *In Practice* 14, 85–90

Cramers, T. Mikkelsen, K.B., Anderson, P., Enevoldsen, C. and Jensen, H.E. (2005) New types of foreign bodies and the effect of magnets in traumatic reticulitis in cows. *Vet Record* 157, 287–289.

Davies, I.H., Bain, M.S., Munro, R. and Livesey, C.T. (1996) Osteochondritis dissecans in a group of rapidly growing bull beef calves. *Cattle Practice* 4(3), 243–245.

Divers, T.J. (2013) Urolithiasis in Large Animals. MSD Manual Veterinary Manual. Urinary system. Available at: https://www.msdvetmanual.com/urinary-system/noninfectious-diseases-of-the-urinary-system-in-large-animals/urolithiasis-in-large-animals.

Eddy, R.G. (2004) Alimentary conditions. In: Andrews, A.H., Blowey, R.W., Boyd, H. and Eddy, R.G. (eds) *Bovine Medicine Diseases and Husbandry of Cattle*, 2nd edn. Blackwell, Oxford, pp. 828–834.

Erdogan, H.M., Cetinkaya, B. Green, L.E., Cripps, P.J. and Morgan, K.L. (2001) Prevalence, incidence, signs and treatment of clinical listeriosis in dairy cattle in England. *Vet Record* 149, 289–293.

Gordon, P.J. (2004) Rumen acidosis: treatment and prevention. *Cattle Practice* 12(3): 209–212.

Greenough, P.R. (2015) MSD Veterinary Manual. Laminitis in cattle – musculoskeletal system. Available at: https://www.msdvetmanual.com/musculoskeletal-system/lameness-in-cattle/laminitis-in-cattle.

Guyot, H. (2011) Case report: two cases of ocular form of listeriosis in cattle herds. *Cattle Practice* 19(1), 61–64.

Nagaraja, T.G. and Lechtenberg, K.F. (2007) Liver abscesses in feedlot cattle. *Veterinary Clinics: Food Animal Practice* 23, 351–369.

Orpin, P. and Harwood, D. (2008) Clinical management of traumatic reticuloperitonitis in cattle. *In Practice* 30, 544–551.

Penny, C., Bradley, S. and Wilson, D. (2017) Lameness due to toe-tip necrosis syndrome in beef calves. *Vet Record* 180, 154.

Sargison, N. (2008) Neurological disease In: *Sheep Flock Health A Planned Approach*. John Wiley and Sons, Hoboken, NJ, pp. 329–331.

Thomas, H.J., Miguel-Pacheco, G.G., Bollard, N.J., Archer, S.C., Bell, N. J., Mason, C., Maxwell, O J., Remnant, J.G., Sleeman, P., Whay, H.R. and Huxley, J.N. (2015) Evaluation of treatments for claw horn lesions in dairy cows in a randomised controlled trial. *Journal of Dairy Science* 98(7), 4477–4486.

Weaver, A.D. (2004) Lameness above the foot. In: In: Andrews, A.H., Blowey, R.W., Boyd, H. and Eddy, R. G. (eds) *Bovine Medicine Diseases and Husbandry of cattle*, 2nd edn. Blackwell, Oxford, pp. 453–454.

Whay, H.R., Webster, A.J.F. and Waterman-Pearson, A.E. (2005) Role of ketoprofen in the modulation of hyperalgesia associated with lameness in dairy cattle. *Vet Record* 157, 729–733.

Chapter 15

Disease and production failure in the heifer replacement

Even in a well-managed suckler herd, a percentage of cows will be culled every year. To maintain numbers, replacement breeding animals are needed; for maximum longevity, these should be heifers, hence the term 'heifer replacements'.

DISEASES OF THE RESPIRATORY SYSTEM

Fog fever

Fog fever is a respiratory disease of cattle typically over 2 years old that have been on a low plain of nutrition and are then suddenly introduced to lush pastures, such as silage aftermaths, or *fogs* as they are called in some parts, in the mid to late summer. The animals, as a group, are generally quiet and slow and on close inspection usually have an elevated respiratory rate. More severely affected animals present with a rapid onset of respiratory distress: air hunger, neck outstretched, excess salivation and, in some cases, an inability to move. Coughing, interestingly, is not a common clinical sign. The condition results from the ingestion of large quantities of L-tryptophan, a naturally occurring amino acid, that exists in large quantities in lush pasture. L-tryptophan is converted, in the rumen by rumen microbes, to 3-methyl indole, a metabolite that unfortunately enters the bloodstream and at sufficiently high levels is damaging to certain cells in the lungs (Andrews and Windsor, 2004). Usually more than one animal is affected. Death can result in severe cases.

There is no diagnostic test for fog fever, a diagnosis is based on the history and clinical signs of the affected animals. The presentation of an animal with fog fever can be confused with that of lungworm but lungworm commonly presents with an associated cough, which is not the case with fog fever.

Treatment involves removing animals calmly and quietly from the offending pasture. Severely affected animals require treatment with corticosteroids under the direction of a vet.

Prevention involves anticipating the problem and introducing cattle to new fresh pasture gradually, a few hours a day, over a period of 2 weeks.

Lungworm (husk)

The clinical signs associated with lungworm infection can range from a slight occasional cough to an animal who holds its head down, is reluctant to move, is in severe respiratory distress or simply collapses and dies. The disease is caused by a thread-like white worm called *Dictyocaulus viviparus* that occupies the upper airways of the lungs. The adult worms live in these airways and lay eggs that are carried up to the throat in phlegm which is then swallowed. The eggs pass through the gastrointestinal tract developing into larvae as they go. They are passed out in the faeces as first-stage larvae.

These larvae then develop into second and third-stage larvae inside dung pats on the pasture and then cunningly hitch a ride on a fungus known as *Pilobolus* that grows on the dung and has a mechanism of popping and firing its spores all over the pasture at distances of up to 3 m. The disseminated third-stage larvae then wriggle up blades of clean grass which are more attractive to the grazing cattle than the grass splattered with dung pats. The ingested larvae burrow through the gut wall into the bloodstream or the lymphatic system and make their way to the lungs where they once again burrow and enter the airways of the lung to set up home (Figure 15.1). It takes three weeks from an animal eating a third-stage larvae to first-stage larvae being passed in the same animal's faeces; a time span known as the prepatent period. The time it takes for development of the larval stages on the pasture varies depending on the weather, it can be as little as one week.

Most surviving cattle will mount an immune response to lungworm, recover and shed the infection. A small population of carrier animals persist from year to year, however, so the presence of the parasite in herds persists. Furthermore, some larvae will survive the winter months in the deeper protective layers of the pasture and dung remnants. Both of these strategies of persistence ensure lungworm survives in herds and pastures from year to year, amazingly on pasture alone for as long as 6 years.

Clinical cases are most commonly seen from July onwards as conditions promote an increasing larval challenge.

Benzimadazole, levamisole and macrocyclic lactones (Chapter 26) are all anthelmintics that are effective against lungworm. There is, to date, no know resistance of lungworm to any anthelmintics (McLeonard and van Dijk, 2017). These anthelmintics are available in different preparations, with different routes of application, and with activity that persists for variable amounts of time. Anthelmintics will kill lungworm in diseased animals and carrier animals. The duration of action of some products exceeds the time that the majority, but not all, of the larvae survive on the

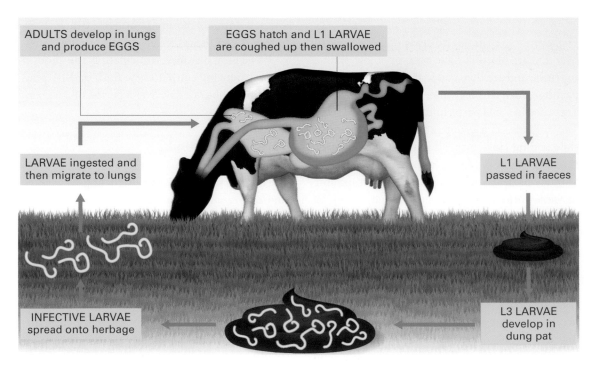

ADULTS develop in lungs and produce EGGS

EGGS hatch and L1 LARVAE are coughed up then swallowed

LARVAE ingested and then migrate to lungs

L1 LARVAE passed in faeces

INFECTIVE LARVAE spread onto herbage

L3 LARVAE develop in dung pat

FIGURE 15.1 The lungworm life cycle

pasture. The strategic use of anthelmintic treatments is useful as part of a lungworm control programme, but the incorrect timing of anthelmintic treatment is a problem. Anthelmintics alone are not enough for cattle to enjoy long-term recovery and protection from lungworm; immunity is essential, and, aside from help from vaccination, can only come from exposure to the worm. Where anthelmintic use blocks exposure to the worm, immunity will not develop and that is a very real problem as the cattle are left vulnerable to reinfection at a later date.

There are two types of immunity to lungworm infection.

1. Immunity to the larval stages – which lasts only a matter of months. If the animal is not exposed to larvae regularly, they lose this immunity in a relatively short period of time (McLeonard and van Dijk, 2017).
2. Immunity to adult worms – here the immune system works to stop adult worms establishing, and also to reduce the egg output from worms that do manage to become established, despite the immune system's best efforts. Immunity to adult worms lasts up to 2 years (McLeonard and van Dijk, 2017).

An oral larval vaccine is available that provides immunity to the larval stages of the disease, which then allows the development of immunity to adult worms in a controlled manner. Two doses of the vaccine are required 4 weeks apart and the course should be completed 2 weeks before the cattle are turned out to the threatening pasture. The animals must not be under the effect of anthelmintics from the time the vaccine is administered through to when the cattle are actually being challenged by the larvae – otherwise the vaccine larvae will be killed and also the natural larvae, both of which are essential in the stimulation of the all important immunity. The importance of natural immunity needs stressing. If the cattle do not experience ongoing exposure to larvae during the grazing season, either because they are under the influence of long acting worming preparations or because they have been moved to clean grazing, then immunity will be inadequately stimulated and the effect of vaccination alone will be insufficient, and will need to be repeated before turn out the following year. The vaccine is not just designed for use in calves; any animal that is not thought to have developed or not thought to have maintained immunity to lungworm can be vaccinated. This may be first-calvers that received a long acting wormer as a heifer or bought-in cattle that have never been exposed to lungworm.

Lungworm can present differently depending on the age and previous exposure of the cattle. Two classic syndromes are as follows.

1. Cattle that have never seen lungworm larvae before – these are unvaccinated animals that have never been exposed to infective larvae. In these animals exposure causes disease and the rapid establishment of an adult population of egg laying adult lungworm.
2. Cattle that are immune to adult worms but through lack of exposure or repeat vaccination have lost their immunity to larvae. This is a bad scenario; if they graze pasture heavily contaminated with larvae (for example, pasture that has been grazed recently by animals in their first grazing season) there will be a mass die-off of worms as they reach adulthood and in so doing become susceptible to the immune system. This mass die-off causes the cow's immune system to overreact to the disintegrating worms and death can result, this allergy-like reaction is referred to as *reinfection syndrome.*

Many farms are unaffected by lungworm and the problem does not receive the attention it deserves in parasite control programmes. Grazing management, vaccination and anthelmintic treatments should all be considered in the context of lungworm as well as other parasites in the control plan.

In the case of a sick animal where lungworm is suspected or in the case of an outbreak; diagnosis in the live animal is problematic. A blood test is available to detect antibodies; however, antibodies are only detectable from 3 weeks post-larval infection. At the same point first-stage larvae become detectable in the faeces, that is, 3 weeks after infection; a technique called the Baermann test. First-stage larvae do not last very long in the faeces sampled so they need to be processed quickly (MacLeonard and van Dijk, 2017). There are two challenges to obtaining a diagnosis of lungworm.

First, the clinical signs occur from 14 days post-infection, this is a full week before the blood test or Baermann test are of any use to obtain a diagnosis.

Second, cattle suffering from reinfection syndrome and are immune to adult worms will not shed eggs and are often negative on the antibody test too. A PME or bronchoalveolar lavage (Chapter 13) are, in these cases, invaluable in obtaining a diagnosis. Often the decision making on one or more affected animals is based on the history and clinical presentation. IBR (Chapter 13) and fog fever have similar presenting signs to lungworm. In cases of IBR often the animal has a very high temperature and in cases of fog fever the animal has been grazing lush pasture and typically does not cough.

If lungworm is suspected, then treatment of the affected animals and the rest of the group with an anthelmintic is required. Coughing may continue for a number of weeks after treatment due to the presence of dead and dying worms in the airways and due to the associated inflammatory response in the airways. Depending on the severity of disease the affected animals may require an antibiotic course for the treatment of secondary bacterial infection, and, in the case of reinfection syndrome a corticosteroid treatment will probably be justified but this should only be carried out after a discussion with a vet.

DISEASES OF THE SKIN AND UDDER

Bovine viral papillomatosis (warts)

Bovine viral papillomatosis is, as the name suggests, caused by a virus and results in pedunculated, hairless skin growths cropping up in various sites around the body. Some animals are more severely affected than others but other than being unsightly they usually, with some notable exceptions, cause few problems. The animal produces an immune response and the condition is self-limiting and resolves over a period of a month or so (Jackson, 1993). The condition is common in younger animals due to their previous lack of exposure and immunity; heifers often have warts on their teats, but they usually and hopefully resolve before calving.

The notable but reasonably rare occasions that the lesions cause problems are:

- when they are severe and extensive and affect the sale value of the animal
- when they attract flies and/or become infected
- if they occur on the prepuce of a bull they may interfere with extrusion of the penis and consequently the animal's ability to mate
- if they are still present on the teats at point of calving and interfere with the ability to suckle or to be milked, or if they attract flies and consequently increase the risk of mastitis.

On occasions intervention is required. Depending on the location and size of the lesion then suture material or a lamb castration ring can be applied around the stalk, effectively ligating the mass which then drops of a few weeks later. In some cases, surgical removal may be warranted. Autogenous vaccination (Chapter 26) is also a possibility where parts of the papilloma are sampled and used to make a vaccine specific for that animal and farm. After the appropriate safety specifications have been adhered to, the vaccine is administered by injection; usually two doses are required.

This increases the animal's immune response to the virus and results in resolution of the papilloma.

Chapped teats

Cows suckling calves often have chapped teats caused by the calf's teeth and by repeated wetting of the teat with saliva. It can be a sign that there is inadequate milk supply from the cow causing the calf to suck overzealously. If this is a herd-wide problem, nutrition on the lead up to calving needs to be reviewed. In the case of a single cow the reason for her poor milk supply needs to be established; genetics, age, concurrent disease all being possible explanations. Lesions on the teats of cows suckling older calves suggest the calves need to be weaned. Teat lesions attract flies and hence increase the chance of summer mastitis.

Blind quarter

There are two reasons why a heifer would calve and not produce milk from a quarter. She may have had summer mastitis pre-calving. Alternatively, she may have a congenital teat obstruction. Examples would be failure of the teat to form correctly where a membrane, either at the teat orifice or at the junction between the teat cistern and the gland cistern, effectively blocks the flow of milk. If the obstruction is at the teat orifice, milk is palpable in the teat itself and it may be possible to break down the seal and there is hope of a normal functioning teat. If the membrane exists between the gland and teat cistern then a surgical teat implement is needed to break down the membrane. Mastitis and haemorrhage are common sequels to this intervention; the bleeding usually resolves and precautionary intramammary antibiotics are recommended to control infection.

Summer mastitis

Summer mastitis is the syndrome resulting from bacterial infection of a non-lactating mammary gland, that is, in dry cows or pre-calving heifers. The bacteria involved can be one or more of the following: *Streptococcus dysgalactiae*, *Trueperella pyogenes*, *Peptococcus indolicus*, *Bacteroides melaninogenicus* and/or *Fusobacterium necrophorum* (Blowey and Edmondson, 1995). Sometimes the infection can be relatively mild, and the animal manages to produce an immune response that is sufficient to overcome the infection without exhibiting any outward clinical signs. In these cases, the infection is not obvious until calving, at which point the cow or heifer presents with a blind quarter.

Sometimes clinical signs are obvious at the time of infection:

- the heifer or cows appear lame, 'swinging a leg'
- the heifer or cow is sick, off her food, and isolated from the rest of the group
- the affected quarter/udder is swollen
- thick yellow/red tinged pus can be milked from the quarter
- large numbers of flies congregate around the affected quarter
- abortion can occur up to 2 weeks after the initial infection.

More than one of the causative bacteria can be involved in the infection. They enter the mammary gland after damage to the teat sphincter. It is widely believed to be transmitted by flies from one udder to another; the blood sucking fly *Hydrotoea irritans* is thought to be the culprit. This fly particularly likes damp, sheltered areas, such as fields near water and fields sheltered by trees, so cattle grazing such ground are at higher risk of disease. Cattle grazing wind swept pastures are at lower risk of this disease (Figure 15.2).

Summer mastitis is painful and production limiting; treatment is both costly and inconvenient. The cow or heifer is usually out at grass and needs to be brought back to the steading, which is often easier

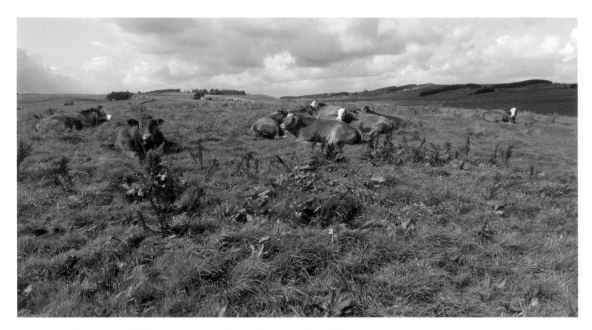

FIGURE 15.2 Pregnant heifers on exposed, wind swept, low risk pasture

said than done. The treatment involves the administration of intramammary antibiotics. Before administering the tube, the teat should be milked by hand to remove as much pus as possible. The hand milking and administration of intramammary tubes can be difficult and dangerous in fractious animals and good restraint is required. A course of injectable antibiotics is also recommended; injectable antibiotics are considered more effective than intramammary tubes (Blowey and Edmondson, 1995) but both should be used where possible though not too much expected of either. The antibiotic needs to be effective against the causative organism, ideally culture and sensitivity should be carried out but in severe infections the prognosis and welfare of the animal is compromised if treatment is not carried out promptly. A penicillin-type antibiotic would be the first line of choice in cases of summer mastitis. The main two causative organisms, *S. dygalactiae* and *T. pyogenes* are susceptible to penicillin (Blowey and Edmondson, 1995). NSAIDs should be administered to reduce inflammation and temperature, which both helps the heifer/cow but also helps protect the unborn calf against fever induced abortion.

Treatment is usually successful in saving the cow, but the affected quarter becomes non-functional. The affected quarter is basically an abscess; a compartment filled with pus which may burst through the skin. If this occurs the area should be cleaned regularly, the abscess flushed out and the hole in the skin kept open to allow the abscess to continue to drain. This often resolves the infection, but, again, the quarter is left non-functional.

An affected cow is infectious to others; the discharging pus from an abscess or teat is the source of spread, made worse by flies or unwashed handler's hands. For this reason, affected animals should be isolated and any area contaminated with pus, for example, the handling facility, cleaned after use. Also, gloves should be worn and disposed of when used.

The difficult nature of treatment and the poor success rate, especially for the functioning quarter, emphasises the need for effective prevention which includes: avoiding fly inhabited pastures; cypermethrin pour-on products or insecticide impregnated ear tags; weaning calves at an appropriate age to avoid teat injury; or sometimes delaying weaning.

A mechanical barrier to physically stop flies

gaining access to the teat orifice should prevent summer mastitis. Stockholm tar and sticky tape have been used effectively but often require repetitive handlings and multiple applications. Internal teat sealants are widely used in dairy cows to prevent infection in the dry period. The use of these sealants is potentially useful in heifers and beef suckler cows but as with dairy cows the procedure has to be done aseptically; if any bacteria are present at the teat end, or on the tube at the point of administration, they are effectively injected right into the middle of a warm sterile udder with a plentiful energy supply, namely milk! Here the bacteria multiply rapidly; a sure-fire way to induce a serious, even fatal, mastitis. If internal teat sealants are to be used a thorough consultation with, and demonstration from, a vet is required; the administration needs to be carried out meticulously under sterile conditions.

Bovine ulcerative mammillitis

This condition is not common and is more of an issue in the dairy herd, but it is worth a mention in the beef context. The disease is caused by a herpes virus, bovine herpes virus type 2. The condition involves characteristic blisters on the teats and the udder that burst to form large ulcers up to 5 cm in diameter. Topical application of udder cream will help to sooth the lesions and NSAIDs should be administered to reduce the pain and inflammation. Calves may develop ulcer like lesions in their mouths from infected cows (Jackson, 1993) but more commonly cows and heifers will be reluctant to let calves suck; as a result, they may develop a secondary mastitis.

Pseudocowpox

This viral infection is rare in the suckler herd, but it is zoonotic and therefore significant. The lesions caused are small pustules on the teats, which rupture leaving a mixture of scabs and pink healing tissue. The lesions lie in a characteristic horseshoe shape. Lesions generally resolve in a month, but immunity is short lived so reinfection may occur.

DISEASES OF THE REPRODUCTIVE TRACT

It is obviously crucial that a replacement breeding heifer has a fully functional reproductive tract. The examination of the heifer as a suitable breeding replacement is discussed in Chapter 8. There are two abnormalities of note, both of which are congenital: Freemartinism (FM) and white heifer disease (WHD).

Freemartinism

Freemartinism occurs when a female and male twin are present in the uterus at the same time. The two placentae of twin calves merge and the mixing of blood means the female calf is exposed to the male calf's hormones.

Approximately 1–2% of all cattle births are twins. Half of twin births have one male and one female (the basic maths here surprises some people!) and 92% of heifer calves born alongside a male are freemartins.

Freemartins vary in how they present. Most freemartins appear externally as no different from their cohorts. Some have an enlarged vulva or clitoris, which causes urine to be passed abnormally, some have extra clitoral hair. The main differences are detected upon internal examination where part or all of the reproductive tract is missing. Some freemartins are almost normal on internal examination but still fail to get in-calf. Good record keeping is essential so that heifers that are twin to a male calf are not retained. The main risk is where heifer replacements are bought in, especially if they are bought through the market, and such information is not available or presented.

White heifer disease

WHD is a genetic condition that results from the same gene that codes for white coat colour. The gene is linked to the development of the reproductive tract (excluding the ovaries). In cases of WHD oestrus behaviour is observed, ovulation occurs, but the egg may not be able to pass into the uterus and the cow does not become pregnant. It may be that only one side of the tract is affected, and pregnancy is then possible but of reduced likelihood. It has been reported to occur in up to 10% of white Dairy Shorthorn heifers (Peters and Ball, 1995), hence the name.

FOETAL LOSS (REABSORPTION, MUMMIFICATION, ABORTION, STILLBIRTH)

Foetal loss, whether the foetus dies in utero and is reabsorbed or mummifies, or whether the heifer is seen to pass a premature or dead foetus, or, whether the foetus is stillborn, is a significant loss to the producer; the calf is lost, the animal's future breeding potential is jeopardised, the animal may pose an infectious risk to others, and she may need treatment – all in all, she is clearly unproductive despite the time and money invested in her. Abortions are relatively easily identified; there is a foetus to see. Reabsorption or mummification, however, is less obvious; cows that were diagnosed as being in-calf, fail to calve.

Foetal loss can be due to a non-infectious cause such as fighting; these are often sporadic one-off events. Abortions and reabsorption can also be caused by infectious agents. These may occur intermittently or there may be several in a short period of time; an outbreak known as an 'abortion storm'. It is generally considered that an abortion rate of greater than 2% of the breeding herd requires further investigation (Caldow et al., 2002), or whenever two or more abortions have occurred in quick succession.

Non-infectious causes of foetal loss

On occasions a mummified calf is retained within the uterus. This is where a calf has died in the uterus and the foetal fluid and membranes have been reabsorbed. As a result, there is a firm, often bony remnant of a calf in the uterus and the uterus is clamped tightly around it. This is palpable on internal examination by a vet and the cow should be culled. Treatment can be attempted if the farmer is keen to try. This involves aborting the mummified calf with a prostaglandin injection; lubrication and aided extraction may be necessary. Breeding potential is reduced.

Twin pregnancies, trauma to the abdomen or the accidental AI of a pregnant female, can all cause abortion. Natural abortions occur with some calves that have genetic abnormalities and malformations – presumably nature's way. Some toxic plants when eaten by the heifer or cow may cause abortion, examples include hemlock and juniper. Ergotism (ergot fungus on the pasture) and nitrate poisoning may also induce abortion but in these cases other clinical signs of poisoning are noted rather than just abortion alone. The ingestion of needles from the ponderosa pine can induce abortion due to a reduction in blood progesterone levels (Cabell, 2007) (progesterone is essential for sustaining pregnancy). Trace element deficiencies can also result in abortions, iodine in particular, which is especially relevant if the cattle are fed a brassica-based diet – brassicas (Figure 15.3) are known goitrogens (inducers of iodine deficiency) (Chapter 10).

Infectious causes of foetal loss

It is important to note that many causes of infectious abortions are zoonotic. The foetus itself, the placenta and the discharges from the aborting heifer or cow all potentially carry infectious pathogens. This is a particular risk to pregnant women. Appropriate protective clothing should be worn

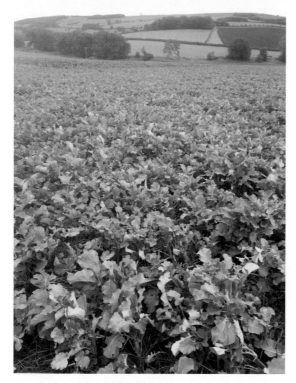

FIGURE 15.3 A field of kale, a brassica crop, ready for the outwintering of spring-calving suckler cows post-weaning; secondary iodine deficiency and associated foetal loss is a risk

along with good personal hygiene measures for all those involved.

There are many infectious causes of foetal loss and they can cause abortion in different ways. The infectious agent can be a bacterium, a virus, a fungus or a protozoan parasite. They may act by affecting the placenta and therefore the nutrient and oxygen supply to the calf. Alternatively, the agent may cause the cow to become ill and abort as secondary consequence – this is often associated with a fever, an example of this would be mastitis.

Brucella abortus

Although not top of the list when investigating an abortion storm, this infection was once a very common and serious pathogen for the UK cattle industry and still is in some parts of the world. It

is a notifiable disease in some countries, including the UK, where *any* abortion should be reported to the appropriate authorities, usually via the farmer's own vet. For the purposes of statutory testing, an abortion is, in the UK, defined as 'an abortion or calving that takes place less than 271 days after service, or 265 days after implantation or transfer of an embryo, whether the calf is born dead or alive' (The Brucellosis (England) Order 2015, No. 364, Article 2).

Bacillus licheniformis

Bacillus licheniformis is a bacterium which lives in the environment and replicates in silage, particularly pit silage, and is one of the most common causes of abortion in the UK. The cow ingests the bacteria and it travels in the bloodstream to the placenta where it causes inflammation (placentitis), which impedes the oxygen supply to the calf. The calf dies and is aborted, usually in the last 2 months of pregnancy. Sometimes the calf will be born alive but dopey; slow to rise and suck. Abortions are often sporadic, and *B. licheniformis* is generally not a herd problem but outbreaks have been reported. It is possible to culture and count the number of *Bacillus* spp. in the silage; good silage making and feeding practices have been proven to decrease *Bacillus* spp. counts (Stevenson, 2017). *Bacillus* spp. can also multiply in water troughs that are contaminated with silage from the mouths of drinking cows; cleaning water troughs out regularly is an additional preventative measure. The sides and top of the silage pit are higher risk and should not be fed to cows in the last third of pregnancy. The feed face should, ideally, be managed with a shear grab to reduce the surface area exposed to air. Also, the time the same feed face is exposed to the air should be less than 5 days. Feed troughs should be cleaned out twice a week to remove stale feed, inside which further multiplication would otherwise be a risk.

Listeriosis

Listeriosis is caused by *Listeria monocytogenes*. Similar to *Bacillus* spp., this bacterium is present in the environment, mainly the soil and water, and it is very at home in silage. As well as abortion it is associated with mastitis, neonatal septicaemia, eye conditions and, most notably, neurological signs.

Salmonellosis

There are many species of *Salmonella* many of which cause problems and are often zoonotic. They cause a range of diseases (Chapter 12) including abortion. The abortion may be a secondary result of the heifer or cow being sick or it may be a primary attack on the foetus or placenta without the mother necessarily appearing ill.

Campylobacteriosis

There are two main species of this bacterium that are of concern: *Campylobacter fetus* subsp. *venerealis* and *C. fetus* subsp. *fetus*. *C. fetus subsp. fetus* is a bacterium that originates in the gastrointestinal tract and causes abortion if it is absorbed into the bloodstream, thus causing a bacteraemia. *C. fetus* subsp. *venerealis* is a sexually transmitted disease and is covered in depth in Chapter 16.

Leptospirosis

Leptospirosis is a bacterial infection that affects animals and humans, that is, it is zoonotic. The bacteria are loosely referred to as leptospires. Many serovars (types) of leptospire exist, several of which can infect cattle but the serovar *Leptospira hardjo* is the most important in the UK. Leptospires favour moisture and warmish temperatures of over 10°C; in these conditions they can last up to 6 months, which provides challenges in its control because

these conditions are quite common especially in temperate regions.

The main source of infection is urine from infected cattle, but the bacteria can also be transmitted via semen and aborted material. Leptospires are burrowing spiral shaped bacteria that are able to penetrate the mucous membranes, that is, the lining surface of the eyes, mouth, nose, udder and genital tract and in the non-immune animal rapid multiplication in the uterus or udder follows. Bacteria are also present in the bloodstream for 6–9 days after infection. The bacteria eventually come to rest in the reproductive tract and kidneys. Following infection, shedding in the urine starts after about 14 days and can persist for months or, intermittently, for years; that animal is now a carrier of the infection. Infected urine is the main source of environmental contamination and further infections. In the dairy herd, personnel are often exposed to cow's urine in the milking parlour and an infected animal shedding leptospires in the parlour is a significant health and safety risk.

Owing to the nature of transmission, and the preferred environmental conditions, most spread occurs during the spring and summer at pasture. Urine-contaminated water sources are a particularly risky source.

Unlike with some strains of *Leptospira* spp., such as the one responsible for human Weil's disease, wildlife such as rats do not carry bovine *L. hardjo* but sheep can carry and excrete it so cattle enjoying mixed grazing are more at risk.

Infection with *L. hardjo* can manifest itself in different ways depending on if the animal is pregnant or lactating.

Lactating cattle infected with *L. hardjo* experience milk drop, otherwise known as 'flabby bag'. This occurs 2–7 days after the initial infection of a non-immune animal and there is a sudden reduction or cessation of milk production, a high temperature, the development of thick colostrum type milk, blood tingeing of the milk in all four-quarters and the development of a soft, flabby udder. The clinical signs resolve over 7–10 days. This form of the disease is reported more commonly in dairy

ction does not always stop infection, but it
does reduce urine shedding of the bug post-infection, it protects against milk drop and it reduces
the incidence of abortion. The vaccine cannot
eliminate existing infections. The vaccines usually
require two doses, 4 weeks apart, and they require
an annual booster. Calves will be protected by
maternal antibodies until 14 weeks of age. Ideally
vaccinating at 1 month old and again before turn
out will provide protection prior to challenge.

The main risk factors for the introduction of
disease are the presence of water courses on the
farm or the practice of buying in cattle (and sheep).
Purchased animals should, therefore, be sourced
from leptospirosis free accredited herds or, failing
that, they should be isolated for 28 days then blood
tested for the absence of antibodies before being
added to the herd. Water provision should be from
mains water wherever possible and it should be
drunk from clean troughs so avoiding the risk of
using contaminated natural sources.

Infectious bovine rhinotracheitis (IBR)

IBR is a viral disease of cattle caused by bovine
herpes virus type 1.1 (BoHV-1.1) a viral pathogen
that causes bovine respiratory disease in all ages of
cattle (Chapter 13) but can also cause abortion up
to 100 days after infection (Cabell, 2007) with or
without the heifer or cow having shown respiratory
signs previously. Animals with IBR often present
with a very high temperature and this alone is sufficient to cause abortion without the virus even
reaching the foetus. Once an animal has been
infected with BoHV-1.1 it can become a carrier
animal and intermittently shed virus in the future
without showing clinical signs. Control is usually
approached through vaccination although CHeCS
herd health certification is available, certainly in
the UK, for IBR testing, culling and vaccination
and this approach can be used to eradicate IBR
from a herd and provide assurance to purchasers.

IBR can be venereally transmitted; the virus can live in semen and consequently all bulls are thoroughly tested for the disease before entering semen collection centres.

Worth a mention is another strain of this virus, bovine herpes virus type 1.2 (BoHV-1.2) which causes a genital disease in females known as infectious pustular vulvo-vaginitis (IPVV). The predominant clinical signs are a brown vaginal discharge and swelling of the vulva with ulceration and sloughing of the mucosa. In bulls the same virus causes infectious balanoposthitis (IBP) resulting in inflammation of the penis and adhesions to the sheath. The virus can be isolated from the lesions to obtain a diagnosis, another option is to blood test three weeks post-infection to look for antibodies as an indication of exposure. More accurate is to take a blood sample at the time of disease and again 3 weeks later to look for a rise in antibodies. The vaccines commercially available for the control of BoHV-1.1 offer some cross protection against other strains but have not been completely effective in controlling disease outbreaks in the field (Cook, 1998).

Bovine viral diarrhoea

BVD is a much talked about viral disease of cattle with a somewhat misleading name – diarrhoea is not a notable feature of this complicated disease. BVD is mostly spread through direct cattle to cattle contact and can linger in the herd in the form of PI animals. The disease presents in several clinical syndromes – reduced fertility, foetal reabsorption, mummification, abortion, stillbirths, congenital disease, poor production and increased susceptibility to other infections through immunosuppression, typically in younger calves and most usually pneumonia, and finally … diarrhoea! The disease is of major financial importance and is the focus of many voluntary and compulsory eradication schemes across Europe and the rest of the world.

BVD is caused by BVDV. There are two strains: BVDV-1 and BVDV-2. BVDV-1 is the common

strain; it is widespread in the UK. A more severe strain BVDV-2 exists and is found in North America. BVDV is related to classical swine fever virus (CSFV) in pigs and border disease virus (BDV) in sheep. These three viruses belong to a group of viruses called pestiviruses. CSFV virus is exclusive to pigs but the two ruminant viruses have an interesting relationship. It is possible to infect cattle artificially with BDV and, conversely, to infect sheep with BVDV. Both viruses can infect the foetus of both cattle and sheep. Under farming conditions within the UK, however, BDV is very rarely isolated from cattle but BVD virus is found reasonably frequently in sheep.

A PI animal has virus permanently circulating in its bloodstream (viraemia) from birth until the day it dies, which it does, at an invariably young age. PI animals shed virus in all body secretions. A PI animal has up to 1 million infectious virus particles per millilitre of blood. Saliva and nasal discharge are also heavily loaded with virus so sharing trough space and nose-to-nose contact hastens the spread of the disease; transmission is less while cattle are at grass. Faeces is not a major source of virus excretion. The virus is transmissible in infected bull semen, naturally and artificially, both fresh and frozen.

The virus is unstable and cannot survive outside the host for long periods of time. It can, however, survive for short periods of time on personnel and equipment and this route of transmission should not be dismissed in designing biosecurity protocols.

BVD disease syndromes

Acute BVD syndrome

This syndrome is seen when previously unexposed animals are exposed to BVDV for the first time. The animals contract the virus rather like any other virus and are transiently (temporarily) viraemic. As with many viraemias this may give the animal a mild fever and mild illness. In the case of acute BVD syndrome the illness may involve dullness, maybe ulcers of the mouth and nose, and transient diarrhoea – hence the original source of the name of the disease. Where older lactating cattle are affected milk-drop is likely. The animal then mounts an immune response as with other viruses and sheds the infection. The animal goes from having no antibodies to BVD to having antibodies to BVD. This is called seroconversion. This occurs within 28 days and the animal should remain immune and antibody positive for years if not for life. Of most interest in acute BVD however, is the immunosuppressive effect the virus has on the immune system. Infected cattle, especially calves, are left significantly more vulnerable to infectious disease for some time afterwards. This results in an increased incidence of diarrhoea, respiratory disease and other infectious diseases – these disease outbreaks can be significant and account for a major contribution to the economic impact of BVD in the national herd.

Infection of females during breeding

When BVDV is introduced to naïve females during the breeding season lower conception rates result and irregular returns to oestrus are seen. In a natural service herd, for example a beef herd, this pattern may not be easily or quickly identified but in herds with a planned compact breeding season a high barren rate may be seen. In herds with a long breeding season less calves are born in the first month of the calving period.

Infection of bulls

BVDV infection in bulls can cause infertility lasting up to 3 months. Semen evaluation reveals poor sperm motility and a high percentage of abnormal spermatozoa. In this time the bull can transmit BVDV in his semen.

Pregnant animals

This is where BVD gets its complicated reputation. When a naïve pregnant female is acutely infected with BVDV and experiences a viraemia, the virus in the blood crosses the placenta and enters the foetus. Depending on the stage of gestation these transplacental infections have different effects.

Infection at 0–110 days of gestation

This can cause foetal death with reabsorption, mummification or abortion depending on the stage of the 110 days of early pregnancy. Any foetus that survives may be born persistently infected with BVDV – the calf will then be a PI. How does this happen? The young foetus does not have a developed immune system at this stage, it fails to recognise the virus as foreign and does not attack it. It instead registers it as 'self' and allows it to stay. This is described as *immunotolerance*. PI calves are, consequently, born viraemic, they have no antibodies to BVDV, and they constantly shed virus throughout their lives. Rather confusingly, despite having no antibodies to BVD of their own they will still absorb antibodies to BVDV from their mother's colostrum. These antibodies achieve nothing other than to confuse the results of testing in these young calves – two complications are (1) the calf testing positive for antibodies, which makes the observer think the calf is not a PI and (2) the colostral antibodies can interfere with some tests looking for the virus itself. The colostral antibodies do dwindle over time after which the calves test correctly as antibody negative and virus positive.

Infection at 111–150 days of gestation

Congenital abnormalities of the calf are more common following infection in the second trimester. These are most commonly eye and brain abnormalities. Calves are usually born blind, weak and wobbly. A calf's immune system develops at around 140 days of gestation and they are then able to mount an immune response to the virus. These calves are normally antibody positive and virus negative but have still suffered the

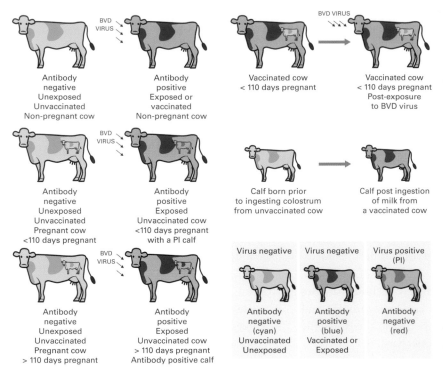

Antibody
negative
Unexposed
Unvaccinated
Non-pregnant cow

Antibody
positive
Exposed or
vaccinated
Non-pregnant cow

Vaccinated cow
< 110 days pregnant

Vaccinated cow
< 110 days pregnant
Post-exposure
to BVD virus

Antibody
negative
Unexposed
Unvaccinated
Pregnant cow
<110 days pregnant

Antibody
positive
Exposed
Unvaccinated cow
<110 days pregnant
with a PI calf

Calf born prior
to ingesting colostrum
from unvaccinated cow

Calf post ingestion
of milk from
a vaccinated cow

Antibody
negative
Unexposed
Unvaccinated
Pregnant cow
> 110 days pregnant

Antibody
positive
Exposed
Unvaccinated cow
> 110 days pregnant
Antibody positive calf

Virus negative

Antibody
negative
(cyan)
Unvaccinated
Unexposed

Virus negative

Antibody
positive
(blue)
Vaccinated or
Exposed

Virus positive
(PI)

Antibody
negative
(red)

FIGURE 15.4 Diagram representing the transmission of BVD virus

permanent ill effects of the virus from the time the infection lasted.

Infection post 150 days of gestation

The well developed immune system of the older unborn calf fights off the virus. As the calf's body is well formed by this stage congenital abnormalities are unlikely. A live, full term calf is usually born, it has BVD antibodies and is virus negative. This is summarised in Figure 15.4.

Abortions can occur following infection at any stage of pregnancy, as is the case with any viral infection, but is, in the case of BVDV not common in the later stages as the virus does not cause much of a fever or illness in the mother, compared, say, to viruses like IBR.

Chronic BVD syndrome (mucosal disease)

PI calves (born PI as the dam was infected with BVD virus before day 110 of pregnancy) eventually develop a syndrome called mucosal disease. The

virus that has been living in the animal suddenly undergoes a change, it spontaneously mutates. In most cases this happens when the PI calf is 6–18 months old. The virus becomes much more damaging, the animal becomes depressed, pyrexic (fever), stops eating and develops the classic signs of mucosal disease that are: severe ulceration of the mouth and nose, salivation, and mucopurulent nasal discharge. The ulceration also affects the gut and they pass diarrhoea often containing shreds of gut lining and blood. There is rapid weight loss in a matter of days, death follows sometimes with secondary pneumonia seeing the calf off. Most PI animals die within the first year of life but some make it to 2–3 years old and in some rare cases they make it to adulthood. PI cows that make it to breeding age have reduced fertility but those that do conceive produce PI calves as the mother's virus gets straight into the young foetus at the earliest opportunity. PI animals, before the onset of mucosal disease, sometimes, but not always, look poorly; they may be stunted and prone to disease. Often, however, these animals look perfectly healthy while unwittingly spreading the virus to all the other cattle around them.

Testing for BVD

There are two tests available.

1. **A test to detect antibody in the blood**. This *usually* shows if an animal has been exposed to BVD virus. This could have been at any stage in its life but is misleadingly negative if the calf was a young foetus (under 110 days of gestation) when infected and has gone on to be a PI animal. Another confusing factor is where calves less than 4–9 months of age still have antibodies to BVD from their mother's colostrum – this will give a misleadingly (false) positive result. Calves need to be over 9 months of age to use this test reliably but still the PI problem exists, so a negative test needs careful interpretation.

2. **A test to detect BVD virus itself**. This can be by testing blood using a PCR or antigen ELISA (enzyme linked immunosorbent assay) test. This test will be positive for any animal that has virus in its blood – this includes PI animals of course but, potentially confusingly, also animals that are transiently infected (TI). TIs only have virus in their blood for a few days after they have been infected, at which point, they fight off the virus in the same way that most viral infections are fought off. BVD virus can also be tested for in tissue, such as a notch of ear or a piece of post-mortem tissue. Ear tag virus testing is commonly used now to test calves to see if they are PI animals as soon as possible after birth. Where a result is positive the calf should be rechecked by taking a blood sample 3 weeks after ear tag sampling. This ensures that the animal is indeed PI and not TI.

Testing for BVD at a herd level

Blood sampling a representative sample of home-bred youngsters for antibody gives an indication of exposure to BVDV within the herd. This is simple, easy and commonly referred to as a *check test*. Typically, five home-bred, unvaccinated animals from a group that are of similar age, between 9 and 18 months, and have been reared together, are tested. This provides evidence of the likely level of exposure for the whole group. If groups of calves are managed separately then five animals from each group need to be tested.

If herd infection is suspected from a positive check test, then a full herd screen for virus is required. Testing the calf crop alone may be sufficient to determine the status of the adult herd without actually testing the adults as well. How does that work? A PI mother will always give birth to a PI calf; if a calf is negative for virus its dam must also be negative. So, by testing the calf crop for virus (using blood or tissue), any infected calves will be found and their mother can then be located and either culled automatically, or tested herself to be sure she is positive before culling. In this approach the bulls and any adults that have not got offspring to test will also need to be tested in addition to the calves.

BVD monitoring, eradication and accreditation

Cattle Health Certification Standards (CHeCS) accredited health schemes exist for BVD alongside national eradication programmes. The testing regime involves either the use of check tests of each separately managed group of calves or blood or tissue tagging each entire calf crop. Generally, two years of negative testing is required to achieve *BVD free* accreditation. Herds can either be *BVD free and non-vaccinated* or *BVD free and vaccinating*, often referred to as *BVD vaccinated monitored free*.

Control of BVD

Strict biosecurity is required to reduce the risk of the introduction of BVD.

- Buying stock only from a herd that is accredited free of BVD.

- Double fencing with a minimum of a 3 m gap is recommended to prevent nose-to-nose contact with other cattle that may be a source of infection, for example, neighbour's cattle.
- Breeding own replacements.
- Avoiding buying in 'set-on' calves.
- When buying from a non-accredited herd new animals should be blood sampled for virus, ideally on the farm of origin before they are moved. Virus positive animals should not be purchased. Once the virus free animals arrive on farm, they should be quarantined for 28 days. This safety period is the time to allow an animal that may have just been infected with BVDV to shake off the transient viraemia before joining the herd.
- Buying in pregnant cows or heifers is the greatest risk as they could already be carrying a PI calf. For extra safety, cows purchased in-calf should be calved in isolation and the calf should be virus tested as soon as possible after birth.
- Where there is a risk that virus may be introduced to a naïve herd, vaccination is strongly recommended. Vaccination is generally recommended in most situations.

BVD vaccination

Vaccination, depending on the type of vaccine, may reduce the risk of an animal becoming infected or becoming viraemic, or reduce the likelihood of a breeding female losing a calf to BVD or giving birth to a calf damaged by BVD or giving birth to a PI calf. This is not, of course, entirely reliable.

There are inactivated and live vaccines commercially available and vaccine schedules and timing vary depending on the vaccine used. The basic principles of vaccination are the same; all animals should be vaccinated well in advance of breeding and boosters are required to ensure that immunity does not wane.

A BVD component is included in some calf pneumonia vaccines, this is to minimise the effects of immunosuppression in a group if virus was introduced. The antibodies from such a vaccine

persist for 3 months. If heifers are being retained as breeding animals and have been vaccinated with a calf vaccine with a BVD component, then they still require a full course of vaccination with a vaccine specifically designed for the protection of breeding females.

Neosporosis

Neosporosis is a disease of several species of animal, including cattle, caused by the protozoan parasite *Neospora caninum*. The disease includes abortion in cattle. While not necessarily the most common cause of abortion in cattle it is nonetheless the most commonly diagnosed cause in the UK. The lifecycle is complicated and involves dogs as the primary host and cows as the intermediate host. As with any parasite with an indirect lifecycle, the spread of *Neospora* spp. is not straightforward.

Faeces from an infected dog contain *Neospora* oocysts. Where contamination of pasture occurs, cattle eat the oocysts which hatch in the gut. If the animal is pregnant the parasite crosses the placenta causing abortion. If a dog then eats the products of abortion, it is eating the intermediate stage of the parasite and the lifecycle then becomes complete. It has been suggested that wild Canidae such as foxes may also play a part in the life cycle by increasing pasture contamination (Toolan, 2003). There are no reports of venereal transmission so infected bulls are not considered to be part of disease transmission (Toolan, 2003).

The exact outcome of the cow becoming infected depends on at what stage of gestation the infection occurs (Figure 15.5). As with everything else involving *Neospora* this is complicated!

If the infection occurs early in gestation, abortion may occur. The foetus may be passed (aborted) many weeks after infection. For example, a cow infected at 3 months of pregnancy may not abort until 5–6 months of gestation. The cow is not usually poorly during this time and rarely retains her placenta (foetal membranes).

Months of gestation								
1	2	3	4	5	6	7	8	9
If a cow ingests *Neospora* oocysts early in pregnancy it is likely an abortion will result			If a cow ingests *Neospora* oocysts later in pregnancy a normal calf may be born OR the calf may have congenital abnormalities usually associated with the brain OR the calf may appear to be normal, but if the animal is female and reaches breeding age she is herself likely to abort					

FIGURE 15.5. Diagram to show the outcome of infection with *Neospora caninum* at different stages of gestation

If the infection occurs late in gestation a normal calf may be born but the calf may be infected with the parasite – known as congenital infection. The congenitally infected calf may appear normal or may be diseased. If the calf is a heifer that goes on to become a breeding animal she may, herself, abort during her first and subsequent pregnancies. A diseased calf may be born with neurological signs: weak, unsteady, dopey and slow to suck.

Neospora caninum can therefore be seen as having a *horizonal mode* of transmission between cattle, but, crucially, via the dog but also a *vertical mode* of infection from cow to the next generation across the placenta.

The most reliable method of detecting disease is the microscopic examination of the brain of the aborted or euthanased calf for the parasite. Blood testing of the dam for antibodies to *Neospora caninum* is another possibility but obtaining a meaningful result is difficult; if a cow aborts and has antibodies to *Neospora caninum* in her blood it might be that the cow had been infected with *Neospora caninum* during pregnancy and has aborted as a result. However, she may have been infected with the *Neospora caninum* long before she was pregnant and has antibodies, but the abortion was due to another cause. If, on the other hand, no antibodies are detected it might be that the cow did have antibodies to *Neospora caninum, Neospora caninum* was the cause of the abortion, but the antibody level has subsequently dropped below a detectable level since the infection – potentially some months ago. Given these complications one approach is to blood test a number of aborted females and a similar random sample of non-aborted females and observe if the aborted group has significantly more seropositivity than the non-aborted group.

The control of disease is focused on preventing completion of the lifecycle. Keeping dog faeces away from the pasture, silage pits, food stores and water supplies is necessary. Dogs should be prevented from eating products of abortion, dead calves or raw beef products.

CHeCS accredited health schemes are available for *Neospora caninum* and testing and culling may be an option for control, although antibody levels fluctuate as discussed and not all antibody positive animals will abort. This means there is a risk of perfectly healthy animals being removed from the herd. If there is a high number of positive animals in the herd and removing them all at one time is not a feasible option, then the testing of replacement heifers and only breeding from the negative animals may be more practical. Another control measure when there are many infected females is to send all calves for fattening and source breeding replacements from a safe source – this, of course, breaches other biosecurity measures. As yet there are no commercially available vaccines in the UK.

Fungal mycosis (mycotic abortion)

Aspergillus fumigatus is the predominant fungal agent causing abortion in cattle; it is found in spoiled silage, straw, hay and brewers' grains and is, consequently, seen more commonly in the winter months when cows are being fed a non-grass diet. The fungi attack the placenta, causing placentitis, which results in abortion; the cow is rarely ill herself.

INVESTIGATING ABORTION IN BEEF CATTLE

It is clear that there are several infectious causes of abortion in cattle, so how do we go about working out which, if any, are causing the problem?

When an abortion occurs, it is important to first isolate the products of abortion; the calf or foetus, the placenta, fluids as far as is practical, and the cow herself. Second, the vet responsible for the farm or local authority should be informed. This is mandatory for Brucellosis surveillance but it is also the start of a consultation as to whether further testing is appropriate in order to identify the possible cause of the abortion. It may be that this is the first abortion and the decision is made to 'wait and see' or there may be a clear reason why the cow has aborted, for example, twins or a known illness or a predictable reaction to certain drugs such as corticosteroids or prostaglandins. If further investigation is required, then the taking of a thorough history should be the first step. In field situations one of the first steps may actually be to remove the aborting calf or foetus from the birth canal! It is surprising how often the heifer or cow is yet to expel the aborting foetus and it is also surprising how difficult this can be – the foetus may be dry and/or the heifer or cow may be poorly dilated.

1. **How old is the aborting female?** A younger heifer may be more susceptible to infectious disease as she is less likely to have come across pathogens and developed immunity than an older cow.
2. **When was she due to calve?** This provides information on the stage of gestation at which the abortion has struck, specific pathogens are known to cause abortion at different stages of pregnancy.
3. **When does the calving period start?**
4. **How many have calved normally, how many have aborted, what is the percentage?**
5. **Have there been any changes or other problems on the farm?** It may be necessary to go back several months in some cases.

6. **What has fertility been like on the farm? What is the barren rate?** Diseases such as campylobacteriosis, BVD and leptospirosis will affect conception rates as well as cause abortions.
7. **Was she served by natural service, AI or is she carrying an embryo calf?**
8. **Is she home-bred or bought-in?** Bought-in animals may not have the same disease status as home-bred animals and may have an uncertain vaccination history. They may have brought the disease in or it may be that she has come in clean and naïve and been exposed to a pathogen that the herd already has but that most members are immune to.
9. **Has she been poorly recently?** Abortions can be secondary to an animal being systemically ill.
10. **What is her vaccination status?** Vaccinations against specific diseases makes that cause less likely but does not rule it out. Has the vaccine been administered in line with best practice? Storage, handling, timing, completion of the course, route of administration, and licensing of the product are all factors to consider
11. **What is she being fed?** Forage-based diets may contain high levels of *Bacillus* spp., *Listeria* spp. and fungal agents.
12. **What condition is she in?** Thin cows may abort due to malnutrition. She may be thin for other reasons of illness that may be relevant.
13. **Is she housed or out at grass?** Grazing animals may be exposed to natural water courses and wildlife.
14. **What is the policy for purchased, incoming and returning animals?** This is a reflection of the biosecurity of the herd and therefore the likelihood of infectious pathogens being introduced.
15. **Are bulls borrowed, hired or shared?** Bulls are the main transmission route for *Campylobacter* spp.

If a foetus and placenta are available, then a PME and appropriate sample collection are the best means of obtaining a diagnosis, although by no means can a diagnosis be promised – a common source of disappointment in the already and understandably frustrated farmer/manager. The reality is that a diagnosis of an infectious cause of abortion is reached in only 35% of all cases in the UK (Cabell, 2007). This rate can be increased through good quality sample collection and, crucially, the submission of placenta with the samples – often the infectious agent does not reach the calf but there is evidence of the agent in the placenta, often sufficient to provide the diagnosis. Even when the actual cause is not identified the testing is helpful as the negative results rule out many of the potential diagnoses – again the frustrated farmer often needs some convincing of this value! Where no diagnosis is reached on a single foetus then any subsequent abortions should still be investigated.

It is rare when examining a foetus that the cause of abortion can be identified just by looking at the gross features of the placenta and foetus; abnormalities may be observed but they are rarely specific to a certain infectious agent. Further sampling for laboratory testing is usually necessary.

Sample collection is fairly standard and includes the following.

- **A sample of placenta**. Smears and stains of the placenta identify some bacterial and fungal infectious agents. When the placenta is preserved in formalin, processed, and then examined under a microscope, certain observed changes can be specific enough to obtain a diagnosis or at least indicate that it was an infectious cause of abortion rather than non-infectious.
- **Foetal stomach contents (FSC)**. The fluid in the stomach of a calf is the amniotic fluid that has been swallowed from that surrounding it in the uterus (Chapter 4, Figure 4.3). It should be completely sterile and contain no bacteria – if the fluid is sampled and cultured and a bacterium present then this is highly likely to be the cause of abortion. A careful sampling technique is required as any contamination from the environment during the sampling process will either mislead, or, risk masking the significant bacterium during the culture. In addition to culture of the FSC, sections of other organs such as liver and lung can also be cultured for bacteria in the same way (Figure 15.6).

- **Foetal fluid**. This is accumulated fluid from anywhere in the body of the calf or foetus itself, for example, within the cavity of the chest, the abdomen, the pericardial sac surrounding the heart or blood from the heart or a major blood vessel. This fluid can be tested for antibodies to key infectious agents such as *Leptospira* spp., *Neospora* spp. and BVD. It is also possible to detect BVD virus itself in such fluid.

In addition to these standard sampling procedures there are more advanced tests that can be used to help obtain a diagnosis.

- **Isolating a virus from foetal organs**. Viral causes of abortion such as BVD and IBR can be detected via PCR, a specialist technique which multiplies specific viral components to detectable levels. This requires small sections of specific organs; spleen and liver are most commonly used for this purpose.
- **Histopathology (microscopic tissue examination)**. Sections of lung, liver and brain can be preserved in formalin, processed and examined under a microscope to look for microscopic changes indicative of certain diseases. For example, microscopic examination of the brain for characteristic changes is required for a definitive diagnosis of neosporosis.
- **Serology**. Blood testing for antibodies to certain agents can be used as part of an abortion investigation. There are three approaches.
- To blood test the cow for antibodies to *Leptospira* spp., IBR, BVD and *Neospora* spp. Here there are caveats. If the result is positive it cannot be assumed that the agent for which there are antibodies was the actual cause of the abortion. The antibodies may be a result of vaccination or previous exposure, and nothing to do with the current abortion under

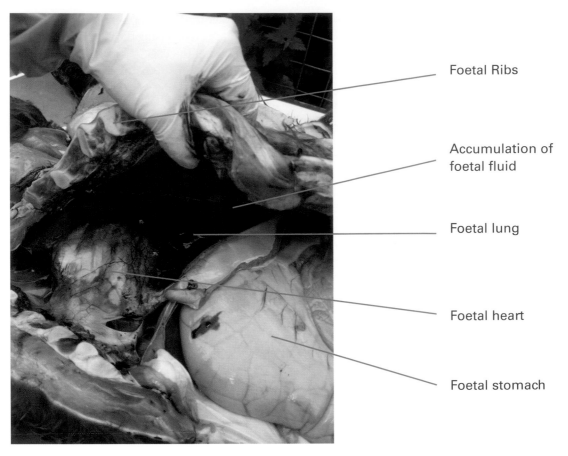

Foetal Ribs

Accumulation of
foetal fluid

Foetal lung

Foetal heart

Foetal stomach

FIGURE 15.6 PME of an aborted foetus with the chest cavity and abdominal contents visible

investigation. On the flip side, a negative result may be important and relevant for ruling out causes but frustratingly a negative result can also be misleading – it is possible that insufficient time has passed for the immune system to produce antibodies against the causal agent.

- Paired blood testing of aborted animals – first, at the time of the abortion and, second, 2–3 weeks later when sufficient time has elapsed for antibody levels for the causal agent to have risen – quite conclusive evidence of infection at the time of the abortion. Again, this is not always straightforward. Sometimes the bug may have struck well in advance of the abortion and the antibody levels may have plateaued by the time of both the first and the second sample.

Sometimes the levels may even be falling from the first to the second sample!

- Blood testing a cohort of unvaccinated home-bred animals between 9 and 18 months of age for IBR, leptospirosis and BVD. This can give an indication of active circulating disease on the farm; if the home-bred calves have antibodies they must have been exposed to the disease on that farm at some point recently in their, so far, short life, Again, this does not necessarily identify the cause of the abortion but it does provide information; another piece of the jigsaw!

Once the cause of abortion has been determined the appropriate control measures and preventative measures can be put in place.

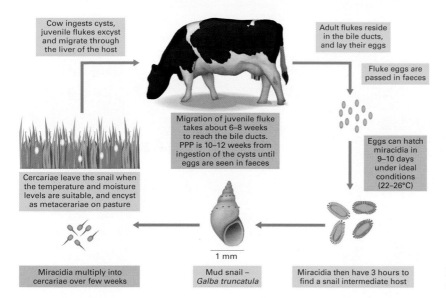

Cow ingests cysts, juvenile flukes excyst and migrate through the liver of the host

Adult flukes reside in the bile ducts, and lay their eggs

Fluke eggs are passed in faeces

Migration of juvenile fluke takes about 6–8 weeks to reach the bile ducts. PPP is 10–12 weeks from ingestion of the cysts until eggs are seen in faeces

Eggs can hatch miracidia in 9–10 days under ideal conditions (22–26°C)

Cercariae leave the snail when the temperature and moisture levels are suitable, and encyst as metacerariae on pasture

1 mm

Miracidia multiply into cercariae over few weeks

Mud snail – Galba truncatula

Miracidia then have 3 hours to find a snail intermediate host

FIGURE 15.7 The life cycle of the liver fluke

DISEASES OF THE GASTROINTESTINAL SYSTEM

Liver fluke (fasciolosis)

Liver fluke (*Fasciola hepatica*) is a type of parasite known as a trematode. It lives within the bile ducts of the liver of cows, sheep, and deer among others such as, occasionally, rabbits and horses. Understanding the complex life cycle of the liver fluke is useful to be able to put the best of control measures in place (Figure 15.7).

Adult liver flukes live, eat and lay eggs in the bile ducts of host cattle. One adult liver fluke can produce 2000–5000 eggs per day. These eggs reach the gut in the bile and pass out in the dung. The eggs hatch on pasture and release a larva called a *miracidium* – an average temperature greater than 10°C is required for hatching. These larvae spread across wet pasture (Figure 15.8) somehow seeking out mud snails (*Galba truncatula*), which also live in wet areas. The miracidia penetrate the mud snails for the next stage of the lifecycle. This must happen within the 3 hours before the miracidia otherwise die (Stevenson, 2016). Inside the snail the miracidia multiply into the next larval stage, a stage called the cercaria. Each miracidium can produce up to 1000 cercariae, which burrow out of the snail. These cercariae metamorphose into metacercariae, which attach themselves to herbage and encyst ready to be eaten by the next bovine host. The development from miracidium to metacercariae (the bit of the lifecycle that happens outside the animal) takes at least 6 weeks but can take several months in less favourable conditions (Stevenson, 2016).

After ingestion by the bovine host the metacercariae penetrate the gut wall, and migrate into the liver where they develop into immature and then mature/adult liver fluke. It takes 10–12 weeks after an animal ingests a metacercaria for the fluke to reach adulthood and start laying eggs for excretion in the faeces.

Acute fasciolosis

Acute liver fluke infection occurs when large numbers of metacercariae on the pasture are ingested over a short period of time. This is usually in autumn and can present as:

- sudden death
- weakness
- pale mucous membranes/anaemia

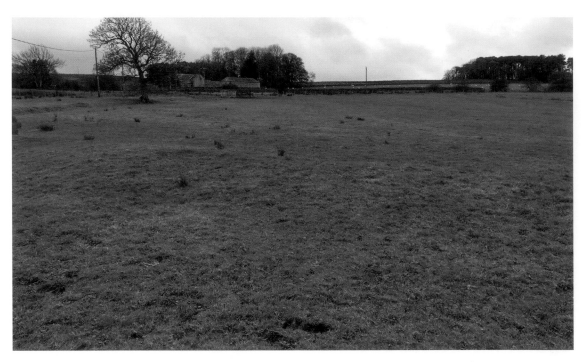

FIGURE 15.8 Poached wet pasture is an ideal habitat for the mud snail (*Galba truncatula*)

- abdominal pain
- liver haemorrhage
- enlarged liver
- low protein levels.

Acute infection is rarely seen in cattle as the bovine liver is very robust and tolerates relatively high levels of infection with few clinical signs (Forbes, 2016); the condition is more common in sheep.

Subacute fasciolosis

Subacute infection occurs when metacercariae are ingested over a longer period of time or in smaller numbers, usually late autumn/early winter and spring. The following clinical signs result:

- rapid condition loss
- pale mucous membranes/anaemia
- swelling below the jaw known as 'bottle jaw' – this is oedema, a result of low blood protein and is not specific to liver fluke infection

- enlarged liver
- possible abdominal pain.

Chronic fasciolosis

Chronic infection involves the residence of adult fluke in the bile ducts over the necessary time period to cause disease, namely months. Disease is usually seen later in winter and/or into spring. The clinical signs include:

- ill thrift
- anaemia (each liver fluke drinks 0.5 ml of blood per day)
- low protein and possible bottle jaw
- emaciation and death if not treated.

There are additional losses or disease, in addition to clinical signs above, that could be due to liver fluke. These include:

- high barren rates due to poor fertility
- liver condemnations at slaughter

- unexplained metabolic disease in cows at the time of calving when the demand on the liver for energy metabolism is high.

The mud snail is essential to maintain the life cycle of *F. hepatica*. The mud snail requires a specific habitat which is slightly acidic with slow moving water, typically fields with clumps of rushes. Permanent habitats include the banks of streams and ditches, and the edges of ponds. During wet years, or after flooding, these temporary habitats extend to include puddles in hoof prints or wheel ruts (Stevenson, 2016). Infected snails can, apparently and amazingly, be carried on the feet of birds which further aids their dissemination!

Other epidemiological considerations

- Eighty per cent of fluke eggs hatch within 1 month but it is possible for eggs to over winter on pasture resulting in early infection the following year; this will only occur if the humidity and temperature are optimal.
- Metacercariae can survive up to 1 year on pasture and can survive 30–57 days in good quality silage (and even longer in poorer crops).
- Most snails become infected in the summer by miracidia developed from eggs deposited in the spring or early summer, resulting in increased numbers of metacercariae on pasture from mid-August. Where eggs or cercariae have overwintered, however, the cercariae get a head

start and new infections and clinical signs due to infection with immature fluke may be seen earlier than expected.

- Given the length of time it takes from initial infection of the cattle with metacercariae to fluke eggs being present in the faeces, a prompt diagnosis (see section on testing below) of fluke infection cannot be relied upon initially from faecal egg counts. A PME is a quick and reliable method of diagnosis – fluke can be seen in the liver and bile ducts. The stage of infection can be estimated by the size of the fluke.
- Black disease, a clostridial disease discussed in Chapter 12, is precipitated by liver fluke infection and deaths may occur due to the clostridial toxaemia even if there is limited fluke damage to the liver.

Testing for and controlling liver fluke

A relatively new test called the coproantigen ELISA is a test performed on faeces that identifies a component of the fluke's saliva. The coproantigen test can detect infection up to 3 weeks earlier than a fluke egg count.

A blood test for antibodies to liver fluke is available and is a useful tool in animals in their first grazing season. Cattle and sheep produce antibodies in response to fluke although they do not develop a great deal of useful immunity after exposure. The antibodies are present from 2 weeks post-infection but last for a number of years. Blood testing an adult cow that has enjoyed

Active ingredient	Age of fluke in weeks													
	1	2	3	4	5	6	7	8	9	10	11	12	13	14
Albendazole										From 10 to 12 weeks				
Oxyclozanide										From 10 to 12 weeks				
Closantel						From 6 to 8 weeks								
Nitroxynil								From 8 weeks						
Clorsulon										From 10 to 12 weeks				
Triclabendazole		From 2 weeks												

FIGURE 15.9 Flukicides licensed for cattle (COWS, 2017)

multiple grazing seasons is, therefore, not useful as antibodies that are detected could be from any point in the historic exposure of previous grazing seasons. Spring-born calves are the ideal animals to blood test. This should be perhaps serially from August onwards to give an indication of whether and when infection with metacercariae is or is not occurring.

Treatment or control of liver fluke involves the use of flukicides of which there are a number of formulations, each one killing fluke of different ages (Figure 15.9) (Chapter 26).

When making a plan to control *F. hepatica* the following should be considered:

- predicted fluke activity forecasts
- previous farm history
- abattoir feedback
- results of any laboratory or PME testing
- known presence of flukicide resistant flukes.

F. hepatica resistance to triclabendazole is widely reported and for this reason it is no longer used on many farms. It is fortunate that cattle are generally fairly tolerant of immature fluke infection so alternative products can be used later in the winter to kill the older stages of fluke. This is not the case in sheep who are very intolerant of immature fluke infection. In mixed sheep and beef farms the use of triclabendazole should be preserved for the use in sheep to delay the rate that resistance develops in the fluke on that farm. There are exceptions; for example, when the treatment of spring-born calves is required because of late summer/autumn fluke activity, then, to maintain growth rates, triclabendazole may be a suitable product to use as soon as 2 weeks post-housing but only when triclabendazole resistance is not suspected on that farm.

Housing obviously abruptly stops the uptake of any more metacercariae from the pasture, so once the cattle have been housed for 8–10 weeks then a faecal sample can be taken from ten cattle in the group for the coproantigen test. If the test is positive a fluke treatment is required, this will kill fluke within the liver and prevent disease but also prevent contamination of the pasture with eggs at turn out. If there are multiple grazing groups, that is, groups grazing different pastures, a sample of ten animals will be required from each group. The laboratory will pool the sample evenly from the ten animals in each group to ensure each individual animal is represented equally.

Alternatively, if it is a high-risk year for fluke, if infection is suspected and if the cattle are in poor condition or suffering from concurrent disease, a treatment at housing with a non-triclabendazole product followed by a second treatment 6–12 weeks later (depending on the product) may be justified, dependent on veterinary advice.

If cattle are not housed then treatments should be scheduled through the winter months as per veterinary advice based on the fluke forecast, the previous farm history, the unfolding weather pattern and any diagnostic results.

Control plans for fasciolosis should be farm specific and reviewed year on year.

Grazing management is vital to reduce the snail habitat, to reduce pasture contamination with eggs and to reduce exposure of stock to metacercariae. Management techniques include:

- drainage where possible
- fencing off snail habitats
- avoiding the grazing of high-risk areas at high-risk times (high-risk areas are those with snail habitats which were grazed by stock earlier in the year – the snail will have been infected and will have released cercariae that become infective metacercariae later in that season)
- introducing ducks, which can help as they eat the snails.

Quarantine treatments are essential to prevent the introduction of liver fluke to a farm that does not already have fluke. Admittedly the farm would also have to have a snail habitat and population. Quarantine is also essential to prevent the introduction of triclabendazole resistant fluke to a fluke population that is otherwise currently susceptible. Quarantine treatment of both purchased and returning animals is very important. Quarantine protocols include sequential treatments:

- treatment with triclabendazole on arrival and closantel or nitroxynil 8 weeks later, or
- treatment with closantel on arrival and nitroxynil 8 weeks later.

In either case animals should be held off pastures with snail habitats for as long as possible but ideally for at least three weeks after the second treatment so if any fluke eggs are shed in the faeces of the animal a fluke population cannot establish.

Rumen fluke

The rumen fluke, *Calicophoron daubuneyi*, is similar to liver fluke in as much as they use the same mud snail (*G. truncatula*), to complete their lifecycle (Forbes, 2016). When the infective stages of the rumen fluke are ingested, they pass through the rumen and attach to the wall of the small intestine. This is the stage of the disease that sometimes causes the animal to become ill: dull, scour, rapid weight loss and anaemia. When the rumen flukes mature, they move back up to the rumen and settle down into adulthood without seemingly causing further disease. These adults shed eggs that can be detected in the faeces but up until then it is very difficult to diagnose rumen fluke in a live animal. A PME is required to see the immature stages in the small intestine.

Disease due to rumen fluke is rare. Rumen fluke eggs are detected in the faeces of many fit, normal animals and are usually nothing to worry about. For this reason, routine scheduled treatments are not required. Oxyclozanide, as it happens, is the only flukicide that kills rumen fluke (Forbes, 2016). It must be noted when designing a combined liver and rumen fluke control plan that oxyclozanide only kills adult liver fluke.

REFERENCES

Andrews, A.H. and Windsor, R.S. (2004) Respiratory conditions. In: Andrews, A.H., Blowey, R.W., Boyd, H. and Eddy, R.G. (eds) *Bovine Medicine. Diseases and Husbandry of Cattle*, 2nd edn. Blackwell Publishing, Oxford, pp. 866–867.

Blowey, R. and Edmondson, P. (1995) Summer mastitis. In: *Mastitis Control in Dairy Herds*, 2nd edn. CABI, Wallingford, pp. 215–219.

Cabell, E. (2007) Bovine abortion: aetiology and investigations. *In Practice* 29, 455–463.

Caldow, G., Buxton, D. and Nettleton, P.F. (2002) Investigating bovine abortion: what samples when? *Cattle Practice* 10(4), 269–274.

Cook, N. (1998) Bovine herpes virus 1: clinical manifestations and an outbreak of infectious pustular vulvovaginitis in a UK dairy herd. *Cattle Practice* 6(4), 341–344.

COWS (2017) Flukicide products for cattle. Control of Worms Sustainably. Available online at: https://www.cattleparasites.org.uk/app/uploads/2018/04/Flukicide-product-table.pdf (accessed 21 September 2020).

Forbes, A. (2016) The biology of fluke and their control in cattle. *Livestock* 21(1), 30–35.

Jackson, P. (1993) Differential diagnosis of common bovine skin disorders Part 1. *In Practice* 15, 119–127.

McLeonard, C. and van Dijk, J. (2017) Controlling lungworm disease (husk) in dairy cattle. *In Practice* 39, 408–419.

Peters, A.R. and Ball, P.J.H. (1995) Reproductive problems in the bull and cow. In: *Reproduction in Cattle*, 2nd edn. Blackwell Science, Oxford, pp. 164–165.

Stevenson, H. (2016) Treatment and control of liver fluke (*Fasciola hepatica*) in sheep and cattle. Technical Note TN677, SRUC. Available at: https://www.fas.scot/downloads/treatment-control-liver-fluke-fasciola-hepatica-sheep-cattle/.

Stevenson, H. (2017) Bacillus licheniformis abortion in cattle. *Cattle Practice* 25(3), 207.

Toolan, D.P. (2003) Neospora caninum abortion in cattle – a clinical perspective. *Irish Veterinary Journal* 56(8), 404–410.

Chapter 16

Disease and production failure in the breeding bull

The bull has always been and still remains an expensive asset in many herds and every effort needs to be made to keep him as healthy, happy and productive as possible, and for as long as possible, if not just for one family of females but for subsequent lines too.

Penny et al. (2001) carried out a survey to establish the average working life of a beef stock bull in the UK and the main reasons for them being culled. The survey included 606 bulls that had been culled, after use, on farm. The most common bull breeds surveyed were the Charolais, Simmental and Limousin. The average age at culling was 5.8 years, and the main reason for culling was musculoskeletal problems. The second most common reason for culling was a management decision on farm, for example, a change in breeding policy or a risk of inbreeding with daughters. Old age and fertility problems were close behind.

For a farm vet, the post-bull-sale period (Figure 16.1) can be fraught with phone calls reporting that the newly purchased bull is failing to get cows in-calf.

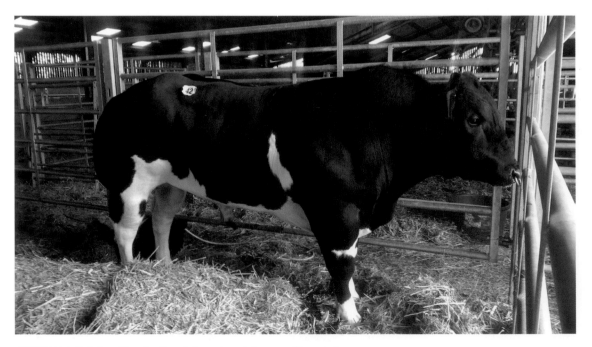

FIGURE 16.1 Belgian Blue bull arriving at new home after a sale

There is, in the UK and other countries, usually a 6 month warranty period post purchase, which adds a certain amount of time pressure to make a decision as to the fitness for purpose of the bull. It is possible to defer the 6 month warranty period and allow the bull to settle into the herd before he is used; this is highly recommended. A bull will not be at his most fertile after being subjected to an intense build up to the sale, 4 days in a market at the bull sale and then a long onward journey. The definition of fertility from a veterinary perspective is that a bull is expected to get 95% of 50 normally cycling, disease-free females in-calf within a 9 week period and 65% of these pregnancies should be achieved within the first 3 weeks of the bulling period. The definition of fertility, by industry standards, however, is that a fertile bull is capable of getting 4 cows or 50% of a group of cows, whichever is the fewer, in-calf by 12–24 months of age (Logue et al., 2005). As you can imagine, these two very different definitions create a large amount of discussion.

When faced with an infertility problem after the purchase of a new bull, it is tempting to jump in and carry out a BBSE on the recently acquired bull as described in Chapter 9. However, some consideration needs to be given to the other factors associated with beef suckler herd fertility; the bull is just a small part of the bigger picture (Box 16.1) yet he becomes the focus of attention as he finds himself the thing that changed most recently!

The main functions of a bull are: to seek out females and therefore need good sight, locomotion and libido; to be able to physically mount a cow; to achieve intromission (penetration); to ejaculate semen of good quality; and not to spread any disease in the process. Problems can arise with each of these functions resulting in the bull failing to get cows in-calf.

SEEKING OUT FEMALES AND LIBIDO

A bull has to be able to see females and to have good enough mobility to get himself over to them. Sight

> **Box 16.1** The five key points to reproductive efficiency in a suckler herd
>
> 1. Management of bulling heifers
> 2. Management of cow condition and nutrition
> 3. Avoidance of difficult calvings
> 4. Bull management for fertility and soundness
> 5. Maintenance of herd health

and mobility are discussed later in this chapter. But the bull also has to want to! He needs *libido*, or, in simpler language, sex drive.

Libido is driven mainly by testosterone and is augmented by sight, sound and smell stimuli, most notably in the case of smell – by pheromones – airborne hormones from other cattle that are detected during a special form of sniffing called the *flehmen reaction* – a curling of the upper lip while sniffing. Although libido has a strong genetic component, it needs to be remembered that young bulls sometimes seem to have to 'learn' how to serve a cow (Chenoweth, 2007). In Chapter 9 we are reminded that young bulls benefit from learning from older bulls and being given a gentle introduction to their work. Problems can be galvanised at this impressionable young age. Any psychological trauma or pain associated with previous mountings or attempts at serving a female will subsequently inhibit a bull's performance.

Libido is not assessed routinely as part of a pre-breeding examination although it is vital in achieving conception. It is no good having testicles full of fertile healthy sperm if this does not get into the cow. To assess a bull's libido, it requires a female to be in heat and then observing the bull with the female. Arranging for the timely heat in a cow or two can be facilitated by hormonal synchronisation of the females using a combination of intravaginal progesterone devices and prostaglandin. The bulls behaviour can then be assessed at a pre-planned appointment.

MOUNTING

The bull needs to be physically able to mount a cow to then achieve intromission. The first factor to be aware of is the size difference between the cow and bull. A small 18-month old bull may not be able to mount a 900 kg cow.

The main reason for a bull being unable to mount a cow is actually due to pain associated with a musculoskeletal abnormality (Figure 16.2). For example, a strained back muscle or a sore leg will be enough to inhibit the bull from mounting a cow. He will be less mobile and he will of course refrain from seeking out cows in the first place (see above)

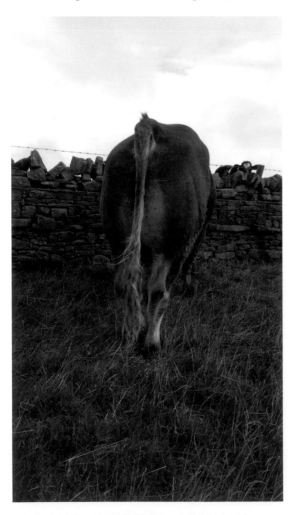

FIGURE 16.2 Limousin bull, lame left hind with significant muscle wastage

and instead choose to lie down for longer. Pain affects spermatogenesis (the production of sperm in the testes) and results in poorer semen quality.

Musculoskeletal conditions affecting mounting in bulls

Conformation and deformities

Poor conformation results in an animal altering its gait and applying forces to joints, ligaments and muscles in a direction they are not designed to handle. Straight hocks or 'post leggedness' applies excessive force to the hock, stifle and hip joint resulting in lameness. A 'sickle hock' conformation where an animal stands with its hocks bent and its feet underneath the body predisposes the bull to overgrowth of the toe horn and collapse of the heel with resultant lameness (see Figure 16.3). Uncontrolled horn growth of the lateral claw of the front limbs occurs when there is a *valgus deformity* of the front legs. Valgus is a term used to describe toes that point outwards rather than pointing forward. *Varus* describes toes that point inwards.

Interdigital skin hyperplasia/fibroma

Commonly seen in bulls with large, splayed hooves are interdigital growths: interdigital fibromas. This is where the digits are far apart and splayed and there is constant irritation of the skin between the digits resulting in excessive skin proliferation and a fibrotic, large, sore lump of skin. Considered a result of poor conformation and, possibly, a heritable trait, these bulls should not be bred from.

Corkscrew claw

Corkscrew claw, seen in both males and females, is the uneven growth of the hoof horn of the inside and the outside digit resulting in a spiral deviation of the claw. The outer wall of the hoof grows beneath the sole. There is a genetic component to this condition and the animal should not be retained for breeding.

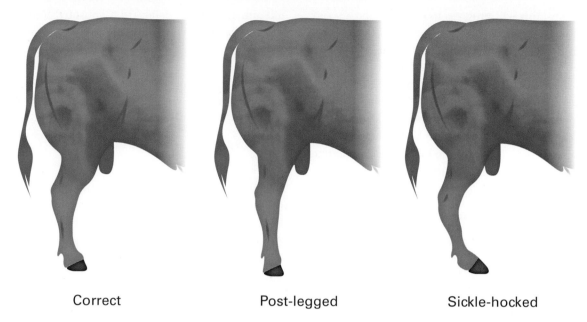

Correct   Post-legged   Sickle-hocked

FIGURE 16.3 Illustration of hind limb conformation

Stifle injuries

Injuries to the stifle joint are common in bulls and this is thought to be related to the extreme forces applied to the joint during the act of mounting and serving a cow. The stifle is held together by a series of ligaments. The *medial and lateral collateral ligaments* lie on the inside and outside respectively and keep the joint in line. There are two ligaments that cross over each other inside the joint, hence the name, *cruciate ligaments*; the cranial and caudal cruciate ligaments to be precise. Any of these ligaments can be damaged, ranging from a complete rupture to small tears in the multiple fibres that they are composed of. All the ligaments are attached to bones and damage can occur at the point of insertion where the bone at the point of attachment is ripped free by the force of the ligament. The cranial crucial ligament is perhaps the most prone to damage. Depending on which ligaments are damaged, how many, and how badly, will dictate the severity of the problem which ranges from emergency slaughter to healing with time and rest. Even when healing succeeds there will always be a weakness and a likelihood

to recur when the bull resumes work. Secondary osteoarthritis is also highly likely. Stifle injuries present as a variable degree of lameness, a swelling of the joint and heat in the area. In the case of complete rupture of the cranial cruciate ligament there is backward-forward instability of the joint and movement of the tibia in relation to the femur may be observed or demonstrated by a veterinary surgeon (Moenning and Sexton, 1972).

Hip dysplasia and hip dislocation

Hip dysplasia is seen in young bulls less than 1 year old. Angus and Hereford breeds seem particularly prone (Weaver, 2004). The hip joint is a ball and socket joint; the ball on the end of the femur should fit snugly into the encapsulating socket in the pelvis. In the condition hip dysplasia, the socket is too shallow and the ball is prone to slipping out of the socket, either partially or completely, resulting in partial, temporary or permanent dislocation. Irregular wearing of the cartilage of the ball and/or socket also results in the premature onset of osteoarthritis. Young bulls appear stiff, with a distinctive 'swinging gate' of the hind limbs; this will progress to lameness and a significant amount of time lying down. There is muscle wastage of the affected side in unilateral cases but in bilateral cases, affecting both left and right hips, which is common, the wastage may be less obvious as it is symmetrical. A partial or complete dislocation is painful, and the bull will be reluctant to weight bear; the toe will be turned out. When a hand is placed over the hip joint as the animal moves a clunking sensation can be felt.

Osteoarthritis (degenerative joint disease)

Osteoarthritis is degeneration of the joint and is seen as a progressive lameness in animals usually 5 years and older (Moenning and Sexton, 1972). Where there has been excessive wear and tear, in the case of injury or poor conformation, the onset of osteoarthritis may be sooner. Lameness will be more obvious after the animal has been at rest but then 'wears off' after a period of mobility. The degeneration of the cartilage surface and inflammation in the joint are a constant source of pain; the animal will become less active, and become reluctant to move which can reduce feeding behaviour so resulting in weight loss. Temporary relief can be achieved with NSAIDs but there is no cure.

Bovine spastic syndrome and bovine spastic paresis

Two diseases that are both rare but very distinctive on presentation are bovine spastic syndrome (BSS) and bovine spastic paresis (BSP). BSS (Figure 16.4), otherwise known as *barn cramps*, occurs in animals greater than 3 years old, is sporadic, intermittent and involves contracture of the musculature of the hind limbs and back, sometimes the whole body, where the muscles uncontrollably contract simultaneously and then release after a variable period of time (Goeckmann et al., 2018).

BSP occurs in animals at any age. BSP is the permanent contracture of the hind limb musculature

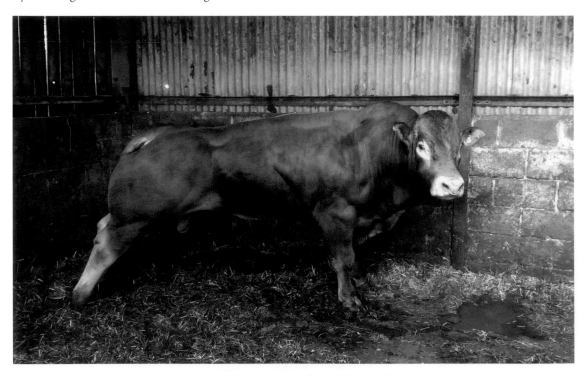

FIGURE 16.4 Limousin bull, 3 years old, with bovine spastic syndrome ('barn cramps'), the bull was euthanased

whereas BSS is slower to develop and is intermittent.

It is possible to treat BSP surgically by cutting the appropriate branches of the tibial nerve, the nerve which supplies the affected muscles. For BSS, however, there is no treatment; the progression of the disease is variable and may take years and, due to its sporadic nature, the animal may have a normal life between episodes. There is possibly a genetic component to both diseases, and it is advised that neither males nor females with the condition are used for breeding.

Dorsal patella fixation

Dorsal patella fixation (DPF) occurs in calves and young cattle when the patella (the kneecap) has slipped from its groove resulting in a leg that cannot bend. The patella can slip back to its rightful place of its own accord and a normal gait resumed; the condition may only be present for a few steps. Surgery can correct DPF by cutting one of the ligaments that holds the patella in place. DPF is intermittent; when the patella is out of position the limb cannot be flexed manually, when it is in position it feels entirely normal.

INTROMISSION

Intromission is the point at which the erect penis enters the vulva of the cow during mating. Immediately prior to this the bull requires an erect penis, which is achieved through the pumping of blood into the penis, thus increasing the pressure in the penis and causing it to straighten and protrude from the sheath (prepuce). There are various reasons why intromission may fail. *Erection failure* can occur if there is a problem with blood flow into the penis, or the penis may be adhered to the prepuce, or a physical obstruction such as an abscess or wart may prevent the penis from extruding from the prepuce or the penis may just be too short. A thorough examination is required to identify the cause.

Deviation of the penis may result in a failure of intromission. The most spectacular deviation is the condition known as 'corkscrew penis'. The erect penis usually appears clearly as a spiral or corkscrew. Diagnosis can sometimes be difficult as the phenomenon may occur intermittently and the bull may be able to get some cows in-calf. The bull may be able to serve normally for a number of years and then develop the condition later in life. It is rarely related to trauma. It is important to note that it is physiologically normal for the bull's penis to twist anticlockwise within the vagina just before ejaculation. Some bulls will corkscrew their penis during electro-ejaculation as part of a bull breeding soundness examination. This does not mean he will corkscrew on natural service and careful interpretation of this finding is required.

A fibrous band attaching the penis to the prepuce exists in prepubertal animals called the *frenulum*. It should break down during puberty but on occasions it persists, causing the penis to deviate downwards. A simple operation is required to cut this band of tissue and resolve this downward deviation of the tip of the penis.

Other than a persistent frenulum and corkscrew penis other deviations of the penis can be a result of scar tissue formation from previous trauma and adhesions. Some bulls learn to adapt and continue to be able to serve cows effectively. Careful observation of the act of service is required and likewise the subsequent monitoring for returns to service; early evidence of failure.

Trauma to the penis during service occasionally occurs and results in rupture of the penis while it is under pressure; associated blood loss into the surrounding tissues, pain and swelling result. The swollen penis will protrude from the prepuce, is then prone to further damage and failure of urination can be a problem. During the healing process adhesions can form between the penis and the wall of the prepuce, which will prevent the penis extruding from the prepuce in future services. Immediate veterinary attention is required in cases of penile trauma.

Sexually active young bulls are prone to prolapse of the prepuce or penis, this is where the pink inner lining of the prepuce and/or the penis fails to retract completely back into the orifice of the prepuce after erection. If the prolapsed tissue is left unattended for more than a few hours the tissues fill with fluid as a result of gravity, and the swelling then means the structures physically cannot retract back into the prepuce. While the preputial lining and penis are exteriorised, they are prone to damage and infection. Treatment involves lubrication of the prolapsed tissue to keep it moist, NSAIDs and body bandages to hold the penis against the abdomen and allow the inflammatory fluid to disperse. The bull should not be around any in-season females while under treatment. Subsequent bacterial infections and associated inflammation are likely. Any purulent smelly discharge from the prepuce is abnormal and if this occurs lavage of the prepuce can be carried out with a mild antiseptic.

SEMEN PRODUCTION

Collecting and assessing a semen sample is an integral part of the PBE of a breeding bull as described in Chapter 9. Once a sample is collected the volume and density are assessed; this is very variable depending on whether an AV or electro-ejaculator has been used to obtain the sample. Little value is obtained from visual examination alone (Penny, 2005) other than noting the presence of blood, urine or pus.

Examination under a microscope for what is called *gross motility* is the next step. Gross motility assesses the concentration of progressively motile sperm and the speed of progression. The sample must be analysed immediately after collection and while being kept warm. The sperm will 'slow down' with time and with a fall in temperature; a chill or cold shock will stop them completely. The gross motility is graded 1–5, 5 being fast moving dark waves to 1 which is sporadic oscillation of small isolated areas of the sample. In a very concentrated

sample, it is possible that a few very active sperm may make the sample look highly motile as they drag a lot of dead, low motile sperm around with them. For this reason, the sample is diluted and observed under a higher magnification; this is to assess individual sperm true *progressive motility* under conditions unaffected by concentration. The grading of progressive motility is expressed as a percentage score, the % of sperm moving in a progressive manor; over 70% is very good, less than 30% is poor. The third and final assessment is *morphology*. This is often carried out away from the farm, back at the practice laboratory as it takes some time and a level of experience. This final step is to assess the percentage of normal sperm. The sample is stained (Figure 16.5) and allowed to dry on a microscope slide and then 100 sperm examined to check they are normal; that is, a normal head attached to a normal mid-piece and a normal tail. It is expected that a proportion of the sperm will be abnormal but over 70% should be of normal shape/morphology. The defects are categorised into whether they are a defect of spermatogenesis within the testicle or if the defect is due to a problem of the final stages of development that occur within the epididymis (Penny, 2005). The terms *compensable* and *non-compensable* defects are used. A

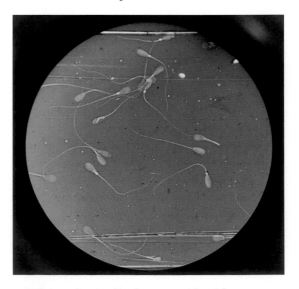

FIGURE 16.5 A sample of semen stained for morphological examination of the sperm

compensable defect is one that can be overcome by increasing the amount of sperm; that is, by multiple ejaculates or by the bull simply having a reasonable volume of semen and density of sperm in each ejaculate. Compensable defects are generally sperm with abnormalities that prevent them reaching the ova, for example a tail defect. Sperm with a non-compensable defect, on the other hand, can reach and penetrate the egg but their abnormality is such that they fail to complete their task while at the same time 'blocking' other normal sperm gaining access to the egg. Such a defect cannot be overcome by increasing the amount of sperm, hence a non-compensable defect. A bull pre-breeding examination or BBSE should be fully documented as detailed in Figure 16.6.

Owners Name and Address:				
Place of examination:			Date of examination:	
Name + ear tag number:	Species: Bovine	Breed: Aberdeen Angus	Age: 18 months	
Fertility history and reason for assessment: Young bull				
General Health Status (eyes, legs, feet, teeth, heart, lungs etc): Good – no abnormalities detected				
Condition Score (1-5):		Rectal Temperature (C): 37.6	Scrotal Circumference (cm): 31	
Testes and epididymes	Right	No abnormalities detected		
	Left	No abnormalities detected		
Accessory glands:				

	Sample 1	Sample 2		
Stimulation level for sampling (1-9)	4	4		
Penis extruded? Description	Yes – no abnormalities detected	Yes – no abnormalities detected		
Semen volume (ml)	5ml	4ml		
Semen appearance	Cloudy yellow	Cloudy yellow		
Gross motility score (Wave Motion) (grade 1-5) Target 3+	2	4		
Progressive Motility % (>30% Pass, pref 60%)	<30%	>60%		
Sperm Morphology	Tally/comments	%	Pass %	Compensable
Normal		84%	>50-70%	No
Proximal cytoplasmic droplets (PD)		24%	<20%	No
Mid piece abnormalities (MP)		1%	<30%	Yes
Tail defects and loose heads (T&H)		8%	<30%	Yes
Pyriform heads (Py)		3%	<20%	No
Knobbed acrosome (KA)		-	<30%	Yes
Vacuoles and teratoids (V&T)		-	<20%	No
Swollen acrosomes (SA)		-	<30%	Yes
Other abnormalities				

On the basis of this examination the above male has achieved a fail for the breeding soundness examination. The male is sub-fertile.

The morphology results of this sample were abnormal with a high percentage of non-compensable defects. I would advise to re-test this bull in 8 weeks time.

This report indicates likely fertility status at the time of testing and is no guarantee of the current or future status of this male. Testing for transmissible diseases (including venereal/congenital disease) is not carried out and the breeding soundness examination does not indicate freedom from these diseases. No assessment of libido or serving ability has been made during this examination.
This report is for the use of the owner only and is not a certificate that guarantees the fertility of this male.

Signature: ....   Date:

FIGURE 16.6 An example of a bull pre-breeding examination report (see appendix for larger version)

Conditions affecting sperm production

Semen is manufactured within the testes and stored within the adjacent epididymis, a coil of tubes sitting attached to the testis within the scrotum. Any disease of the scrotum, testis and epididymis is likely to affect sperm production and fertility. This can be due to damage to the cells and tissues responsible for the production and maturation of the sperm but also any disruption in thermoregulation of the testes will affect sperm quality. Spermatogenesis prefers temperatures below the standard core body temperature, hence the reason the testes in most animals hang outside the body. Interestingly in Brahman cattle in equatorial regions the reverse is true – the testes are retracted up into the body to protect them from the fierce environmental heat. The raising of the temperature of the scrotal contents may be due to something as mild as a scrotal skin infection.

Summary of conditions affecting sperm production

- **Small testes syndrome** is where one or both testicles are small. Terminology gets a bit complicated at this point. *Testicular hypoplasia* is used to describe the congenital presence of one or more small testicles. *Testicular degeneration* is where one or more testicles becomes small but later in life, usually post illness, trauma or infection (Statham, 2010). Degenerated testicles often feel firmer and possibly nodular whereas hypoplastic testicles are more often soft and uniform. It can be difficult to establish when the abnormality occurred, that is, whether the testicles have been like that from birth or from a very young age, unless the bull has been examined and measured at regular intervals throughout his life. Whatever the name of the condition, in these situations the bull will have a smaller scrotal circumference and reduced fertility if for no other reason than a lack of testicular tissue for spermatogenesis.

- **Trauma** to the scrotum and testicles can result from a kick or from slipping or from compression when lying down. The scrotum will appear enlarged, swollen and painful to the touch. The bull will be temporarily or permanently infertile depending on the severity of the injury.

- **Inguinal hernias.** Bulls can suffer from scrotal hernias, similar to humans, where a loop of bowel drops through the channel that the spermatic cord passes from the abdomen, down into the scrotum or at least the inguinal region. This causes an enlargement of the neck of the scrotum and/or the scrotum itself. If the bowel twists and the blood supply is compromised the condition can be fatal; surgery can be performed to correct the defect or if caught early the experienced veterinary surgeon can perform a rectal procedure that involves pulling the intestines back into the abdomen.

- **Inflammation** of the testicle is called *orchitis* and inflammation of the epididymis is called *epididymitis*. Orchitis and epididymitis can result classically from infection with *Brucella abortus* and *Histophilus somni* and then, as a secondary bacterial invader, *Trueperella pyogenes*. One, or occasionally both, testicles are enlarged and hard on palpation. When a semen sample is obtained the motility is poor and the semen have defects of the head of the sperm. Treatment with antibiotics is largely ineffective and if the condition is unilateral, removal of the affected testicle is advised (Statham, 2010). The adjacent testicle will initially be infertile due to the compromised temperature control while its neighbour was infected but there is a small chance normal fertility will resume.

- **Varicocele** is a dilation of the veins within the pampiniform plexus (the network of veins within the neck of the scrotum). The dilation is occasionally palpable and usually significant as the condition invariably affects thermoregulation of the testis.

- **Spermatocoele** is a palpable finding on the epididymis or spermatic cord. They are small, firm, nodular lumps that result from leakage of sperm from their tubes where they are stored and transported, into the surrounding tissue. This could be due to a small blockage caused by orchitis or epididymitis but also could be a result of a congenital malformation where the tubes are not quite sealed properly and leakage occurs. The spermatocoele can block the movement of sperm from the epididymis up into the deferent duct and thus compromise fertility; sometimes there is no real blockage and no effect on fertility – just a notable finding. There is no treatment and they are permanent although they can shrink down and fibrose/scar.

- **Idiopathic angioneurotic oedema** is the name given to a condition where a young bull has been turned out to grazing and the scrotum swells up to a huge size post-turnout (Statham, 2010). The bull is infertile at that time but fertility will resume when the swelling reduces, and a fresh cycle of sperm can be produced. The cause is as yet unknown.

- **Systemic disease.** The scrotum may be affected by some systemic diseases. Liver disease and heart disease cause fluid to sequester in the lower part of the body, due to the effect of gravity, and scrotal enlargement may occur. If a bull has been fevered at any time this will affect spermatogenesis with subsequent temporary infertility. A common question when faced with a sick bull is whether the antibiotics used to treat it will affect the fertility of the bull? The standard answer is that the drug itself probably will not but the condition the bull is suffering from probably will! Any pain or stress will affect fertility. To fully answer the question though, tetracyclines are thought to have a minor detrimental effect on semen quality but there is a lack of evidence for this, and there is no evidence that any other antibiotics have a detrimental effect.

- **Accessory gland disease.** The accessory glands lie adjacent to the urethra within the pelvis and can be palpated via the rectum by a vet. There are four glands as described in Chapter 9. The vesicular gland is the gland most prone to cause problems. Congenital abnormalities of the vesicular gland occur and *vesiculitis* as a result of infection with bacteria is also known to occur in young bulls. Vesiculitis is easily identified on rectal palpation and pus and white blood cells are usually present in the ejaculate; sperm motility is poor as a result. The most commonly isolated bacteria are *T. pyogenes*, treatment with antimicrobials is largely ineffective and the condition is untreatable.

BIOSECURITY THREAT FROM BREEDING BULLS

In some herds the bull may be the only incoming purchase, even if it is on a relatively infrequent basis. This makes the bull the 'weakest link' in terms of biosecurity. It is therefore imperative he does not introduce disease to an otherwise clean herd (see Chapter 9). Conversely, a purchased bull from a high-health status herd that is introduced to a herd that is endemically infected with diseases, such as IBR and BVD, will suffer acute infection on arrival and resultant temporary infertility for some period of time thereafter. This will undoubtedly be the case in many post-purchase bull infertility investigations where the vendor, on these occasions may well get the blame! TBF should also be considered on farms known to have ticks when a bull, from a non-tick infested farm, is introduced.

To prevent mishaps such as this a full history of the bull should be provided by the vendor. The history should include: health status, vaccination status, feeding regime, grazing history and parasiticide treatments. The bull should, where possible, be sourced from a CHeCS accredited herd (Chapter 18) and subjected to a quarantine period incorporating testing and vaccination as appropriate. It is advisable that a bull is purchased at least 6

months in advance of when he is required to work, to allow him to become acclimatised to his new home in the traditional sense and in the *infectious harmony* sense.

The bull is a vector for venereal disease transmission. *Campylobacter* infection is a relatively common bacterial venereal disease passed between bulls and cows during natural service. One species, *C. fetus* subsp. *venerealis* is able to live within the reproductive tract of an infected bull. The bacteria populate the prepuce, the penis and the bottom part of the urethra. Older bulls have more crypts and crevices in the prepuce for the bacteria to hide in and there is a higher incidence of infection in bulls over 5 years old (Taylor, 2002). An infected bull has no outward visible signs of disease, nor ill health, and no immune response is generated; a bull that is infected, treated and recovered can be infected again with the disease. In the cow the bacteria live within the vagina, cervix, uterus and oviducts. Cows are infected by the bull by the physical transfer of bacteria from the penis. The cow may conceive but the embryo dies very early in gestation or is aborted at around 5–6 months (Taylor, 2002). Occasionally a moderate endometritis may be seen post-infection.

Campylobacter infection comes into the herd via a bought-in infected bull (hired bulls or second-hand purchases) or, less commonly, via a bought-in infected female who in turn infects the bull and so on.

The initial signs are a large number of returns to service and/or late abortions. *Repeat breeder* cows who are infected sometimes show a vulval discharge associated with very early pregnancy failure and then eventually develop an immunity and then hold to service 3–6 months after initial infection (Truyers et al., 2014).

A diagnosis can be made from culturing the bacteria from either the bull or infected cow. In the male, *preputial washings*, sometimes called *sheath washings*, are the method of sampling commonly used. The prepuce of the bull is washed with phosphate buffered saline (PBS) and the washings collected and submitted to the lab for testing. Alternatively, the vagina of heifers recently served, within the last 2–3 months, can be washed out with PBS, collected, and again tested by a laboratory.

Campylobacter spp. are difficult to culture and false negatives from a single test are a distinct possibility. Multiple samples should be taken to rule out *Campylobacter* spp. in an investigation into poor fertility – this can be laborious, expensive and frustrating and therefore quite off-putting so it is a concern that many herd infections go undiagnosed.

It is possible to treat infected bulls with antibiotics and the recommended treatment protocol has also been suggested if non-virgin bulls are being added to the herd. Cows do not require treatment, as they develop immunity over 3–6 months after exposure. Bulls entering an AI stud are rigorously tested for *Campylobacter* spp. on introduction and subsequently with annual screen.

Streptomycin is the antibiotic of choice administered by injection and by preputial antibiotic washings for three consecutive days. The combination of local and systemic routes of treatment is recommended as the injectable antibiotics will kill any bacteria that may have migrated up the urethra and are not exposed to the antibiotic infused into the prepuce. After treatment the bull should be re-tested no sooner than 30 days post-treatment. A second sample is required between 3 and 7 days after the first and again 30 days later to ensure the treatment has been effective (Taylor, 2002). Treatment cannot always be relied upon and some studs will simply not attempt it, instead choosing to cull the bull rather than risk it.

The disease can be controlled by a move to artificial insemination instead of natural service. Cows eventually overcome infection and after allowing two normal pregnancies by AI natural breeding can be resumed (Truyers et al., 2014). Bulls, however, stay infected if they are not treated and need to be culled if not treated, and will still need culling if treatment fails which it can do.

It might be possible, with good record keeping, to identify clean and 'infected' animals and run two separate herds with no interbreeding or bull sharing between the two.

A vaccine is available in the USA and has been used to prevent and eradicate disease (Taylor, 2002). It is not licensed for use in the UK but is available under specific licensing and has been used with good success. Autogenous vaccination has also been trialled by some vets (Chapter 26).

TEASER BULLS

A teaser bull is a vasectomised male; intact but sterile, he actively seeks out females in oestrus and is an effective heat detection aid when using AI. A teaser bull will identify cows showing weak heats – heats not obvious enough for a stockperson to detect. They will also hasten the cycling of peripubertal heifers and the cyclicity of cows post-calving (Morgan and Dawson, 2008). An operation (vasectomy) is required to render the bull infertile by removing either the deferent duct or the tail of the epididymis. The result of either operation is that the semen can no longer travel from the testicles through the penis to be ejaculated. The testicles remain and the bull is hormonally and behaviourally normal.

The correct bull needs to be selected as a teaser animal. Ideally the animal should be home-bred to reduce the risk of the introduction of disease, bearing in mind that the bull is still able to achieve intromission and is still capable of passing on venereal diseases. They should be of good temperament and easy to handle. The surgery is easier and less risky in animals less than 300 kg (Morgan and Dawson, 2008). Larger, more mature bulls are more difficult to restrain, may haemorrhage more and take longer to heal. The operation can be carried out in a restrained, standing, sedated animal in a clean environment. The operation needs to be carried out at least 6 weeks before he is expected to be used. This is to allow time for healing but also so that any sperm left within the reproductive tract is passed or dies off before the bull is presented to fertile cows; sensible to ensure there are no accidental pregnancies by an unintended sire. Alternatively, a recently vasectomised bull can be intentionally allowed to serve an oestrus female, perhaps one in the process of being imminently culled, or, if she is staying in the herd, she could be chemically aborted, with an injection of PG, 11 days post service (and checked at a later date to ensure the injection has had the desired effect). This sounds a little unethical but is better than an unplanned pregnancy that does not fit within the production scheme and could therefore result in all sorts of problems for cow and calf and possibly unnecessary culling.

EYE ABNORMALITIES

The bull predominantly uses sight to seek out females in oestrus, closely followed by smell. It is important that he can see from both eyes. The conditions described below can affect both sexes of cattle, not just bulls.

Infectious bovine keratoconjunctivitis ('pink eye')

Infectious bovine keratoconjunctivitis (IBK) is a bacterial infection of the eye by *Moraxella bovis*, a bug transmitted mechanically by flies from eye to eye in the summer months. Young cattle are more susceptible which suggests there is a degree of immunity that develops with exposure. Carrier animals have, however, also been identified; they do not show the disease themselves but carry the bacteria and are a source of infection to others (Bedford, 2004). Outbreaks of disease with a significant proportion of cattle affected is well recognised.

Initially there is tear staining of the face, a partially closed eye followed by a white pussy discharge exuding between the eyelids, matting the eyelashes, and then ulceration of the cornea (the surface of the eyeball). In advanced cases the eyeball becomes filled with inflammatory cells and pus; at this stage the condition is irreversible – and sight is lost in that eye. In severe cases, infection can track up the optic nerve and cause meningitis and death (Bedford, 2004).

Pink eye is a painful condition and even more so when the eye is exposed to direct sunlight. Some cases will resolve without treatment but due to the painful nature of the lesion, prompt treatment is essential. An NSAID is imperative as a painkiller and topical antibiotic cream be applied under the eyelid once or twice daily for 3 consecutive days to kill the *Moraxella bovis* and any additional secondary bacterial infection. It is possible for a vet to inject antibiotic under the conjunctiva, ideally of the sclera (the white of the eye), not the eyelid; this provides a constant diffusion of antibiotic into the tear film covering the cornea. This is an effective treatment but, done properly, is difficult to administer in a fractious or poorly restrained animal. Affected cattle should be housed out of direct sunlight and away from susceptible animals; they themselves are a source of infection. In severe cases the cornea may perforate, and the eye will rupture – prompt veterinary attention is required here – surgical *enucleation* (removal of the eye) may be necessary. Prevention of pink eye is through avoidance of high-risk fly pastures and the use of pour-on insecticides or cypermethrin impregnated ear tags.

Squamous cell carcinoma ('cancer eye')

Squamous cell carcinoma is a cancer of the con junctiva of the eye and is the most common cancer seen in cattle (Figure 16.7). Cattle with white hair around the eyes, such as Herefords and Simmentals, are more predisposed to the condition, usually later in life. Direct sunlight on susceptible cells of the conjunctiva cause them to mutate and proliferate. The condition affects the lower eyelid but even more so the third eyelid which is most exposed to the sunlight. Melanin is the dark pigment in the skin, and it protects the cells from

UV exposure; in unpigmented skin there is no such protection. The condition is seen in the UK but is more common in countries with more sunshine and higher UV levels, especially those that have imported Herefords and Simmentals from the less sunny UK and the Alps.

The tumour does not affect the animal until it reaches such a size where it irritates and causes physical damage to the surface of the eye. In the early stages the tumour can be surgically removed from the eyelid, in more advanced cases it may require removal of the whole eye; enucleation. Culling should be considered as there is some evidence that the tumour can spread via the lymph system to the lungs, heart, liver and kidneys (Bedford, 2004).

Enucleation can be used more as a salvage procedure in cases of advanced squamous cell carcinoma but also in any *end stage eye*; this is an eye that has not responded to treatment and remains uncomfortable causing pain and discomfort. The surgery can be carried out on the restrained standing animal with mild sedation and infiltration of local anaesthetic, but it is kinder to perform the procedure under general anaesthetic when the cow is oblivious. It is important that the animal is left with a functional eye on the other side so that it retains some sight – if this is not the case the operation should not proceed and the animal should be culled.

Bovine iritis (uveitis) ('silage eye')

This condition is seen more commonly during the winter in cattle who are fed baled silage. It is associated with infection by the bacterium *Listeria monocytogenes*, which exists at high levels in poorly preserved silage. Infection can occur via two routes: (1) direct infection of the conjunctiva of the eye; or (2) the bacterium penetrates the gums of the mouth and travels up a nerve to the eye. Another theory is that the infection does not actually enter the eye but rather the immune system reacts to infection elsewhere in the body and the structures inside the eye react to immune factors in the bloodstream. Whatever the mechanism, the following is observed. Initially the eye is sore and may be only partially open with tear staining of the face. The cornea becomes opaque and behind the cornea the iris is inflamed and swollen (*uveitis*). Ulceration is not, in the early stages, a typical feature unless there has been physical damage resulting in infection, for example a fibrous piece of forage or straw causing abrasion to the cornea. The condition is painful and even more so when exposed to strong light. An injection of antibiotic and steroid under the conjunctiva, ideally the scleral conjunctiva, is effective and an NSAID is also required to alleviate

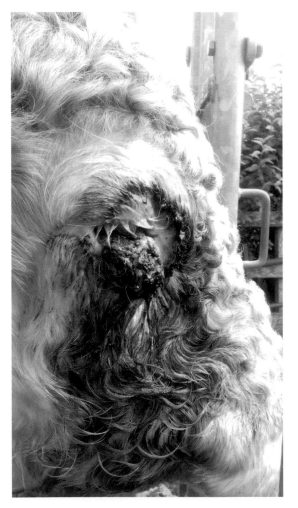

FIGURE 16.7 Squamous cell carcinoma of the eye in a White bred Shorthorn bull

pain. Subscleral conjunctival injection is superior to injecting the eyelid but is difficult, requires a vet, and good restraint is essential. Prevention is through good silage making and preservation as discussed in Chapter 25.

Foreign bodies

Hay seeds, grass seeds, straw, silage and herbage are common FBs affecting the eye. The animal may present with a sore eye and initially it is thought to be silage eye or IBK (pink eye) but on closer examination there is damage to the surface of the eye due to foreign material. The foreign material can be lodged behind the third eyelid and careful examination, following the application of local anaesthetic eye drops, is required to identify and remove it. Farms that blow chopped straw over the cows to bed them are particularly affected by this problem.

Entropion

Entropion is the correct term for an in-turned eyelid, almost always the lower lid. This is a problem particularly in the Charolais breed, where there are copious amounts of skin around the eye. It is surmised that an event occurs that causes the eye to sink back into the eye socket slightly which allows the skin and associated hair to curl inwards, towards the eye, and consequently irritate the cornea with the haired surface of the skin. This results in irritation and a spiralling of the problem, that is, further *scrunching* of the eye. Ulceration eventually occurs. The retraction of the eye may be due to loss of condition, dehydration or irritation due to a dusty environment, or an initially mild conjunctivitis. The problem can be temporarily resolved by administering a large quantity of antibiotic suspension (up to 35 ml) into the skin of the lower eyelid, to make the lower eyelid so distended and bulbous that it is no longer physically able to roll inwards. This effect usually lasts long enough for the problem to resolve. If the condition is persistent then an operation to remove the excessive skin can be performed – essentially a *nip and tuck* of the lower eyelid!

REFERENCES

Bedford, P.G.C. (2004) Ocular disease. In: A.H. Andrews, R.W. Blowey, H. Boyd and R.G. Eddy (eds) *Bovine Medicine Diseases and Husbandry of Cattle*, 2nd edn. Blackwell Publishing, Oxford, pp. 919–922.

Chenoweth, P.J. (2007) Bull libido/serving capacity. *Veterinary Clinics of North America: Food Animal Practice* 13, 331–344.

Goeckmann, V., Rothmanner, S. and Medugorac, I. (2018) Bovine spastic syndrome: a review. *Vet Record* 216, 64–71.

Logue, D.N., Williams, E.J. and Crawshaw, W.M. (2005) Problems with the bull. *Cattle Practice* 13(3), 189–198.

Moenning, L.E. and Sexton, J.W. (1972) Bovine lameness. *Iowa State University Veterinarian* 34(1), 44–48.

Morgan, G.L. and Dawson, L.J. (2008) Development of teaser bulls under field conditions. *Veterinary Clinics: Food Animal Practice* 24, 443–453.

Penny, C.D., Faulkner, G., Boreland, J., Doyle, B., Wilson, A., Gibson, D. and Ballard, D. (2001) A survey of the longevity and reasons for culling in UK beef stock bulls. *Cattle Practice* 9(1), 55–56.

Penny, C. (2005) Practical semen collection and examination techniques for breeding soundness evaluation of bulls. *Cattle Practice* 13(3), 199–204.

Statham, J. (2010) Differential diagnosis of scrotal enlargement in bulls. *In Practice* 32, 200–206.

Taylor, A.J. (2002) Venereal Campylobacter infections in cattle. *Cattle Practice* 10(1), 35–42.

Truyers, I., Luke., T. and Sargison, N. (2014) Diagnosis and management of venereal campylobacteriosis in beef cattle. *BMC Veterinary Research* 10, 280.

Weaver, A.D. (2004) Lameness above the foot. In: A.H. Andrews, R.W. Blowey, H. Boyd and R.G. Eddy (eds) *Bovine Medicine Diseases and Husbandry of Cattle*, 2nd edn. Blackwell Publishing, Oxford, pp. 453–454.

Chapter 17

Disease and production failure in the suckler cow

The average suckler cow spends more time in the herd than any other age cohort of female and in most cases longer than the breeding males. Inevitably the long productive career of the cow inevitably involves a number of disease and production pitfalls that will be discussed in this chapter. As with other chapters there is inevitably some overlap between the conditions of the different age and sex classifications of cattle.

JOHNE'S DISEASE

Johne's disease (JD), named after Dr Albert Johne (pronounced *yoh-ne*), a German pathologist from the 1800s, is an infection of cattle with the bacterium *Mycobacterium avium* subsp. *paratuberculosis* (MAP) and as the name suggests the bug is closely related to the tuberculosis bacterium with which it shares some features. It is an important chronic wasting disease of cattle that also affects sheep, goats, rabbits and deer, all of which can be a source of infection to cattle. It generally presents as an individual case, although for every clinical case within a herd there are generally 10–25 subclinically infected animals.

The clinical signs often occur after a period of stress, such as calving, and are usually seen in animals over three-year-old although it can be seen as young as 1 year old. The signs of the disease in an infected animal towards the end of the disease process are chronic diarrhoea (liquid and occasionally, but certainly not always, the famed 'bubbly') and emaciation in an animal that is generally bright and eating. There is a decreased milk yield, and due to the loss of protein from the bloodstream, an oedematous swelling under the chin, *bottle jaw,* is often seen. There is no treatment and the animal will eventually die. Infected animals with no clinical signs are currently allowed to enter the human food chain but recent concerns of a potential link with Crohn's disease in humans attracted some controversy to this arrangement; no solid evidence for a link has been established. In a clinical case of JD, euthanasia is warranted.

Infection is acquired at an early age, 80% occurring in calves less than 4 weeks old, but infections can occur up to 6 months of age. Experimentally calves have been infected up to 12 months of age and even adult cows are reported to have been infected from another adult cow in situations of very high environmental contamination. The major route of transmission is the faeces from infected, and shedding, cows being ingested by calves. Calves can also be infected via colostrum from an infected cow and on some occasions the calf can even become infected in the uterus before it is born. This in utero infection occurs in 20–40% of clinically affected cows, that is, those losing weight and scoured, while it occurs in only 9% of cows that are subclinically infected – yet to show clinical signs. A calf is six times more likely to suffer from JD if it is born to a cow infected with JD, but equally important, calves born to an unaffected mother can become infected if they are exposed to MAP in an environment contaminated with faeces from infected cows other than the mother. There are no signs of disease in the calf when it is initially infected. It has been shown, however, that the newly infected calf will itself shed the bacteria for a short period after infection adding to the bacterial environmental load. It is possible that one infected calf could infect another 3 calves all by itself without the need for an adult shedder.

The Johne's bacterium, MAP, can survive a long time outside of the cow. It has been demonstrated to last 55 weeks on pasture, 48 weeks in contaminated water and more than 26 weeks in stored slurry. MAP does not, however, survive as long in muck heaps (straw mixed with faeces) due to the heat generated through decomposition/composting. Muck is a less risky medium for MAP than slurry when it comes to spreading on pastures, but only if it has been allowed to 'heat' for long enough. Controlling JD is aimed at preventing young calves coming into contact with MAP. The testing and removal of infected animals alone will fail to completely remove the infection and disease from the herd. Testing and culling, alongside management practices to eliminate calves becoming infected, will, however, in theory at least, eventually result in the elimination of JD from within the herd. Owing to the long incubation period this can take years and as some animals will not test positive until ten years post-infection or more, it will remain almost impossible to guarantee that a herd is completely MAP free until improved diagnostics or control measures come along.

The following critical control points should be borne in mind.

1. Identify positive animals through regular (at least annual) blood and, if required, faecal screening followed by removal of these animals from the herd as soon as practically possible. If there is a time delay between identification and removal the animal should be isolated and any faecal material, that is, bedding and slurry, be considered highly infectious and disposed of accordingly; never spread on pasture. Calves from the positive animal's last two pregnancies should not be retained or sold as breeding heifers or bulls.

2. Keep the calving area as clean as possible with minimal faecal contamination.

3. Prevent the contamination of water and feed troughs with faecal material. Mains water should be supplied and in modern, cleansable, dedicated troughs where possible. Natural water courses should be fenced off (Figure 17.1).

4. Avoid co-grazing with sheep as this poses a risk of cross infection between the species (Figure 17.2).

5. Do not source slurry and muck from other farms as they may contain MAP. Home generated slurry should not be spread on land that is going to be grazed within 55 weeks of application. Muck should not be spread on to fields that are going to be grazed within 6 months of application. Silage ground is usually a safe place to spread home generated muck and slurry depending on the future schedule for the pasture.

Diagnosis of Johne's disease

There are several diagnostic tests available to confirm the presence of MAP infection. A faecal smear stained with Ziehl–Neelsen (ZN) stain and viewed microscopically will detect MAP in the faeces of a *shedding* animal in 36% of cases. A more sensitive test to be carried out on faeces is the PCR with a sensitivity of 48%. PCR involves amplifying the MAP DNA to a more detectable level, which is then picked up in the lab by special techniques. The most sensitive test to detect MAP in the faeces of an infected cow is the combined *culture-PCR test*. The faeces are incubated for 6 weeks and the liquid from the culture then tested by PCR. This test will detect MAP in 86% of animals that are shedding. The disadvantage of culture-PCR test is that the process takes 6 weeks which is slow, especially for the quarantine testing of incoming animals.

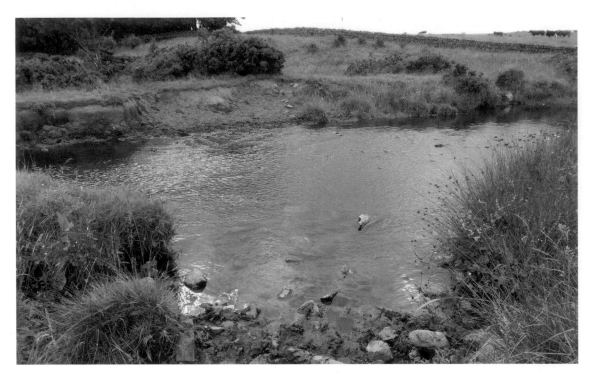

FIGURE 17.1 Poached area, contaminated with faeces, around a drinking hole in a natural water course

An antibody blood test is most commonly used in herd situations to screen animals for MAP infection or to test a suspected case. In the early stages of infection, the animal will not have mounted an immune response to the bug and there will be no detectable antibodies in the blood nor any bacteria in the faeces. As the disease progresses, however,

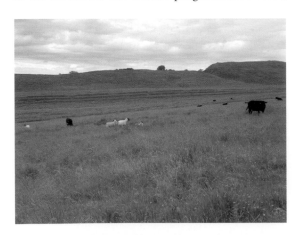

FIGURE 17.2 Autumn-calving suckler cows calving at grass and grazing with sheep

antibodies become evident as do bacteria in the faeces, although shedding can be intermittent, especially initially. Herds can choose to control and monitor MAP infection through a CHeCS health scheme (Chapter 18). This involves adhering to strict biosecurity and management measures as well as annual blood testing of all animals over 2 year of age. The number of animals in the herd testing positive on the annual screen dictates which risk level the herd is awarded. Risk level 5 is an infected herd with a high number of positive animals and poor control measures in place. Risk level 1 herds have two or more years of clear testing.

Biosecurity is important to prevent infected animals entering the farm. Where possible any replacements should be sourced from a CHeCS accredited, low risk herd that is undertaking annual testing and management practices to maintain freedom from JD. If the situation arises where cattle are not sourced from a risk level 1 herd or the status of the herd is unknown, the animal should be isolated, and blood and faeces tested for the presence of MAP. Individual negative results, however, do not provide a high level of assurance of freedom from infection due mainly to the very long incubation period.

Some points of note, first, false positive MAP antibody blood test results can occur for up to 3 months after a bTB test. This is due to similarity between MAP and the bTB bacterium, especially the avian variant which manages to stimulate the production of antibodies that are indistinguishable from MAP antibodies.

Second, there is a vaccine available for JD that does not succeed in eliminating infection but does reduce the number of bacteria shed in the faeces of infected animals, and also decreases the severity of clinical signs of JD so allowing the animal to remain productive in the herd for longer. Once vaccination of a herd is initiated, blood testing to monitor infection can no longer be carried out as a vaccinated animal will have antibodies. In addition, there are concerns that the close relationship between the Johne's bacterium and bTB may cause problems when interpreting the bTB skin test; the authorities need to be informed when this is the case.

THE 'DOWNER COW'

A 'downer cow' is an often-misused phrase used to describe a cow that is, simply, *down* but the veterinary industry defines it more precisely as a cow who is *recumbent and unable to rise despite treatment*. The cow is often bright and eating, sitting up, but unable to stand. The longer the cow is recumbent the more muscle and nerve damage occurs to the legs on which the cow is lying. This damage can occur after only 6 hours of being down on a hard surface and the situation progressively worsens. Ultimately this secondary complication may be the reason why the cow fails to rise, rather than the primary condition.

There are four *primary* reasons for a cow becoming recumbent in the first place.

1. **Trauma**, usually associated with a fall, bulling behaviour, a collision with machinery. A fractured pelvis, broken leg or joint dislocation, may result in a cow collapsing and staying down.
2. **Metabolic disease** such as milk fever (hypocalcaemia) and staggers (hypomagnesaemia) are classic causes of collapse.
3. **Neurological dysfunction**, for example, nerve damage following calving, or central nervous disease such as listeriosis. Damage to the nerves supplying the hind limb is a relatively common presentation in cows that have had a difficult calving.

The obturator and sciatic nerves can be affected due to the position of these nerves on the lining of the birth canal. They can be affected at the same time or independently of each other. Non-steroidal anti-inflammatories can be used as pain relief and/or steroids to reduce bruising/swelling around the nerve which may help speed recovery if administered in the early stages, that is, soon after the dystocia has occurred.

The sciatic nerve is the hind limb nerve most commonly affected (Hartnack, 2017). When this is the case cows *may* become recumbent but on most occasions, they are able to walk but with a characteristic gait. They are still able to extend the stifle, as those muscles are supplied by a different nerve, but they *knuckle over* on their fetlock joints. The sciatic nerve passes down the back of the hind limb; if intramuscular injections are administered in the back of the thigh, damage to the nerve may occur – another possible cause of this condition. Over time the condition will resolve but care needs to be taken to ensure that abrasions to the skin on the front of the fetlock do not result. Soft bedding or careful protective bandaging may help but great care with bandaging is needed as, the bandages are prone to digging in and making the situation worse.

The obturator nerve is responsible for keeping the leg *adducted*; underneath the body of the animal rather than splaying out to the side (Hartnack, 2017). Obturator nerve paralysis is characterised by cattle in a splay legged position, unable to stand. They require regular lifting and are usually able to stand once they are lifted to their feet. The injury also occurs when a cow has 'done the splits', typically on slippery concrete which tears the adductor muscles and possibly damages the obturator nerve too.

4. **Toxaemia** from bacterial disease such as acute *E. coli* mastitis, acute metritis or peritonitis, all of which are post-calving complications as discussed later in this chapter.

The initial cause of recumbency should be identified and treated as quickly as possible to reduce the likelihood of a true 'downer cow' ensuing. Thereafter nursing and 'TLC' is required as follows.

- Immediate movement of the cow to a clean, well-bedded lying area such as a well established straw yard or, if the weather is suitable, a paddock (simply spreading a covering of straw on clean concrete does not help – the cow still slips – the surface should be soft and comfortable to prevent abrasions and to allow sufficient grip to facilitate attempts to rise).
- Provision of ad lib good quality forage, water, and limited concentrate feed within easy reach of the recumbent animal.
- Turning of the patient every 3 hours to alternate which hind limb is bearing the weight. Once turned the limb that has been lain on should be massaged and manipulated (for example, repeatedly flexed and extended) to help stimulate blood flow to the muscles involved.
- Administration of anti-inflammatory drugs to reduce pain and inflammation in the affected muscles/tissues.
- Lactating downer cows should still be milked twice daily to reduce the discomfort of milk engorgement and to reduce the risk of *retention mastitis* – an udder infection resulting from stretching of the udder and teat and the dribbling of milk through an open teat sphincter which can therefore allow bugs to travel in.
- The cow should be kindly encouraged to rise occasionally if she is making no attempt herself. The cow can be encouraged to rise by mechanical means if she has made no attempt herself after 24 hours. A hoist or cow sling are most commonly used but floatation tanks are also available for hire and work very effectively. The operators, regardless of method, must be competent with the technique and the equipment used so as to ensure the welfare of the cow; an incorrect technique can do more harm than good. The operator also needs to ensure they take into consideration their own safety while working around the animal and during the lifting process. A cow should be lifted until she finds her feet and then gently lowered until she starts to weight bear. The legs can be massaged to restore blood flow, the bedding repositioned or changed and the cow milked as required. The duration the cow is lifted for depends on how well she tolerates the procedure and how comfortable she is. If she is distressed or making no attempt to move her legs or hold her own weight, she should be lifted for only the absolute minimum period of time to allow a quick bed change and massage. Where it is clearly painful the cow should be immediately lowered back down and veterinary advice sought. If good nursing and a clean, dry, comfortable environment cannot be provided, or if pain cannot be controlled, the cow should be euthanased before she is allowed to suffer further.

There are several factors associated with a poor prognosis, they include:

- hip lock at calving (especially if prolonged)
- 'doing the splits'
- hind limbs fully extended forwards (touching elbows)
- down on bare concrete for more than a few hours

- unable to stay sitting up, repeatedly falling back down on one side or other
- no attempts to rise
- attempting to rise on forelimbs only
- recumbent for 10 days or more with no clinical improvement.

Where one or more of these poor prognostic indicators prevail then euthanasia may well be warranted. Where a downer cow is comfortable, not displaying poor prognostic indicators, appears to be making progress and is able to receive good nursing and treatment as described above, then, under veterinary approval, the allowance of a reasonably long recovery period may be acceptable – in the authors' experience it is quite common for cows under these circumstances to rise after three weeks of recumbency.

METABOLIC DISORDERS

In the last trimester of pregnancy, through calving and into the early post-parturient period, cows are at risk of metabolic disease. Metabolic diseases are loosely defined as *chemical imbalances* in the body and in this context shall include *milk fever* (hypocalcaemia), *staggers* (hypomagnesaemia) and *ketosis* (slow fever, acetonaemia).

Milk fever (hypocalcaemia)

Milk fever is a metabolic disorder characterised by low blood calcium (hypocalcaemia). Calcium is required for muscles to function and as a result cows initially present with muscle twitching and irritability followed by weakness and then recumbency. The myometrium, the muscle of the uterus, is also weak and a prolonged calving or retained foetal membranes (RFM) may result from what is called *uterine inertia* (see later in chapter). The cow may fail to eructate (belch) and consequently becomes bloated, there may be a large amount of faeces in her rectum as a lack of rectal muscle

tone causes a failure of defaecation. The levels of calcium within the blood can be measured and hypocalcaemia confirmed although there is much debate on the type of test used and exactly which form of calcium to measure, that is, ionised calcium or total calcium. Treatment involves administering calcium borogluconate intravenously. This must be administered slowly as rapid administration may cause the heart to slow, sometimes to the point of stopping; some vets monitor heart rate during calcium administration for this reason. In mild cases administration under the skin *may suffice* but absorption is slow and according to some evidence simply inadequate. To aid absorption of subcutaneous calcium as much as possible, therefore, the bottle should be warmed and the large volume, typically 400 ml, divided between three separate sites. Low blood calcium results from the huge demand on calcium supply from the growing calf, muscular activity and the production of milk in late pregnancy through to early lactation. There is, actually, adequate calcium within the skeleton that can be mobilised, but it is the hormonal control of this mobilisation that may be at fault. Hormonal pathways under the influence of, principally, Vitamin D3, limit calcium excretion from the kidneys, increase gut absorption of calcium and increase calcium mobilisation from bone. The problem arises when the hormonal pathways are interfered with or cannot keep up with demand, this is usually not due to lack of production but a reduced sensitivity to the circulating hormones. Interestingly it is the exposure to high levels of dietary calcium in the dangerous build-up to calving that renders the cow less sensitive to the hormones and the Vitamin D3 so the cow is essentially 'starving in the face of plenty'. Older cows are more susceptible as they are less able to mobilise calcium but confoundedly produce more milk. Magnesium is also involved in the production and release of one of the hormones involved in calcium regulation, so hypomagnesaemia and hypocalcaemia are often interlinked. As alluded to, the mainstay of prevention of milk fever is to restrict dietary calcium intake in the prepartum period. This negative feedback loop then strongly activates the calcium raising hormone pathways so maintaining blood calcium levels at a time when they are prone to fall (Husband, 2005). Guidelines on calcium supplementation are provided in Chapter 10. Being a common condition in the dairy cow much work has been carried out to find other control measures. A fairly recent development was realising that changing the acidity of the cow's blood to a slightly acidic pH level causes an increase in the production of the calcium raising hormones and an increased sensitivity at the hormone binding sights – this is known as the *dietary cation–anion balance* (DCAB) concept (Husband, 2005). Adding certain salts to the diet is how the manipulation of blood pH is achieved in DCAB, but it can have serious consequences if mismanaged and needs to be supervised by a vet and nutritionist. The demand on the suckler cow is not sufficient to warrant calcium regulation at this level but the science exists to do so.

Staggers (hypomagnesaemia)

Staggers is a metabolic condition characterised by low blood magnesium – hypomagnesaemia. Magnesium has an essential role in nerve function so low magnesium levels result in neurological signs that are often very acute; staggers is a true veterinary emergency. Cows are initially depressed and dull followed by excitability, stiffness, twitching and salivation followed by collapse, spasms, seizures/convulsions ('fits') and death (Foster et al., 2007). If an animal is found alive, immediate treatment is required with magnesium sulphate administered subcutaneously and, often, calcium borogluconate administered intravenously. Magnesium sulphate must not be administered intravenously as it can cause a cardiac arrest and death. It was used as a lethal injection in the distant past, but its failure to reduce consciousness deemed it a cruel method and its use was rightly outlawed.

Blood magnesium levels can be easily and reliably tested but there is not usually enough time – diagnosis and treatment need to be decided on immediately. Cows do not store magnesium like they do, say, calcium, so they rely on a daily intake of magnesium from their diet. The complexity of magnesium intakes and absorption are discussed in Chapter 10. Often an *outbreak* of clinical cases will occur, frequently with a number of deaths. It may be difficult to establish a diagnosis from a dead animal as there are no distinguishing features of the condition on PME. Fluid extracted from the eye of a dead animal within 12 hours of death is, however, a good indicator of low magnesium levels and is useful in establishing a diagnosis (the magnesium levels in this fluid do not change after death as they do in the blood).

Where clinical cases of hypomagnesaemia or hypocalcaemia have occurred, it is likely that *subclinical disease* is present in the rest of the herd and they may be just 'teetering on the edge'. Blood testing 5–10 animals in the group to confirm a diagnosis of the subclinical state and, therefore, the prompt introduction of preventable measures, is advised.

Ketosis (slow fever, acetonaemia)

Ketosis, otherwise referred to as slow fever or acetonaemia, is a metabolic disease involving a fall and a change in type of metabolic energy levels in the body; it is very similar to twin lamb disease seen in sheep. Clinical signs are non-specific; cows present dull, depressed, inappetent and have poor rumen fill, that is, they appear empty. Neurological signs can be a feature of the disease with excessive salivation and licking of inanimate objects. Some people, but not all, can detect the smell of *pear drops* on the cow's breath. Ketosis arises when the cow's dietary intake is not supplying sufficient energy to satisfy her demands and she has to mobilise body fat to release energy. This process relies heavily on the liver which, somewhat ironically, itself then becomes clogged with the mobilised fat in the bloodstream – so called *fatty liver syndrome*. The fat is not an easy, readily usable form of energy for the body, so the fat is broken down into products which are. These products are called ketones or *ketone bodies* and include acetate, acetoacetate and beta-hydroxybutyrate. These ketones do perform as metabolic energy sources, but they are designed to be a temporary emergency supply only. Their presence in the bloodstream for any length of time does, sadly make the animal ill; this combined with the fatty liver syndrome leaves the animal with the overall syndrome of ketosis. It is commonly seen in dairy cows post-calving; cows who are producing huge volumes of milk and are unable to eat as much as they need to match their energy demand. The energy demand placed on the suckler cow is not as great and although there will be some fat mobilisation this can usually be tolerated by the liver and ketosis is not seen under normal circumstances. Cows with an extreme body condition score, however, scoring 1 or 5, are more likely to suffer from ketosis. Very thin cows are extremely energy deficient so end up relying heavily on ketones released from what little fat they have (usually abdominal). Very fat cows have so much fat that mobilising even a small percentage of it releases significant amounts of ketones and to add to her problems the high bodily fat levels tend to equate to high levels of fat in the circulation which we know clogs up the liver in fatty liver syndrome. For this and other reasons, every effort should be made to achieve target condition scores at key points in the production cycle (Chapter 10).

Sickness is another risk factor in ketosis. If a cow is sick with metritis, mastitis or peritonitis post-calving and goes off her food, she will need to mobilise body fat, produce a high level of ketones and again display signs of ketosis. Here we are reminded that ketosis is a problem that is a clinical sign of other problems, it is secondary to an illness or nutritional shortfall and not in itself a primary disease.

Treatment of ketosis involves supplying alternative energy supplies that are safer than ketones, for example, oral propylene glycol, or, alternatively, or additionally, encouraging the body to try and produce its own glucose as it normally would – this can be achieved with glucocorticoid injections. The primary cause of inappetence or energy shortfall needs to be identified and corrected and an appropriately balanced diet needs re-establishing to restore normal energy balance.

Ketosis in an individual sick animal is an acute and extreme indication of energy deficiency usually secondary to inappetence. When a problem in the herd overall it is an indication of poor nutritional management which needs correcting. A longer-term consequence of poor nutritional management is poor fertility. A cow will not be fertile, ovulate or conceive, if her energy balance is incorrect. She may not return to oestrus at all, this is called *anoestrus*. Hormonal treatment can be used to induce oestrus such as intravaginal progesterone devices. If, however, a cow is in deep anoestrus and getting in-calf is not 'on her agenda' as she is not metabolically stable enough to do so because of poor nutritional management then the management system has failed her; using artificial hormonal manipulation is a sticking plaster for the bigger problem created by management. Ovarian cysts are a similar warning of metabolic energy dysfunction, that is, ketosis. Ovarian cysts result when a cow starts to come into oestrus but fails to ovulate properly and the follicle remains on the ovary and enlarges to become a cyst. An in-depth explanation of the oestrus cycle is included in Chapter 10. Cysts are defined as a structure present on the ovary, greater than 2.5 cm in diameter, and in the absence of a corpus luteum. There are two classifications of ovarian cyst; a follicular cyst and a luteal cyst. A follicular cyst is a fluid-filled cyst that secretes oestrogen. High oestrogen levels prevent the development of new follicles but also induce the cow to display bulling behaviour out of her normal cycle and sometimes persistently – referred to amusingly as *nymphomania*. A luteal cyst contains solid tissue that produces progesterone. This progesterone suppresses the release of LH and prevents oestrus and ovulation. Hormonal injections and implants can be used to treat cows with cysts but again there should be a focus on why the cow was unable to ovulate normally. Cystic ovarian disease is not often encountered in suckler cows and again is predominantly a production disease of the dairy cow.

VAGINAL/CERVICAL PROLAPSE

Vaginal and cervical prolapse is a condition mostly seen in late pregnancy, but cases can occur at any time. The vagina and/or cervix everts and protrudes from the vulva appearing like a large, red, smooth football (Figure 17.3). When the cervix is involved the appearance changes – a prolapsed cervix looks like a large, red, swollen, flower head. The condition is seen late in pregnancy as the ligaments of the pelvis relax and the soft tissues of the perineum can no longer hold the vagina behind the vulva. Fat cows are predisposed, and it has been suggested that there is a hereditary component to the condition. The vagina may only protrude when the cow lies down as the weight of the

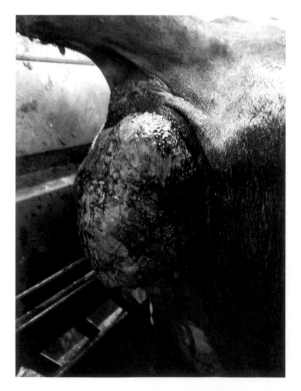

FIGURE 17.3 A vaginal prolapse in a suckler cow 3 weeks pre-calving

calf presses back into the pelvic area, only for the prolapse to slip back into the cow when she stands up. In this case it does not require any further attention. Where the vagina remains outside of the cow for periods longer than those lying down then reasonably prompt veterinary attention is required albeit not an emergency as would be a uterine prolapse. The cow may be unable to urinate when the vagina is prolapsed as the exit of the urethra may be occluded. The vagina is also susceptible to damage when outside the cow. Where either is scenario applies the situation is more urgent.

The attending vet will, first, administer an epidural anaesthetic, to prevent the cow from straining when the vagina is re-introduced back through the vulva, and also as a very effective form of pain relief for during the procedure. The vagina will be cleaned and examined for damage. With the application of a lubricant the prolapse is then gently pushed back through the vulva and *re-everted* so it lies in the correct anatomical position. A purse string suture, called a 'Buhner suture', is then applied to the deep base of the vulval lips to prevent the vagina from re-prolapsing (Momont, 2005). There is absolutely a right and a wrong way to suture a vulva – it is often done wrong – the correct method must be pursued or the procedure will fail; the prolapse will recur and the vulva will be irreparably torn. Mattress or simple sutures must not be used, it has to be a purse string suture. If the cow is in late gestation, she requires careful monitoring as calving approaches as the suture will need to be removed pre-calving.

There can be several complications subsequent to a vaginal prolapse. Incomplete cervical dilation at calving is a common sequel as the cervix is likely to have been traumatised when outside the cow and inflammation and the resulting scar tissue will prevent compete dilation. Abortion is more likely than normal following vaginal prolapse as the cervix, which usually forms a tight seal protecting the calf, has been stretched and partially opened so allowing bacteria to enter the uterus and cause a placentitis. Cows that have suffered from a vaginal prolapse should not be re-bred as not only is poor future dilation of the scarred birth canal a likelihood but the prolapse tendency may be genetically propagated through subsequent generation.

DYSTOCIA (ABNORMAL OR DIFFICULT BIRTH)

Dystocia, defined in terms of cows giving birth, is a calving requiring human intervention because of a prolonged first- or second-stage labour.

This can be due a variety of reasons.

- Malpresentation, where the head and two forelimbs of the calf are not present in the birth canal and manipulation is required to correct it.
- Feto-maternal disproportion, where the calf is simply too big for the cow to 'push out' on her own and additional force is required (Figure 17.4).
- Calf deformity. A deformed calf may prevent itself from passing through the birth canal. A *schistosoma reflexus* calf is an example. This deformity is an extreme curvature of the spine resulting in four legs and a head all bent backwards to the point of being in close proximity with each other and with a failure of the belly wall to fuse, meaning that the organs of the calf are not enclosed within a body cavity and are clearly hanging out and visible (Figure 17.5).
- An abnormality of the birth canal preventing passage of the calf, such as a tumour, a bony mass, an abscess or most commonly a failure of the cervix to dilate and/or a twisted uterus.
- Uterine inertia, where the myometrium of the uterus fails to contract, and labour does not progress. This can occur in older cows or where there has been damage to the uterus. It also occurs in hypocalcaemia or any situation of illness, weakness, exhaustion, or old age.

It could be said that dealing with dystocia, whether as a vet or as a farmer is inevitable, just

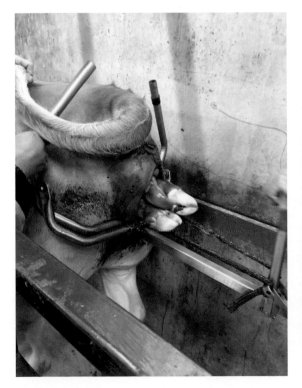

FIGURE 17.4 Calf receiving traction to assist with delivery

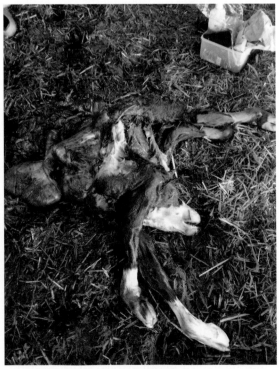

FIGURE 17.5 *Schistosoma reflexus* calf

part of the job … calve the cow and move on to the next one! Dystocia, however, is not normal, it is a significant welfare issue for the cow and the calf and it incurs significant costs: cow and calf mortality, consequent infertility, consequent poor milk yield, reduced longevity, higher cull rates, poor growth rates in the calf, increased neonatal disease incidence and veterinary costs for the initial intervention and then all the many knock-on problems. All for a bigger calf? It is simply not acceptable. There will, of course, always be a proportion of calvings that require human intervention, for example, a leg back or a set of twins, but the vast proportion of assisted calvings are due to feto-maternal disproportion, the calf is simply too big to pass through the mother's pelvis and severe traction or a caesarean is required. 'Hard pulls' or caesareans are largely preventable. Where they occur more than just the odd time, they are very likely to signify a failure of management and strategy on the farm. Recommendations to avoid dystocia due to feto-maternal disproportion are discussed in Chapters 10 and 11. To monitor the success of any management changes and intervention rates there needs to be continuous monitoring. A suggested calving grading score could be: Grade 1 – no assistance; Grade 2 – mild slight corrections usually carried out by the stockperson; Grade 3 – heavy traction with calving aid or extensive correction, or caesarean section (Dobson et al., 2008). There have been attempts to calculate the cost of a difficult calving for the dairy herd. A study carried out from a survey of dairy farms using beef semen suggested that the cost of a slightly difficult calving was £110 and a seriously difficult calving between £350 and £400 (McGuirk et al., 2007). The cost of a caesarean in the UK in 2020 can range from £400–450 for necessary medicines and the procedure alone. That is without the additional time commitment of aftercare labour, the risk of calf and cow mortality, and subsequent reduced fertility, health and lifetime productivity. In other words, the true cost of a caesarean is much higher than the £400 quoted for an average grade 3 calving, much higher!

Regular supervision of calving cows is required to detect any problems promptly; the Konefal method of daytime calving has been adopted by some to increase the number of daytime calvings when they can be observed more closely. Konefal, based in Manitoba, reported that feeding twice daily, once at 11 am–12 noon and again at 9.30–10 pm, resulted in 75% of his cows calving between 7 am and 7 pm. This somewhat inexplicable regime would, were it to be tried, be started 1 month pre-calving and continue through the calving period (Herring, 2014).

When does a birth turn from normal to abnormal and require assistance?

It is difficult to know just when to intervene in a calving and many texts quote a time from the water sac being present at the vulva – but this is not always visible and may rupture inside the cow. In the authors' opinions, if a cow is actively straining with strong frequent abdominal contractions for 1 hour with no progress, an internal examination is required. If upon internal examination the problem is not readily identified and corrected a vet should be called for. The prognosis for the cow and calf is better if intervention occurs sooner rather than later and more so if in the hands of trained personnel.

Malpresentation

Most calves are presented in a forward direction (anterior) with the nose resting on top of the front legs. On occasion this is not the case and there will be an unexpected part of the calf in the birth canal, or, none at all. The calf can, hopefully, be carefully and skilfully manipulated within the cow into the correct presentation before gentle traction is applied to complete the calving process. The person providing the assistance should clean and disinfect their hands and arms before entering the cow, and should preferably wear arm length disposable obstetric gloves. Care should be taken not to cause damage to the cow, it is quite feasible for a calf's foot to tear the uterus and enter the abdomen if a correction is mismanaged. This does happen occasionally and when it does it causes peritonitis that carries a poor prognosis; euthanasia should be considered or an attempt made to repair the hole surgically through a flank incision (rather like a caesarean). Often, however, the hole is in the area of the uterus in the pelvic cavity and therefore inaccessible, so, it would be common for the attending vet to advise against this difficult course of action. Before attempting to apply traction to the calf it is important the cervix is fully dilated. If a calf is pulled through a partially closed cervix it may tear instead of stretch/dilate and worse still the tear may extend back to the uterus. Worst of all the un-dilated cervix can be partially or entirely ripped off the body of the uterus leaving a massive hole into the abdomen/peritoneal cavity. These detachments are normally the top half of the attachment of the cervix to the uterus, that is, running from 9 o'clock to 3 o'clock but, as stated, it can be a full circumference detachment. If this occurs or if a cervical tear extends to the uterus, peritonitis will occur and in the case of large tears and detachments death is guaranteed and no attempt should be made to 'hope for the best' – euthanasia should be employed.

Lubrication always helps to get a large thing through a small hole! It helps the cow, and it helps the operator. In the authors' experience lubrication is massively under-utilised on farm and could make such a difference. Powdered lubricants exist – these mix with water or uterine fluid to become a mucoid lubricant. Powder can be useful as it can be carried in the hand to the point in the birth canal where it is needed. Liquid lubricants are also very good. Standard liquids or powders made into liquid can be delivered into the uterus or birth canal using a stomach tube and hand pump.

What's the difference between a vet and a farmer? ... Lubricant! (Anon.)

Common malpresentations demonstrated in Figure 17.6 include the following.

- **Backwards (posterior presentation)**. Two back legs and a tail are present in the birth canal. This does not require correction; the calf can be pulled backwards from the cow. The complication here, however, is that the umbilical cord is often wrapped around one back thigh, and even when it is not the cord still tends to get compressed during delivery. This means a slow or difficult backwards delivery is more likely to result in a hypoxic or dead calf.

- **Leg or legs back**. There is only the head and one, or neither, leg present in the birth canal. Care should be taken to reach into the uterus and locate the missing leg(s). It/they may be just slightly retracted, bent at the knee (Figure 17.6b), or right back alongside the calf's body (Figure 17.6a). A calf should not be pulled from a cow with either or both legs back; the presentation should be corrected to avoid unnecessary friction and unnecessary traction.

- **Malposition of the head**. This can be difficult to correct; the head may be pointing downwards (Figure 17.6e) and the nose tilted below the rim of the pelvis, or, the calf may have its head turned to the side looking back at its tail (Figure 17.6d). The head needs to be skilfully guided and flipped round into position with an appropriately positioned hand on the side of the head or nose. Once in a better position a head rope is nearly always useful. A head rope or head wire, formed into a loop, should be passed over the back of the head of the calf and placed behind the ears – that should usually be enough for the rope or wire to grip the back of the neck. Some operators complete the loop and place the knot in the calf's mouth – this is controversial as it may damage the calf's jaw and it reduces the streamline nature of the head with an otherwise closed mouth. The argument that closing the noose in the mouth prevents the rope from slipping is misleading as the rope only slips when it is not correctly placed behind the neck in the first place; were an incorrectly placed noose able to grip only because it was in the mouth would imply the noose is compressing

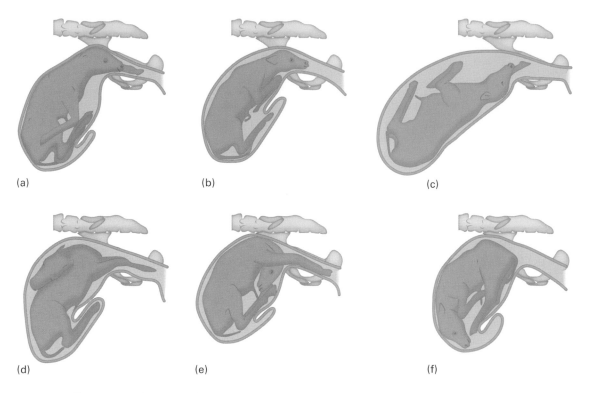

(a)　　　　　　　　　(b)　　　　　　　　　(c)

(d)　　　　　　　　　(e)　　　　　　　　　(f)

FIGURE 17.6 Common malpresentations

the cranium or possibly even the nose/upper jaw, which would be very dangerous for the calf. Traction should always be applied to the calf's legs at the same time as the head, the calf should never be pulled by the head alone; this risks neck injury and makes extraction more difficult as the legs concertina rather than slide streamlined with the head. Conversely, if only the legs are pulled, and not the head, in a situation where the head needs a little traction too, then it is the head and neck that concertina rather than the legs again making delivery difficult if not impossible.

... What's the difference between a vet and a farmer apart from lubricant? ... A head rope! (Anon.)

- **Breach (Figure 17.6f)**. A breach presentation is where there is a tail only in the birth canal, the calf is coming tail first with its hind legs

tucked underneath it. This can be corrected by pushing the rump of the calf forward to create space behind the calf and then reaching down, locating the hock, drawing the hock up towards the cervix and then one leg at a time extending the hock so the hind foot is present in the birth canal. This is tricky and the risk of uterine rupture, from the point of the calf's hoof, is high. Once both hind feet are successfully present in a dilated birth canal the calf can be calved in posterior presentation.

- **Upside down**. A calf, whether forward or backward, may be upside down in the uterus (Figure 17.6c). The calf needs to be rotated along its long axis, that is, as if it was on a spit! In a cow with a large pelvis where the calf is not too big this can sometimes be relatively easy, it can, however, be very difficult. It is very important to mention here that in many cases of so called 'upside down' calf presentations, the problem is actually one of uterine torsion which has gone

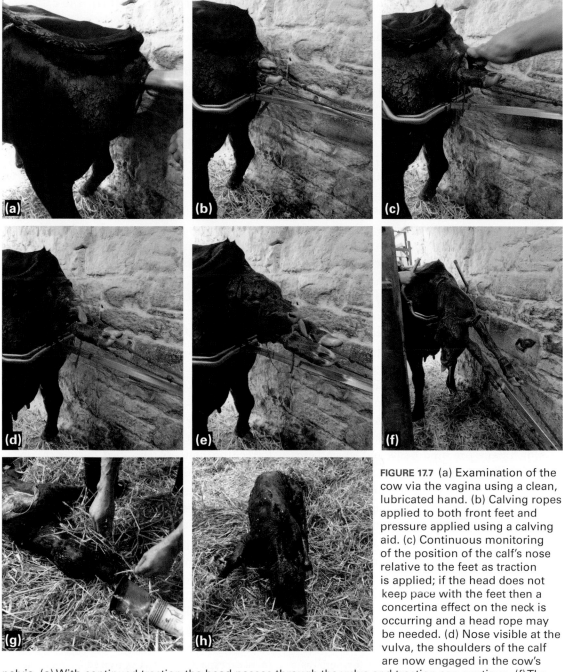

FIGURE 17.7 (a) Examination of the cow via the vagina using a clean, lubricated hand. (b) Calving ropes applied to both front feet and pressure applied using a calving aid. (c) Continuous monitoring of the position of the calf's nose relative to the feet as traction is applied; if the head does not keep pace with the feet then a concertina effect on the neck is occurring and a head rope may be needed. (d) Nose visible at the vulva, the shoulders of the calf are now engaged in the cow's pelvis. (e) With continued traction the head passes through the vulva and traction can continue. (f) The calf hips are now engaged in the cow's pelvis at this stage and traction continues and may need to be increased a little. Rotating the calf slightly off the vertical plane may help at this stage. Pushing the bar of the aid down at this stage can also help but the best approach is to alternate the bar up and down a little to see which works best. The bar can be pushed too far down and cause the calf to jam at the hips or stifles. (g) The calf is born on to a clean, dry, straw bed and is stimulated to breath using a stem of straw to tickle the inside of the nostrils. An aspirator/resuscitator designed to both remove birthing fluid from the calf's airways and to inflate the lungs can be employed but requires care and training. (h) Calf has been licked by its mother and is now attempting to stand.

unnoticed by the stockperson, that is, the 180 degree twist has not blocked the cervix sufficiently to prevent a hand passing through. The corrective action in both cases is, however, really the same – to *swing the calf* back round to the correct orientation and in doing so the uterus, if twisted, usually follows. What can go wrong? When the calf truly is 'upside down', in the absence of a uterine orsion, the correction of the calf can sometimes actually create a uterine torsion – that is a headache and it is probably time to call the vet. *Swinging calves*, whether part of a uterine torsion or just simply upside down is a knack that vets learn and may be able to pass on to the stockperson – it is considered by some to be extremely difficult. Proprietary devices exist to help with this – these calf twisters attach to short ropes applied to the calf's legs and apply rotational torsion force to the calf via the ropes and legs. Care is needed in their use and should only be attempted by trained personnel – they can break the legs of the calf.

- **Twins (or triplets)**. Multiple foetus births can be born normally but occasionally are tangled up and need unravelling for delivery. This is a case of working out which limbs are fore limbs, which limbs are hind limbs and which heads and limbs belong to which body. It cannot be stressed how important it is to take great care over establishing this – pulling on the wrong parts is disastrous for obvious reasons. The first thing to practice is knowing a front leg from a back leg – this can be practised on a calf at leisure. The rule of thumb is that a front leg's last two joints bend the same way, in a back leg they don't! Care needs to be taken not to mistake a hock for an elbow. There are two joints below an elbow, one below a hock. The next thing to practice at leisure on a live calf (or perhaps a dead calf before it is taken away) is being able to follow legs up to the body and back down the other legs so as to establish when legs belong to the same body and when they do not.
- **Foeto-maternal disproportion**. The most common (and avoidable) form of dystocia is

foeto-maternal disproportion. The calf is too big, or the cow's pelvis is too small. This requires additional force to extract the calf from the cow. This may just be a matter of force; ropes are placed above the first main joint of both legs and pulled by hand, lever, pulley or by way of a mechanical calving aid. A calving aid is a metal frame attached to a pole with a ratchet mechanism, seen in Figure 17.4. It can apply significant force to a calf and cow and should be used with caution. Figure 17.8(a–h) shows the use of a calving aid. If the force required seems too strong, that is, hard work for an averagely strong person, then providing lubrication and head ropes have already been employed, a caesarean section is needed.

CAESAREAN SECTION

A caesarean section is the surgical removal of the foetus, at term, from the uterus via the abdominal wall. Contrary to popular belief Julius Caesar was *not* born by this means; *caesar* is Latin for *dissection*. In those days caesareans were crudely performed on mothers who died during childbirth – hence dissection. Such children were described as *not having been born* and it was decided that to *not have been born* was, for reasons best known to them, befitting of a Roman Emperor! So, bizarrely, the name was pinched for Julius, or so the story goes! These days the aim of a caesarean section is to achieve a safe and pain free delivery of the foetus where normal delivery is not possible and to achieve a full recovery of the mother. The aim with the foetus is to preserve life but the foetus may already be dead before the operation commences, especially if an attempt to correct a severe dystocia was persevered with. The operation is still occasionally performed in haste in the event of the death of the mother where the aim simply becomes to extract a live calf before the failure of the placental circulation kills the foetus. In practice this period does not seem to be very long, if it exists at all, as the processes leading to the death of the mother usually kill the foetus also. One situation where the chances of foetal survival improve is when the mother, the cow, is euthanased by shooting and an emergency caesarean section immediately performed.

Deciding on whether and when to do a caesarean section is not an easy decision. If too much force is applied to a calf during obstetrical traction, then it may cause irreparable damage to the cow and/or the calf and there is a risk to the life of both. Calves can suffer fractured legs, spinal injuries, nerve damage of the hind limbs, bruised or fractured ribs and liver rupture, all from excessive traction. The calf may get stuck in the birth canal, this usually happens as the hips fail to pass through the pelvis and is known as *hip lock*. The calf soon dies as a result and then has to be cut into pieces to be removed from the cow, by which time the cow has suffered severe trauma to her pelvis and birth canal and pressure on the nerves that supply the back legs; she is likely to be unable to rise and will therefore become a downer cow; many of these cows are euthanased. A caesarean may be the obvious solution but let's keep this decision in perspective; it is a major operation with the risk of mortality to the cow from peritonitis and she will be less fertile if she is required to rebreed. An old cow who has fulfilled her expected lifetime quota of calf production could be argued as definitely warranting a caesarean for this one last calf prior to culling. A more difficult decision is the young cow or heifer who has a lifetime of calf production ahead of her – a caesarean may leave her infertile and prevent the future birth of several calves, a delivery solution that loses the life of the calf that is stuck may actually preserve the life of the heifer and furthermore the potential lives of several subsequent calves. This is a difficult area for debate involving economics, welfare, animal rights and ethics. The starting point in any 'on-the-spot' decision making will be the immediate welfare of the animals involved.

An experienced stockperson usually knows what force can safely be applied with a calving aid,

and when to call for veterinary assistance; they may also be very good at knowing when a caesarean is needed. The vet will, nevertheless, through professional obligation, examine the cow and offer an opinion having assessed the birth canal and the size of the calf. There are subtle indications a caesarean may be required: if the head is not able to engage in the birth canal with gentle traction from a head rope, if the forelimbs of the calf are crossed in the pelvis due to compression of the shoulders, if the calf is under mild traction and a hand cannot be passed around the elbows and shoulders of the calf once it is engaged in the birth canal.

Once the decision has been made to carry out a caesarean operation, preparation should be made for surgery, calmly but fairly swiftly, depending on the exact circumstances.

The cow needs to be adequately restrained for the safety of all personnel and for the cow (Figure 17.8). The operation is usually carried out with the cow standing; the incision will be made in the left flank, just behind the ribs. The surgeon can carry out a better job if he or she is not in constant fear of being kicked or even worse knocked to the ground and stood on. A calving gate or crush with bars or a solid side between the cow's legs and the surgeon is preferable. The cow's left flank needs to be clipped and thoroughly cleaned with warm, clean water and detergent and then skin disinfectant. Local anaesthetic is then injected into the skin and musculature or a 'nerve block' is performed which numbs the nerves supplying the left flank nearer where they exit the spinal cord. The surgery itself involves incising the skin and muscle layers, accessing the uterus and, after careful positioning, incising the uterus and removing the calf. The uterus, muscle layers and skin are then stitched back together (Figure 17.9). NSAIDs are administered to provide pain relief and if, as is usual under farm conditions, infection is considered a risk, antibiotics will be administered. These drugs are best given before surgery commences so they have time to work.

The survival of the cow after a caesarean is largely down to the quality of the surgery on the

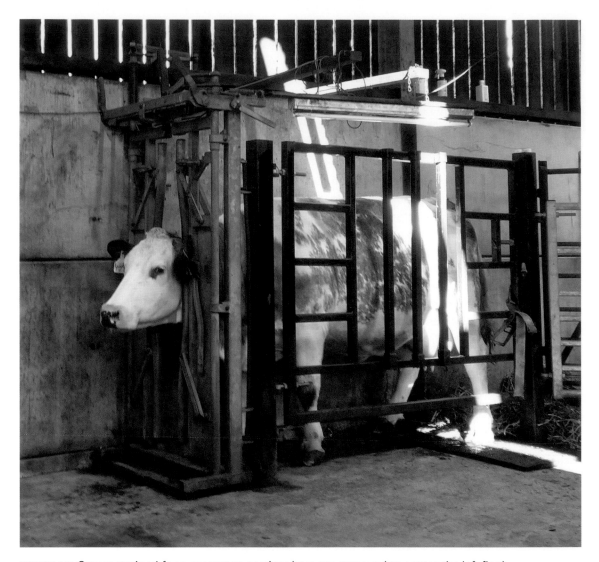

FIGURE 17.8 Cow restrained for a caesarean section; bars are removed to access the left flank

day and this can be affected by many factors. There are, however, critical actions on the lead up to surgery that can make a huge difference to survival rate.

1. **Not waiting too long**. If there is a calving difficulty that cannot be rectified easily then veterinary assistance should be called for without undue delay. A cow that has undergone a long stressful labour with multiple dirty hands within the uterus is far less likely to survive a caesarean section than a cow that was promptly

and hygienically attended to by a vet. On first examination if the calf is unresponsive, is dry and has a swollen head and tongue, these are all indications that second-stage labour has been going on for a long time and the prognosis for the cow and calf is already compromised.

2. **Cleanliness**. The crush, surrounding area, personnel, water, buckets and equipment need to be spotlessly clean. Caesarean sections carried out in a dirty environment and without clean equipment and water are at a high risk of

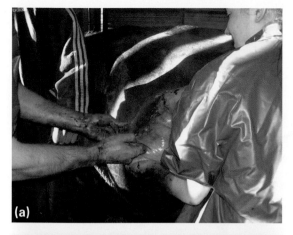

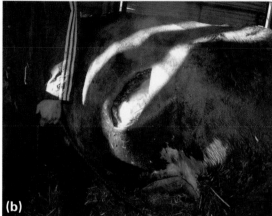

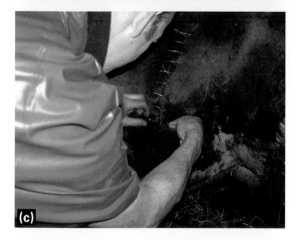

FIGURE 17.9 A series of photographs from a caesarean operation performed on the left flank of a standing cow: (a) the uterus is exteriorised from the abdomen and the hole where the calf passed through is stitched securely; (b) the uterus is returned to the abdomen; (c) the muscle layers and skin are stitched

post-operative infections due to direct contact with bacteria and those in the air and dust.

3. **After care**. The cow has undergone major abdominal surgery after a prolonged labour. She needs to be looked after and nursed; free access to clean water, a deep clean straw bed, easy access to fresh appetising food, timely administration of medications, and some peace and quiet to allow the cow and calf to bond and suckle (Figure 17.10).

There are occasions when the calf is dead within the cow. It can, in the early stages, be difficult to tell if the calf is dead or alive and this can influence decision making. A live calf may fidget about in the uterus, have tone in its anus, its tongue may move, it may retract a limb or have a pulse in its tail; some live calves will, however, lie completely still making it difficult to tell. Sometimes the placenta separates from the uterus and is pushed past the calf, and placenta and cotyledons are visible at the vulva, this is a good indication the calf is dead. A calf that has been dead for a period of time will be smelly, distended with gas and the hair will start to come away from the skin. A caesarean can be performed on a freshly dead calf but bacterial multiplication and putrefaction occur very quickly after death; performing a caesarean in these cases causes bacteria to be released into the abdomen of the cow causing peritonitis and a very grave prognosis, so grave that surgery is rarely attempted in these cases. If a calf is dead it may be possible instead to cut the calf up within the cow; a procedure described often as an *embryotomy* but more correctly a *foetotomy*. This is performed using an instrument called an *embryotome* or *foetotome* – a pair of fused copper/stainless steel barrels rather like a shot gun barrel or, a DIY version being, usually, a single tube, threaded with a cutting wire. This is best carried out by a vet as there is great risk to the cow from wire damage if it is not performed correctly.

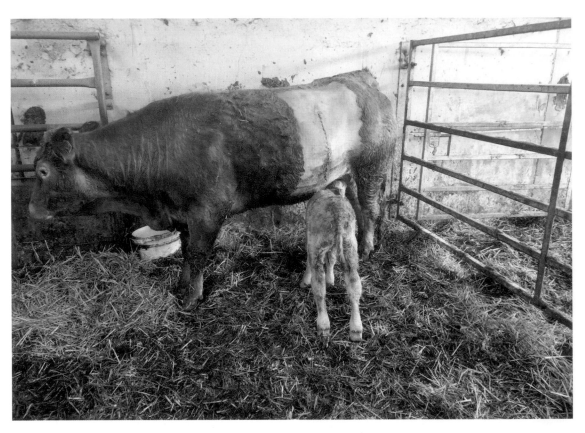

FIGURE 17.10 A cow post-caesarean section allowing her calf to suck

ABNORMALITIES OF THE BIRTH CANAL RESULTING IN DYSTOCIA

Inadequate vulval dilation

Stricture or tightening at the vulva, where the soft tissues and musculature of the vulva have failed to relax, can be a problem even though there is room for the calf to pass through the pelvis and the cervix. A veterinary procedure called an *episiotomy* can be used to allow passage of the calf. An episiotomy involves making an incision in the vulva either to the left or right of the anus. If the perineum were a clock face, and the anus was 12 o'clock, the incision would be at either 10 or 2 o'clock. An epidural injection is administered to numb the perineum before the incision is made. After the calf is removed the incision is stitched so

the normal conformation of the vulva is retained. In contrast, if a cow calves, assisted or unassisted, it is possible, if the vulva has not relaxed, for the vulva to tear in an uncontrolled manner. If the tear occurs and it extends into the anus and rectum then there is a risk of continual faecal contamination of the vagina with faecal material. Tears such as this are difficult to repair as the tissue is bruised, swollen and heavily contaminated with faecal material. They are often better left to heal alone without stitches, a decision best made by a vet. The cow may need to be culled and not re-bred.

Uterine torsion

Uterine torsion is defined as where the uterus has twisted within the cow on its longitudinal axis, which results in a twist just before, at, or just behind

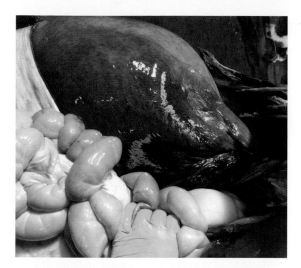

FIGURE 17.11 Post-mortem examination of a cow that died due to a twisted uterus – note the purple colour of the uterus as it had a reduced blood supply; sequestration of blood, shock and toxaemia would be the fatal factors

the cervix, known as *pre-cervical* or *post-cervical*, respectively. This twist inevitably constricts the birth canal and prevents passage of the calf. In addition, the twist reduces the blood supply to both the uterus and the calf (Figure 17.11). Calf mortality is typically high when associated with uterine torsion as it represents prolonged labour and a lack of oxygen. This condition is seen more commonly in dairy cattle; with an estimated prevalence of 0.24% accounting for up to 22% of all veterinary attended dystocia (Lyons and Gordon, 2013). It is thought that there are two factors that predispose a cow to a uterine torsion; the first is anatomical, how the uterus is suspended in the abdomen, and the second, relates to how the cow rises to her feet, first rising on her hind limbs and then her knees allowing the uterus the freedom to swing with the weight of the calf in only one uterine horn (Noakes, 2009). A torsion can be diagnosed by examination of the vagina where spiral folds are palpated. It may be possible to reach the calf through the twisted cervix, creating a feeling rather like putting ones hand down a toilet, but in some cases where the uterus has twisted more than 360° the vagina is a 'dead end' and the calf cannot be reached. A

uterine torsion is much more likely to be anti-clockwise (when the cow is viewed from behind) than clockwise. Correction can be achieved in the standing cow via the vagina if the calf can be felt. A hand is placed against the shoulder of the calf and after gaining some momentum the calf is 'swung' clockwise and the twist corrected. This is often facilitated by spontaneous movements of the calf and is far harder to achieve if the calf is dead. If the calf is large, the uterus is dry or there is little room within the abdomen of the cow, the correction may not be possible in the standing cow. An alternative approach is to 'cast' the cow. Casting involves applying ropes to the cow in a specific manor such that pulling on them results in the cow lying down. The vet lies behind the cow and, per vaginum, *holds the calf still* while the cow is then rolled left or right, depending on the direction of the twist. Techniques are described where external forces applied to the flank of the cow may aid in rotating the uterus, in the authors' experience this is usually unsuccessful and may even risk ruptur-ing the uterus so should probably be best avoided. Tools mentioned above for the upside down calf, such as a 'calf twister' or 'detorsion rod' have been designed to help in correcting a uterine torsion and are the preferred method of correction for *some* vets. Immediately post-correction it is unlikely the cervix is sufficiently dilated to allow parturi-tion as the cervix has not been stimulated by the calf's head and front feet. At this point the tempta-tion to rush and pull the calf through this poorly dilated cervix must be resisted. This is a common scenario for tearing of the cervix and possibly the uterus – both described earlier in this chapter. The cow should, instead, be allowed time to continue to calve as normal, as, aside from the torsion, there is likely to be no other reason for calving not to proceed (the administration of calcium boroglu-conate may, however, be appropriate). If, however, a reason becomes apparent why, aside from the poorly dilated cervix, a normal calving will not proceed, or, a reason for urgent extraction of the calf exists, then an immediate caesarean would, despite all the hard work, become appropriate. In the former case of the cow being allowed time to calve normally then, if there has been no progress within an hour or two, the cow should be examined again and assisted accordingly.

POST-CALVING COMPLICATIONS

Haemorrhage

Even a normal calving is quite bloody; there may be a fair amount of blood from the lining of the cow's uterus and from the placenta and the calf following rupture of the umbilicus. The more traumatic the birth the more bleeding is likely from the lining of the uterus, that is, from the damaged placentomes, but the haemorrhage in its own right is not usually a problem – as the uterus constricts post-calving, the blood vessels constrict and the bleeding stops; this process can be artificially augmented by the administration of oxytocin in severe cases where it is considered necessary (Momont, 2005). Haemorrhage associated with rupture of the vaginal artery, however, is a life-threatening condition. There are two vaginal arteries, they run along the left and right wall of the vagina and in close association with the cervix. If the cervix is not fully dilated when traction is applied to the calf and the cervix tears, or if the vagina is overly stretched and torn during delivery, there is a risk that one or both of these arteries will also tear. If this occurs, large quantities of blood will gush from the vulva; within minutes the cow becomes weak and wobbly and immediate action is required. Veterinary attendance should be summoned immediately but while waiting a hand should be inserted into the vagina and through calm and patient feeling, the source of the hot pulsing blood found. It will hopefully be appreciable that the blood is coming from a small, 5 mm diameter, pulsing tubular structure that is the bleeding end of the torn artery. The artery should be pinched shut with thumb and forefinger while waiting for the vet. If the operator is unable to appreciate the finer details of the structures then blunt pressure can be applied to what is thought to be the haemorrhaging area, maybe using a wad of cloth. If even that area is not locatable then a bath towel should be pushed into the vagina which will apply pressure until the vet arrives. The vet will use forceps to clamp the artery; it may be impossible to ligate the artery in which case the forceps may be left in place for up to a week to ensure there is clot formation and fibrosis before they are removed. The vet may apply a leash to the forceps and suture them to the skin near the vulva so that if the forceps detach, the farmer will be alerted by them hanging from the leash. It also means the expensive forceps are not lost! Depending on the amount of blood loss, the cow may require additional supportive therapy and in some cases a blood transfusion may need to be performed using blood from a healthy herd compatriot.

Uterine prolapse

The uterine prolapse is a life-threatening condition that usually occurs immediately after or within a few hours of calving. It involves the large post gravid uterus everting itself, inside out, through the still open cervix and birth canal, to hang outside the vulva of the cow; the cotyledons that were on the inside of the uterus now appear on the outside (Figure 17.12).

There are many theories as to what causes the uterus to prolapse. Hypocalcaemia increases the risk of prolapse three-fold, probably related to lack of muscular tone or floppiness of the uterus, and any hypocalcaemia suspected or detected should be corrected as part of the treatment of a uterine prolapse. Some vets will give calcium boro-gluconate routinely to cases. It is something the farmer may be wise to do while waiting for the vet to arrive. The birth of a large calf also increases the risk of uterine prolapse; it is thought that air is unable to pass by the calf and therefore suction is created beyond the calf that essentially pulls the uterus out with the calf or at least some way out, at least enough to evert the tip of the horn as far

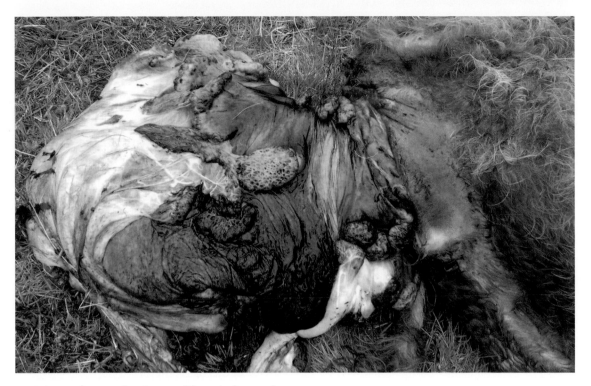

FIGURE 17.12 A recumbent cow with a uterine prolapse

as the cervix, which is then stimulated to trigger off further contractions and straining to push the uterus out fully. Older cows are predisposed to uterine prolapse, possibly due to their increased incidence of hypocalcaemia but also due to them having weaker perineal musculature and wider birth canals. Prevention is based on preventing hypocalcaemia and reducing dystocia in the herd.

It is important that a uterine prolapse is distinguished from a vaginal prolapse. A vaginal prolapse is smaller, smooth (see Figure 17.3) and more often, but not always, occurs pre-calving. A uterine prolapse is large, there are cotyledons visible and is a post-calving event. A vaginal prolapse requires vet attention but is not usually an emergency whereas a uterine prolapse requires immediate treatment and veterinary attendance. The attending vet will need several buckets of clean warm water, and a strong empty glass bottle (sparkling wine bottles are the strongest). Some vets like to use a clean feed bag or sheet to help support the uterus during replacement. If the cow is down, a

pair of ropes will be needed to position the cow's hind limbs in a 'frog' position. If the cow is standing, she must be restrained as calmly as possible to minimise damage to, or contamination of, the uterus. If the cow is lying down, she should be left in position until the vet arrives but other animals in the vicinity should be carefully removed to avoid damage to the uterus.

On arrival, the vet will administer an epidural injection – this is an injection of local anaesthetic given into the space surrounding the nerves from the spinal cord at the tail head. The local anaesthetic numbs these nerves, which supply the perineum, vulva and anus. This provides the cow with pain relief but also, to some extent, stops her pushing during the procedure which involves the vet packing the uterus back into the cow through the vulva. Before replacement, and while waiting for the epidural to work, the vet will meticulously clean the uterus with the buckets of water and remove as much placenta as will readily detach. Following replacement of the uterus the bottle is usually used (as an 'arm extension') to ensure that the whole uterus, all the way to both ends of the uterine horns, is back in the correct position and is fully re-inverted – if a portion of uterus remains everted the whole process of prolapse will recur. Antibiotics and an anti-inflammatory drug are usually given following replacement and more calcium may be given if the cow is still showing signs of hypocalcaemia – if the cow was suspected of having hypocalcaemia at the outset and the farmer had not yet given calcium then the calcium should be administered before replacement commences, as the stress of the procedure during a state of hypocalcaemia would add to the risk for the patient.

In straightforward cases cows usually do well following replacement, but occasionally replacement is not possible and in some cases death may result. Death may result before or during attempts to replace the uterus – this can be due to haemorrhagic shock. The *broad ligaments* that suspend the uterus in the body get extremely stretched during a prolapse and can tear; this causes fatal haemorrhage every time. Sometimes this is well underway when replacement commences, and death coincides with an otherwise successful completion. The other cause of death which seems to coincide with a successful replacement is thought, by some, to result from the returning to the circulation of a large volume of cold stagnant blood from the uterus when it is finally replaced and circulation is restored.

The prognosis in the case of a uterine prolapse depends on the time between the prolapse occurring and its correction, the degree of trauma to the uterus, the extent of stretching of the uterus (some say if the uterus is hanging as low as the cows hocks then the uterine arteries are likely to have torn) and any associated conditions, such as hypocalcaemia or another source of haemorrhage such as the uterus itself.

A previous case of uterine prolapse in a cow does not increase the risk of her experiencing the same at the next calving (unlike vaginal prolapses that do tend to recur) so cows that recover do not need to be culled for this reason. Cows that have had a uterine prolapse and survived should, however, be examined by a vet 3 weeks pre-breeding to check for endometritis ('whites') which will otherwise prevent the cow from getting back in-calf (see later in this chapter).

Retained foetal membranes

The third stage of labour involves the passage of the foetal part of the placenta – the cotyledons and membranes that sometimes get called the *cleansing* or *cleaning*. RFM is the failure of third-stage labour; which should occur within 12 hours of the calf being born. Instead the membranes remain attached to the uterus and are usually clearly visible, hanging from the vulva of the cow, or sometimes remain in the uterus and are not externally visible. The membranes decompose over time and there is a distinct smell that follows these cows around. Cows that have suffered RFM generally take longer to get back in-calf, on average by 25 days (Cooper, 2014) as endometritis usually follows an incidence of RFM. RFM has occurred because the caruncles on the lining of the uterus have failed to 'unlock' from the cotyledons, thus leaving the placentome intact – the placentome being the combined structure (Chapter 4). There are between 100–150 placentomes distributed unevenly across the lining of the uterus – more in the pregnant than non-pregnant horn. In addition, during RFM, the myometrium, the muscle of the wall of the uterus, has not contracted sufficiently to expel the membranes post-calving. The reason that RFM occurs is not fully understood but is thought to have hormonal, immune and mechanical involvement. Abortion, dystocia, twins, caesarean and prematurely induced calving are all factors that increase the risk of RFM. Forty-three per cent of twin births are associated with RFM (Peters and Ball, 1995). Hypocalcaemia, resulting in weak myometrial contractions is likely to lead to RFM. Selenium and Vitamin E deficiencies have also been suggested as contributory factors although the evidence is variable.

Treatment of this condition varies between vets. The use of hormonal injections, such as prostaglandin and oxytocin, have been used to try and restore myometrial contractions and expulsion of the placenta but studies suggest this is futile (Peters and Ball, 1995). More recent studies in dairy herds have suggested that oxytocin or carbetocin injection given at the point of calving may reduce the subsequent incidence of RFM. On occasions, it is just closure of the cervix and hence a gripping of the cleansing, that is holding the membrane within the cow. Some vets will try to manually remove the placenta from the uterus but there is a risk of damaging the uterine wall, so reducing subsequent fertility, and also releasing the toxins from bacterial decomposition into the circulation which can make the cow ill. Uterine lavage with a very weak iodine solution is used but it is possible there is retrograde movement of the solution up the ovarian tubes, which may cause them to narrow and block, preventing further conceptions. Antibiotics, in the form of a paste or pessary, have been advocated although there is very little evidence behind the effectiveness of this treatment and little to support its ongoing practice (Cooper, 2014). In the authors' opinions, if the cow is well, no intervention is required until 5–7-days post-calving at which point systemic injectable antibiotic therapy may become necessary if the cow is becoming ill. Vaginal examination is important at this stage as sometimes the membranes are attached by very little and can be easily dislodged without damaging the lining of the uterus as it can earlier post-calving.

Metritis

Metritis is inflammation of the full thickness of the uterine wall, nearly always caused by infection, and nearly always within 3 weeks post-calving, and usually within the first 10 days. Poor immune function, faulty nutrition and poor hygiene at calving are all related risk factors for the occurrence of metritis. Metritis is more common in cases of twins, abortions and dystocia and is often associated with RFM. The cow will be unwell, weak, fevered and inappetent. On examination of the vagina there is a hot, smelly, red, watery discharge. The infection is usually by one or more of the following bacteria: *Escherichia coli*, *Trueperella pyogenes* and *Fusobacterium necrophorum*. The treatment involves NSAIDs, injectable antibiotics and in some cases, where the cow is very sick, due to the associated toxaemia, intravenous fluids or in less severe cases fluids by stomach tube.

Endometritis

Endometritis is inflammation of the lining of the uterus, usually caused by infection and nearly always within 3 weeks post-calving. The cow does not appear unwell and the discharge from the vagina ranges from mucus mixed with globules of pus through to pure yellow/white pus, unlike the red watery discharge seen in cases of metritis. Owing to the nature of this discharge, endometritis is often referred to as 'whites'. As the cow is not unwell, this condition often goes unnoticed until the next pregnancy diagnosis is carried out several months post-calving. A cow cannot get in-calf while she has endometritis and most affected cows will not come into heat. Endometritis can be a sequel to RFM and metritis but can occur after any infection is introduced through the cervix and where the immune system has failed to shake it off. There often lies the problem – these low-grade infections will usually be overcome by the healthy, well nourished, non-stressed cow – where endometritis is occurring these herd health factors may need addressing.

There are two options for the treatment of endometritis. If a corpus luteum is present on an ovary, prostaglandin can be used to induce oestrus. During oestrus the raised levels of oestrogen stimulate the white blood cell activity in the lining of the uterus and this helps clear up the infection and the uterus is returned to normal without the need for antimicrobial therapy. Alternatively, buffered antibiotic suspension can be administered into the uterus via a catheter passed through the cervix – these licenced treatments are to be administered by a vet.

Mucometra and pyometra

These conditions involve the accumulation of mucus and pus, respectively, in a uterus with a tight closed cervix. The conditions are always associated with an absence of bulling (anoestrus) and the abnormally persistent presence of a corpus luteum on one of the ovaries. Here the cow's reproductive cycle finds itself in stalemate – the condition of the lining of the uterus causes abnormal mucus/pus production which in turn stops the lining of the uterus manufacturing natural endogenous prostaglandins that are normally needed to knock out the corpus luteum, start a new heat, open the cervix, and spill out the mucus and pus – a vicious cycle. The solution, once diagnosis is made by scanning, is simple – an injection of artificial prostaglandin to set a normal cycle away.

Contagious bovine pyelonephritis

Contagious bovine pyelonephritis is an infection of the urinary tract of cattle caused by a specific bacterium called *Corynebacterium renale*, although other bacteria may also be present in the urine of affected animals. Cases appear sporadically, usually in animals over 3 years old.

The bacteria travel from the urethral opening, into the bladder and then ascend the ureters to the kidneys. Females are much more commonly affected as the distance between the bladder and the outside of the animal is much shorter and the urethra is wider in cows than in bulls. Some cows will be carriers of the bacteria and shed it in their urine, contaminating the environment, while being unaffected themselves. There is also a possibility that bulls may transmit infection.

Decreased flow of urine allows the infection to become established and this can be due to water deprivation or kidney stones or a pregnant uterus causing temporary or permanent obstruction of the urinary tract.

Affected cows present with a gradual loss of condition, a slowly declining milk yield, fluctuating appetite and the intermittent passage of blood-stained urine. Intermittent blood-stained urine may be seen in an apparently healthy animal for a few weeks before the other signs develop. The disease progresses to cause more frequent and painful urination with the characteristic passage of small amounts of urine. Death occurs due to a combination of kidney failure, blood loss and a progressive loss of condition/energy.

The disease may be suspected from the clinical signs alone, but a definitive diagnosis can be made by a vet through palpation of the kidneys, a blood sample to assess kidney function and a urine sample for visual examination and, if necessary, culture.

C. renale is sensitive to penicillin and a full 10 day course is required. The prognosis is fair to good if treatment is commenced during the early stages of disease, before damage to the kidneys has occurred. In advanced cases only a temporary recovery may be achieved, or the animal may not recover at all. The affected animal should be isolated with thorough cleansing and disinfection of the contaminated environment to prevent spread of the contagious bug.

Post-calving mastitis

Mastitis in a suckler cow during lactation usually only occurs in the immediate post-partum period when the cow's resistance is low, the udder is distended with milk, she is lying around more than usual, often in contaminated conditions, and the calf is not yet avidly stripping milk from her. After this time the calf will be sucking effectively and around eight times a day so clearing any bacterial infection from the udder. The next risk period for mastitis is then at drying off and throughout the dry period, often called 'summer mastitis' (discussed in Chapter 15).

Mastitis post-calving is started by bacterial contamination of the teat orifice that then travels up into the gland cistern (see Chapter 8). This does not happen easily as the udder has its own in-built defence mechanisms, for example: the teat orifice is usually tightly sealed and cells of the immune system patrol the area. The bacterium most commonly associated with mastitis post-calving is *E. coli*, found in the environment. If the cow is in good health with a strong immune response and the calf is suckling all four teats effectively it is rare that mastitis will establish. If this is not the case the bacteria replicate, the udder becomes firm and hot and the milk becomes watery and tinged yellow or brown. The cow is often very sick, inappetent, fevered, sweaty and recumbent with sunken eyes and brick red mucous membranes. This type of mastitis can be fatal. It is not the bacteria that is causing her to be so ill, but the toxin released into the circulation from the *E. coli* within the udder. Treatment needs to be administered promptly and NSAIDs are the mainstay of treatment. There is debate over the effectiveness of antibiotic treatment and intramammary tubes have been suggested not to be effective, although often used.

Antimicrobial injections are still probably advocated in severe cases as there is likely to be translocation of bacteria into the bloodstream and secondary infection as a result (Suojala et al., 2013). Intramammary antibiotics will also often be prescribed despite the lack of evidence for efficacy – the rationale here being that when given early in the disease process they will stop multiplication of the *E. coli* and therefore reduce the amount of toxin produced so reducing the severity of the disease. The prevention of this type of post-partum mastitis involves good nutritional management to maintain cow resilience, good environmental hygiene (minimising faecal contamination of the calving area) and good facilitation of the cow-calf bond for good suckling.

REFERENCES

Cooper, R.L. (2014) Retained foetal membranes in cattle: the knowns and unknowns. *Cattle Practice* 22(1), 17–25/

Dobson, H., Smith, R.F., Bell, G.J.C., Leonard, D.M. and Richards, B. (2008) (Economic) cost of difficult calvings (in the UK dairy herd): how vets can alleviate the negative impact. *Cattle Practice* 16(2), 80–85.

Foster, A., Livesey, C. and Edwards, G. (2007) Magnesium disorders in ruminants. *In Practice* 29, 234–539.

Hartnack, A.K. (2017) Spinal cord and peripheral nerve abnormalities of the ruminant. *Veterinary Clinics: Food Animal Practice* 33, 101–110.

Herring, W.O. (2014) Calving difficulty in beef cattle. Agricultural MU Guide, University Extension, University of Missouri-Columbia.

Husband, J. (2005) Strategies for the control of milk fever. *In Practice* 27, 88–92.

Lyons, N. and Gordon, P., (2013) Clinical forum: bovine uterine torsion: a review. *Livestock* 18, 18–24.

McGuirk, B.J., Forsyth, R. and Dobson, H. (2007) Economic cost of difficult calvings in the United Kingdom dairy herd. *Vet Record* 161, 685–687.

Momont, H. (2005) Bovine reproductive emergencies. *Veterinary Clinics of North America: Food Animal Practice* 21(3), 711–727.

Noakes, D.E. (2009) Maternal dystocia: causes and treatment. In: D.E. Noakes, T.J. Parkinson and G.C.W. (eds) *Veterinary Reproduction and Obstetrics*, 9th edn. Elsevier, London, pp. 232–246.

Peters, A.R. and Ball, P.J.H. (1995) Parturition and lactation. In: *Reproduction in Cattle*, 2nd edn. Blackwell Science, Oxford, pp. 134–135.

Suojala, L., Kaartinen, L. and Pyorala, S. (2013) Treatment of bovine Escherichia coli mastitis – an evidence-based approach. *Journal of Veterinary Pharmacology and Therapeutics* 36, 521–531.

Part IV

Measuring and monitoring health, disease, production and efficiency in the beef herd

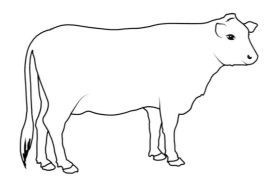

Chapter 18

Measuring and monitoring health in the beef herd

WHAT IS HEALTH?

Health is classically defined as 'the state of being free from illness or injury' (*Oxford English Dictionary*). This is obviously the state in which anybody or any animal wants to be. And as vets and farmers, when we multiply the individual's state of health up to a whole herd or a whole region of cattle then we clearly have the opportunity to influence the health of many individuals whose combined health is everything in terms of production and, most importantly, welfare. But is that an assumption? Maybe we need to prove that health is worth having. We can easily imagine that health is desirable. In people we link it to well-being, in animals we tend to link it to welfare and productivity. Some concerning language, perhaps of yesteryear is the notion that health comes at a price: Is it too expensive to try to have too much health? Is there an affordable amount of non-health that is acceptable? Sadly, there may actually be some truth to this in a purely economic argument, but as we constantly evolve into a future where welfare is paramount then maybe we can refuse to accept an amount of disease as economically optimal, and hope we can show that *total health* is realistically a state worth pursuing at an economic level and not just at a welfare level.

WHY DO WE NEED TO MEASURE HEALTH?

Dairy farmers are in the fortunate position of having data at their fingertips; any UK dairy herd has a daily measure of yield, butter fat and somatic cell count. Any change in health or nutrition or environment quickly throws up changes in yield and quality, usually within days, sometimes even hours, and the change is promptly reflected in their monthly milk payment too.

For beef herds we have to look a little harder at what can be measured, why it is worth measuring and how we are going to measure it. Many businesses still function adequately by measuring their bank balance alone. If the sum of the money in the bank in a particular month is similar to what it was 12 months ago it seems that everything is just about ok! When working to improve any herd, however, whether it be health related or not, there is a need to monitor 'performance' (health, productivity and profitability) to enable cost-effective decisions to be made and to assess the response to these decisions over time; to know if the decisions that were made were right or wrong.

WHAT DO WE NEED TO MEASURE?

It all starts with 'data'. What is data? Answer: facts and statistics collected together for reference or analysis. On farms there is a lot of data – in diaries, white boards, scraps of paper, veterinary invoices, abattoir reports and mart sale receipts to name but a few. Which of this data needs to be measured to help decision making? How do you go about it?

Data, when put into a context useful to help business decision making, is referred to as a KPI. KPIs are measures that demonstrate whether a business is achieving its objectives.

Collecting data to calculate KPIs can be time consuming and daunting. Initially, it is easier to start using the data that is easily obtainable and measures only a few relevant KPIs. The method of calculating the specific KPIs should be consistent, so allowing comparison over time.

Within any given industry, standardising how this data is collected and presented allows a comparison between different units, in our case farms. This process is often referred to as 'benchmarking'. Benchmarking can and should be refined, for example, by farm type, geographic area or even clients of a specific veterinary practice! Such refinement ensures comparisons of 'like for like' are being made, rather than comparing apples with pears!

In England the Agriculture and Horticulture Development Board (AHDB) is the government levy board that represents farmers, growers and others in the supply chain. In the beef division of the AHDB a document called the Stocktake Report is produced annually. This report consists of data that has been collected from hundreds of beef enterprises around England. Over time these annual figures have become industry standards by which English beef producers can benchmark their physical and financial performance against each other thus seeing where there is potential scope for improvement. The Agri Benchmark Beef and Sheep Network is a global, non-profit making network of agricultural economists, advisors, producers and specialists in key sectors of the agricultural and horticultural world. This network provides a forum, in our case, to compare beef farms internationally – maybe not fitting the 'like for like' model but potentially interesting and useful.

There have been numerous attempts to develop so called 'cloud-based' programmes to standardise data collection, analysis and its presentation. These cloud-based programmes collect data electronically across the internet and the resulting analyses are then available to be viewed across the internet – they are stored in servers at some organisation but are described as cloud based, as they can be accessed by anyone with the appropriate permission. Some of these programmes are available to purchase; others are available through providers, such as AHDB. There are many advantages of cloud based systems for recording data.

- Data can be updated by uploading 'in real time', that is, immediately, using, for example, a mobile phone application ('app'). Examples may include the recording of a calf's birth or a case of pneumonia.
- The data is continually 'backed up', that is, a copy created so rendering the data 'safe'. Pieces of paper or diaries, on the other hand, or even non-backed up computer data on a farm can easily be lost or damaged.
- Systems can be linked to increase efficiency, save time and eliminate human error in copying data from one system to another.
- Calculations within the programme are quick and easy and standardised so aiding benchmarking.

As with any system, however, the information still needs entering in the first place – correctly and accurately. The quality of data that goes in is reflected in the quality of data that comes out.

It is mandatory in the UK to record all calf births and all movements of cattle on and off a holding. The BCMS is the database that handles this. Access to the database can be achieved with the relevant permissions, and records can be extracted for further analysis of things like the number of calves tagged, the spread of calving dates, the age distribution of the breeding herd and the number of cattle purchased and sold. It does, however, have its limitations; there is no information on dead calves that are not tagged.

One of the ways in which vets get involved in data collection, analysis and the subsequent measurement of health is in the process the industry calls herd health planning. Much of this is actually herd health reviewing but *planning* for improvement is the sensible end objective.

WHAT ARE HERD HEALTH REVIEWS?

Herd health reviews, historically referred to as herd health plans, have long had an association with farm assurance and have been on some occasions more of a tick box exercise; a form that has to be filled in! However, vets have tended to look on these reviews as an opportunity to engage with farmers, talk about things that are working well, things that are not, and then the establishment of measures to put in place to improve the herd's health, welfare and productivity (Oliver et al., 2014).

Health reviews take many different forms depending on the vet involved but generally they look at disease incidence, production data, preventative treatments, standard operating procedures and a biosecurity review.

1. **Disease incidence**. This is covered in depth in Chapter 19 but in summary is a measure of disease over a set period of time in a given, defined, population. This allows the vet and the farmer to assess objectively what has worked well and what health aspects require more attention. A template to record disease incidence is shown in Table 18.1.
2. **Production data**. This is covered in depth in Chapter 19 but in summary is data that assesses the herd's productivity allowing informed decisions to be made relating to the results of controlling, eradicating and preventing disease as well as modifying management practices such as nutrition, bull fertility and heifer rearing. Initially, this may start as paper

exercise compiling data from the previous calving period as shown in Figure 18.1, the data can then be entered into a digital application for further analysis.

3. **Preventative treatments**. This involves a discussion about anthelmintics, flukicides, trace element supplementation, ectoparasitacide treatments and vaccination. These treatments are commonly displayed in a calendar format as depicted in Table 18.2. This process promotes the discussion of 'best practice' in the use of each product; its timing and the target groups of stock to be treated. It may involve further discussions about diagnostic testing that may be needed to confirm the nature of disease present or to confirm it is actually present as opposed to guessing, for example, fluke or worm egg counts. Online calendars with built-in automatic reminder systems are useful so key management tasks or routine treatments are not forgotten.
4. **Standard operating procedures (SOPs)**. These are clearly agreed, accurate written protocols that can be established at herd health reviews and then communicated to all farm team members for implementation. Displaying SOPs on the wall in an appropriate place on the farm is a commonly employed method of SOP reinforcement. This may include protocols for all sorts of frequently encountered situation (or perhaps infrequent ones too) such as downer cows, retained placentas, calf castration, calf diarrhoea, colostrum supplementation and so on.
5. **Biosecurity review**. Biosecurity is defined as 'safety from the transmission of infectious disease'. In the beef farm situation, it refers to keeping the herd safe from the introduction of infectious cattle disease. Certification of a herd health status for specific infectious diseases, such as bTB, BVD, IBR, leptospirosis, neosporosis and JD, can add financial value to the stock, so benefitting the vendor while providing assurance for the purchaser. The principles of biosecurity are not new to the cattle industry but have been less stringently implemented when

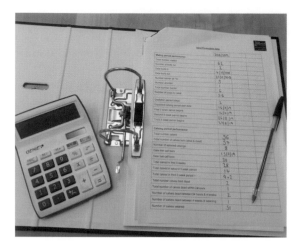

FIGURE 18.1 A set of production data in progress

compared with the poultry and pig sectors. A study carried out which interviewed 56 cattle farmers in the north west of England (Brennan and Christley, 2012) suggested that although certain biosecurity practices were acknowledged they were carried out infrequently or not at all.

The FMD epidemic of 2001 highlighted the need for better biosecurity to prevent the spread of a highly infectious disease. Disinfectant foot baths, wheel washers, tractors barricading farm entrances, and closed footpaths were common-place across the UK countryside during the erad-ication programme. Most animal movements (not all – for example, those animals going direct to

TABLE 18.1 Disease incidence template

Condition	No. cases	No. dead	Farmer diagnosis	Vet diagnosis	Interference level
Infectious diseases					
BVD					
Leptospirosis					
Johne's					
TB					
IBR					
Parasites					
Liver fluke					
Worms					
Cow specific					
Abortion					>2%
Prolapse					>2%
Difficult calving					>5%
Barren					>7%
Mastitis					>3%
Still birth					>2%
Ill thrift					>10%
Metabolic disease					
Lameness					
Calf specific					
Pneumonia					>5%
Scour					>5%
Ill thrift					>5%
Navel infection					

TABLE 18.2 Example calendar of herd events

Month	Stock	Drug/action	Disease targeted
January	Cows	Blood sample	Trace elements
	Cows	Blood sample and BCS	Johne's, IBR & Lepto
February			
March	Cows & heifers	Dairy cow mineral lick	Hypomagnesaemia
	Cows & heifers	Scour vaccine	Calf scour
April	Cows & heifers	Calving	
May	Bulls	Pre-breeding exam	
	Heifers	Pre-breeding exam and pelvimetry	
June			
July	Cows and youngstock	Pour-on insecticide	Flies
August			
September			
October	Calves	Pour-on anthelmintic	Worms
	Calves	Pneumonia vaccine	BRD
November	All stock	Housing	
December	Cows & heifers	PD and BCS	
	Cows, heifers & bulls	BVD vaccine	BVD
	Youngstock	BVD check test	BVD
	Cows, heifers & bulls	IBR vaccine	IBR
	Cows, heifers & bulls	Flukicide	Fluke
	Youngstock	Flukicide	Fluke

slaughter) were ceased in an effort to contain the highly contagious virus and so protect the UK's cloven hooved population of livestock. Although the extreme measures eventually ended, they left a raised awareness of the importance of biosecurity. One of the legacies of the 2001 FMD outbreak was the '6 day rule'. The '6 day rule' enforces that if cattle or sheep are moved on to a holding, the subsequent movement of sheep or cattle off the unit (except directly to slaughter) is forbidden for the ensuing 6 days. It was introduced to limit the rapid movement of livestock over long distances – a factor that was considered particularly to blame in the rapid and widespread dissemination of infected stock in the 2001 epidemic. In a repeat disease outbreak, the disease would spread more slowly allowing detection and control measures to 'keep up' better.

Infectious disease may be viral, bacterial, fungal or parasitic. Parasitic diseases are often not classed as infectious diseases but, essentially, they are and are best considered as such. Some examples of our broader definition of infectious disease to be aware of include:

- BVD
- leptospirosis
- IBR
- JD
- ringworm
- bTB
- liver fluke
- salmonellosis
- campylobacteriosis.

SPREAD OF INFECTIOUS DISEASE

Infectious disease can be spread by:

- infected animals, known as the host, for example a ewe infected with FMD virus

- another animal that is not the primary host of the disease but carries it – known as vectors; an example would be the midge when transmitting blue tongue virus (Chapter 28)
- an inanimate object that is contaminated with the infectious agent – known as *fomites*.

Disease spread can therefore take many routes. The following lists a few examples of disease spread between cattle farms:

(a) cattle
  - purchased cattle
  - neighbouring cattle
  - returning cattle from shows or summer grazing
  - escaping cattle
(b) personnel
  - vets
  - breeding technicians
  - foot trimmers
  - visitors (Figure 18.2)
  - other farmers
  - contractors
  - farm staff
(c) equipment
  - slurry tankers
  - foot-trimming crates
  - veterinary equipment
(d) other animals: wildlife, dogs, vermin and co-grazing with sheep
(e) watercourses.

The risk of the introduction of specific disease should be discussed during a biosecurity review. Knowing the activities on farm and the routes of disease transmission each activity can be classified as either high risk (red), medium risk (amber) or low risk (green), see Table 18.3.

Once herd activities have been classified into high, medium and low risk, recommendations can then be discussed to decrease the risk, especially for the riskier activities.

The recommendations must be practical and cost-effective; building a Berlin-style wall around the farm would not be cost-effective or practical. Recommendations should also take into account the herd's existing health status. For example; if a herd is known to be BVD free and not currently vaccinating then the introduction of the

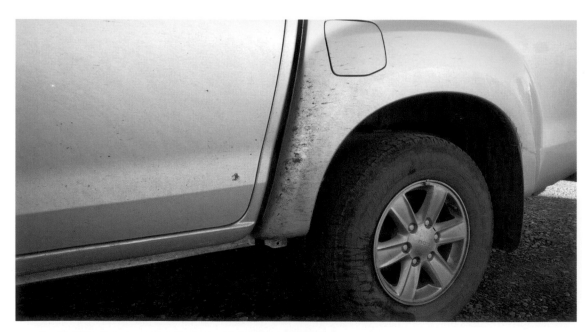

FIGURE 18.2 Wheel arch contaminated with faeces and mud

TABLE 18.3 Diseases risk attributed to each farm activity: high risk = red; medium risk = amber; low risk = green

	Cattle	Personnel	Equipment	Other animals	Water courses
Farm activities	Replacement heifers and bulls purchased Neighbouring cattle have nose-to-nose contact	Son works on the neighbouring farm Vet and foot trimmer attend No contractors	No shared equipment with other farms	Cattle grazed 5 months of the year No sheep	Water courses in 2 fields Flow from a neighbour's field Cows with calves at foot graze here
BVD					
Venereal campylobacter					
Ringworm					
Fluke					
Leptospirosis					

virus is potentially devastating and extremely costly.

The recommendations should take into account the objectives of the enterprise. For example; the introduction of JD into a beef fattening herd is of little consequence and therefore no further action is required.

The recommendations are often a compromise between cost, practicality and the consequence of introducing the disease in question. Figure 18.3 illustrates the recommendations based on the risk assessment in Table 18.3

A bespoke biosecurity assessment forms part of a robust herd health review for any specific farm but there are general principles that can be applied to any herd.

Cattle

- Buy in as few cattle as absolutely necessary and, if possible, operate a closed herd where no cattle are purchased and all breeding replacements, including bulls, are home-bred. The bull stipulation seems difficult for many farms so AI is an alternative solution – biosecure and a great opportunity for ambitious genetic progress.
- Find out as much as possible about the herd of origin when purchasing cattle (Figure 18.4) and visually inspect the cattle for body condition (fluke, worm, JD and bTB), skin lesions (ringworm, mange), lameness (digital dermatitis) and nasal discharge (respiratory disease, for example, IBR, mycoplasma, RSV).
- Buy from a herd certified free of specific diseases, for example, bTB, BVD, IBR, leptospirosis.
- Avoid purchasing breeding cattle through livestock marts. Farm-to-farm movements are less risky.
- Avoid mixing differently sourced cattle during transportation, for example, when using a commercial haulier.
- Avoid sharing or hiring bulls – this poses a particularly significant disease risk.
- *Showing* (competitive exhibition) is a high-risk activity: returning cattle should be treated as newcomers and subjected to the quarantine procedure on farm. Vaccination for specific diseases may lower the risk. Where possible, a

BVD
- Vaccinate all breeding animals – there is significant risk from neighbouring cattle, water courses and personnel.
- Fence off natural water courses.
- Replacement heifers and bulls should be purchased from CHeCS accredited BVD free or vaccinated monitored free herds.
- If this is not possible:
  - Don't purchase in calf animals,
  - Isolate purchased or returning cattle and blood test after 28 days for BVD antigen and antibody. Once negative results have been obtained and BVD vaccination complete animals can be released from isolation.

Venereal campylobacter
- Do not purchase non-virgin bulls.

Ringworm
- Ensure cattle are free from lesions on purchase.
- Isolate purchased or returning cattle for a minimum of 4 weeks before mixing with the herd.
- All personnel attending the farm to have farm-specific waterproofs and wellies and that clothing should remain on the farm.

Leptospirosis
- Vaccinate all breeding animals – there is significant risk from neighbouring cattle, water courses and personnel.
- Fence off natural water courses.
- Replacement heifers and bulls should be purchased from CHeCS accredited leptospirosis free herds.
- If this is not possible:
  - Isolate purchased or returning cattle and blood test after 28 days for antibody. Once negative results have been obtained and vaccination complete animals can be released from isolation.

Fluke
- Purchased or returning cattle should be treated with an appropriate flukicide and housed or grazed on land not known to be inhabited with the mud snail. A second flukicide may be required depending on the active ingredient of the initial product that was administered.
- Fence off natural water courses, wet patches of land and minimise poaching of land so as to avoid wet pockets for snail inhabitation.

FIGURE 18.3 Biosecurity recommendations based on the risk assessment in Table 18.3

show 'team' could be housed separately to the main herd during the show season and for 28 days after the last attended show.
- Quarantine any purchased or returning cattle for a minimum of 28 days after arrival in a designated isolation facility. If cattle are not sourced from a health certified herd then the necessary testing can take place during this

period. Delaying the testing until day 21 of isolation can be discussed. Quarantine anthelmintic and flukicide treatment can be carried out. Stock can be inspected for signs of disease such as ringworm or lameness. Vaccinations can be administered to ensure stock joining the herd are vaccinated to the same standard.

- An isolation area can be a field or a building. There must be at least a 3 m gap from other stock and no shared air space. A completely separate building is, of course, ideal. Any drainage, effluent or manure from the isolation facility should not come into contact with any other livestock. Farm personnel should wear separate overalls while handling the stock in isolation. A footbath should be at the entry/exit of the isolation facility.
- Manure from the isolation facility should not be spread on fields that are going to be grazed by other cattle within 12 months. An isolation

paddock should not be grazed by other cattle for 12 months in the case of JD control and 3 months where BVD, IBR and leptospirosis are the focus of the control measure.

- Farm boundaries should be sufficiently sound and elaborate enough to prevent straying and nose-to-nose contact with neighbouring stock. BVD and IBR accredited flocks require a 3 m gap, at least, between accredited and non-accredited stock. Studies have demonstrated both BVD and IBR can be transmitted over distances as far as 5 m (Crawshaw et al., 2002), so the bigger the gap, the better. Single electric fence wires are useless in preventing nose-to-nose contact between cattle! Hedges, unfortunately, also offer poor boundary security, but, well-spaced fences, one each side of the hedge, would be ideal. In other words, do not pull the hedges out!

Cattle Purchasing Disease Checklist

Date:.. No. of animals:.....................

Name & address of farm where cattle are to be purchased from:
....
....
.... Tel:...............

Vendor's vet name & address:
....
....
.... Tel:...............

Bovine Tuberculosis – A notifiable bacterial disease of cattle which can also affect people.

- Have the cattle to be purchased been tested recently? ☐ Yes ☐ No
- Has the source herd had a clear herd test recently? ☐ Yes ☐ No
- What is the testing frequency imposed on the source herd? ☐ Annual ☐ Biannual ☐ 4 Yearly
- Does the source herd have a history of bovine tuberculosis? ☐ Yes ☐ No

Johne's Disease – An invariably fatal disease of cattle with insidious onset after a long incubation period.

- Does the source herd have Johne's disease free accreditation? ☐ Yes ☐ No
- Has the source herd had any confirmed or suspect cases? ☐ Yes ☐ No
- Does the source herd vaccinate? ☐ Yes ☐ No

BVD – A viral disease of cattle that causes a multitude of clinical signs including infertility, abortions and the production of deformed or persistently infected calves. Persistently infected calves invariably die.

- What is your herd's status? ☐ Clear ☐ Vaccinated ☐ Infected
- What is the source herd's status? ☐ Clear ☐ Vaccinated ☐ Infected
- Are the animals to be purchased persistently infected? ☐ Yes ☐ No
- Are the animals to be purchased pregnant? ☐ Yes ☐ No

Leptospirosis – A bacterial disease of cattle causing reproductive failure and milk drop. It can affect people.

- What is your herd's status? ☐ Clear ☐ Vaccinated ☐ Infected
- What is the source herd's status? ☐ Clear ☐ Vaccinated ☐ Infected

IBR – A viral disease of cattle causing respiratory disease, reproductive failure and milk drop. A carrier status often exists following infection and apparent recovery.

- What is the status of your herd? ☐ Clear ☐ Vaccinated ☐ Infected
- Are the animals to be purchased antibody positive? ☐ Yes ☐ No
- If antibody positive, have the animals to be purchased ever been vaccinated? ☐ Yes ☐ No
- If so which vaccine was used? ☐ Conventional ☐ Marker

DairyCo

Bluetongue

- Are the cattle to be purchased being sourced from a BTV endemic area? ☐ Yes ☐ No
- If so, which are the relevant strains of BTV? ....
- Have the cattle to be purchased been vaccinated against BTV? ☐ Yes ☐ No
- If so, with which vaccine and when? ....
- Have the cattle to be purchased been tested for the bluetongue virus (PCR test) or for antibodies to the virus (ELISA test)? ☐ Yes ☐ No
- If so, when and what were the results? ....
- Have the cattle to be purchased been treated with a pour-on insecticide which is active against midges? ☐ Yes ☐ No
- If so, when and with what? ....

Campylobacter foetus venerealis – A sexually transmitted bacterial disease of cattle that can cause infertility and abortions.

- Do you use any natural service in your herd? ☐ Yes ☐ No
- Are the animals to be purchased virgins? ☐ Yes ☐ No
- If the animals to be purchased are not virgins and they are female, were they run with a bull? ☐ Yes ☐ No

Salmonella – A reportable disease with human health implications.

- Is there any evidence of salmonellosis in the source herd? ☐ Yes ☐ No
- If so, what? ....

Brucellosis – A disease that can affect people and which causes cattle to abort.

- Have the cattle to be purchased been imported from outside GB? ☐ Yes ☐ No

Neospora caninum – A protozoal parasite that can cause cattle to abort.

- Have the animals to be purchased been tested? ☐ Yes ☐ No

Parasites – Purchased cattle may harbour a variety of parasites including gut worms, lung worms, liver flukes, lice and mites.

- Has the parasite status of the animals to be purchased been assessed? ☐ Yes ☐ No
- Have the animals to be purchased been vaccinated against lungworm? ☐ Yes ☐ No
- Has any treatment been given to eliminate parasites? ☐ Yes ☐ No

Digital Dermatitis – The most common infectious cause of lameness currently affecting particularly dairy cattle in the UK.

- Is digital dermatitis present in your herd? ☐ Yes ☐ No
- Is digital dermatitis present in the source herd? ☐ Yes ☐ No
- Have the animals to be purchased had their feet lifted, cleaned, inspected and treated? ☐ Yes ☐ No

Mastitis – A common multifactorial disease which can cause significant economic loss.

- Are the animals to be purchased cows or maiden heifers? ☐ Cows ☐ Heifers
- Have the source herd's cell count and mastitis records been seen? ☐ Yes ☐ No
- If cows, have the cell count and mastitis records of the animal to be purchased been seen? ☐ Yes ☐ No

FIGURE 18.4 A cattle purchasing disease check list to aid in obtaining a thorough history from the vendor on the health of the animals (BCVA and DairyCo) (see Appendix for larger version)

- Where biosecurity cannot be maintained then vaccination against specific diseases should be considered as an insurance policy. The choice of diseases against which to vaccinate will depend on the herd's own disease status, the risk posed from its activities and the consequences of the disease being introduced.

Personnel

- The number of visitors to the farm should, ideally, be restricted to essential personnel. Dedicated overalls and footwear should be provided.
- Alternatively, visitors who have had contact with other stock can be requested to wear clean protective clothing and a cleaning and disinfection procedure applied to the vehicle at the entrance to the farm.
- Access to farm livestock areas should be restricted to the farm's own vehicles.
- A fallen stock collection point should ideally be located at the farm boundary and be amenable to cleansing and disinfection.
- A clean footbath containing a disinfectant should be placed at all exit and entry points to the farm (Figure 18.5). Dirty, contaminated footbaths act potentially as an infectious 'soup' and can actually spread disease rather than stop it (Figure 18.6).

Equipment

- Equipment should be farm specific; if shared, it should be thoroughly cleansed and disinfected before use.

Other animals: wildlife, dogs, vermin and co-grazing

- Minimise contact with other species. For example; sheep can pose a risk of JD,

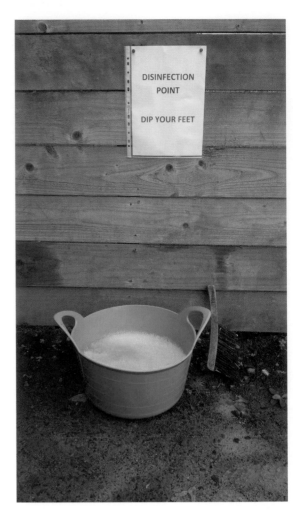

FIGURE 18.5 Clean footbath

leptospirosis, BVD, digital dermatitis and drug resistant fluke. Rented ground may pose a risk from infections, such as JD, where the causative bacteria can survive for up to 12 months on pasture.
- A rodent control policy should be in place. This can be important for leptospirosis and salmonellosis.
- Access by vermin to feed and bedding should be prevented where possible, for the same reasons as above.
- Reputable suppliers should be used to source feed and bedding.
- Uneaten or spilled feed should be removed.

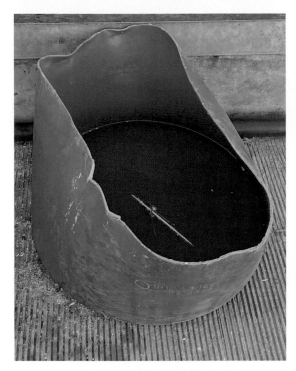

FIGURE 18.6 Contaminated footbath 'infectious soup'

- Feed should be stored in sealed containers to prevent access by vermin.
- Dogs should not have access to bovine carcases including calves, placentas or aborted calves and they should not be allowed to defecate on pasture, forage or concentrate. This is to prevent *Neospora* spp. transmission – the dogs become infected by eating infected bovine tissue and the dog completes the life cycle of the parasite by defaecating the eggs out for cows to then ingest so starting the cycle all over again.

Watercourses

- Piped mains water rather than natural water sources should be used wherever possible. Natural water courses may be contaminated with faeces and urine from other animals, including humans (Figure 18.7).

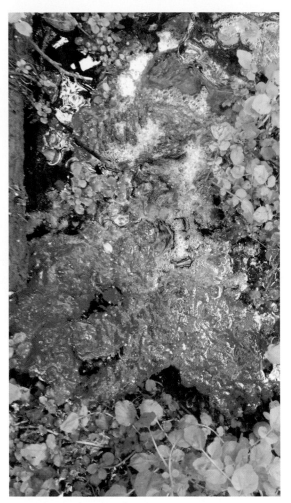

FIGURE 18.7 Water course contamination with human waste from an overflowing domestic septic tank

HERD HEALTH CERTIFICATION

Herd health certification is available for several infectious diseases of cattle. It is regulated in the UK and Ireland by CHeCS. CHeCS was established in 1999 by industry stake holders as a non-trading organisation to facilitate the eradication of certain diseases through the establishment of standards by which to do so. Standards have been set for the four most important non-statutory/non-notifiable diseases prevalent in the beef and dairy herds of the UK and Ireland, namely BVD, IBR,

JD and leptospirosis. Control and eradication of these diseases is documented in the CHeCS technical manual – publicly available online at https://www.checs.co.uk/. Advice and guidance are also available for *Neospora* spp. and bovine tuberculosis control.

CHeCS is not a provider of health schemes itself but sets the standards for those who do act as licensed health scheme providers.

What are the advantages of joining a health scheme?

- It is an extra motivator to reduce disease on farm so increasing health, welfare and productivity.
- Reducing disease decreases the use of antibiotics and promotes the beef industry favourably to the public.
- Strict biosecurity for the four main diseases standardised within the CHeCS technical document will also prevent the introduction of other diseases.

- Certification of the absence of disease facilitates trade and adds value to stock by giving the buyers confidence they are not buying in disease.
- Many European countries have either eradicated or embarked on national control programmes for BVD, IBR, JD and leptospirosis. The UK and Ireland need to compete with the rest of Europe in trade.

REFERENCES

Brennan M.L. and Christley, R.M. (2012) Biosecurity on cattle farms: a study in North-West England. *PlosOne* 7(1), 0028139.

CHeCS (n.d.) https://www.checs.co.uk/ (accessed 15 April 2019).

Crawshaw, M., Caldow, G., Rushbridge, S. and Gunn, G.J. (2002) Herd biosecurity for cattle. Technical Note T502. Scottish Agricultural College, Edinburgh.

Oliver, L., Scott, R. and Eaglesham, L. (2014) Implementing health planning in beef suckler and sheep enterprises. *Livestock* 19(2), 110–115.

Chapter 19

Measuring and monitoring disease in the beef herd

MEASURING DISEASE INCIDENCE

Having defined disease as any 'abnormal state or condition' then *disease incidence* is the extent to which such an abnormality prevails in the population in question. One could, for example, talk about the incidence of pneumonia on a farm or the incidence of pneumonia in Canada. It could be expressed as a percentage of the population that currently has the disease, or *has had* the disease at some point in its lifetime or during a fixed time period, for example, the last 12 months. It could be expressed as the number of cases per 100 animals in the last chosen time period, for example, 12 months and in this case allowance is made for the possibility of one animal getting the disease more than once.

We usually talk about disease as classic 'illnesses' but remember – a 'broken leg' is, by our definition, a 'disease'.

CLASSIFYING DISEASE

Diseases can be classified into two groups.

1. **Endemic disease**. These diseases exist in the population on an ongoing basis. It may be an infection that lives in the environment or possibly even inside the animal itself without always causing harm. This would include, for example, pasteurella pneumonia or calf scour. An interaction, with some form of balance/imbalance, exists between the animal, its environment, and the level of challenge from the infectious agent. The balance between challenge and immunity can often be adjusted. The challenge can be reduced through managemental techniques such as ventilation, and immunity can be boosted through good nutrition and vaccination.

2. **Epidemic disease**. These diseases are not normally present in the population and have to be introduced. These are classically infectious diseases, FMD being a famous example. Other epidemic diseases could be something less obvious such as obesity in non-westernised kids suddenly introduced to a poor-quality westernised diet of highly palatable and digestible burgers.

There are other ways of classifying disease.

The cost of disease

Disease is a direct cost to producers; it has been linked consistently with reduced output, increased replacement costs, increased veterinary costs and increased labour requirements.

Detailing the cost of specific diseases has been attempted by economists for years. There are many studies published focusing on one or two diseases but generally the studies are not comparable as the methodology used varies between studies. Calculating the cost of disease can be a simple 'fag packet' exercise or a complex evaluation using computer simulations of different disease scenarios and production systems. For the beef industry many costs are extrapolated from the dairy industry; any assumptions or inaccuracies which may result should be taken into consideration.

The cost of disease can be reported in different ways. Commonly it is presented as the 'cost per cow'. These are quite easy to visualise. For example, a case of summer mastitis in a beef suckler cow is estimated to be £140/cow. Costs are also reported at a national level for example: 'It is estimated that parasitic gastroenteritis in cattle costs UK farmers £84 million a year.' Such huge national figures can be difficult for the individual producer to grasp or visualise but they become important at a governmental level or at national industry stakeholder level.

There may be considerable bias in the way that statistics are presented. Certain questions need to be asked when interpreting estimates of the cost of disease.

- **In which country were the figures sourced to work out the cost of disease?** Each country potentially has its own unique economy and its own systems of industry. For example, the assessment of the cost of disease in the USA is going to be different from the UK – currency and production systems are different.
- **Who did the calculations?** For example, a company selling a flukicide may tend to overestimate the cost of fluke per cow – it is not about being dishonest necessarily but being a little selective over which data to publish!
- **When were the costings done?** To calculate the cost of any disease it involves estimating the current market price of the output be it by kilogram of meat or litres of milk and naturally the market value varies enormously over time.
- **How are the costs of a disease calculated?** Bennett et al. (1999a) conducted a study

standardising the methodology for calculating the direct costs of 30 endemic diseases/conditions of farm animals in Great Britain; 13 were diseases affecting cattle.

Bennett et al. calculated the direct costs of a disease as follows.

$$C = L + T + P$$

C = COST = direct cost associated with the disease
L = LOSS = value of the reduction in expected output and /or cost of resource wastage due to the disease
T = TREATMENT = treatment costs incurred in trying to mitigate the effect of the disease on the population
P = PREVENTION = the costs associated with the specific disease prevention measures

For example, imagine an IBR outbreak in a fattening unit. The cost associated with IBR would be summated as follows.

L = value of the reduction in expected output and/or cost of resource wastage due to the disease:

- reduced DLWG of animals infected with IBR that survive compared to those unaffected
- mortality from IBR.

T = treatment costs incurred in trying to mitigate the effect of disease on the population:

- veterinary time
- veterinary medicine
- farmer time.

P = the costs associated with specific disease prevention measures:

- vaccination
- biosecurity.

This model includes the cost of losses due to a disease and the cost of preventative activities but it must be remembered that the more focus there is on preventing a disease, the lower will be the losses due to the disease.

Other impacts of disease may be the effect on human health, animal welfare or environmental pollution. These are often hidden costs not acknowledged in disease cost calculations.

Bennett et al. (1999b) concluded in a follow-on study of this initial work that mastitis followed by lameness, lungworm, summer mastitis and liver fluke were the costliest diseases in terms of monetary sum per animal at risk in the UK. The study used data across all cattle production systems and was not specific to beef.

Cost–benefit

Up to now we have focused on the cost of a disease. Cost-benefit is achieved when an intervention such as a new disease prevention measure reduces the cost of the losses and treatments associated with the disease more than the cost of implementing the new measure. The process of working out whether or not a cost benefit is to be had or not is called a *cost benefit analysis* (CBA).

In Bennett's formula the cost of the disease prevention measure (P) is used to calculate C so adding to the cost. What we need to know is does the loss associated with the disease (L) and the cost of treatment (T) drop by more than P when the measure is applied? There are therefore two calculations to perform in the CBA:

$$C1 = L1+T1+P1$$
$$C2 = L2+T2+P2$$

where C1, L1, T1 and P1 are the total costs, the losses, the treatment costs and the prevention costs in the process before the measure is implemented, and C2, L2, T2 and P2 are the total costs, losses, treatment costs and prevention costs after the new measure is implemented.

In a favourable CBA P2 may be higher than P1 but thanks to the new measure L2 and T2 are reduced sufficiently to make C2 less than C1. This is the maths that hopefully proves that 'prevention is better than cure'! But without the maths you will not actually know for sure when it is, or, when it is not; some preventions are simply not worth the cost. Or even then are we sure? In simple financial terms it may not 'stack up' but it is worth remembering that in an industry affected by the emotional motivational drivers of the consumer, simple economic arguments are not always enough – a preventive measure which does not withstand a simple CBA may well be proven beneficial when the whole bigger picture is assessed. A lighthearted illustration to demonstrate this principle would be, for example, providing all cows with fluffy scarves to keep them warm in winter. Health, fertility and calf production figures may fail to show a response, in other words losses (L) are not reduced, but the cost of the scarves (P) is significant. The CBA here will fail to demonstrate a positive benefit, but, meanwhile, beef consumption in the local town has shot up thanks to the photograph on social media of the cows wearing the scarves!

Less silly examples exist. Sometimes the intervention, the P measure, brings some additional benefits that are rational and could have been predicted but may not have been factored into the maths of the CBA. Are there gains being made somewhere that we did not expect, notice or acknowledge? Are the control measures somehow, directly or indirectly, actually bringing about additional, rational, tangible, financial gain? For example, the disease under consideration may be neonatal diarrhoea and the disease prevention measure may have been to improve colostrum management. Not only did this decrease the costs endured from neonatal diarrhoea but also reduced the costs associated with navel ill and BRD and brought about a significant improvement in calf growth rates.

This could be thought of as *cost super benefit*!

The study performed by Bennett et al. (1999a) was used to focus attention on national resource allocation for the control of endemic diseases but, whether used at a national level or at farm level, a CBA is a most useful exercise, as it is to any industry or business process.

For example, a 100 cow suckler herd which breeds its own heifer replacements is infected with JD. The farmer is contemplating whether to embark on a JD 'test and cull' control programme. This would involve the vet blood-sampling 100 cows annually and arranging for the bloods to be tested for JD antibody. The costs are predictable, the benefits are that cows infected with JD are detected early while they still retain a cull value rather than dying on farm and incurring a fee for carcase disposal. It does not reduce the replacement rate, at least not in the short term; it may well increase it.

New prevention costs P2 per annum:
Vet time £240
Laboratory fee £550
Farm labour £100
Total P2 £890 = £8.90 per cow
New losses L2 per annum:
Cull value of one infected cow still in good condition rather than a death at zero cull value £900.
Avoidance of disposal of one carcase from the the dead cow -£120
1020 = -£10.20 per cow
New treatment costs T2:
Avoidance of wasted treatment for cow -£100
Total T2 -£100 = -£1.00 per cow
New costs associated with JD
C2 = P2 + L2 + T2
= £8.90 + (-£10.20) + (-£1.00)
= -£2.30 per cow (a saving)

A very basic calculation concludes that if one positive animal is detected and culled while still in good body condition there is a net C benefit of £230 divided over 100 cows, that is £2.30 per head. If more than one positive animal is detected and culled the net benefit increases.

Not all L and T costs have been included – the overall costs and benefits of JD control, are harder to evaluate.

- The cow can be culled from the herd before there is contamination of the environment with JD bacteria, which otherwise carry the potential to infect other animals.
- If the herd is registered with a cattle health certification provider then they may, if successful with their measures, be able to market the herd as certified low risk.
- Cattle subclinically infected with JD, in other words, not yet showing outward signs, do actually have reduced fertility and will have, on average, fewer calves born than uninfected cows.
- Herds infected with JD have to cull animals younger as *forced culls* and have an overall reduced herd productivity with a higher herd replacement rate in the long run (although short-term replacement rate may be higher in a herd introducing control measures).

Researchers have attempted to model JD in the beef suckler herd and design user friendly software to aid decision making, which would factor in all the considerations above (Bennett et al., 2012). This type of model, a step beyond the basic Bennett formula, is known as a computerised decision support systems (DSS). These models allow different scenarios to be 'tested' and the outcome to be calculated at the 'touch of a button'! (http://www.fhpmodels.reading.ac.uk/models.htm).

For example, using the basic JD calculation above, the software would allow us to change the size of the herd and it would automatically calculate the cost–benefit using the formulas already established. Computer DSS have, for most part, not been successfully implemented in practice. There may be a number of reasons for this. Maybe the programmes are not as user friendly as they set out to be, maybe the data they require is not easily available, maybe there is insufficient commercial gain from bringing such a product to market, and maybe there is distrust of the data and costing used to 'do the sums'? It is a start though; they do, if nothing else yet, raise awareness and stimulate discussion on management practices.

WHY RECORD DISEASE INCIDENCE?

Recording data enables it to be inspected and to be measured. Measuring disease information is useful for observing trends within a population, and, of most interest to the farmer, the population in question is the farm unit itself. In a seasonal calving suckler herd this usually involves observing the trend from one year to the next, and then compiling a trend over several years. For example, number of cases of dystocia one spring compared to the year before, and so on for subsequent years. This can allow for reflection and the targeting of resources to tackle emerging problems before they would have otherwise become apparent and perhaps before they become too significant.

The existence and then the incidence of disease and any observed trends can then be compared between farming enterprises locally or against national industry targets. This often demonstrates what is realistically achievable in 'the real world'. For example, if the barren rate in a herd has been in excess of 8% year on year, until it is known that some herds consistently achieve less than 4%, it is not necessarily perceived as a problem. Conversely, if a farmer is being self-critical of, say, a lameness incidence only to find that neighbours are having even more problems, then factors common to the area can then be investigated but also the farmer can get his or her own problem into perspective; it may be the local flint stone pathways and not a bad stockperson! Not that sharp stone pathways do not need addressing of course!

Benchmarking disease data across farms within vet practices or farmer discussion groups is useful. Unless unanimous consent is obtained it is usually done anonymously. For example, to be able to discuss the level of calf mortality anonymously each farm is allocated a letter of the alphabet; only they know the letter they are allocated. This is depicted in Figure 19.1. In this example the mortality rate ranges from 0 to 12%. The group average is 3.76%. Each farm can clearly see where it stands.

Figure 19.2 illustrates the group average in

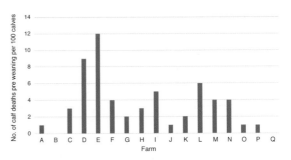

FIGURE 19.1 Benchmarking calf mortality

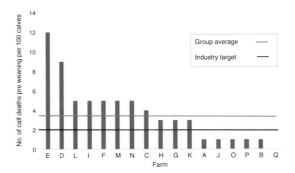

FIGURE 19.2 Benchmarking calf mortality when sorted by incidence from highest to lowest and shown in relation to the group average and the established industry target

orange, which is above the industry target in red. Only 5 out of 16 farms are below the industry target for calf mortality. This quantifies the problem and sets a goal that can be achieved.

HOW DO WE CALCULATE THE INCIDENCE OF DISEASE?

The incidence of a disease can be measured as the number of cases of the disease per 100 animals in a defined population.

$$\text{Disease incidence per annum} = \frac{\text{Number of cases of disease}}{\text{Number of animals in the population}} \times 100$$

Sometimes the population is easier defined as the number of breeding units as opposed to the number of young which may be very variable – especially in the case of say, pigs. So, in a suckler herd it may be done per 100 cows instead of per 100 calves. For example, if a 180 cow suckler farm had 8 cases of calf scour in a 12-month period then the incidence may often be quoted as 4.4 cases of calf scour per 100 cows per year. Alternatively, disease incidence can be quoted as a percentage but the 'percentage of what' needs to be defined.

Expressed as a percentage of cows whose calves are affected:

$$\text{Incidence of calf scour} = \frac{8 \text{ cases}}{180 \text{ cows}} \times 100 = 4.4\%$$

If it was expressed as a percentage of calves affected instead of cows with calves and the 180-cow herd has only 164 calves born then the denominator would be 164 rather than 180 and the incidence of disease is now 4.9%.

Expressed as a percentage of calves affected:

$$\text{Incidence of calf scour} = \frac{8 \text{ cases}}{164 \text{ cows}} \times 100 = 4.9\%$$

This is an example of how calculations need to be standardised when they are used for comparison either between years on the same farm, between farms or with national industry standards.

To complicate matters further there are certain diseases such as pneumonia, lameness and mastitis where there may be recurrence of the disease so the incidence of disease may be high but there may only be a few individuals affected. Here the percentage of the herd affected is calculated; in which case we can change the numerator.

$$\% \text{ of animal affected} = \frac{\begin{array}{c}\text{Number of animals} \\ \text{with 1 or more cases} \\ \text{of a disease}\end{array}}{\begin{array}{c}\text{Number of animals} \\ \text{potentially affected}\end{array}} \times 100$$

For example, a 180 cow suckler herd has 25 cases of lameness recorded but one cow has been lame 4 times and another 3 times.

$$\% \text{ of animals affected} = \frac{20}{180} \times 100 = 11.1\%$$

Disease incidence is often used to determine an *interference level* – the level of incidence of a disease which when reached warrants further investigation and probable action.

Using calf mortality as an example, the interference level for a pre-weaning population has been proposed as 3% (AHDB, n.d.). Once the incidence of calf mortality exceeds 3% further investigation is required. Further analysis of the data can then help with the next step which may be to find out at what stage losses are occurring.

Commonly used time based data subsets here would be the following.

- Death within 48 hours of life – this is commonly associated with dystocia. Here efforts would be focused on cow nutrition, heifer management, bull EBVs, and supervision at calving.
- Death between 48 hours of life and 4 weeks of age – here this would be an indication of neonatal diseases such as calf diarrhoea and septicaemia. Efforts would be focused on the time it takes calves to stand after birth (to 'foot'), hygiene in the calving shed, colostrum management, and cow nutrition.
- Death between 4 weeks of age and weaning – here deaths would be commonly associated with bovine respiratory disease. Calf housing, immunity, BVD control, parasite programmes, trace element supplementation and vaccination would be investigated.

Surveillance

Surveillance is the attempt to record disease over large areas, for example, regionally, nationally or even across continents and the world generally. This is done for a variety of reasons, the reasons being most obvious when done nationally, such as, setting government policy, targeting national resources, improving the country's welfare

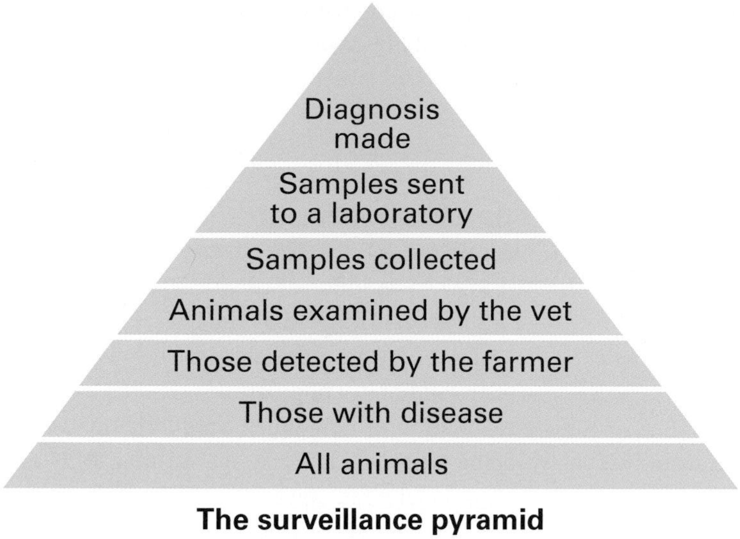

The surveillance pyramid

FIGURE 19.3 The surveillance pyramid

reputation, research, disease modelling or to assess the efficiency of enterprises within that country's overall economic performance. Unfortunately, however, there can be poor correlation between what is actually happening on farm and what is being recorded by government agencies. This is depicted in Figure 19.3 as a pyramid.

There are a large number of animals on farm that will have a disease, some of which are observed by the stockperson, some of which are not. Of those cases observed some will be inaccurately diagnosed. Then only a small number of these disease incidents will be reported to a vet, many will not be. And even when the vet gets to know, there is no obligation for the vet to report the disease to anyone else, unless of course it is a suspected case of a *notifiable disease*, in which case the vet has a duty to let the state veterinary service know. Where a vet decides to carry out further investigation into an undiagnosed disease, by submitting samples to a laboratory, then some laboratories report the diagnosis to a central database; some do not. In the UK the database is called the Veterinary Investigation Diagnosis Analysis (VIDA) system. In the UK it is some of the private laboratories that do not submit disease information to VIDA. The net result is that very few of the disease incidents that occur on farm make it to the VIDA database. For the incidents that do make it, however, the data is available online and filters can be used to look at different diseases and their incidence across the regions. For example, the number of beef cows with a diagnosis of JD in England in 2018 can be looked up; it would be seen there were 19 cases in the North East of England, and there were 1138 cases nationally (APHA, 2019).

Measuring antibiotic usage on farm

The mandatory requirement of antibiotic reviews by farm assurance providers in some countries, such as the UK, has helped vets and farmers identify units with high usage so allowing them to focus their attention on underlying problems, be that high disease incidence or injudicious use of the drugs, or both. This is especially helpful when disease data is not accurately recorded; the drug usage essentially gives the game away. Calf pneumonia incidence provides a good example here. In this 100 cow spring-calving herd example, individual cases have not been recorded.

The farmer has purchased 10 × 100 ml bottles of 20% oxytetracycline antibiotic.

Facts:

Oxytetracycline 20% antibiotic has a dose rate of 1 ml per 10 kg.

The average weight of a spring-born calf through the housing period is 300 kg.

The correct dose for a 300 kg calf is 30 ml.

The farmer has bought enough oxytetracycline to correctly treat 33 average calves.

Assumption:

The farmer has had an estimated 33 cases of pneumonia.

There are actually several assumptions in this calculation.

- All the purchased antibiotic has been administered. There may still be some unused on the farm or a bottle may have been dropped.
- The antibiotic was solely used for the treatment of pneumonia and not another condition in the calves or another condition in a different class of animal such as a lame cow or sheep!
- The correct dose rate has been used and the assumed average weight of the calf is correct.
- A single calf may have been injected more than once.

Although antibiotic annual reviews have been beneficial to estimate disease incidence, they were designed to focus the attention of the farmer and the vet on the responsible usage of antibiotics on farm at a time when the issue of bacteria developing resistance to antibiotics is becoming a huge concern to the combined medical professions and industries. The problem is popularly referred to as AMR and is of global concern (Mills et al., 2018). Targets were set by several governments across the world, the UK being one of them, to reduce antimicrobial usage in the livestock industry. To achieve this, antimicrobial usage has to be measured, and measurements have been developed to enable this to happen.

Two commonly used measurements are milligram/population correction unit (PCU) and defined daily dose (DDD). Both measures can be used at farm level or nationally.

Milligram/PCU

The milligram/PCU is a unit of measurement developed by the European Medicines Agency (EMA) to monitor antibiotic use across Europe; this has been adopted by the UK.

The EMA has standardised the average weight of an animal in a population – the PCU – to enable calculation of how much antibiotic on average is being given to each 'average' animal. PCU examples: slaughtered cows 425 kg, slaughtered heifers 200 kg, slaughtered young cattle 140 kg.

$$\text{mg/PCU} = \frac{\text{mg of antibiotic used}}{\text{Number of animals in the population} \times \text{EMA std. av. wt.}}$$

Traditionally pharmacists measure the concentration of an active ingredient as grammes per 100 ml of liquid or ointment, or grammes per 100 g of solid mixture, tablet or powder. This concentration is often expressed as a percentage where preferred. For example, if a medicine contains 1 g of active ingredient in 100 ml of the suspension or solution the medicine would be described as 1%. In many medicines the quantities of active ingredient are small and they are measured in milligrammes and often expressed as mg/ml. A 1% medicine would actually contain 10 mg of active ingredient per 1 ml – a little confusing!

Defined daily dose

DDD is defined by WHO as the average dose of a drug used for its intended purpose in mg per day for a standardised weight of target patient. For example, paracetamol in humans: it is given at 1000 mg four times a day to an adult with a persistent headache. The DDD would be 4000 mg in this calculation.

DDD is commonly used in human medicine; it helps to overcome the issue of total milligram and milligram/kilogram measurements not accounting for different dose rates in different antimicrobials (Mills et al., 2018).

The medicines used on the farm can be entered into standardised automated spreadsheets and for each drug the usage will be converted into either milligram/PCU or DDD. This data can be benchmarked between farms, regions, nationally and internationally.

The outcomes from an antibiotic review on farm are not just numbers. It is an opportunity to discuss with a vet the responsible use of antimicrobials for the greater good of all, not just the farm in question.

REFERENCE

AHDB (n.d.) AHDB Beef KPI Calculator online. Available at: http://beefandlamb.ahdb.org.uk/returns/tools/kpi-calculators/.

APHA (n.d.) http://apha.defra.gov.uk/vet-gateway/surveillance/scanning/disease-dashboards.htm (accessed 19 April 2019).

Bennett, R., Christiansen, K. and Clifton-Hadley, R. (1999a) Preliminary estimates of the direct costs associated with endemic diseases of livestock in Great Britain. *Preventive Veterinary Medicine* 39, 155–171.

Bennett, R., Christiansen, K. and Clifton-Hadley, R. (1999b) Modelling the impact of livestock disease on production: case studies of non- notifiable diseases of farm animals in Great Britain. *Animal Science* 68, 681–689.

Bennett, R., McClement, I. and McFarlane, I. (2012) Modelling of Johne's disease control options in beef cattle: a decision support approach. *Livestock Science* 146, 149–159.

Riddell, I., Caldow, G., Lowman, B. and Pritchard, I. (2017) *A Guide to Improving Suckler Herd Fertility*. QMS, Midlothian.

Mills, H.L., Turner, A., Morgans, L., Massey, J., Schubert, H., Rees, G., Barrett, D., Dowsey, A. and Reyher, K.K. (2018) Evaluation of metrics for benchmarking antimicrobial use in the UK dairy industry. *Vet Record* 182, 379.

Chapter 20

Measuring and monitoring production and efficiency in the beef herd

Accepting that the term 'production' is quite specific to an industry, for example tonnes of beef produced, the term 'performance' allows a broader appraisal of the industry. Any aspect of performance can usually be measured in some form or other and the measurable bits of performance get called parameters or sometimes, and annoyingly, these days … *metrics*! Examples of parameters would be goals scored, lap time, number of hot cakes sold. The performance parameters detailed in Table 20.1 are considered to be beef industry standards in the UK and the targets stated are agreed as realistic and achievable by the best performing beef herds. The ultimate challenge is to achieve these performance targets not for just one year but every year.

There are many computer systems and apps developed to analyse production data. A basic home-made spreadsheet can often be a simple but effective alternative. Table 20.2 is a basic template of the information that can be collected to measure production. Table 20.3 is the same data analysed and compared to industry targets. This sort of exercise can be, and often is, used to promote discussion as part of a veterinary herd health review.

Explanation of table headings in Table 20.2 and 20.3:

- total number mated = number of cows and heifers, females, put to the bull
- number of bulls run = number of bulls used to serve the cows
- date bulls in = date on which the bulling period starts
- date bulls out = date on which the bulling period ends
- number barren at PD = number of cows and heifers identified as not in-calf at pregnancy diagnosis
- number aborted = number of cows and heifers that were diagnosed as being pregnant but failed to calve or were known to have aborted a calf
- total number barren = number barren at PD + number aborted
- number of cows and heifers to calve = total number mated – total number barren
- gestation period = agreed number of days gestation, in this case 286 days
- expected calving period start date = date bulls in + 286 days
- first 3 week period begins = expected calving period start date
- second 3 week period begins = first 3 week period start date + 21 days
- third 3 week period begins = second 3 week period start date + 21 days
- total number calved = number of females that calve
- total number of calves born (alive and dead) – this may not be equal to the total number calved if there are twins to be accounted for
- number of assisted calvings = number of

TABLE 20.1 Performance targets. Industry Standard Performance Targets for the UK beef herd (adapted from AHDB Beef KPI Calculator online)

Category	Target
Female to bull ratio	<40
Percentage of females confirmed in calf	>96%
Bulling period for females	9 weeks
Percentage barren females	<6%
Percentage females calving in the first three weeks of the calving season[a]	65%
Percentage calf mortality from birth to weaning	<3%
Percentage calves reared per female put to the bull	>94%
Percentage female mortality	<2%
Percentage females requiring assistance at calving	<5%
Breeding female replacement rate[b]	<15%
Calf daily liveweight gain (DLWG) from birth to 200 day weaning (kg)[c]	1.2
Calf weight as a % of female weight at 200 day weaning	>50%
Percentage of females culled	<6%

Notes: [a]Sixty-five per cent of females should calve in the first 3 weeks of the calving period. The start of the calving period is taken as 285 days after the bulls were introduced to the breeding females. Given that there is a natural variation in gestation length, of approximately 10 days, any calves born before this date are added to the first 3 week block of the calving period.
[b]Also known as herd replacement rate = (number of female deaths + number of females culled) × 100 / total number of females put to the bull. Any breeding females sold should be included in the numerator.
[c]DLWG birth to weaning = (weaning weight – birth weight)/age of calf at weaning. In some situations, the birth weight may not be known due to practical difficulties in weighing suckled calves especially when born at grass. Where a birth weight is unknown a standard of 40 kg is used.

calvings that required assistance; this may be farmer or vet assisted calvings
- date first calf born = start of the calving period
- date last calf born = end of the calving period
- total calved in the first 3 weeks = number of females calved in the first 3 weeks from the start of the calving period
- total calved in the second 3 week period = number of females calved in the second 3 week period of the calving period
- total calved in third 3 week period plus = number of females calving after the second 3 week period of the calving period has ended
- total number of calves born dead = number of calves born dead or still born
- total number of calves dead within 24 hours = number calves born alive but dying within 24 hours after birth
- number of calves dead between 24 hours and 4 weeks = number of calves that died between 24 hours old and four weeks old
- number of calves dead between 4 weeks and weaning = number of calves born dead between 4 weeks old and weaning
- total number of calves weaned = total number of calves born – total number of calves born dead – total number dead within 24 hours – number of calves dead between 24 hours and 4 weeks – number of calves dead between 4 weeks and weaning.

Table 20.3 shows the raw data in Table 20.2 presented as percentages.

- Female to bull ratio = total number females mated/number of bulls run. Target < 40%
- Barren rate % = total number barren females x 100/total number mated. Target <6%
- Calving period (weeks) = date bulls out – date bulls in. Target <9 weeks
- % Total females calved in first 3 weeks = total females calved in first 3 weeks × 100 / total number females calved. Target >65%
- % Total females calved in second 3 week period = total calved in second 3 week period × 100 / total number calved
- % Total calved in third 3 week period plus = total calved in third 3 week period plus x 100 / total number calved
- Still birth rate % = total number of calves born

TABLE 20.2 Spreadsheet of raw data from an example herd calving season

	2015	2016	2017
Mating period performance			
Total number mated	60	65	75
Number of bulls run	3	3	2
Date bulls in	30/04/2014	30/04/2015	30/04/2016
Date bulls out	30/08/2014	30/08/2015	30/08/2016
Number barren at PD	0	0	0
Number aborted	1	1	2
Total number barren	2	2	1
Number of breeding females to calve	57	62	72
Gestation period (days)	286	286	286
Expected calving period start date	10/02/15	10/02/16	10/02/17
First 3 week period begins	10/02/15	10/02/16	10/02/17
Second 3 week period begins	03/03/15	02/03/16	03/03/17
Third 3 week period begins	24/03/15	23/03/16	24/03/17
Calving period performance			
Total number calved	57	62	71
Total number of calves born (alive & dead)	59	67	72
Number of assisted calvings	3	5	4
Date first calf born	12/02/2015	07/02/2016	08/02/2017
Date last calf born	11/05/2015	30/04/2016	20/05/2017
Total calved in first 3 weeks	36	41	43
Total calved in second 3 week period	15	16	20
Total calved in third 3 week period +	6	5	8
Total number calves born dead	1	3	2
Total number of calves dead within 24 hours	1	0	1
Number of calves dead between 24 hours & 4 weeks	0	1	0
Number of calves dead between 4 weeks & weaning	1	0	1
Number of calves weaned	56	63	68

dead × 100 / total number of calves born. Target < 3%

- Death in the first 24 hours % = total number calves dead within 24 hours × 100 / (total number of calves born – total number of calves born dead). Target < 1%.
- Death between 24 hours and 4 weeks % = total number calves dead between 24 hours and 4 weeks × 100 / (total number of calves born – total number of calves born dead–total number calves dead within 24 hours)
- Death between 4 weeks and weaning % = total number of deaths between 4 weeks and

weaning × 100 / (total number of calves born – total number of calves born dead – total number calves dead within 24 hours – total number of calves dead between 24 hours and 4 weeks)

- Calf mortality birth to weaning % = total number of calves born – number of calves weaning × 100 / total number of calves born. Target < 3%
- Calves reared per female put to the bull % = number of calves weaned × 100 / total number mated. Target >94%.

TABLE 20.3 Analysis of raw data from example herd calving seasons and comparison with industry targets

	2015	2016	2017	Target
Female to bull ratio	20	22	38	<40
Barren rate	3%	3%	1%	<6%
Calving period (weeks)	17	17	17	9 weeks
Total calved in first 3 weeks	63%	66%	61%	>65%
Total calved in second 3 week period	26%	26%	28%	
Total calved in third 3 week period +	11%	8%	11%	
Still birth rate	2%	4%	3%	<2%
Death in first 24 hours	2%	0%	1%	<1%
Number of calves dead between 24 hours & 4 weeks	0%	1%	0%	<1%
Number of calves dead between 4 weeks & weaning	2%	0%	1%	<1%
Calf mortality birth to weaning	4%	6%	4%	<3%
Calves reared per female put to the bull	93%	97%	91%	94%

Managing a herd's reproductive performance can be one of the easiest ways to improve the productivity and consequently the profitability of a unit. Box 20.1 provides an example showing how the number of calves born and their weight at weaning can make a difference to the farm's 'bottom line'.

There are five key points to consider when improving reproductive efficiency in the suckler herd.

1. Management of the bulling heifers.
2. Management of the cows' condition and nutrition.
3. Avoidance of difficult calvings.
4. Management of the bulls' fertility and soundness (especially non-lameness).
5. Management of the herd's general health.

The production data collected does not have to be linked to reproductive efficiency. Calf performance alone can be analysed. For example, data can be collected purely to identify the calves with the highest DLWG from birth to weaning. To compare calves which will be at slightly different ages on a fixed date of weaning, the weights of the calves therefore need to be standardised to a set number of days; typically, 200 days is used. This calculation can be done using a spreadsheet. For each calf it requires a calf identification number, a date of birth, a weight at birth, a date of weaning and a weight at weaning. The DLWG from birth to weaning is then calculated and can be colour coded using the traffic light system. Below target (red) less than 0.7 kg/day, moderate (amber) 0.7–1 kg/day and above target (green) >1.2 kg per day.

To take this performance assessment further the calf weight at weaning can be analysed as a percentage of the cow's body weight. This does become a measure of overall herd efficiency as it is assumed larger cows eat more feed. The target is for a calf to weigh at least 50% of its mother's weight at a 200 day weaning weight. A similar spreadsheet can be used, and the additional information required is dam identification and dam body weight. Less than 40% is below target (red), 40–50% is moderate (amber), and greater than 50% is above target (green).

Herd reproductive performance example

A common measure of output from a unit is number of kilograms of calf weaned per female bred.

$$\text{Number of kg calf weaned per female bred} = \frac{\text{Total weight of all calves weaned}}{\text{Number of cows put to the bull}}$$

This is obviously influenced by two primary factors: the number of calves weaned and their weight at weaning.

The number of calves weaned is, however, influenced by the number of barren cows/heifers, calf mortality and dam mortality. Furthermore, the weight of calves at a fixed point of weaning is dependent on their DLWG and their age at weaning, and that in turn depends on when they were born in the calving period.

TABLE 20.4 Example breeding herd performance, 100 cows, rearing 88 calves

Parameter	Current performance
Percentage calves weaned	88
Average weight per calf at weaning (kg)	285
Average calf weight per cow put to bull (kg)	251
Average selling price of calf (£/kg)	3
Gross financial output per cow	£753

Table 20.4 shows a 100 cow breeding herd that rears 88 calves. The calves weaned on a fixed date irrespective of their age and the average age at weaning is 285 kg.

So, 88 calves weighing 285 kg equates to 25,080 kg of calf weaned but this has to be divided by the number of females that went to the bull. In this example, 12 females did not rear a calf, either because they were barren or the breeding female or calf died. The number of kilogram of calf weaned per breeding female equates to 251 kg. At a value of £3 per kilogram this is an output of £753.

In Table 20.5 the same 100 breeding females has reared 94 calves instead of 88 and they achieve the same weaning weight but there are more of them. This equates to an output of £804 per breeding female.

Table 20.6 illustrates the effect of both increasing the number of calves born from 88 to 94 and increasing the average calf weight at weaning by 20 kg from 285 kg to 305 kg. This increases the financial output per breeding female from £804 to £861.

To increase the calf weight at weaning requires good growth rates, which are dependent on the cow's milk supply, genetics and nutrition but, also, the older the calf is at weaning the more days it has had to gain weight. Table 20.7 divides the calving period into 3 week blocks. It is assumed calving starts 15 March, weaning 1 November, birth weight is 40 kg, and DLWG is 1.1 kg/day.

Over a 12 week calving period there can be a 70 kg weight difference at weaning between the first and last calf born. This highlights the benefits of a compact calving period with as many calves as possible being born in the first 3 week period.

TABLE 20.5 For performance comparison, output from same herd with improved weaning percentage of 6%

	Current performance	Improve % reared
Percentage calves weaned	88	94
Average weight per calf at weaning (kg)	285	285
Average weight per calf at weaning per cow put to bull (kg)	251	268
Average selling price of calf (£/kg)	3	3
Gross financial output per cow (£)	753	804
Change in gross financial output per cow (£)		51
Financial improvement for 100 cow herd (£)		5100
Financial improvement for 100 cow herd over 10 years (£)		51,000

TABLE 20.6 Performance of the same herd, 100 cows, rearing 94 calves at an average weaning weight of 305 kg

	Current performance	Improve % reared	Improve weaning weight
Percentage calves reared	88	94	94
Average weight per calf at weaning (kg)	285	285	305
Average weight per calf at weaning per cow put to bull (kg)	251	268	287
Average selling price of calf (£/kg)	£3	£3	£3
Gross financial output per cow (£)	£753	£804	£861
Change in gross financial output per cow (£)		£51	£54
Financial improvement for 100 cow herd (£)		£5100	£5400
Financial improvement for 100 cow herd over 10 years (£)		£51,000	£54,000

TABLE 20.7 Weight at weaning depending on birth week within the calving period

Three week calving periods	Age at weaning days	Weaning weight (kg)
1st	221	283
2nd	200	260
3rd	179	237
4th	158	214
5th	137	191
6th	116	168

REFERENCES

AHDB (n.d.) AHDB Beef KPI Calculator online. Available at: http://beefandlamb.ahdb.org.uk/returns/tools/kpi-calculators/.

FURTHER READING

Riddell, I., Caldow, G., Lowman, B. and Pritchard, I. (2017) *A Guide to Improving Suckler Herd Fertility.* QMS, Midlothian.

Part V

Beef business management and development

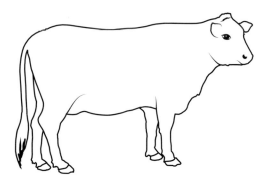

Chapter 21

The balanced scorecard approach to the beef farm

An inevitable and critical factor in the long term viability of most *for-profit* businesses is financial viability. The long-term *financial viability* of a beef business, or put in more farming terms, the long-term financial viability of a farm which farms beef cattle, sounds like a subject that does not really belong in a veterinary book for beef farmers. It maybe does not, and is, instead, likely to belong in a book specifically on farm business management and one written by someone with the appropriate expertise. But any sensible holistic approach to assessing the long-term success of a beef business will not just be a financial approach; it will not just be about bottom line accountancy, it will be about many factors, and given that the cattle themselves are a big factor in this story then maybe as vets we *are* allowed to talk a little about 'the business' and if nothing else someone needs to encourage a broad overarching approach to the way we look at long-term farm success. Here we have an opportunity to do just that. We will do it through what business analysts call the *balanced scorecard* approach.

WHAT IS THE BALANCED SCORECARD?

The balanced scorecard (BSC), was the result of a piece of work in the 1990s by Harvard Business Professor Robert Kaplan and his business consultant friend David Norton. In building this concept of the, soon to be named, 'balanced scorecard'

they first demonstrated that businesses benefit from having a clear *vision* of where they want to get to and an *objective strategy* by which to achieve it. The vision will, ideally, take the form of *goals* or *objectives*. The strategy is the implementation of what is known as the business *mission* – 'what the business does' – and this should be founded on what are referred to as *values* – 'the things that are important in the delivery of this mission' – the things that are important to the staff, important to the stakeholders, important to the customers and, finally, important to the public. These values may take the form of behaviours, principles, morals, aspirations, standards and, no doubt, other things. Look around at other businesses, especially on their websites, and you will see it is very common for businesses to publicise their *vision*, their *mission* (often called a *mission statement* or *purpose*) and their *values*. Kaplan and Norton then went on to demonstrate further that the delivery of the mission to achieve the vision successfully was heavily influenced by four key areas, areas they called *key perspectives*. One of these key perspectives was indeed financial, but all four were deemed very important, probably equally important, in their own rights. The four key perspectives are as follows.

1. **The financial perspective**. This is the money side of the story – the amount of cash in the bank, the business turnover, the net profitability, the return on investment, the prediction of

cash flow; all the usual things you would expect from a reasonably in-depth financial analysis.

2. **The business process perspective**. Sometimes referred to as the **internal process perspective**. This is about *how things get done within the business*, for example, manufacturing, processing or, in our case, the actual *farming*, and how logically and efficiently these things are being done.

3. **The customer perspective**. Sometimes referred to as the **external perspective**, this is about how the customer *sees* what you are doing. Are you giving the customer what they want? Do they like the way they are getting it? How satisfied are they overall?

4. **The people perspective**. This often gets described as the **learning and growth perspective** or the **organisational capacity perspective**. Does the business have the right people? Are they in the right positions? Are there enough of them? How well trained are they? How well is the innovation of new ideas being cultivated and nurtured? Are your people happy? Are you happy? How is everyone's *well-being*?

Figure 21.1 shows these four perspectives influencing the *central theme* that is the *strategy* in such a way as to achieve the long-term vision, or not! A wheel and hub model has been used to demonstrate that the wheel needs to be *balanced*, and the wheel revolves around the central theme that is *the hub*. Taking a long-term view is deliberate and crucial here. Short-term gains in a business often have no relationship with long-term success.

The goals or the objectives of the vision can then be allocated to one or more of these four perspectives. You can then see how well balanced, or not, the scorecard is. Do you have at least one objective in each area? Do you have a similar number of objectives in each area? The theory is you probably should have; that is why they call it the *balanced* scorecard.

These objectives influence each other – the way they influence each other can be demonstrated by simply connecting them with arrows – this produces what is known as a *strategy map* (Figure 21.2) and this finishes off the model, the scheme, that hopefully shows the balanced scorecard not only in balance, but as a dynamic flow chart.

So how does this model fit with a beef farm? Are you still reading?! Stick with it! Your scorecard will be very much yours but let us have a go at a trial version; an imaginary one.

Let us imagine you are planning to retire in 5 years and you have nobody to inherit the business on your rented farm. Table 21.1 is an attempt at your BSC.

This is obviously a very simple one and is intended to be lighthearted. But it is easy to see that this points in the direction of what could be bigger issues.

THE MODIFIED BALANCED SCORECARD FOR LIVESTOCK FARMING

Is farming a little unique compared to other businesses? Most business consultants seem very resolute on the notion that all businesses are the same; 'business is business' whether it's selling apples from a barrow or Apple Macs from an Apple store

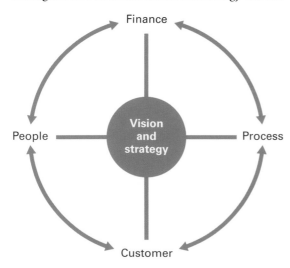

FIGURE 21.1 The balanced scorecard for business – the wheel and hub model

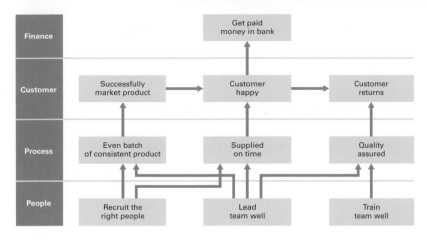

FIGURE 21.2 The balanced scorecard based strategy map

or producing suckled calves for the autumn sales. If they all say it, they are probably right. But ... if we took a balanced scorecard approach to the very thing that is the balanced scorecard, but in this case – beef farming, or any livestock farming for that matter, what would it look like?

- **The financial perspective**. Fair enough, it is hard to argue with figures, with money. They are right, business is business!
- **The business process perspective**. Are living, *sentient* animals (animals with feelings) a business process? They are really, but is that really right? Feeding processes may be processes, as may be water supply, bedding systems, housing and so on. But are the animals really just a unit? Are they really just a commodity? Thinking that they are may in itself be a faulty strategy. Read on!

- **The customer perspective**. Your immediate customer may actually see animals as a business process – let us face it, in this context, they are. But do the supermarkets see it like that? They listen to the public. Do the public see animals as a business process? According to supermarket research they absolutely and passionately do not! Do you see animals as a business process? Does your family? Do your friends? Possibly not. Probably not.
- **The people perspective.** Are farmers different? They are at risk of lacking ongoing education (CPD – continuing professional development – as other industries call it). They are at risk of relative isolation, lack of social connection in the workplace. Their jobs are linked to an increased risk of mental health disease. So maybe it is a little different for farmers?

TABLE 21.1 A simple example of a balanced scorecard

Perspective	Objective
Financial	Enough cash to pay off debts
	Retirement fund
Business process	Switch from bull to AI for safety concerns
	Non-replacement of culls to reduce investment
Customer	Smaller store calves for local fattener who deals directly with you and wants small cattle to suit his system
	Disbud when young – the buyer has stopped tolerating horns
People	Organise some future career advice for your one young worker
	Join a bowling club in time for your retirement!

So, in summary might it just be possible that farmers could do with a modified approach to the balanced scorecard? At risk of upsetting the business world let us be brave and suggest our modified version, it needs, in our opinion, five, not four, perspectives:

1. **The financial perspective**. There is still no getting away from this one!
2. **The business process perspective**. Let us make this one about the *inanimate processes* in place on the farm: the machinery, the feeding systems, the handling systems, the drug storage and usage, the computers and so on.
3. **The customer perspective**. We really are listening now! Not just what the next guy in the supply chain wants but what the supermarkets want and what the public want.
4. **The people perspective**. We are definitely thinking more about this these days – education, community, leisure, *well-being* – not just for you but for the whole farming workforce.

And last but most definitely not least …

5. **The animal perspective**. Should the animals not be allowed their own cornerstone in the balanced scorecard? The people in the workforce do, so why not the animals? Let us think about the animals. Are they genetically suited to the system, are they the right size, the right age, the right breed, the right health status but most importantly, and, in summary *are they happy?* Is their welfare satisfactory? Is satisfactory good enough? The term animal welfare is slowly being transformed into *animal well-being*; they deserve, they are entitled to, they have a right to, the physical and mental health that we too yearn for.

AN EXAMPLE MODIFIED BALANCED SCORECARD FOR THE BEEF BUSINESS

Imagine Bob and Diedre Hall on their fully owned inherited 400 acre hill farm in Yorkshire. They have an 80 cow spring-calving Simmental cross suckler herd living in traditional stone straw yards modified from old stall byres. The farmer and his wife, in their 50s, work on the farm with their son, Jason; he is 23 years old, has a level 3 diploma in agriculture and plans to take on the family business one day. His sister is a nurse at the local hospital and has left home but helps occasionally. They have a farm worker Alan, who is 60; he has been asked to reduce his hours from full time to 2 days a week, but he still turns up for work every day and has said he does not mind if he only gets paid for 2 days. The family are worried about Alan's state of mind. They sell their calves at 12 months old in the spring suckler calf sales at the local market. They have no sheep because Grandpa did not like sheep. Bob has not been speaking much recently, he argues with Jason all the time, he has told Diedre he is getting chest pains.

Their business consultant friend draws up a balanced scorecard for them but chooses the new modified model that she read about in *The Veterinary Book for Beef Farmers*. The consultant realises that it is a three-step process. First,

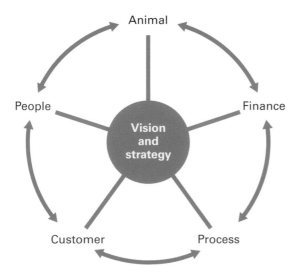

FIGURE 21.3 The modified balanced scorecard for livestock farming

identify the agreed vision and strategy for the farm business. Second, identify the problems that are holding the farm back (Table 21.2). Third, identify the objectives the business needs to achieve the long-term vision and strategy (Table 21.3). This three-step process will be conducted under the scheme of the balanced scorecard so nothing is missed and the view is balanced.

What is the vision and strategy of the Hall family farm?

Vision

1. Continue to own the farm.
2. Continue to farm beef cattle.

TABLE 21.2 Initial scoping out of balanced scorecard problems

Perspective	Problem
Financial	Bob, Diedre, Alan (part time) and Jason all *need* paying monthly
	Bob and Diedre have made little provision for retirement
	Jason is keen to do more training as he disagrees with Bob on some matters and is keen to be sure
	Jason wants the money to build a new shed
Business process	Mucking out the old buildings is difficult; Bob insists on doing much of it by hand
	Lack of head room in some of buildings, hence pressure to keep mucking out
Customer experience	They do not have a regular buyer at the spring calf sale
	They seem to be given a late slot in the sale each year
People	Bob has chest pain and argues with Jason
	Jason is frustrated and not talking about it
Animal	The cattle seem too big for the buildings
	The calves do not seem to be in demand at the sale

TABLE 21.3 Balanced scorecard objectives

Perspective	Objective
Financial	Make enough money to pay Bob, Diedre, Alan (part time) and Jason
	Invest some money for Bob and Diedre's retirement
	Make enough money to fund extra training for Jason
	Raise money to build a new shed? Proving difficult
Business process	Jason has seen a small machine that will muck out the small buildings. It is quarter the cost of a new shed
	Head room will be kept reasonable by regular use of the new machine
Customer experience	Jason has been on a beef marketing course and met a local owner of a beef fattening unit who is interested in a local direct contract for store calves
	The local fattening unit is forming a relationship with a second abattoir who have a preference for smaller carcases
People	Bob is seeing the doctor. Things have improved since getting the new machine. He is on stress management exercises
	Jason has enrolled on a Herdsman's Certificate course and already seems a lot happier
	Alan was given a National Trust membership for his birthday and has taken a few days off
Animal	Decision made to use a smaller breed of bull and move as quickly as practicable into a smaller breed of cows to cope better with the smaller buildings and to please the buyer

Strategy

1. Earn enough money to keep the farm and pay all existing stakeholders.
2. Continue to breed calves and sell stores at 1 year old.
3. To stay together as a team.

Again, this is a rather trivialised approach but it illustrates the point. Objective thinking can seem such common sense but, so often in reality, seems to get by-passed.

BUILDING YOUR OWN BALANCED SCORECARD

When, or if, you come to working on your own balanced scorecard you may wish to seek help with it. Colleges, universities, and national agencies may be able to help, as may broad based consultants and advisors. If you need help with more specific perspectives, then the following suggestions may be of use.

Financial

Many commercial banks offer the balanced scorecard as a process they will happily take you through, some bank managers now even recommend it.

Business process

Advice in specific areas of farming process abounds. Nutrition, housing, handling, machinery, grassland management, advanced breeding, and so on, are all readily accessible industries that come to us with masses of marketing, support and advice behind them and this can be extremely useful. It is, however, in this area that balance becomes of paramount importance. It is

here where a disproportionate amount of time, resource and money can be allocated. You, or someone, needs to take time to balance this perspective with the others. In the above example a new shed would have been, to many, irresistible, and may not have been challenged as perhaps not the best solution. Buying machinery, mineral mixes, the latest semen from America, will be made very easy for us; we need to balance this up with some of the less 'easy' perspectives of the business.

Customer experience

The obvious people to talk to here are, of course, the customers. This may be the local auctioneer, the abattoir or butcher you supply, or the finisher that that you are dealing with, perhaps directly. But what about the more remote customer – the supermarket, the public? Here it is very important to remain aware of what is wanted. That may be in terms of whether people want lean meat or marbled meat, but it may be, and is more likely to be, welfare orientated. How were the animals kept, housed, fed? How far were they transported, how old were they? A large part of the customer experience perspective of the balanced scorecard is the huge subject that is *marketing* – a separate chapter has been devoted to this subject (see Chapter 23).

People

This is also a rapidly developing area. When did you last go on a training course? When did you last send someone on a training course? How do you view training? You may think it is over-rated, not for you, a waste of time, overpriced. It may be, on the other hand, that because you are reading this book then you are already fairly tuned into the idea of further education. Reading is certainly great but there is nothing quite like going on an interactive or practical course with a group of like-minded people to refresh knowledge, exchange ideas or learn something new. Only by doing it do you realise how energising and enthusing it can be and if nothing else it lets you see you are not the only one with problems. Again, the colleges and universities can help here, as can private training organisations or training laid on by your local veterinary practice. Technical CPD is the type of training that most springs to mind here but in broader industry the concept of *personal development* has also become a highly valued process. In most walks of life now – care, finance, manufacturing, commerce, communication, professional services and so on – personal development is avidly laid on for the workforce. This can sound like a real turn off – especially to the traditionally tough, hardened society of farming, but it is now officially recognised as valuable and the likes of farmers may indeed be one of the sectors most standing to benefit – remember the aforementioned factors – loneliness, lack of social contact, loss of confidence and the development of excessive risk aversion.

Personal development can be sourced in various forms and from many different sources. It may take the form of team building – fun stuff like high wires, organised walks, skiing trips or raft building. These activities are designed to help people be more courageous and less risk averse. It may be classroom sessions on personality profiling, stress management or, again, just fun things like pottery or cocktail making! The idea? Simply to build confidence, enhance social skills, facilitate teamwork and to help people better understand the behaviour and personalities of others, for example, why their farm worker, or worse still, their son, is not talking to them. The aim is a happy team made of happy individuals. Happy businesses have been shown to be more successful than unhappy ones (Lencioni, 2016). The expansion of one's horizons and the expansion of the learning environment has been observed to improve not only personal development but the development of the organisation in which the learner works (Fuller and Unwin, 2004) (Figure 21.4).

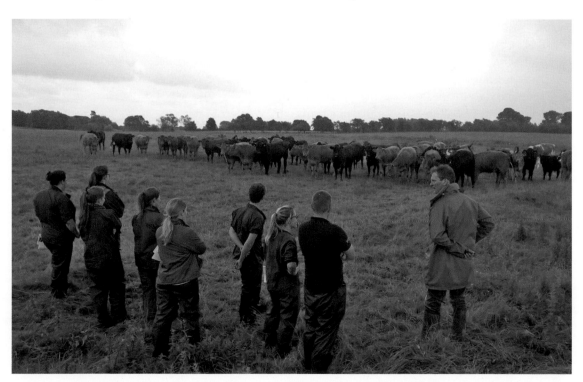

FIGURE 21.4 A learning environment – usually a very healthy one for both people and livestock

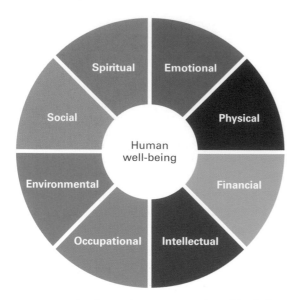

FIGURE 21.5 A schematic representation of holistic thinking for human well-being.

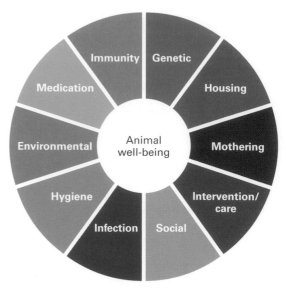

FIGURE 21.6 A schematic representation of holistic thinking for farmed livestock well-being

Animal

A holistic view of animals is what this perspective about. What does holistic mean? Holistic is a popular word these days. The philosophical definition of holistic is *the belief that the parts of any entity are interconnected and the entity is only explicable when viewed as a whole*. In medicine and veterinary medicine, we use the phrase to remind us all that a person or an animal or a herd of animals is affected by all factors, be they genetic/intrinsic or environmental/extrinsic and that only by considering all of these factors can we fully understand the health, well-being and disease of these people or animals. And that is a definition we solidly believe in; we also solidly believe that vets working with farmers and other industry partners can collectively, as a team, develop a fuller, more intelligent understanding of what our animals need and deserve in order to be healthy, content and productive and, in turn, profitable for the farm – dare we say it … the business process perspective? No, the animal perspective!

The Figures 21.5 and 21.6 schematically represent a view of holistic well-being in terms of people and then in terms of farmed animals. After reading this book a good exercise would be to draw one's own version of this scheme – maybe not just for your livestock, but for yourself too!

REFERENCES

Fuller, A. and Unwin, L. (2004) Expansive learning environments. In: Fuller, A., Munro, A. and Rainbird, H. (eds) *Workplace Learning in Context.* Taylor & Francis, Abingdon, ch. 8.

Kaplan, RS. and David Norton (1992) The balanced scorecard: measures that drive performance. *Harvard Business Review* 70(1), 71–79.

Lencioni, P. (2016) *The Truth About Employee Engagement: A Fable About Addressing the Three Root Causes of Job Misery.* Jossey-Bass, San Francisco, CA.

Chapter 22

Motivational theory for the beef farm

Rather like a discussion on the balanced scorecard the subject of motivation may not really seem to belong in a veterinary book for beef farmers. And that may well be so, but given that farmers, not specifically beef farmers as it happens, but farmers generally, have an above-average incidence of mental health disease and, tragically, an above-average suicide rate, then, once again the better question may be – why not have a discussion on motivation? Motivation, after all, is almost certainly connected with *well-being* and is often loosely defined as 'what gets you up in the morning'. Not wanting to get up in the morning is, for sure, a bad sign – yes, of course, it may be due to physical illness but very often is associated with mental illness – so it is probably safe to say it is definitely worth talking about it!

A BASIC PERSPECTIVE ON MOTIVATION

A person has *needs* or *wants* which *cause* or *drive* the person to *behave* in a certain way so as to achieve those needs or wants; the person then feels a sense of *satisfaction*. Once satisfied, that person then either stops feeling the need or experiences an intensification of that need. That might be needing more of the same – referred to as a *primary need* or it may be moving onto needing the next thing – referred to as a *secondary need*.

People's needs vary. Not everyone values the same things; not everyone wants the same things. Theories of motivation try to understand, to categorise, and to model, groups of people who want the same thing and why they want it. This is quite difficult!

An early and long-standing theory was established by Abraham Maslow in 1943. He was convinced that we were actually quite simple and more similar to each other than we realise. He decided that our needs were ordered, or ranked, in importance or immediacy, and that one need had to be satisfied before you would give much thought to the next need in the rankings. He established his famous *hierarchy of needs* (Figure 22.1).

Maslow tells us that first we have to satisfy our basic *physiological needs,* namely food, water, rest, warmth and sex. We then move onto our *safety* needs such as shelter from the elements, protection from predators and safety from assailants or enemies. Our next priority, he proposes, is the sense of *belongingness* – to be part of a family or a community, to have friends and/or an intimate, loving relationship. The penultimate of Maslow's needs is *esteem* or *self-esteem* as it is often referred to. This is about feeling accepted and approved of by those you belong to, to feel confident. The final need, the ultimate need, is what Maslow calls *self-actualisation* and by this he means fulfilling your talents and potentials, for example, with education or training, or repeated practising (or all three usually!).

On first inspection Maslow's theory seems obvious – you need the basics before you get the

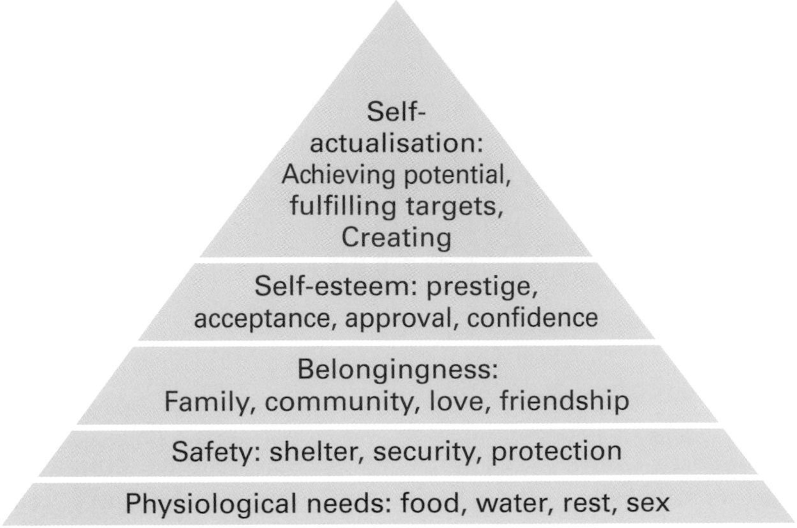

FIGURE 22.1 Maslow's 'hierarchy of needs' pyramid

higher brow stuff. And it is the higher brow stuff that people really vary on. This is a good enough theory for an overview and it remains a very popular one. So, it leaves us then to think about what motivates the self-actualisation of all of us, in our case, what drives the way we live our lives as farmers or vets. But before we move on, it's worth noting that Maslow has his critics. Maslow has religion in the self-actualisation section but evidence from around the world frequently demonstrates that many people put religion before anything else, sometimes their own lives. So, his critics challenge whether Maslow sufficiently taps into the deeper interpretation of *values* – what people *believe in*, sometimes to a seemingly irrational extent. And he has sex in the most basic of needs! It is sort of true but that would suggest that you could not go on, say, a training course if you had not first had sex! A little extreme perhaps?! Some may disagree, some may not – that is the difficulty in motivational theory!

MORE DEVELOPED THEORIES ON MOTIVATION

McClelland attempted to refine Maslow's theory. He accepted that we have basic needs but he tried to separate out our *higher needs*. He suggested the following three categories:

1. need for achievement; to accomplish something difficult
2. need for affiliation; to form relationships
3. need for power; to control others.

It was then separately pointed out, in the Cognitive Evaluation Theory of Motivation, that motivation comes either from within, known as *intrinsic motivation*, or from elsewhere, *extrinsic motivation*. Intrinsic motivators are the things already mentioned like achievement, or a sense of responsibility or competency. Extrinsic motivators are things like money, feedback, environment. People tend to be more one than the other and can even be *demotivated* by the wrong thing. Money, for example, has been shown to reduce the quality of work produced by fine artists and by rock musicians! Herzberg (1964) similarly talked about two factors at play: *hygiene factors* and *true motivators*. Hygiene factors are another way of describing the things in life that are basic needs – they do not particularly motivate, you maybe do not even notice them, but taking them away would de-motivate you. Examples are, once again, money, poor working conditions, unfriendly colleagues. True motivators, in contrast, do exactly that – their presence motivates but their absence is not necessarily disastrous. Examples are, again, things like job satisfaction and achievement. So, in summary, hygiene factors dictate dissatisfaction, true motivators dictate satisfaction. The two things are different, you can experience both, neither or one or the other!

Now, if you are a bit confused, so was everybody else! Dan Pink made a pretty good job of simplifying things in his 2009 book *Drive*. In our practice and in our training courses we, the authors, take Pink's summary and overlay it with McClelland's theory to produce a working motivation model that seems to work well in understanding the motivation of our farm clients, and ourselves as members of a veterinary team serving the needs of farmers.

This Pink/McClelland hybrid model proposes that the *higher motivational needs* of people fall into four areas and while people can be motivated in all or some of these ways they tend to fall into one particular category.

1. **Mastery**. These are the people who like to be the best! The farmer who likes to win the Christmas show, the farmer who likes to have the calf with the biggest backside! The farmer who gets the top price in the sale every week.
2. **Autonomy**. These are the people who like to be in charge! The farmer who likes to be the boss, who likes to decide what is going to happen next, who does not particularly like to do what they are told to do, but instead likes to tell others what to do!
3. **Purpose**. These people like to do something that really needs doing. The farmer who likes to produce an even batch of calves for sale, not necessarily the biggest or the best, but alive, healthy and edible!
4. **Affiliation**. These are the people who like to have other people around them. The farmer who goes to the market every week even when there is nothing to sell or buy; they have their lunch in the market canteen; they keep the vet talking at the farm gate; they take them in for a cup of tea; they go to every meeting.

HOW ARE YOU MOTIVATED? IS IT IMPORTANT TO KNOW?

We think it is important to know what motivates each of us. It helps us design health plans and schemes that will appeal to the user; so, the end result gets achieved – the end result which we, as advisors, believe will benefit you and be satisfying for us to deliver – a win–win where both the farmer and the advisor are motivated, are satisfied.

The problem is that depending on whether you are motivated by mastery, autonomy, purpose or affiliation, the desired end result will vary accordingly. That is where advisors often have to vary their offerings depending on the type of client they are trying to help.

THE ADOPTION OF NEW PRODUCTS AND TECHNIQUES BY FARMERS

Quite how a population of farmers take on a new piece of advice, such as the use of a new product, taking up a new service or adopting a new method, is exactly the same as any population taking on anything new. For example, when pregnancy diagnosis was introduced by the veterinary profession not all farmers took to it at the same time as others, but, eventually, most did. Similarly, when mobile phones were introduced in late 1980s by Vodaphone not all the people in the world took to them; not initially at least, but eventually most people did. Marketeers and economists sum this up in the diffusion of innovation curve as shown in Figure 22.2.

This curve demonstrates that a new idea is first adopted by a keen group called the *innovators*. These people are presumably very motivated by the idea for some reason – one of the reasons given above, that is, mastery, autonomy, purpose

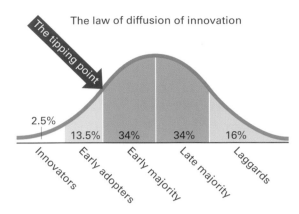

FIGURE 22.2 The 'diffusion of innovation' curve

or affiliation. But which is most likely? Innovators are usually very driven, fairly happy with risk and their key driver is often … mastery. So, if the innovation was the introduction to the marketplace of, say, the iPhone then these innovators typically want the best phone! The autonomous types do not like to be told anything by marketeers or advisors, the purposeful ones want to see if it works or if they have a genuine use for it, and as for the affiliators? They are just waiting to see what their friends do!

The next group on the curve are the *early adopters* – these folk are like innovators; just a little more moderated.

Next come the *late adopters* – some of the types described before who hold back or are not initially motivated. These are often the affiliators who are affected by peer pressure; doing what their mates are doing.

And finally, … the beloved *laggards*; the least motivated of all. These are often the autonomous types but not always. Sometimes these folk are the smartest of all – they may have worked out that the change simply is not beneficial. Sadly, though, the real truth is so often that they are just laggards! But is that their fault? They may have been poorly motivated; others may not understand their values, the marketeers have failed on them.

Sales teams, advisors and even governments are concerned with how to drive this diffusion of innovation as effectively as possible (Garforth, 2015). The idea is, hopefully, that it is in everyone's interest to get the new, supposedly beneficial, change happening. The change may not, however, be beneficial. It may be beneficial to the sales team but not the farmer, it may make money for the advisor but not the farmer, it may be an ill-fated government scheme that does not benefit the farmer but keeps civil servants in work. When this happens, the innovation fails. In fact, the theory shows that if a product taken to market does not succeed in crossing the point called *the chasm* or *the tipping point* then the product, or the service or the scheme will fail. And it is often thanks to the wisdom of the farming community that non-beneficial change does fail. The most frustrating situation arises when a *known beneficial change* fails. For those who do cross the chasm the change goes on to be adopted and it is a success. What can then frustrate sales teams, advisors and governments is the *speed* of innovation.

How do we as advisors speed up the adoption of sensible change? Like we say, we need to make it *motivating*. As for governments, when they are really struggling, what do they do? They legislate. It is a great way of catching the laggards! For example – the 'clunk-click every trip' campaign in the UK in the late 1970s got most people to use their car seat belts, but it was the introduction of a law in 1983 that got the laggards to comply. Funnily enough, farmers featured heavily in the seat belt laggard group, see Figure 22.3!

There has been a fair bit of research and market research into how to speed up the diffusion of innovation into the farming industry. It can be quite frustrating for good quality advisors, consultants and indeed government departments who know they have a recommended change that has been clearly demonstrated to be beneficial to the industry only to see it ignored by too many. Research by Garforth (2015) supports the notion that the advisors need to understand motivation and to go slightly deeper into motivational theory by understanding the values and beliefs held by the farmer for it may well be these that are blocking the adoption of the change.

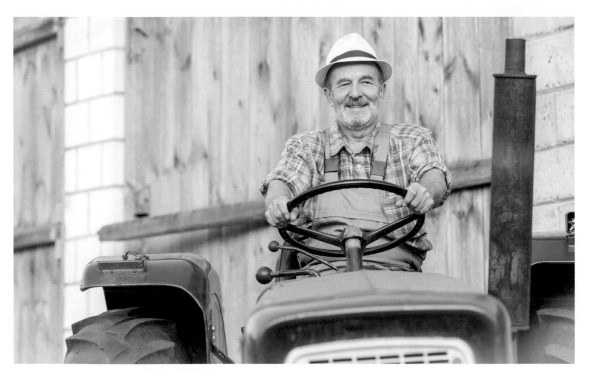

FIGURE 22.3 Farmers were late to adopt seat belt technology! Adobe Stock: Moodboard

Before leaving this subject, there is one more branch of thinking that fits in here, and that is the concept of *the mindset*. Carol Dweck (2006) has introduced huge changes into the world of children's education and subsequently student and adult education through her *growth mindset theory*. She has demonstrated that people tend to belong to a fixed mindset or to a growth mindset. Those with a fixed mindset believe they are born the way they are; they cannot change, they cannot improve and that is that. Those in the growth mindset, however, believe they can improve through effort and learning. One of the key differences between the two groups that Dweck demonstrated was that of *fear of failure*. Those with a fixed mindset seem to fear failure, those with a growth mindset do not; they see failure as just another way of learning – a signal to try harder or do it differently next time. That is all very well, we may think, but, what can you do about it? You have either got a fixed mindset or a growth mindset, right? Well here is the interesting bit. Dweck has shown that you can voluntarily change your mindset with just a bit of self-discipline and determination, a bit of effort. School educators have adopted this approach; the growth mindset is now *taught* as part of the national curriculum in many countries of the world. The fixed versus growth mindset is summarised in Figure 22.4.

SUMMARY OF MOTIVATION FOR BEEF FARMERS

If we all, and that includes farmers, improve our understanding of motivation, values and mindsets we will surely be in a better position to take full advantage of any beneficial new changes in the industry rather than get left behind.

- Advisors could better understand the motivation, values and mindsets of others.
- Farmers could benefit from a better understanding of their own motivation, values and mindsets and those of their team.

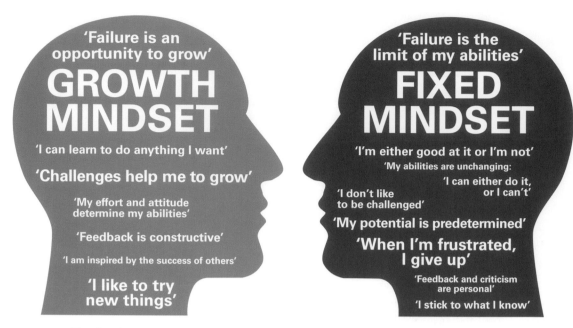

FIGURE 22.4 The fixed versus growth mindset, courtesy of Meopham Community Academy

- Farmers could benefit from a shift to a growth mindset.
- Farmers could then adopt beneficial change where they would previously not have done.
- Farmers could then adopt beneficial change faster than they would previously have done.
- The farming industry could then keep pace with other industries.
- All industry partners (farmers, advisors, vets and responsible suppliers) could thrive.
- Our beef cattle could then also thrive more, and be seen to thrive more by the public; more so than they would have done in the absence of the change and to everyone's mutual benefit, not least of which their own.

BUSINESS THRIVING

Business theory suggests that growing and thriving are essential to long-term business survival, that is whether you are a new *start-up*, in the earlier years of *growth*, in the later years of *scaling up* or in the fortunate stage of reaching business *maturity* or *prime*. Business theory also shows that businesses tend to go through these phases in an S-shaped curve fashion and at the end of each S phase the crucial crossroads crop up – choose to thrive, choose to stagnate or choose to fail (see Figure 22.5). Choosing to thrive is part of the growth mindset, it is helped by understanding motivation, by balancing your business scorecard (with particular attention to marketing) and by striving for good teamwork and team leadership (see Chapter 24). Armed with a growth mindset much of this necessitates continuous learning – continuing professional development as industry call it.

BUSINESS FAILURE

It is easy to say all we have said about ensuring a business thrives but with the best will in the world, some businesses will fail – is it always for the above reasons? A study of small business failures in the USA suggested that 19% of failed businesses are beaten by competition, 23% are deemed to lack

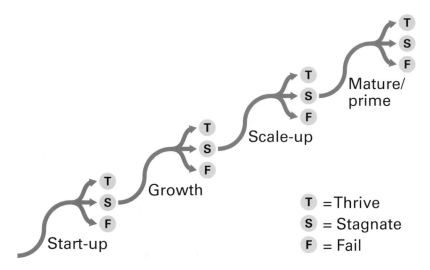

T = Thrive
S = Stagnate
F = Fail

FIGURE 22.5 S-curves of business growth

team structure and skill, 29% run out of cash and a massive 42% fail through lack of market need for their product or services (Figure 22.6) (Desjardins, 2017).

So sometimes it is finance, sometimes it is customer perspective (marketing), sometimes it is people. The only part of the balanced scorecard not alluded to is business process that, funnily enough, was suggested as the one part of the balanced scorecard that tends not to get neglected – the other areas clearly do – that is why we all need balanced scorecards!

REFERENCES

Desjardins, J. (2017) Entrepreneurship. *Visual Capitalist.* Available at: https://www.visualcapitalist.com/why-do-businesses-fail/ (accessed 1 February 2020).

Dweck, C.S. (2006) *Mindset: The New Psychology of Success.* Random House, New York.

Dweck, C.S. (2012) *Mindset: How You can Fulfil your Potential.* Constable & Robinson, London.

Garforth, C. (2015) Livestock keepers' reasons for doing and not doing things which governments, vets and scientists would like them to do. *Zoonoses and Public Health* 62(Suppl 1), 29–38.

Herzberg, F (1964) The motivation-hygiene concept and problems of manpower. *Personnel Administration* 27, 3–7.

Maslow, A.H. (1943) A theory of human motivation. *Psychological Review* 50(4), 370–396.

Pink, D. H. (2009) *Drive: The Surprising Truth About What Motivates Us.* Riverhead Books, New York.

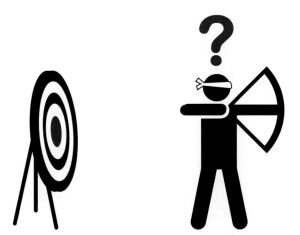

FIGURE 22.6 Common reasons for business failure – missed market

Chapter 23

Marketing theory for the beef farm

What do farmers not know about marketing?! Did they not invent it!? Markets were indeed invented by farmers as a place to take their crops and animals, a place where they could show them off and sell them. They still do; that is marketing. While only a tiny fraction of finished cattle go through markets these days the majority of breeding stock still do (Figure 23.1). Plenty of farmers still go to a market to buy bulls, breeding heifers and sometimes breeding cows. A large percentage of store cattle are also marketed conventionally. So, we know about marketing? Sadly, for many beef farmers we maybe do not know enough about true marketing, marketing in the broader sense of the word, marketing to the end user, the ultimate customer. And in beef farming that is the consumer. However, between the farmer and the consumer there is a supply chain, a chain in which there are several links, in each of which the customer must still be remembered (how it should be) or, unfortunately forgotten (how it should not be).

DEFINITION OF MARKETING

A loose abbreviated version of the definition of marketing as proposed by the American Marketing Association (AMA) is 'the activity and process of creating, communicating, and delivering offerings that have value for customers and society at large'.

It seems that the beef industry frequently falls down in all of these steps, not always, but frequently.

Creating an offering

The initial creation of an offering is surely the first key step. The offering needs to be something the customer wants. To create an offering that the customer wants is to fully *understand* what the customer *wants*. It may even be to understand *what the customer thinks they want* as opposed to *what they actually want* – they may not know that! Or to take things a step further it may be to understand what the customer wants when the customer does not actually realise what they want, at least not consciously – the fascinating world of *subliminal marketing*!

Does the farmer know what the customer wants? Are they being told? Are they asking? Is it the case that farmers will often produce something that they themselves want to produce as opposed to what the customer actually wants; an animal they like the look of, a breed they have always had a fancy for. Does that necessarily convert into the meat the consumer wants? And is it just about meat? Many consumers may be more interested in the welfare of the animal before it died than the meat itself and certainly more than what the animal looked like or what breed it was.

To understand what the customer wants is to be fully aware of the 'market research'. And market research has to be very good to get to the truth. Who do you ask? What questions do you ask? Good market research will obviously get answers to relevant questions from a large number of

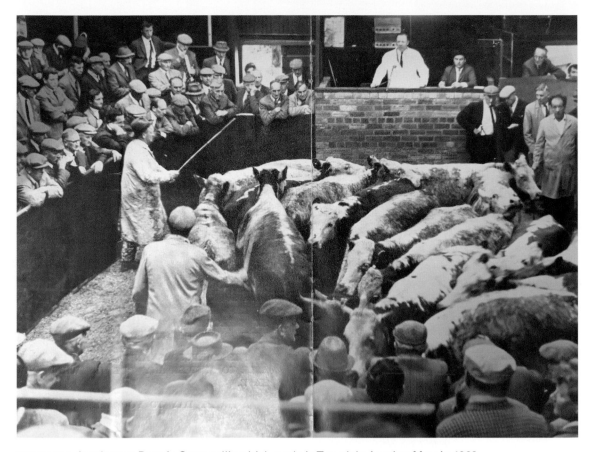

FIGURE 23.1 Auctioneer Dennis Scott selling Irish cattle in Tynedale Auction Mart in 1968

consumers, and from a diverse range of customer types – different ages, sexes, socio-economic groups, ethnicities and so on.

The best people to find out these truths are the supermarkets – it really matters to them; they are big businesses and generally very well run. So, the best people the farmers can ask about the *creation of the offering* are the analysts at the supermarkets. And how do you go about asking someone what they think, what they know, what they want? This is a good time to raise the matter of communication, and of *listening*.

Communication of the offering

As is so often the case, communication here is crucially two-way. Communication is a lot about asking good questions and listening. Getting this good communication from the consumer helps you design your offering and then, when you have created your offering, making sure you effectively communicate its availability back to the consumer. There are obviously many ways that this communication can operate within the supply chain – the links that sit between the individual farmer and the final consumer.

The individual farmer can communicate his offering directly. This could be the promotion of home-bred bulls or breeding females to other breeders. It may be the promotion of home-bred store cattle to beef fattening customers. It may be the promotion of home reared meat to the consumer via a local farmers' market stall or by advertising the farm name on the menu of a restaurant that serves the product.

The offering may not be communicated directly; it may be done through an agent or a members' organisation. Classically the agent would be an auctioneer – a brokering service still widely practised. At this point the science of marketing then, to some extent, becomes their problem but for the primary producer, the farmer, to relinquish the responsibility for a contribution to the marketing chain would clearly be unhelpful. In terms of members' organisations, they may be something like a national meat marketing board who promote the product on behalf of the industry. Again, that is their job, but is the primary producer contributing? Is the primary producer actually complying with the offering that has been agreed on or is the primary producer still, instead, producing what *they* want to produce? That would, again, break the consistency of the supply chain.

Delivering the offering

One of the key elements of successful marketing is to deliver what you say you are going to deliver; to deliver the product or service as described, to the quality expected, in sufficient quantities to satisfy demand and in a logistically satisfactory way – quick enough, not damaged, in a way that is convenient to the customer, and, very importantly these days, not too many 'food miles' away.

An offering that represents value for customers

Value could be defined as the state of mind the customer finds themselves in on receipt of the product or service; *good value* would be a feeling of reward and contentment and an absence of negative feelings such as being 'ripped off'. This feeling of value takes many forms: loving the taste, loving the smell, loving the sight, proudly carrying the bag out of the shop with their favourite logo on it, knowing the animal enjoyed a high welfare life, knowing it came from just up the road, knowing it never had antibiotics. Value is a personal thing; we are not all good at understanding other people's 'values'; the things they attach importance to; the things that hold emotional value to them, but, when it comes to good marketing we have to try.

The AMA definition talks about value not just to the individual but to society at large. This leads onto consideration of societal trends and fashions. Value to the individual is supposedly a personal thing but it is very evident that much, so called, *personal value* is hugely influenced by societal pressure; by social influence, variously described by terms such as peer pressure, keeping up with the Joneses, fashion, trend. In the recent history of first world beef consumption we can think of some positive trends and negative trends.

Examples of positive *trends and fashions* in beef consumption:

- the American burger boom of the 1950s
- the arrival of the American burger in the UK in the 1970s
- Aberdeen Angus steak houses in the UK in the 1970s
- Argentinian steakhouses in Europe in the 2010s
- Wagu meat in Europe in the 2010s.

Examples of negative *trends and fashions* in beef consumption:

- concerns over links between BSE and Creutzfeldt–Jakob disease (CJD) in the 1990s
- concerns over links with bowel cancer in the 2000s
- vegetarianism and veganism in 2010s.

That is our amateurish overview of marketing in the beef industry. How would the real marketing industry sum up the subject?

THE 4Ps AND 4Cs

Marketeers like to consider the 4Ps and the 4Cs of marketing.

The 4Ps of marketing

1. **Product**. Define your product or service.
2. **Price**. Set a price for the product or service.
3. **Promotion**. Advertise your product or service.
4. **Positioning**. Sell your product or service in a marketplace where the customer can easily access the offering.

The 4Ps were revised into the 4Cs as it was realised that they did not *start with the customer* and as we know the *customer always comes first!* And that meant all the other factors had to start with C also!

The 4Cs of marketing

1. **Customer**. What do they want?
2. **Cost**. Not just the price. What is the real cost of a product when producing it and when selling it? How much does it damage other *values* such as the environment? The welfare of the animal? And, of course, how much is the customer prepared to pay? How much do they really value it?

3. **Communication**. Promotion and advertising alone do not do justice to the concept of great communication; two-way communication at all levels, listening to the customer, hearing them, what they really want, and only then getting the customer to hear you. Advertising is therefore just a small part of communication, but it is an important part. Advertising is all around us, even in nature. Peacocks are a great example of advertising; they are advertising their own genes! Marketeers know this – that is where the marketing term 'peacocking' comes from (Figure 23.2).
4. **Convenience** – Convenience is what we are ultimately defining when we are talking about positioning. For example, positioning coffee vending machines on train platforms, or embarrassing personal items on the internet instead of in a public shop. What is most convenient to the customer is what is most likely to happen.

To satisfy both models, marketeers combine the Ps and Cs into the following standard marketing checklist, the **5PCs of marketing** we will call them.

1. Customer and Product
2. Cost and Price
3. Communication and Promotion

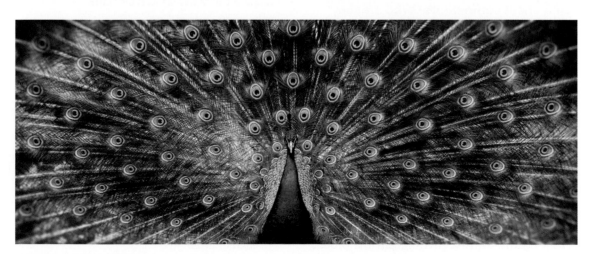

FIGURE 23.2 'Peacocking' or advertising is all around us. Adobe Stock: Baranov

4. Convenience and Positioning

and this time, a fifth consideration:

5. Competition and Pressure in the marketplace – being aware of what others are doing, be that successful or unsuccessful.

CUSTOMERS, COMPETITORS AND CAPABILITY

Much of marketing science is about understanding the impediments to the successful marketing of a product, in our case, beef. To help think through this area here comes yet another marketing model and yet again all the words start with C!

1. Customers
2. Competitors
3. Capability

Customers

We have already talked about the customer and the importance of putting *them*, not ourselves, first. Competitors are next on this list.

Competitors

What about competitors? Who are they?

- Businesses selling the *same type of product* that you sell.
- Businesses selling an *alternative to the product* you sell.

Businesses selling the same type of product – commoditise or differentiate?

Beef farmers may take a view they do not want to compete with their colleagues; they may feel that 'we are all in it together'. That is the foundation of movements like cooperatives and meat marketing boards. In this environment the producers are actually *commoditising* their product – it is

all meat, meat is meat, we all produce it, it is all the same.

On the other hand, some producers may take the approach of *differentiating* their product. It is not just meat:

- it is grass-fed beef
- it is slow reared beef
- it is Hereford beef
- it is beef reared by its mother, reared as nature intended, not by a machine.

In either case, commoditising or differentiating, the response to competition is actually to minimise 'head on competition', to avoid a fight.

Businesses selling an alternative to your product – similar but different, or completely different

A 'similar alternative' would be products that are not beef but are still meat of some sort – obviously things like lamb or venison, close red meat alternatives, or something a little further removed, that is, white meat, or, further still, fish meat. Then there are the non-meat alternatives such as Quorn, tofu, seitan and tempeh, some of which are processed to actually *look like meat* while some are deliberately prepared to look nothing like meat so as to achieve a complete dissociation from any animal connection. Here the response to the competition is more like 'head on competition'.

Categorising competition

Whether comparing one beef producer with another, or comparing beef producers to non-beef producers, the marketing world classifies competitors into four types.

1. **Laidback competitors**. These competitors are slow to respond to competition, they enjoy the fact they have loyal clients, they are rather lacking resource should any sort of response be needed or attempted.
2. **Selective competitors**. These competitors

respond to some forms of competition but never price.
3. **Tigers**. Tigers respond quickly and aggressively to competition.
4. **Stochastic competitors**. These competitors respond to competition in an unpredictable way.

Which one are we as an industry and which one are you as an individual producer?

Responding to competition

As with other business activities, responses to competition take the form of a long-term view, known as a strategy, and of short-term responses, known as tactics. It is interesting to note that these terms are military in origin. The word strategy actually comes from Greek and means something along the lines of 'leading an army' and the word tactic also stems from the Greek for 'arranging in battle formation'. Let us face it, marketing strategy and tactics seem to be based on winning; not just a fight, but a war!

Know your enemy! Know your competition!

Porter's generic strategies for tackling competition

One of the key things a general does is stand on a hill to view the enemy forces, to know them, to understand them, to develop a strategy to deal with the competition. Porter (2008) suggests businesses, in our case beef producers, can adopt one of four generic strategies to gain a competitive advantage.

- **Cost leadership**. Being the cheapest. This often equates to a large scale of production, maximum efficiency, running at high capacity, having buying power, being happy with a standard 'no-frills' offering, having good logistics, making full use of technology. Warning – only one producer/supplier can be the cheapest. This may involve changing suppliers to save money. Are you in a position to do this? Supplier power may be a problem here.
- **Differentiation leadership**. Being different, specialising. This often equates to a premium

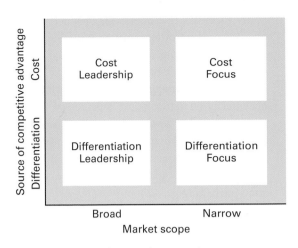

FIGURE 23.3 Porter's generic strategies

offering. The premium product may be produced through exacting regulations or qualifications so making the market difficult for others to enter. It may be that the product succeeds at being premium through good branding, good advertising, a large nationwide availability, a household name.
- **Cost focus**. Being the cheapest but only to smaller markets, those who are happy with a non-premium product, a generic, an economy line, a *white label* product.
- **Differentiation focus**. A niche product, a high price tag, different, specialist, a smaller market with less competition. This means fewer customers and the fewer customers you have the more customer power they develop so it is essential the offering is genuinely special, and valid, and, difficult to copy.

Specific ways to get a competitive advantage in the beef industry

There are specific ways a beef producer or a supplier could gain a competitive advantage over their adversaries in business:

- **Superior product or service**. Having noticeably better beef is quite difficult. Meat quality is very variable, and this variation is subject to many factors (see Chapter 7). Producers may need to explore other ways of being superior; superior packaging for example, added value such as a marinade or dressing.

- **Perceived advantage**. The product may not necessarily be better, but it is perceived by the customer to be better. That can come from long-standing reputation (existing brand value) or the quick creation of new brand value which may come from good advertising or, again, good packaging.
- **Low cost**. Being the cheapest budget option can work but there can only be one and there may be a race to the bottom.
- **Legal advantage**. The possession of a licence or a patent or a copyright can be very advantageous. For example, a Melton Mowbray Pie.
- **Superior contacts**. A good third-party relationship can be helpful. You may have a Royal Appointment or you may have a contract with Harrods of Knightsbridge.
- **Superior knowledge**. You may be a specialist supplier. You may supply a special type of meat that requires specialist advice in its cooking, for example, carpaccio.
- **Scale advantage**. You may be a huge producer able to satisfy a bulk contract that others cannot.
- **Offensive attitude**. Offensive in terms of attack rather than unpleasant – although you may be both! In other words, a very eager approach which manages to get you the sale.

Capability

The third and final impediment to successful marketing is the potential lack of capability a producer may have to deliver the product. But not literally to just deliver it. Capability here refers to the ability of the producer to design a good offering, to develop it, to sell it, to distribute it and, often neglected by many producers and service providers, to offer good customer support, be that pre-sales or post sales ('after care'). It may not be the producer who is primarily failing in this capability – it may be collaborators,

support industries upon whom the producer has misguidedly chosen to rely, say, for example, to handle distribution logistics. But at the end of the day the customer will see it as the producer who has failed in the overall provision of satisfaction.

MARKET DEVELOPMENT AND PENETRATION

Market development is all about expanding your existing market, whereas market penetration is about entering a new one. If you want to improve success in these manoeuvres, then marketing theory recommends adopting the technique of market segmentation.

Market segmentation

Market segmentation is all about dividing up your marketplace into different types of customer and focusing on each of them in a more tailored fashion. Much of this relates to motivational theory as described in Chapter 22 where different types of people are understood to be differently driven, differently motivated, but there are other, and often easier, ways of subdividing a marketplace:

Market segmentation is often based on the following four subdivisions:

1. **geographic** – such as county, region or country
2. **demographic** – such as age, gender, lifestyle, socio-economic group
3. **psychographic** – such as activities, interests, hobbies, opinion, values
4. **behavioural** – such as loyalty, usage, benefits sought, occasion.

A market segment needs at least one, preferably more, of the following characteristics to be worth pursuing:

- accessible
- substantial

- unique
- appropriate
- predictable
- stable.

CONCLUSION

This rather detailed summary of marketing aims to, at least, generate more awareness and further thinking on the subject. We are widely believed by other industries to have a need to be better at marketing. Taking the broader view, we need to remember that marketing is just part of the *customer perspective* portion of the balanced scorecard; that's one of the perspectives that seems to be neglected and, in which case, most definitely needs 'balancing up'.

REFERENCE

Porter, M. (2008) *On Competition.* Harvard Business School Publishing, Boston, MA.

FURTHER READING

Kotler, P. and Armstrong, G. (2008) *Principles of Marketing*, 12th edn. Pearson Education, Upper Saddle River, NJ.

Chapter 24

Leadership, followership and team theory for the beef farm

LEADERSHIP

Leadership is a much talked about concept. It is talked about every time there's an election – who is the best leader for the party? Who would be the best leader for the country? Industry talks about leadership and spends millions of pounds a year on *training* people in the discipline; training people to lead departments and to lead organisations. Sports analysts talk about leadership – whether leadership from the captain, leadership from the coach, or leadership from the club owner. It seems to be important. So, what exactly is leadership? Is it important on a farm? Is it even relevant to a farm?

One definition of leadership is that it is 'a process of social influence in which one person is able to enlist the aid and support of others in the accomplishment of a common task or objective' (Chemers, 1997). That fits with things we have talked about previously, for example, the importance of being objective, of having a 'why', and the importance of motivation; being motivated towards the common goal. So, the definition of leadership makes it sound like something an organisation would *want* and it seems most people are agreed on that. Perhaps the next questions are:

- Who is the right person to lead?
- How does that person lead?

Who leads?

For a long time, it was thought, and is still thought by many, that leaders are born – you either are or you are not. But the current view is different; you can learn to be a leader, you can be trained to be a leader, and that is exactly why industries spend so much time and money on it. But, like most things in life it does seem there is still an innate element, a genetic component to leadership qualities, as well as a learnt part. The balance between the two remains uncertain but it does seem to help if you have the right personality for a bit of natural leadership, a headstart. But for those who lack that, behaviours, skills and actions can be honed to make a big contribution to the ability to lead. The thing is, particularly on, say, a small farm, you may have little choice but to just get on and *lead*, so you may as well do the best job possible. How?

How to lead?

Some traditional leaders used force and coercion to lead – like the sergeant major shouting at the troops or the threat of the firing squad being enough to get you to follow orders. Others did it the *softly softly* way.

Let us take a look at some considered views on what is right on *how to lead*. Stephen Blakesley who ran a recruitment agency in the USA studied his own business and, perhaps even more interestingly, he also studied the businesses that he recruited staff for. He wrote a book on his findings. He feels that leadership is about six key elements.

Self-awareness

Blakesley reminds us that leadership is actually *defined by the people who are being led* (the *followers* – see later), they decide whether to be led by you or not, and that depends on *how they see you*. And if you cannot see what they see, that is, if you have not got a fair idea of what you are really like then you are going to struggle, especially if you are seen to be an *imposter*, someone who lacks *authenticity*. So, self-awareness is important, self-honesty, seeing your behaviour and your values and your skills for what they really are. This is the first element of leadership and it, for one, can be taught – you can practise self-awareness and you can be coached in it.

Perspective and context

Helping your team members to *know the objective of the organisation*, and equally important, *to know how they contribute to it*, is very helpful. This can also be taught. For example, being taught how to write a good *vision statement* and a good *mission statement* for your organisation, for your farm. And, providing a team member with *context* can also be taught. For example, by learning to write a good *job description* will help that person see clearly and constructively how they are contributing to the goal; or simply telling a team member how they make a difference.

Knowing and understanding the team

Blakesley observes that you have to genuinely get to know your team and get to know their trials and tribulations, their interests, their hobbies, their families, their problems. This just takes time and effort. It needs to be authentic though.

Building trust

According to Kouzes and Posner (1995) *trust is built* and this is achieved through:

- **integrity** – being honest and morally sound
- **reliability** – doing what you say you are going to do (and that means not over-committing – and that takes a bit of thought and planning)
- **listening** – listening more than talking, making eye contact, taking notes and thanking people for talking to you
- **accountability** – taking the blame (but not the credit!)
- **respect** – being grateful and respectful of the team
- **loyalty** – standing by the organisation, the team and their decisions – but only within reason, only if it does not compromise the integrity factor.

Much of these can be worked on, improved, taught, learnt.

Goal *getting*, not just *setting*

Goal setting alone is very powerful: a study of Harvard graduates revealed that those who left college with a *written goal plan* ended up earning a staggering ten times more money than those who did not have a goal (McCormack, 1984). But *goal getting* is even better; being seen to succeed sounds very elitist but it is true – it inspires a team. Blakesley's tips are as follows.

- Writing down a goal and the date by which it is to be achieved (Maltz, 1960).
- Picking something you are genuinely passionate about.
- Recognising the cost, both financial and human, and still wanting it!

Emotional intelligence

Emotional intelligence is all about understanding emotions, '*feelings*', your own and those of others, and, how then to manage them. This is perhaps one trait that is least teachable, it's fairly innate, but it can be worked on. Mayer et al. (2000) recommend improving emotional intelligence through the following steps.

- Make notes of your emotions (feelings) and what triggered them.
- Delay decision making and creativity to when you are in a calm mood.
- Learn to understand emotions; yours and those of others. Know that you feel either *secure* or *insecure* – life really is that simple!

But what makes you feel secure or insecure? It seems to boil down to understanding the SCARF model (Rock, 2008).

- **S**tatus – how important or unimportant does the situation leave you feeling?
- **C**ertainty – how sure are you about what is about to happen in the situation?
- **A**utonomy – how much control do you feel you have over the situation?
- **R**elatedness – how socially connected and accepted do you feel in the situation?
- **F**airness – how fairly treated do you feel in the situation?

We all have our own SCARF profile – our own mix of the *emotional domains*. Which are more significant to you? It helps you to know your own SCARF profile, and then you can get to work on thinking about other people and theirs. Once we grasp the SCARF concept we can then think about *how we can behave* to best influence someone else's SCARF response, that is, *their emotional response to you*. It is very powerful stuff and worth taking seriously. It is obviously instinctive for some people. For those for whom it is not, once again it is something that can be worked on (see Figure 24.1).

Learning to manage emotions seems more than worthwhile, for example, learning to stay calm when things are going wrong on farm – that alone is thought to calm those around you. But do not be

Emotional state	Behavioural influence
Status	Respect
Certainty	Reliability
Autonomy	Empowerment
Relatedness	Sociability
Fairness	Integrity

FIGURE 24.1 SCARF emotional states and behaviours that influence them

scared to also show when you feel good, when you manage to calve the cow that someone else could not, as long as it does not involve gloating!

FOLLOWERSHIP

Followership is a little-used word, that is until now.

> An intentional practice on the part of a team player to enhance the synergistic interchange between team and leader. (Uhl-Bien et al., 2014)

We have talked about leadership and how being able to do it well, or learning to do it well, positively influences and motivates the team to succeed in achieving a common objective or goal. But we were also reminded that *followers*, that is, team members, *hold the power* to some extent – *they define the leaders*, in some cases they choose them, they appoint them, and again, to some extent, they choose how much or how little to be led by them. Followership is, it seems, a form of leadership! And sure enough, the *discipline* of followership is now being looked at by industry. It is seen as something that can be done well for positive benefit and it is something, like leadership, that can, to a large extent, be taught.

Followership theory seems to have come from the military world. Military organisation has always been heavily based on very strict *chain of command* structures. The leader tells the followers what to do and the followers do it. But increased openness and transparency in the investigation of military failures has shown that bad decisions by leaders can lead to loss of life and that sometimes the advice coming from the ranks could have saved lives. The military have adopted the concept of followership, and it is something they now *teach* operatives to do properly; they call it *loyal and professional dissent*. In 2012 the US Army defined good followership as learning loyalty, subordination, respect for superiors, but also *when and how to lodge candid disagreement*. And the advice from Lt. Col. Mark Cantrell (1998) is for team members 'to get their facts straight, be certain the boss is wrong before calling any attention, bring the correct information and guidance to the boss for everyone's good, and to always work with the boss rather than going over the boss' head, unless absolutely necessary'.

Is this really relevant to a farm environment? Almost certainly. A farm team leader has to try to get on and lead as best they can but the team members are also leading in their own way in that they define the leader, they are the ones who actually deliver the objective and they are entitled to disagree. But the advice is clear – do it properly, do it constructively and do it by talking to the leader, the boss, and not someone else, in just the same way the leader, the boss, should be talking to the team members, the stock persons for example, instead of moaning to someone else.

Followership key skills

Eight key skills in followership, skills that can be taught, learnt and developed, have been proposed (McCallum, 2013).

Judgement

It's right to take direction from leadership, but is the direction ethical and proper? Simply disagreeing may not be evidence enough to object but a moral judgement may be. This reminds us of the old saying: 'Good judgement comes from experience; experience comes from bad judgement.'

Work ethic

Making the effort is always the starting point. Moaning and objecting holds no water when the team member in question shows no diligence, commitment or attention to detail.

Competence

The team member needs the skills and competencies to do their job, but it is of course leadership that is to blame when this is not the case. The leader must ensure training and skill is in place, if that still fails then there is a problem.

Honesty

A team member needs to be honest and forthright with feedback to the leader when a strategy or tactic seems flawed. Respect and politeness remain important, however, to keep the debate constructive. Remember, either party can be wrong, both can be wrong, both can be right.

Courage

Honest confrontation with leadership can require courage – it may be a serious challenge with consequences but when judgement and honesty backed up with a track record of competency and work ethic lead to a necessary challenge then a deep breath and courage is needed. As Churchill once said: 'Courage – the foremost of the virtues, for upon it, all others depend.'

Discretion

Discretion, put bluntly, is about keeping your mouth shut when faced with the temptation of saying something inappropriate, insensitive or confidential. It should be easy but some team

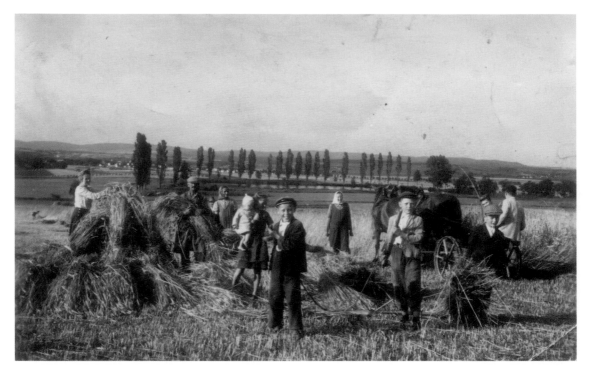

FIGURE 24.2 Farm teamwork is not a new concept. Adobe Stock: Vitezslav Halamka

members (and leaders) seem to find it next to impossible. We all have a duty of care; indiscretion is not care, it is careless.

Loyalty

Loyalty is perhaps best seen as allegiance and commitment to the cause and objectives of the organisation, of the farm business. It is not synonymous with being a lapdog to a leader. Disloyal team members are considered a source of difficulty, they compromise the team goals, they waste team time and energy, they are distractors.

Ego management

Good team members have their ego under control. They are all about team performance and goals over and above personal recognition and self-promotion. These people usually have good interpersonal skills and define the true team player.

So, while a good leader ultimately takes the blame it is pretty clear it will not be entirely down to him or her. The team members have an enormous responsibility in the overall achievement of the team objectives.

However, teaching followership is a tricky one – who wants to be taught to be a follower? It does not sound very appealing or ambitious. It is far more palatable to see it as being a good team member, being good at *teamwork*, or to use another made up word, *teamship*!

Team theory on the beef farm

> None of us are smarter than all of us. (Jim Rohn, 1930–2008)

You may well be part of a 'team' if you happen to work on a medium- or large-sized beef enterprise. You may, on the other hand, may be a team of one! Is it possible to have a team of one? Probably

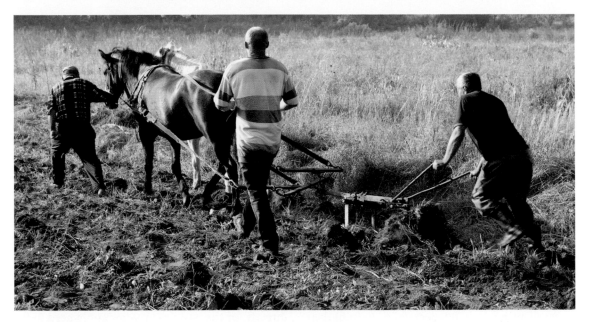

FIGURE 24.3 Farm teams include animals. Adobe Stock: Pavlofox

not. But are you really a team of one? What about the lad down the road who helps every now and then? What about your neighbour's daughter who helps at calving time? And your spouse who helps with a calving in the middle of the night? Or your aunty who does the books? You may even consider outside suppliers, technicians and consultants as part of your team – they are really, or at least they should be! (Figures 24.2 and 24.3)

There is much theory on the construction of an effective team; the building of what is popularly referred to nowadays as a 'high performing team'. There is nothing new in this. Team structure has, for decades, been fiercely debated every week on sports programmes and in every pub around the country on a daily basis! Indeed, football provides a great model for the study of team building and team structure. It is clear, listening to the football pundits, that the following requirements need satisfying.

- Fill every position – the team simply cannot manage without a goalkeeper for example.
- Each position should be filled with an appropriate person – you would not pick the big solid fullback for the wing.

- The team needs a captain – someone to confidently step forward and toss the coin and dish out the orders.
- The team needs a coach – someone to guide them, to see the team from the outside as well as the inside.

All nice simple stuff. But let us take a closer look at team theory.

In 1969, Dr Meredith Belbin began a study of team behaviour. Belbin was a highly respected academic/industrialist. Belbin recruited Bill Hartson, a mathematician and international chess master, Jeanne Fisher, an anthropologist who had studied Kenyan tribes, and Roger Mottram, an occupational psychologist, and together they began what was to be a 9 year task playing business games with eight teams, each team performing like pretend businesses. They then studied the different kinds of contribution from each individual team member.

Those participating were judged on their 'high level reasoning ability', their smartness, using a test called the critical thinking appraisal. Teams of various designs were composed on the basis of these individual test scores. The contribution of team members was recorded and classified into one of seven categories by trained observers. At the end of the exercise, which ran for a week, the results of each team (business) were presented in terms of *financial success*. This allowed the more effective and less effective 'businesses' to be compared with each other.

As well as critical thinking ability, team members were also compared on personality type (using the Cattell personality inventory) and their own personal motivation (using a personal preference questionnaire developed specifically for the purpose).

It was expected that the high-intellect teams would succeed where lower intellect teams would not. The outcome of this research was pleasantly surprising – that some of the teams, predicted to be excellent based on intellect, failed to fulfil their potential. It became apparent by looking at the various combinations that it was not intellect, but what they called *balance*, which enabled a team to succeed. Successful 'businesses' were characterised by the compatibility of the roles that their members played while unsuccessful companies were subject to *role conflict*. Starting afresh using new information from psychometric tests, predictions could then be made on the roles that individuals would play and ultimately on whether the business would be more likely to succeed.

One interesting observation from the experiment was that individuals reacted very differently within the same broad situation and that commonly individual differences caused the group to fall apart. Some people just do not fit in, it seemed. Conversely, variation in personal characteristics was seen as a strength if they were recognised and taken into account. So, as stated earlier in this chapter, understanding the nature of these differences is an essential first step in the leadership and management of people, providing one can recognise what is useful for a given situation and what is not.

The most successful companies tended to be those with a balanced mix of different people, that is, those with a range of different behaviours. Nine discrete clusters of behaviour turned out to be distinctive and useful. These were called 'team roles'. Belbin's team roles have been used in organisations and teams across the world ever since (Table 24.1)

So, if a good business needs all these team positions filled how can you expect a small farming business to achieve that? Well it may be that one person has to cover more than one role. For example, asking the fullback to double up as goalkeeper when the team has had three players sent off! It may be that you look outside the core business to fill some of the roles – for example, using the farm accountant, a trusted friend, or who knows, maybe even your vet!

For the bigger farming unit with over 10 members of staff it may well be you can fill each role with a different person and they may all work directly for the business. You may only need to fill one role yourself, your preferred role. If you have got gaps in your team your business performance *will suffer*, it is essential to get this right, to get those gaps filled, even if it means out-sourcing.

Try filling in a Belbin team sheet for your farm business – the following mocked up example in Table 24.2 may help.

HOW DO TEAMS GO WRONG?

The sending off of a player in a football match significantly reduces the results performance for the sanctioned team (Červený, 2018). This fact supports what is said above – fill every position on the team. What else goes wrong?

The five dysfunctions of a team

Patrick Lencioni talks about the five dysfunctions of a team and in doing so seems to capture much of the essence of leadership, followership and team theory.

1. **Absence of trust**. Lack of willingness on the part of team members (leaders and

TABLE 24.1 Belbin's team roles

Team Role	Contribution	Allowable weaknesses
Plant	Creative, imaginative, free-thinking. Generates ideas and solves difficult problems	Ignores incidentals. Too preoccupied to communicate effectively
Resource-investigator	Outgoing, enthusiastic, communicative. Explores opportunities and develops contacts	Over-optimistic. Loses interest once initial enthusiasm has passed
Co-ordinator	Mature, confident, identifies talent. Clarifies goals. Delegates effectively	Can be seen as manipulative. Offloads own share of the work
Shaper	Challenging, dynamic, thrives on pressure. Has the drive and courage to overcome obstacles	Prone to provocation. Offends people's feelings
Monitor-evaluator	Sober, strategic and discerning. Sees all options and judges accurately	Lacks drive and ability to inspire others. Can be overly critical
Teamworker	Co-operative, perceptive and diplomatic. Listens and averts friction	Indecisive in crunch situation. Avoids confrontation
Implementer	Practical, reliable, efficient. Turns ideas into actions and organises work that needs to be done	Somewhat inflexible. Slow to respond to new possibilities
Completer-finisher	Painstaking, conscientious, anxious. Searches out errors. Polishes and perfects	Inclined to worry unduly. Reluctant to delegate
Specialist	Single-minded, self-starting, dedicated. Provides knowledge and skills in rare supply	Contributes only on a narrow front. Dwells on technicalities

followers) to be vulnerable, open and human with each other.

2. **Fear of conflict**. Team members seeking artificial harmony over constructive, passionate debate.

3. **Lack of commitment**. Team members feigning (faking) agreement with group decisions and in doing so creating confusion and ambiguity throughout the team.

4. **Avoidance of accountability**. Ducking the responsibility to call-out peers on poor attitude, behaviour or performance or refusing to accept the same in return.

5. **Inattention to results**. Focusing on personal success, status and ego rather than the overall performance of the team.

Any of this sound familiar?

The five stages of tribal team player development

Lencioni's fifth point leaves us something to finish on: the five stages of tribal team player development (Logan et al., 2008). This thinking is based on the evolution of pack-like behaviour in human teams and is quite interesting. Where are you in this?

Stage 1 'Life Sucks!'

Stage 2 'No, it's actually just my life that sucks!'

Stage 3 'I am great! I now believe in myself. I speak the language of "*I, me, mine*".'

Stage 4 'We are great! I can see clearly now; I have had an epiphany! We are better together; we are a team. I now speak the language of "*we, us, ours*".'

Stage 5 'Life is great.' This can be a magic phase

TABLE 24.2 Example Belbin team sheet

Plant	Bob, your slightly eccentric but clever friend in the pub who is fascinated by your farming business. He used to work in industry albeit a totally different one to farming. He makes unusual suggestions.
Monitor Evaluator	Your rather introverted son who doesn't say much but is very interested in the details.
Coordinator	Maybe that's you?
Shaper	And you again?
Resource Investigator	Maybe your spouse who is well connected and brings great ideas back from the bowling club.
Team Player	Jim; he's worked for the farm for years, he only does 3 days a week now but often works longer and without any expectation of overtime payments.
Completer Finisher	Your sister, who happens to be a school teacher, always checks any letters or reports you write. She's great at spotting spelling mistakes and typing errors. She's quite fussy and pedantic.
Specialist	You use an Agricultural Consultant who is very knowledgeable about grassland management, an accountant who's great with the finances and your vet who does some very in-depth health planning with you. You suddenly realise you're well off for specialists!
Implementer	That's Jim again, he is very good at making a start with anything that needs doing when everyone else tends to hold back a bit. He keeps at it 'til the jobs done.

of greatness but is usually unrealistic and unsustainable and is at risk of being the *fat cat stage* and at great risk of collapse. Go back to stage 4!

Let us finish teamship with the Jim Rohn quote we began with: 'None of us are smarter than all of us.'

SUMMARY OF LEADERSHIP, FOLLOWERSHIP AND TEAM THEORY FOR THE BEEF FARM

We have now heard all about these overlapping disciplines but a frequently raised dilemma has not been fully addressed. Scenario 1: Does a good leader roll their sleeves up and muck in at the coal face? Scenario 2: Does a good leader sit with their feet on the desk scanning the horizon for problems and opportunities?

Given that we have decided leadership is as much about followership and that both are even

more about teamship, is that dilemma any easier to answer? Certainly, mucking in at the coal face ticks some boxes but to tick the *empowerment of a team* box is it not best for a leader to back off from the coal face? To some extent this will get back to how clearly defined the job descriptions and team roles are, but what else is at play here? What can go wrong in either scenario?

Scenario 1: Let us take the old farmer, Jack, who has very much been the leader, the boss. He insists on still doing the dehorning, doing the difficult calvings, and always selecting the cattle for sale. Jack sees this as very helpful, and quietly he thinks to himself he is actually the only person who can do it properly. The daughter, Annie, wants to do the calvings and more of the farm administration. The long-standing team member, Dave, wants to select the cattle for sale and to do the dehorning. They feel disempowered and disengaged. One day Jack gets a head injury during dehorning and is left in a coma. Annie and Dave are not up to speed with the jobs Jack used to do. Things are very difficult on the farm, Annie feels depressed, Dave is anxious.

Scenario 2: Jack sits in the office. No one's entirely sure what he does but he seems to make phone calls and send emails. Dave loves doing the dehorning and has progressed to castration too. He selects the sale cattle and even gets to go to the mart. Annie does the calvings and has taken over most of the farm administration. Annie suggests Jack takes a holiday. 'But how will you manage?', asks Jack. 'It's fine Dad, we don't really need you now', replies Annie. Jack has delivered what most analysts would describe as good team empowerment and good leadership. Jack, however, suddenly feels terrible, he does not want to go on holiday, he feels redundant.

Both scenarios show a lack of team development. In scenario 1 the team members were not trained or empowered. In scenario 2 Jack was not coached for retirement and he was unclear on the expectations of his changing role and certainly had not explained his changing role to the rest of the team. All of which leads to scenario 3: Jack, Annie and Dave are all given a book on leadership, followership and team theory and they are booked onto some training courses. Everyone will get there eventually but with education, coaching and planning some of this could have been avoided.

But still, have we actually decided which approach is best for a leader – coal face or not? It seems that the coal face is best left to the empowered team whose job descriptions and skills are designed for that role; it is their role. It seems that maybe stepping back is the right thing for a leader, *but*, when the need arises, surely a good leader will jump straight back in until the team bring the problem under control. But what do you think?

REFERENCES

Belbin, R.M. (2010) *Management Teams, Why They Succeed or Fail,* 3rd edn. Butterworth-Heinemann, Oxford.

Blakesley, S.J. (2013) *Performance at the Highest Level P: Leadership = Followship.* CreateSpace Independent Publishing Platform, Scotts Valley, CA.

Cantrell, M.E. (1998) The doctrine of dissent. *Marine Corps Gazette* 82(11), 56–57.

Červený, J., van Ours, J.C. and van Tuijl, M.A. (2018) Effects of a red card on goal-scoring in World Cup football matches. *Empirical Economics* 55, 883–903.

Chemers, M.M. (1997) *An Integrative Theory of Leadership.* Lawrence Erlbaum Associates Mahwah, NJ.

Kouzes, J.M. and Posner, B.Z. (1995) *The Jossey-Bass Management Series. The Leadership Challenge: How to Keep Getting Extraordinary Things Done in Organisations,* 2nd edn. Jossey-Bass, San Francisco, CA.

Logan, D., King, J. and Fischer-Wright, H. (2008) Corporate tribes: the heart of effective leadership. *Leader to Leader* 2008(49), 25–30.

Maltz, M. (1960) *Psycho-Cybernetics.* Simon & Schuster, New York.

Mayer, J.D., Salovey, P. and Caruso, D.R. (2000) Models of emotional intelligence. In: Sternberg, R.J. (ed.) *Handbook of Intelligence.* Cambridge University Press, New York, pp. 396–420.

McCallum, J. (2013) Followership: the other side of leadership. Ivey Business Journal. Available at: https://iveybusinessjournal.com/publication/followership-the-other-side-of-leadership/. (accessed 1 February 2020).

McCormack, M.H. (1984) *What They Don't Teach You at Harvard Business School.* Bantam, Toronto.

Rock, D. (2008) SCARF: a brain-based model for collaborating with and influencing others. *NeuroLeadership Journal* 1, 1–9.

Uhl-Bien, M., Riggio, R.E., Lowe, K.B. and Carsten, M.K. (2014) Followership theory: a review and research agenda. *The Leadership Quarterly* 25(1), 83–104.

Part VI

Miscellaneous

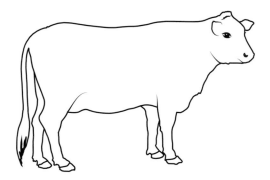

Chapter 25

Forage conservation

Forage, also referred to as fodder or provender, is herbage, principally grass, grown in the growing season for immediate feeding, or as was traditionally practised, preserved for use in the winter months by the relatively simple, but often thwarted, process of drying. The preserved product, hay, lasted well enough for use throughout the winter and is a practice still popular in many parts of the world and not just for cattle but for sheep, goats and horses.

Ensilage is the process of preserving grass, and other forage crops, not through drying but through *fermentation* much the same way as cheese, wine, beer and salami-type sausages, to name but a few, are processed to keep. The product resulting from the ensilage of grass is called *silage*.

SILAGE

The nutritive value of grass silage at the end of the ensiling process is influenced by the stage at which the grass is cut more than by any other factor. The grass should be cut when at an appropriate stage in leaf development to suit the type of livestock that would ideally be eating it at pasture. Different grasses have different *heading dates*: the stage in the season the seed heads of fertile tillers emerge. Where crops are mixed, as they usually are, having species of grass with the same heading dates helps. Typically, there is a choice between low yields of highly digestible young grass, or, higher yields of grass with seeds/flower heads, which are more stemmy and have a lower digestibility.

The silage making process relies on fermentation of the sugar within the crop by naturally occurring bacteria that happen to produce relatively large amounts of lactic acid in the process. As soon as the grass is cut sugars and protein within the crop start breaking down as plant respiration continues in the early stages of decomposition. Undesirable bacteria increase in numbers at this stage. A short, rapid wilt minimises this complication. A certain amount of wilt is actually necessary as a little decomposition is necessary for the process to begin. The optimum time for wilting is between 24 and 48 hours; grass digestibility decreases by 1% unit per day in the field (Wilkinson and Chamberlain, 2017). Using a mower with a conditioner lays the grass out over a larger area thus exposing it to the air and, hopefully, sunshine, both of which facilitate a quicker wilt. The grass needs a sugar level of 2–3% for good fermentation to occur. Higher sugar levels are present in the afternoon so cutting after lunch is advantageous (AHDB, 2015). The crop should, ideally, be dry when it is cut, even waiting for the dew to lift is important; wet as well as lower sugar crops often undergo what is known as secondary fermentation producing the undesirable butyric acid (Wilkinson and Chamberlain, 2017). Soil contamination of the silage should be avoided as *Listeria* bacteria live in soil and thrive in silage, especially certain types. Cutting the crop too low and/or the presence of mole hills will increase soil

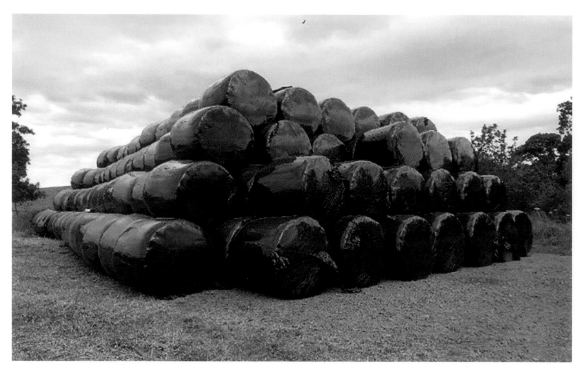

FIGURE 25.1 Freshly stacked round bales of silage

contamination. As a guide the remaining stubble should, optimally, be 5 cm in height.

Once wilting is complete the grass is 'raked' into larger swaths for rapid collection.

Silage can be baled or packed in a silage pit, essentially a hole in the ground, or a clamp, a three-sided box or building with a plastic sheeting roof and front wall. Bales, Figure 25.1, use a vast amount of plastic which is costly, environmentally damaging and must be disposed of appropriately, but this method does allow smaller areas to be cut and collected at different times, such being the case when harvesting residual grass growth in a rotational grazing system. If grass is cut from grazed ground, however, contamination with faecal material needs to be avoided as far as possible. Having less grass cut and wilting is advantageous when the weather is temperamental – cutting it all at once is a risky gamble! Storing bales is relatively easy and avoids the capital tied up in constructing a silage pit or clamp. When bales are stacked, they should be marked and allocated to different types of stock

to make best use of what is inevitably a variable crop. DM losses in baled silage are less than they are for clamp silage, effluent results from both, albeit much more from a clamp, and this contaminant must be managed appropriately for environmental reasons. It also represents a nutritive loss, so retention is desirable, to a point.

The forage harvester, especially used in the case of pit silage, will chop the silage. A shorter chop length is required for high DM crops (2.5–5 cm), a longer chop length (8–10 cm) for wetter crops. Shorter chop lengths in dry silage help with compaction and consolidation which helps eliminate air from the silage pit – this is necessary for fermentation, which is best when *anaerobic*. Forage boxes or forage wagons have a longer chop length, and this can cause problems with compaction and excess air remaining in the pit – this allows *aerobic* fermentation, which facilitates the growth of undesirable bacteria such as spoilage bacteria and worse still, *Bacillus* and *Listeria*, both of which can cause abortion and other diseases. Some balers are also able to chop silage, which again increases the density of the bales and helps fermentation.

As soon as the crop is in the silage pit and sheeted or baled the bacteria use up the remaining oxygen in a brief period of aerobic fermentation.

The silage pit should be filled in thin layers because the weight of the tractor rolling the pit will only compress to a depth of 15 cm (Wilkinson and Chamberlain, 2017). Silage pits are sheeted, and two layers of plastic sheet are better than one, generally a thin flexible layer first, covered by a thicker top layer. Where a standard polyethylene sheet is used oxygen will penetrate over time and cause some aerobic spoilage of the top layer of silage. The spoilage is anticipated to be at least three times the depth of the visibly affected silage. This is an area of rapid development and new materials are being developed to minimise oxygen permeation.

Bales should be wrapped as soon as possible after forming; a minimum of four layers of wrap at 50% overlap and 70% stretch (Wilkinson and Chamberlain, 2017). If bales are of low DM care should be taken when stacking and moving so they are not distorted, which can allow the airtight seal to be breached.

Sheeted pits and wrapped bales need to be protected from birds and vermin to prevent them damaging the plastic which would obviously allow air to enter.

Once there is no oxygen left fermentation proper begins and lactic acid is produced creating a more stable environment. Once fermentation is complete the crop is stable providing air is not subsequently introduced through damage to the pit walls, cover or bale wrap. As soon as the pit or bale is opened for feeding, and exposed to the air, aerobic spoilage will occur. Minimising the surface area of the pit exposed, and the time taken to feed across the open pit face is important to ensure aerobic spoilage is kept to a minimum. Figure 25.2 shows an adequately managed pit face compared to Figure 25.3 where the feed face is poorly managed – there is a large surface area exposed. The width of the face of the pit should be fed in a maximum of 5 days (Cooper and Hutley, 2010).

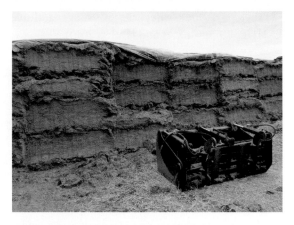

FIGURE 25.2 Adequately managed silage pit; collected with a sheer grab

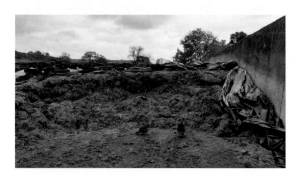

FIGURE 25.3 Poorly managed silage pit; collected with a non-shear grab resulting in a large surface area being exposed to the air

SILAGE ADDITIVES

Additives can be mixed with the grass when it is harvested. The efficacy of additives has been questionable but European Union legislation now governs the efficacy and safety of animal feed additives and efficacy claims need to be supported by reasonable scientific evidence.

Additives can be utilised to:

- help with fermentation
- increase the feed value of the crop
- reduce production or loss of silage effluent
- reduce the rate of spoilage at feeding. (Cooper and Hutley, 2010)

There are four categories of silage additive (AHDB, 2015; Cooper and Hutley, 2010).

1. **Acids**. Generally used for wet and low sugar crops to speed up the establishment of an acidic environment for *Lactobacilli* spp. to thrive and produce more lactic acid. Formic, acetic and propionic acid are commonly used. Propionic acid is also known to help reduce spoilage at 'feed-out' by inhibiting mould and yeast growth.

2. **Sugars**. Usually in the form of molasses, give the bacteria a substrate to ferment and encourages their survival and ongoing lactic acid production. These additives are difficult to apply evenly, and a large amount is needed.

3. **Enzymes**. Enzyme additives specifically digest fibre into sugar for bacteria to then ferment and produce lactic acid.

4. **Bacterial inoculants**. Consisting of two types.
   - *Homo-fermentative agents* that contain bacteria that convert sugar to lactic acid to speed up fermentation.
   - *Hetero-fermentative agents* that contain bacteria that produce acetic and propionic acid and are not designed to help with fermentation but to create stability at feed-out.

PHYSICAL APPEARANCE OF SILAGE

Although a chemical analysis is required to give accurate details on the nutritive and fermentation characteristics of silage, a visual assessment is invaluable in assessing the likely feed quality of the silage.

Touch

Well compacted silage should not be easily compressed by a thumb or fist when force is applied to the face of an open pit. Chop length should be less than 8 cm otherwise cows will be able to 'sort' their ration and it may have been too long for adequate compaction leaving some air behind which will have resulted in aerobic fermentation.

If the silage is stemmy it will have lower digestibility than a leafy silage. The silage should not be warm to the touch as this indicates that secondary fermentation and nutritive loss has occurred.

The DM content of silage can be estimated by the *squeeze test*. When silage is pulled from the pit, and squeezed, water will run from the hand if the silage is 18–20% DM or less. When the hand is simply wet after squeezing the silage then this would indicate a DM of 25–30%. A silage greater than 30% DM falls apart after squeezing when the hand is relaxed.

Smell

The silage should be sweet smelling and not repulsive as is the case with butyric silage. Silage should not smell burnt or tobacco-like as this is a sign of overheating from secondary fermentation.

Colour

The silage may, acceptably, be dark in colour, but any blackened areas or mould indicate poor fermentation or secondary fermentation and should not be fed to animals. A greener silage is likely to have a higher CP value. A yellow or light green silage will tend to have a lower CP.

Taste

Observing the cows' response to silage when fed gives a good indication of its appeal. Refusal rates and intakes will drop if the silage is not appealing and this tends to be linked with poor quality of the silage.

SAMPLING SILAGE

Ideally silage should be sampled and analysed in advance of feeding so as to allow rations to be formulated accurately and the likely longevity of the feed supplies to be calculated. In the case of pit silage, quality will vary throughout the pit, so several representative samples are required for analysis (Wilkinson and Chamberlain, 2017).

In a sealed pit, typically five core samples are required from different areas of the pit and each at a depth of 1.5 m. When a pit is open the silage should be sampled on a dry day when the pit face is relatively dry. Seven to eleven fist-sized samples taken in a 'W' pattern across the face of the pit should be taken into a clean dry bucket. The samples should be mixed well in a bucket. The bucket is then tipped out and the heap split down by halving it and then halving it again so that the sample size is a mixture of all the samples but the

correct amount for the laboratory to work with (Wilkinson and Chamberlain, 2017).

In the case of bales, samples from five bales from each batch should be pooled to get a representative sample (AHDB, 2015).

The samples should be placed in a polythene bag, the air squeezed out and the bag sealed tightly. They can then be submitted to the laboratory for further analysis.

SILAGE ANALYSIS

There are two techniques used for silage analysis. Biochemistry using traditional laboratory techniques is now the less popular method. Near-infrared reflectance spectroscopy is more commonly used these days, and results can be obtained within 24 hours (Wilkinson and Chamberlain, 2017). An example of a silage analysis report is presented in Figure 25.4.

Fermentation quality	
pH (NIR)*	4.3
Lactic acid (g/kg DM)	61.2
VFA (g/kg DM)	40.2

Feeding value	
Dry Matter (g/kg)*	165
D-value (%)*	65.1
ME (MJ/kg DM)	10.4
Protein(g/kg DM)*	105
SIP (gDM/kgLW^0.75)*	74
NDF (g/kg DM)*	570
Sugar (g/kg DM)	42
Oil (g/kg DM)	30
Ash (g/kg DM)	79
TFA (gJ/kg DM)	101.5
PAL (meq/kg DM)	1074

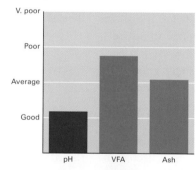

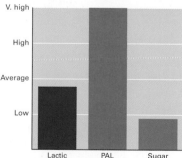

Degradability characteristics	s	a	b	c
Dry Matter	0.16	0.32	0.43	0.034
Nitrogen	0.51	0.65	0.24	0.066

*The above silage results were produced using the Forage Assurance Analysis Models on fresh silage material

FIGURE 25.4 Typical silage report for grass silage intended to be fed to spring-calving suckler cows

Nutritional analysis

Dry matter

DM is reported as a percentage or g/kg of fresh weight. Dry silages, a high DM, are difficult to compact and limited water and sugar content may limit good quality primary fermentation. Wet silages are difficult to conserve as a large amount of acid production is required to lower the pH (Wilkinson and Chamberlain, 2017). Rain or poor wilting will decrease the DM. A target DM for pit silage is around 30%, baled silage 35–45%.

Crude protein

Silage CP of 14–16% is ideal. CP estimation includes non-protein nitrogen. In some analyses it is broken down into ERDP and DUP. Research carried out by SAC suggests that the CP levels in silage are decreasing year on year. There are a number of reasons for this. Newer grass varieties are more nitrogen-efficient, so less nitrogen is being applied resulting in lower CP silage. In general, less nitrogen is being applied to agricultural land, this also resulting in lower CP silage. Sulphur is required to produce some grass proteins. There is a reduction in sulphur being applied to grass land so as to reduce environmental pollution. There is also less sulphur in the atmosphere these days thanks to environmental control measures and this is consequently being reflected in reduced grass sulphur levels.

Digestibility

Digestibility or D-Value should be between 55–75%. This is assessed by measuring the loss of silage organic matter over 72 hours in ruminal fluid or, more artificially, in a detergent and enzyme medium (Cooper and Hutley, 2010).

Metabolisable energy

ME is the energy in the silage that can be used by the cow and is reported in units of MJ/kg DM. A high energy silage would be above 12 MJ/kg DM, a typical suckler cow silage would be around 10 MJ/kg DM. It is calculated from the D-Value. The earlier the crop is cut the higher the ME. The D-Value decreases by 0.5% per day during seed head emergence, which is the equivalent to a decline of ME of 0.5 MJ/kg DM (Wilkinson and Chamberlain, 2017).

Neutral detergent fibre

NDF is the fibre content of silage. Reported as a percentage or g/kg DM. More mature crops have a higher NDF. A normal range for NDF is between 350 and 600 g/kg DM. Higher NDF silages are generally lower in ME.

Ash

Ash should be less than 7%. Ash is the mineral content of the silage and levels will be raised if there is excessive soil contamination (soil increases the risk of diseases such as listeriosis).

Fermentation characteristics

pH

pH is a measure of the acidity within the silage and therefore its stability. Target pH is dependent on the dry matter but should generally be between 3.7 and 4.7. Greater than 5 suggests instability but drier silages can have a higher pH and still be stable. Lower values indicate an overly acidic silage that may adversely lower the cow's rumen pH.

Potential acid load

PAL is a combination of the acidity of the silage and the acid production from fermentation within the rumen. Normal values are between 600 and 1200 mEq/kg. Over 1100 mEq/kg would need consideration when formulating the ration so as not to affect rumen pH adversely (Cooper and Hutley, 2010).

Ammonia

Ammonia nitrogen (NH_3-N) is a measure of secondary fermentation. The higher the value the more protein loss that has occurred during ensilage.

Lactic acid

Lactic acid is the main acid produced in good fermentation. Low lactic acid levels may be due to secondary fermentation or a lack of fermentation in very dry silages. The target range is between 80 and 120 g/kg DM (Cooper and Hutley, 2010).

Volatile fatty acids

VFA is a measure of unwanted volatile fatty acids. Low levels are indicative of good fermentation. High values are indicative of nutrient loss and protein breakdown and may reduce cows' intakes. The target is less than 20 g VFA/kg DM.

Sugars

The higher the better. High sugar silages have either had a high sugar content to start with or fermentation has been restricted. High sugar silages contain energy that is readily available to the rumen microbes. The target is greater than 100 g/kg DM.

REFERENCES

AHDB (2015) Making Grass Silage for Better Returns. Beef and Sheep BRP. Manual 5. Agriculture and Horticulture Development Board, Stoneleigh.

Cooper, R. and Hutley, B. (2010) Guide to the assessment and analysis of silage for the general practitioner. *In Practice* 32, 8–15.

Wilkinson, J.M. and Chamberlain, A.T. (2017) Silage for veterinary surgeons – making, feeding and understanding silage. *Cattle Practice* 25(2), 82–91.

Chapter 26

Medicines for beef cattle

The use of medicines in any animal is, quite rightly, highly regulated; there are tight controls on research and development, manufacturing, marketing, storage, labelling, packaging, supply, prescription, administration, record keeping and handling of the product. This all adds to the cost of medicines. The development of a new medicinal product is a particularly time consuming and costly endeavour. It involves expertise from many specialists from organic chemists, analytical chemists, pharmacologists, manufacturing/ process experts right through to the trialists and end users, often involving farmers and vets. The development of a truly novel product incurs a degree of risk as the market return may not exceed the cost of development. Although science is evolving all the time so too are the regulatory requirements. For all these reasons new products in the animal health field are few and far between. For this reason alone, we need to preserve the medicines already available so as to ensure they remain effective for future generations.

MEDICINE CATEGORIES

Medicines that are administered to food producing animals are classified into different legal categories. The categories change periodically in line with changes in the legislation but loosely speaking there are medicines that can only be prescribed by veterinary surgeons, medicines that can be prescribed by veterinary surgeons and *suitably qualified persons* (SQPs), individuals who have undergone training and passed an examination, and medicines that do not need a prescription and can be sold by anyone with an appropriate retailing licence.

Whoever prescribes a medication, whether it be a vet or an SQP they are required to ensure that the medication is used responsibly. Any medication should be used only for the animal, or group of animals, it was prescribed for and in accordance with the 'data sheet' or 'summary of product characteristics' (SPC). A data sheet or SPC is a document proving the specifications for a particular product; it includes important information such as the strength of the drug, other additives, licensed indications (permitted uses of the product), dose rate, route of administration, precautions, contraindications, storage instructions and food withdrawal periods. A food withdrawal period is the time that must elapse before the meat or milk of a treated animal can be used for human consumption. This stated time relies on all the rules of the data sheet having been applied, as the residue testing of the meat and the milk will be based on the correct use of the medicine. When using any medicine, it must be safe for the animal, the administrator, the consumer and the environment – the data sheet sets out to uphold these important requirements.

OFF-LICENCE USE OF MEDICINES AND THE CASCADE

A veterinary surgeon may recommend the use of a particular medicine, dose or route of administration of a medicine that is not in accordance with the data sheet or SPC. This is termed 'off-licence' or *cascade* use and automatically means that the food withdrawal period stated in the data sheet or SPC is no longer valid. The prescribing veterinary surgeon should advise on the correct withdrawal period. Cascade use of medication is not undertaken lightly but is necessary in some situations. Veterinary surgeons are permitted to prescribe cascade use of a medicine as long as they adhere to strict secondary guidelines specified in the legislation, rules referred to as 'the cascade'. The rules are called the cascade because the prescribing veterinary surgeon is expected to cascade down the steps of the rules and stop as soon as able so as to stray as little as possible from the primary guidelines.

CONCURRENT USE OF MORE THAN ONE MEDICINE

There are very few products that are licensed to be administered to an animal at the same time as other medicines, often referred to as 'concurrent use'. Some vaccines and mastitis treatments produced by the same manufacturer have a licence for concurrent use. This is where the manufacturers have proven that there are no adverse effects and that the products can be administered concurrently with no detriment to the efficacy of either product or risk to the patient. This is, however, the exception rather than the rule. Concurrent use should generally be avoided unless the data sheet or SPC specifies that is acceptable to do so. If two products not licensed for concurrent use are administered at the same time the food withdrawal periods of each separate product no longer apply and an extended withdrawal period for the food will be advised by the prescribing vet.

SAFETY MARGINS

Different medicinal products have different safety margins. The safety margin is the multiplier by which the normal dose rate can be increased before the appearance of adverse side effects in the target animal. For example, for a product that has a safety margin of 1.5 and the dose rate is 10 ml/kg then if the dose rate exceeds 15 ml/kg then adverse effects may occur. Products with higher safety margins are desirable as there is less risk of causing harm from inaccurate dosing.

STORAGE OF MEDICINES

There are health and safety considerations in the storage of veterinary medicines. All medicines whether or not required to be stored in a refrigerator need to be in a secure, locked space away from public and domestic areas (Figure 26.1).

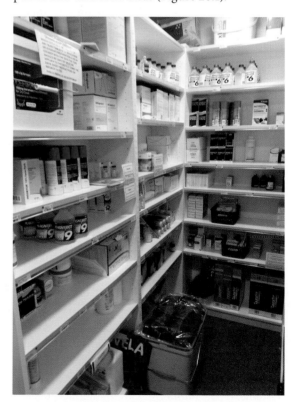

FIGURE 26.1 Veterinary pharmacy

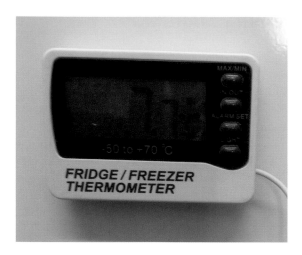

FIGURE 26.2 Refrigerator thermometer

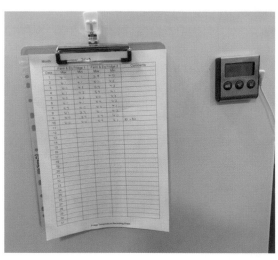

FIGURE 26.3 Refrigerator temperature monitoring

Medicines that require refrigeration should be kept in a designated refrigerator and not one used for food storage as veterinary medicines should not come into contact with human or animal food or drink. If refrigerated products are exposed to temperatures outside their recommended temperature range then they may not be effective or may, at least, have reduced efficacy when administered. Vaccines are the most common veterinary medicine that require refrigeration, the temperature range that is commonly stated being a consistent temperature between 2°C and 8°C (Figure 26.2).

Fluctuations in temperature should be minimal. This emphasises the need for a non-domestic refrigerator where the door is not opened and closed multiple times a day. Refrigerator temperatures should be monitored daily and recorded either manually (Figure 26.3) or with a digital data logger. Data loggers continually monitor temperature at specific intervals and are an easy and effective way of keeping track of cold storage. Refrigerated products are transported between the manufacturer, wholesaler and veterinary practice via a monitored 'cold chain'. The cold chain should be upheld when a product is transported, post purchase from the pharmacy, back to the farm. This can easily be achieved through cool packs and portable refrigerators. Research suggests it takes 20 minutes for a refrigerated product to equilibrate with the ambient temperature (Williams and Paixao, 2018). Vaccine should only be removed from the fridge immediately before use or some means of ongoing refrigeration needs to be used adjacent to the handling facilities. This again may be a cool box or bag (Figure 26.4). The effectiveness of a cool box or bag is improved with the use of a proprietary re-freezable ice pack.

Product should not be left in direct sunlight during use. There are vaccines on the market that need to be brought up to 15–25°C before use, this is stated in the data sheet or SPC of the specific product (Cresswell et al., 2019). A farmer questionnaire focusing on the use of vaccines within the UK cattle population with 266 respondents suggests as few as one in three farmers refer to the data sheets or SPC before administering a vaccine (Cresswell et al., 2014).

EXPIRY DATES

There are two dates of note when storing and handling veterinary medicines: the expiry date and the shelf life once broached.

The expiry date is clearly printed next to the batch number on all veterinary medicines. The efficacy and safety of the medicine cannot be guaranteed

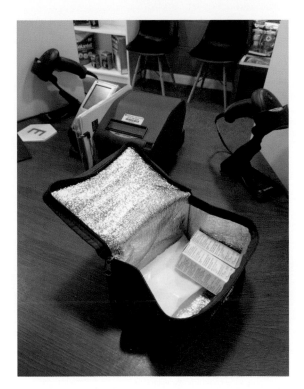

FIGURE 26.4 Vaccine dispensed in a cool bag with ice packs

after this date. Any medicines past their expiry date should be disposed of; it is illegal to administer an out of date product to a food producing animal.

The shelf life of a medicine after the vial has been broached varies depending on the product and is stated on the SPC or data sheet. For many vaccines it is a number of hours, some antibiotics may be up to 28 days from the day the bottle is broached. Once this time has been exceeded the medicine should be disposed of.

CONTAMINATION OF MEDICINES

Care should be taken when administering medicines that the bottle does not become contaminated. For injectable preparations only a newly opened sterile needle should be inserted into a bottle to draw up the medicine. A needle that has been used to inject an animal, or indeed used for anything, should not be inserted into a medicine bottle. The use of multi-dose injection guns prevents contamination of medicine bottles but raises issues over the cleanliness and sharpness of the needle with respect to its use on subsequent animals.

ADMINISTRATION OF MEDICINES

It is important that any medicine is administered via the route for which it is licensed. If a medicine is administered incorrectly it may not work and/or it may cause adverse effects; perhaps local inflammation, as may be the case when an intramuscular injection is given subcutaneously, or vice versa. More worryingly, incorrect routes of administration can cause illness or death, such as the administration of an intramuscular or subcutaneous suspension into a vein. A medicine administered by a route outwith the data sheet or SPC guidelines will need a reconsideration of the milk and meat withdrawal period.

DIFFERENT ROUTES OF ADMINISTRATION

- **Topical or transdermal** (applied to the skin). Topically applied medicines may be designed to work on the surface of the animal, or to be absorbed into the skin. Some topical medicines are designed to penetrate right through the skin and enter the animal's bloodstream. These medicinal preparations are sometimes referred to as transdermal or, more simply, as 'pour-ons'. Some transdermal medications are given by a new method of application based on a high-pressure pulse of gas which punches the preparation straight through the skin. Some transdermal medications contain solvents to help 'carry' the drug through the skin, an example being dimethyl sulfoxide.

- **Oral**. Given by mouth so as to be swallowed. Some oral medications require a gastro-protective coating to resist acid damage in the stomach.
- **Sublingual**. Given under the tongue so as to be absorbed through the lining of the mouth.
- **Intravenous**. Administered into a vein. This should only be performed by a veterinary surgeon or registered veterinary nurse. These products are nearly always clear solutions and will hardly ever take the form of suspensions of any sort.
- **Intramuscular**. Injected into a muscle. The hindquarters are often the most convenient site to inject medicines intramuscularly but given the high value of meat cuts of this area of the carcase the neck region is recommended. The neck also has superior circulation and is less likely to suffer an injection reaction. The neck, however, is sometimes less accessible and injection here seems to be met with slightly more resentment. These products are often suspensions, not exclusively solutions.
- **Subcutaneous**. Injected under the skin. This is often performed in the neck region, over the shoulder or over the ribs. Care should be taken that the needle is under the skin and not in the underlying muscle layers. Care should also be taken that the needle has not entered a tent of skin and re-exited through the other side of the skin tent. These may be suspensions or solutions.
- **Intraperitoneal**. Injected into the abdominal cavity. Care, skill, or luck is needed here to avoid injecting into an abdominal organ or into the lumen of the intestine or bladder. These products are usually solutions, not suspensions.

Irrespective of the route of administration the animal needs to be adequately restrained to avoid injury to the operator and animal. When an injection is administered through any route the skin should be clean and dry. When dirty needles, contaminated medication or dirty injection sites are used there is a possibility of bacteria entering the

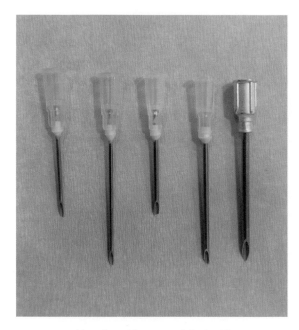

FIGURE 26.5 Needles: 18 gauge, 1 inch; 18 gauge, 1½ inch; 16 gauge, 1 inch; 16 gauge, 1½ inch; 14 gauge, 1½ inch

body either into the muscle, under the skin, into the bloodstream or into the abdominal cavity. Infection can result and sepsis can follow or abscesses can form either at the site of injection or at remote sites; commonly the heart, lung and liver.

The correct needle size should be used. Needles are measured in diameter and length (Figure 26.5). If administering an intramuscular injection to an adult cow a 1½ inch long needle would be appropriate whereas a subcutaneous injection may require only a 1 inch needle. As a general rule a 16 gauge needle is required for thick or oily based suspensions, commonly the case with antibiotics. An 18 gauge needle is suitable for thinner/water based solutions such as most anti-inflammatory medicines. A 14 gauge needle is recommended for the administration of calcium and magnesium preparations when the typically large volumes are administered subcutaneously and administration through a narrow needle would simply take too long, no other reason for such a wide needle!

Automatic injector guns (Figure 26.6), can be useful for speedy administration although it is

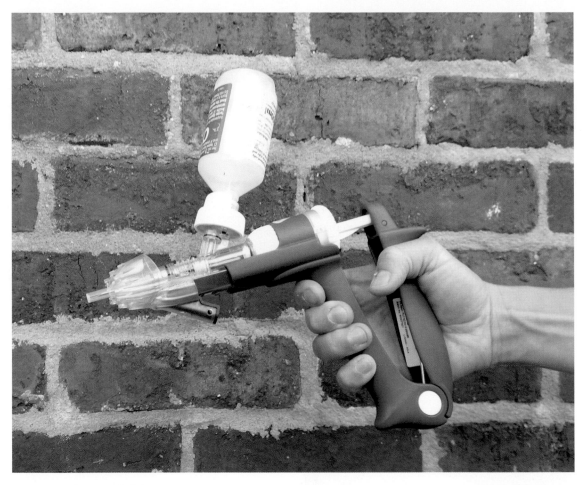

FIGURE 26.6 Automatic injector gun

essential they are regularly calibrated and maintained. It is important the chamber fills up fully with the medicine to be dispensed before the gun is discharged and only then should the gun should be discharged, which should be done fully. There is a risk of underdosing if this is not given adequate attention.

When large volumes of medication are required intramuscularly (for example, if an antibiotic that has a dose rate of 1 ml/10 kg then a 700 kg cow requires 70 ml) such a dose should be administered in two to three different sites. The maximum volume to be injected in one site is often stipulated on the data sheet and typical values would be 15–20 ml, but sometimes less.

Some medicines have a fixed dose irrespective of the weight of the animal; most vaccines fall into this category. The dose of antibiotics and anti-inflammatories are calculated on a milligram per kilogram basis. For example; a drug may be of a concentration of 100 mg per ml and an animal requires 10 mg/kg of body weight. This would equate to a dose rate of 1 ml/10 kg of body weight. Knowing the weight of animal is essential to administer the correct amount of medication. This is best achieved by using calibrated weigh scales, second best would be a weigh tape. Some medicines are dosed according to the surface area of the animal, the reason being that surface area is closely correlated with metabolic rate. Metabolic rate influences the speed at which some drugs are cleared from the body. The authors are unaware of any cattle medicines that are licensed this way but such products are likely to appear in the future as this is considered a far more accurate method of dosing for certain classes of potentially toxic drugs, a notable example being cancer chemotherapy.

DISPOSAL OF MEDICINES

All needles, empty bottles and unused medicines should be disposed of appropriately (Figure 26.7); a service usually offered by veterinary practices, but beware, usually chargeable! Immediately upon use, needles should be placed in a proprietary approved sharps bin (Figure 26.8). This is a safe receptacle for needles that are not only sharp but potentially contaminated with drug and, what could be, infected blood – a recipe for potentially dangerous accidental self-injection. Sharps bins when full have irreversibly locking lids, once locked they should be disposed of by an approved handler along with empty medicine containers and waste medicines.

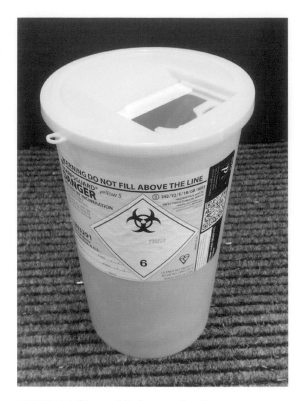

FIGURE 26.8 Sharps bin for needle disposal

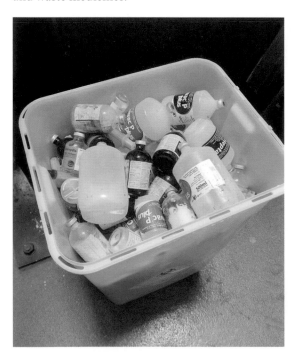

FIGURE 26.7 Waste medicine disposal for incineration

RECORDING MEDICINE USAGE

As food producers, farmers have a responsibility, both moral and legal, to the consumer to ensure the meat is safe to eat; that includes freedom from drug residues. Regulations exist to help producers ensure such safety. When an animal is treated with a medicinal product the following information should be recorded in a proprietary record of medicinal product administration (hard bound book or permanent electronic format): official identification of the animal, the date(s) of administration, the proprietary name of the medicine, the amount administered, the route of administration, the batch number, the expiry date, the food withdrawal period and the name of the food product to which the withdrawal period applies, in our case, meat. The meat withdrawal period is the period of time from when the last dose of a veterinary medicine is administered to when the level of residue in the tissues is lower than or equal to the maximum residue limit (MRL). The MRL is the maximum concentration of the residual administered molecule from the administered medicine that is legally permitted within food. The licensed withdrawal period for a product is calculated through various studies and is the **minimum** time required between the last treatment and the slaughter of the animal. The period of time, usually in days, is stated on the data sheet and/or SPC. If the product is used according to the cascade, this period changes and the new withdrawal period is set by the prescribing vet. The consequence of not observing withdrawal periods is that medicine residues are detected in meat at the abattoir, which has potentially serious consequences to human health and as a result is taken extremely seriously by the authorities. It is important to note that the withdrawal period does not relate to the duration of activity of a product – that is a very different matter – duration of activity relates to the concentration of drug in the target tissue being of a sufficient level to have the desired effect, and, for it to remain so for the appropriate length of time.

ADVERSE REACTIONS

Any *suspected adverse reaction* (SAR) in either the animal or the operator should be reported to the Veterinary Medicines Authority. This is normally something that would be carried out by your vet; they have the relevant paperwork, terminology and contacts to see this through. An SAR is a response to a drug or a vaccine that is not detailed in the data sheet. An extreme example would be death post-vaccination but a myriad of less severe effects can inadvertently occur. Examples could include local swelling, seizures/convulsions, extreme pain at the injection site, abortion. These situations are often subjected to a thorough investigation but not if the drug has been misused – the case is likely then to be dropped on the basis of 'no case to answer'!

MEDICINE GROUPS ACCORDING TO USE (INDICATION)

A medicine when used legitimately is used for its intended and described therapeutic effect, also known as its *indication*. Medicines can be classified or grouped according to these indications. The following groups will be discussed.

Antiparasiticides:

- endoparasiticides
  – anthelmintics
  – flukicides
- ectoparasiticides.

Anti-infectives:

- antibiotics/antibacterials
- antifungals
- antivirals
- anticoccidials/coccidiostats.

Anti-inflammatories:

- steroids
- non-steroidal anti-inflammatories (NSAIDs)

Antiparasiticides

Endoparasiticides

This broad class of drug kills, controls or prevents infestation of the host with internal parasites; parasites in the gut, respiratory tract, blood and so on. The two main subclasses in cattle are anthelmintics and flukicides, both of which shall be discussed separately.

Anthelmintics

Anthelmintics, or anthelminthics, as they are sometimes called, are the classic wormers known so well to the farming industry. These medicines are used to treat and prevent infections with helminths such as gutworms, lungworms, sometimes tapeworms and, sometimes, liver fluke. Tapeworms and flukes are not actually helminths, so this stretches the definition a little. Tapeworms are a different type of worm known as *cestodes*, and flukes belong to a very different class of the animal kingdom; *trematodes*. The main species of gut worm causing clinical disease and reduced growth rates are *Ostertagia ostertagi,* within the abomasum, and *Cooperia oncophora,* within the small intestine (Chapter 13). The main species of lung worm affecting cattle is *Dictyocaulus viviparus*. The main liver fluke of cattle (and sheep) is *Fasciola hepatica* (Chapter 15).

After an anthelmintic is administered, either orally, by injection or as a pour-on preparation, the active ingredient is absorbed into the bloodstream and transported to different parts of the body, including the liver. The liver breaks down the active ingredient (most drugs and unwanted chemicals in the body are broken down by the liver) and the metabolic by-products are then excreted either in the faeces, the urine or both. Some pharmaceutical active ingredients need to be broken down by the liver to actually become active – these products, sometimes referred to as *pro-drugs*, may not be effective in animals that have liver disease. Similarly many of the flukicides rely on the liver to, if not activate the pharmaceutical ingredient, then at least excrete it in the bile so subjecting the flukes within the bile duct to high levels of the drug. Anthelmintics that are administered orally may kill parasites by direct contact in the gut lumen but the parasites, despite being in the gut, are also exposed to the anthemintic from the bloodstream via the lining of the gut, particularly effective when the parasite is attached to the lining. Not all active ingredients can be administered orally. Nitroxynil, for example, is a flukicide that is broken down by the rumen bacteria so it can only be administered by injection (Barragry, 1994).

Anthelmintics have been the corner stone of worm management for nearly 50 years. Using an anthelmintic preparation on any stock should not be undertaken lightly, but worryingly they are among the veterinary medicines that are least regulated. Parasites over the years have developed resistance to anthelmintics, and farmers and prescribers have a responsibility to preserve the efficacy of these products for future generations. Worm control should not rely on anthelmintic treatment alone; it is important to have a working knowledge of the worm life cycles and seasonality so that grazing strategies can be effectively deployed to lessen the dependence on drugs. Every 6 months a parasite plan should be discussed with a vet or SQP, accurately documented and adhered to. A parasite plan needs to take into consideration: knowledge of the farm, local parasite risks, stocking density, grazing patterns, seasonality and the age profile of the stock. The immune status and health of an animal are crucial factors to consider. Undernourished, poorly animals are more likely to be parasitised as they are less able to 'fight off' infection. Young animals are also vulnerable as they will not yet have established immunity.

Anthelmintics are broken down into three main groups and are available in a range of preparations: oral drench, injectable, pour-on and ruminal bolus.

- **Benzimidazoles** (BZ) ('white wormers'). This group includes albendazole, oxfendazole and fenbendazole. The mode of action is to disrupt the energy metabolism of the worm. They are available as oral drenches or boluses. They are effective against gut worms and lungworm. They can, at higher dose, be used in the control of liver fluke. The efficacy of BZ relies on the contact time between the parasite and the drug; the longer the period of contact the more efficacious the product; BZ that are less soluble and reside in the rumen for longer are more efficacious. Newer BZ products such as oxfendazole, fenbendazole and albendazole were designed with this in mind. When BZ bypass the rumen, via the oesophageal groove, they are eliminated from the gut and body quicker and are less efficacious. They are suspensions, they are usually white!

- **Levamisoles** (LV) ('yellow wormers'). This group is effective against gut and lung worms. The mode of action is to affect the neurological system of the worm and cause paralysis. They are available in oral drench, pour-on and injectable forms. They are usually solutions; they are usually yellow!

- **Macrocyclic lactones** (ML) ('clear wormers') This group includes ivermectin, doramectin, moxidectin and eprinomectin. They have no activity against liver fluke. They have some activity against ectoparasites. MLs are available in injectable and pour-on forms. Their mode of action varies between chemicals, but they are highly lipophilic (absorbed by fat) and following administration are stored in the animal's fat tissue from where it slowly diffuses. The products can, consequently, have a persistent effect. This duration of activity varies depending on the chemical, its distribution in fat tissue, its metabolism by the body and its excretion from the body (Taylor, 2000). They are usually solutions and guess what? They are usually clear!

Some products on the market contain an anthelmintic and a flukicide; these are called combination products. They are a convenient method of administering two medications at the same time but should only be used if both an anthelmintic and a flukicide are actually required; surprisingly rare as it happens. Being on 'special offer', for example priced cheaper than the single component products, is most certainly not a reason to use them! Such a commercial manoeuvre these days could almost be seen as negligent merchandising.

Oral drench and boluses

Oral drenches and boluses are administered over the back of the tongue into the back of the animal's mouth and, actually, and ideally, straight into the oesophagus. Bypassing the swallowing reflex ensures the product goes straight into the rumen rather than the abomasum (up to 6 months of age swallowing activates the oesophageal groove taking the product past the rumen and straight into the fourth stomach instead – as occurs with milk.) Being in the rumen or in the abomasum will affect the absorption and availability of the product – the rumen is the preferred destination for these products as they are less designed for an acidic abomasal environment. Patience, skill and experience are needed when dosing to ensure there is no damage to the mouth or throat of the animal from either incorrect or rough technique or from sharp edges on poorly maintained or over-used dosing guns.

There are two types of oral anthelmintic bolus; sustainable release and pulse release, both of which are administered with a bolus gun (Figure 26.9).

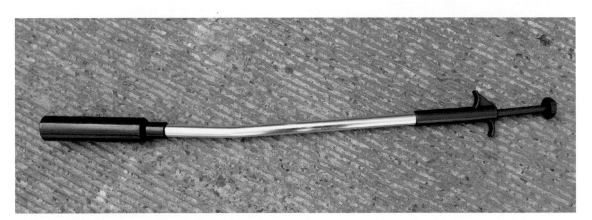

FIGURE 26.9 Example of a bolus gun

Sustainable release boluses

These boluses continually release a constant level of anthelmintic for a set period of time as stated on the data sheet. They are a convenient way of providing anthelmintic treatment to cattle during the grazing period but the downside is that they do not allow for any natural exposure to gut or lung worms so the host is not given the opportunity to develop natural immunity for future grazing seasons.

Pulse release devices

These boluses are made up of separate tablets threaded on a central core and as the architecture of the bolus corrodes in the ruminal fluid a tablet is released approximately every three weeks (Figure 26.10). The number of tablets dictates the number of pulses of anthelmintic released (Taylor, 2000). These products *do* allow the host some natural exposure to lung and gut worms, so stimulating

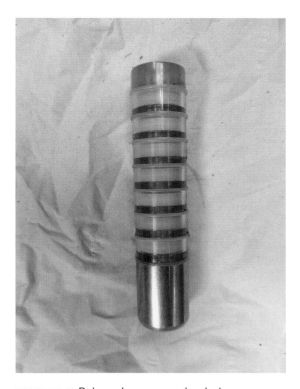

FIGURE 26.10 Pulse release worming bolus

the development of natural immunity, but while still ensuring parasite burdens are not allowed to reach a critically high level where they would affect growth rates or cause clinical disease.

Anthelmintic resistance

Resistance is the ability of a worm to survive a dose of anthelmintic which would normally be effective. It could also be described as 'drug tolerance' in worms. Anthelmintic resistance in a worm is heritable, it is genetic. A worm is said to be resistant if it survives exposure to the standard recommended dose of the anthelmintic and can then pass this ability on to its offspring (SCOPS, 2019).

There are reports of *Cooperia* spp. demonstrating resistance to ML for a number of years in the UK but while overt clinical disease has not been a result of this there is likely to be a negative impact on DLWG as a result of failure to kill the worm. Interestingly, non-resistant, normal strains of *Cooperia* spp. are hard to kill regardless and easily survive an anthelmintic treatment if the animal was not quite given the required amount. They are also less likely to be killed by ivermectin pour-on preparations, even at the normally dictated dose rate. In contrast, however, there is no known resistance within the *O. ostertagi* population in the UK although resistance has been reported in other countries. *O. ostertagi* can, consequently, and currently, be treated effectively with all three classes of anthelmintic (COWS, 2014).

How does anthelmintic resistance develop?

There are naturally occurring worms in any population that are resistant to anthelmintics. Quite why or how they have the genetic make-up to enjoy this status is not understood, but appears to be an example of nature's ability to adapt to change and in doing so survive. When the whole population of worms in an animal's gut is subjected to an anthelmintic these naturally resistant or tolerant worms survive. The normal, susceptible worms die, the resistant ones do not and unless partially damaged, which is possible, they continue to shed eggs on to the pasture. In doing so they are populating the pasture with a new generation of resistant worms; the survivors, the populators of the new world, the 'refugees' or *refugia*, as they are rather inaccurately referred to. These survivors carry the genes for resistance; they represent a new population of worms that have an ability to survive the use of that particular anthelmintic. These worms survive in the gut and for the time being have no other worms to breed with apart from other resistant worms, that is until the animal ingests some more eggs, hence worms, from the pasture. This leaves them with a great advantage in the gut over and above the other worms – the survivors get all the food! Worse still these well-fed survivors are breeding with other survivors to create a new super race. The more times the animals are treated with this anthelmintic the more the resistant worms gain the advantage. We can make things even better for the resistant worms by using a long acting anthelmintic; the animal takes longer to get re-infected with normal worms and therefore the resistant worms continue to get all the food, and breed with each other, for longer. We can help a resistant worm population even more by treating cattle and then moving them to a clean pasture; the once popular 'dose and shift' policy. The cattle are on clean grazing, they are not ingesting normal, non-resistant worms, the resistant worms once again have the advantage, they get the food and they breed with each other, and, what is more, the eggs dumped on the clean pasture have no non-resistant eggs to dilute them, to compete with them. The super race takes the lead.

How is anthelmintic resistance detected?

The simplest, but inaccurate, way is to notice disease and poor growth rates in treated animals. More accurately, however, anthelmintic resistance can be detected by using a method called faecal egg count reduction test (FECRT). This involves taking a group of animals, in our case, cattle, and performing individual faecal worm egg counts on each of them. The cattle are identified, weighed and dosed with the correct amount of anthelmintic. A specified time period after treatment, the period depending on the product, the individual faecal worm egg counts are repeated. For a worm population to be classified as being susceptible to an anthelmintic treatment there needs to be a 95% reduction in eggs within the faeces between the pre and post treatment worm egg count. Unfortunately, however, this technique is not actually considered to be all that reliable in cattle because of the phenomenon of *intermittent shedding* of eggs by resident gut worms; the natural fluctuation that occurs under any circumstances, treated or untreated, that is not fully understood. This simply means that a snapshot bovine faecal egg count is not always reflective of the host's gut worm population numbers. The effect of this can be minimised by sampling large numbers of cattle but this is costly, time consuming and not practical in commercial farming operations. In summary, proving resistance is not that easy.

Responsible use of anthelmintics

1. Seek advice from a vet or suitably qualified person on the correct product to use in that scenario and, how to administer it.
2. Use the correct product for only the parasite that needs to be controlled or killed; a product with as narrow a spectrum of activity as possible but obviously still including the target parasite. For example; if there is no need to kill immature liver fluke, a narrow range flukicide would be nitroxynil, a drug which only kills adult fluke. A product containing albendazole, on the other hand, will kill adult fluke but it also kills gut worms, this makes albendazole a broader spectrum choice and therefore not the right choice.
3. Use the correct product at the right time of year. Again, using liver fluke as the example, it is inappropriate to use a product that only kills adult fluke in grazed cattle in the autumn

when there is a high risk of immature fluke. Here nitroxynil would not be the drug of choice.

4. Always read the data sheet before administering the product and use the product in accordance with the guidelines – a simple notion: read the instructions! Calculate the amount required to be administered by weighing the animal. Ensure the dosing/injecting equipment is clean and calibrated so the animal is actually receiving the amount you think it is receiving. The gun should be calibrated by pumping known doses into a graduated measuring cylinder or syringe. By using the actual medicine then any differences generated by viscosity or stickiness of the preparation can be allowed for.

5. Store the anthelmintic correctly and do not use medicines exceeding their broach date or expiry date. Do not subject medicines to extremes of temperature, such as frosts, or direct sunlight or hot vehicles. Ensure the product is shaken before use so the active ingredient is evenly distributed in the solution or suspension.

6. Do not mix products. For example, do not mix mineral drenches and anthelmintics. They have a tendency to separate and overdosing and underdosing is a common consequence.

7. Do not use more than one product at the same time unless the two products are licensed to be used concurrently.

8. Record the identity of the animal, the product name, the route of administration, the quantity of product administered, the date of administration and the meat withdrawal period.

9. For most pour-on medications animals should not be treated when the hair is wet or when rain is anticipated within 2 hours of treatment. The area to which the product is applied will be stated in the data sheet and this stipulation should be adhered to. Pour-on products should not be applied to broken skin and the skin should be clean; free of mud or faecal soiling.

Flukicides

Flukicides are anthelmintics that kill flukes, either liver, rumen or both. They should normally be used as part of a pre-planned parasite control programme, a programme that should be reviewed every 6 months with a veterinary surgeon or SQP. Emergency tactical use of flukicides in cattle is less often needed; cattle cope quite well with a light infection of liver fluke and flukicides are largely used to kill adult flukes and prevent contamination of the pasture for the coming season. Grazing management is an integral part of a fluke control program.

There are several active ingredients that kill liver fluke and rumen fluke. They are available in a range of preparations – injectable, oral drench and pour-on. Each active ingredient kills a different range of fluke. Table 26.1 details the flukicides commonly used to treat liver fluke.

Triclabendazole is the only product effective against very young fluke, from 2 weeks of age, as well as older, and adult fluke. There is, however, and unfortunately, widespread fluke resistance to triclabendazole and while this is usually reported in sheep rather than cattle, it must be remembered that liver fluke in cattle and sheep are the same species so where triclabendazole resistance is noticed in the sheep of a mixed grazed farm the product will also have limited efficacy in cattle too.

Flukicides have no persistent activity so they only kill the fluke that are in the animal at the time of administration. If the cattle are housed after treatment, they will not ingest any more metacercariae (the infective stage of fluke), however, if they are returned to a high-risk pasture then they may require subsequent treatments. Cattle attempt to develop an immune response against liver fluke but largely fail; fluke have techniques to evade immune system attack.

When cattle or sheep are purchased or returned to a farm there is a risk of introducing fluke and if the fluke happen to be triclabendazole resistant then that trait too will be introduced. Quarantine treatments should avoid triclabendazole products

TABLE 26.1 Flukicides available in the UK

Active ingredient	Age of liver fluke killed
Triclabendazole	2 weeks onwards
Closantel (often in combination with an ivermectin)	6–8 weeks onwards
Nitroxynil	8 weeks onwards
Clorsulon (often in combination with an ivermectin)	Adults only, 10–12 weeks onwards
Oxyclozanide	Adults only, 10–12 weeks onwards
Albendazole	Adults only, 10–12 weeks onwards

but other products will not kill fluke less than 6 weeks of age so a second treatment will be required. The interval between the two products depends on the stage of fluke that the active ingredient kills.

Rumen fluke

The significance of rumen fluke infestation is discussed in Chapter 15. Routine treatment of rumen fluke is not generally considered necessary where clinical disease has not been experienced. If treatment were to be required, oxyclozanide is the only drug that kills rumen fluke, both the immature and adult stages. It must be remembered when designing a combined liver and rumen fluke control plan that oxyclozanide only kills adult liver fluke.

Controlling liver fluke is not about flukicides alone. Grazing strategies are an integral part of a control program and are discussed in Chapter 15.

Ectoparasiticides

Ectoparasiticides are drugs that kill, control or prevent infestation of the host with ectoparasites – parasites that live on the surface of the host, parasites such as lice, mites, ticks, flies and larvae (maggots). Ectoparasiticides include topical synthetic pyrethroids such as deltamethrin, alpha-cypermethrin, cypermethrin and permethrin, all of which kill lice but only permethrin has a licence to kill both lice and mites. Ear tags impregnated with cypermethrin exist to control flies. There is a variation in their duration of action and withdrawal periods. ML, which are also anthelmintics, control lice and mange mites. The injectable forms are less effective against surface living species such as chorioptic mange mites (Chapter 13) (COWS, 2014).

Vaccines

Vaccines are known as biologicals rather than drugs. Drugs are usually used to kill something or modify the chemistry of an animal in some way. Vaccines, however, are used to increase an individual animal's or a population of animals' immunity to disease. Some vaccines produce such a strong immunity that the animal is pretty much fully protected from that disease, such is the case with modern BVD vaccines where disease eradication relies on protection of the individual. Some vaccines, however, induce an antibody response that does not completely prevent disease but helps reduce the clinical signs of the disease or the subsequent shedding of the disease-causing organism. The latter of these two mechanisms, the reduction of bug shedding, is important with some vaccination programmes such as salmonella, leptospirosis and ringworm as the vaccine is indirectly helping to reduce human exposure to these bugs that are carried by infected, or, so called, carrier cattle.

How do vaccines work?

Vaccines trick the recipient's immune system into thinking it is being attacked by the bug in question. This trick involves giving the recipient a dose of one of the following.

- A milder form of the disease, what is known as an *attenuated strain* of the disease, for example, live IBR vaccine where the administered strain of IBR is one that cannot multiply in the warmth of the lower airways thus rendering it relatively safe. Live vaccines produce a rapid and strong immune response in the face of a disease outbreak and often just require a single dose. They are often, however, very delicate and susceptible to damage from poor storage, for example, fluctuating temperatures (Paton, 2013).

- A similar disease that is less harmful but provides cross protection to the more serious disease, for example, using a cowpox virus vaccine to protect humans against smallpox virus.

- A killed or inactivated bug that is intact enough that the immune system can still recognise it, for example, killed IBR vaccine. Generally, they produce a weaker immune response and produce less antibodies and the protection it provides does not last as long. Multiple doses are often required to achieve an adequate immune repose (Paton, 2013). A method of increasing the immune response to inactivated vaccines is to use an *adjuvant*. An adjuvant is a chemical incorporated into the vaccine which slows the dispersion of the vaccine from the site of injection and so stimulates the immune system for a longer period and more strongly. Aluminium oxide, Quil A and mineral oils are commonly used adjuvants (RUMA, 2007).

- A subunit, recombinant, polysaccharide, or conjugate vaccine. These biologicals use specific pieces of the bug – like its protein, sugar, or capsid (a casing around the bug) that are enough of a target on the bug for an attack by the immune system to successfully denature the bug.

- A toxin produced by the bug rather than the bug itself, for example, tetanus toxin. These vaccines tend to be very effective but usually multiple doses are required.

A small quantity of a vaccine is all it takes to trigger the immune system. The immune system learns what the bug, or at least the target, looks like, it is then 'primed' and ready to respond quickly and effectively when next exposed to the real thing.

The immune response

The immune system responds to a bug or toxin usually in one of two ways.

1. **Humoral response**. This is where special cells in the immune system, B-lymphocytes, release antibodies. These antibodies, or immunoglobulins, are proteins that lock-on to the recognised part of the bug, or toxin, and stop it from working.
2. **Cell mediated response**. In this case the immune system releases special cells, *killer cells*, T-lymphocytes, that directly attack the bug or toxin and again stop it from working, usually by engulfing and digesting it – very sci-fi!

The bug, the disease-causing organism, may be a parasite larva, a virus, a bacterium, a mycoplasma or a fungus, or, as already mentioned, it may be a toxin; a harmful chemical released by the bug.

Usually a full response to the vaccine is not maximised until 10–14 days after administration and sometimes two doses are required to elicit a satisfactory response; the two doses are referred to as a primary course. The timing between these two injections is quite specific and stated on the data sheet for each particular vaccine. The full response will not be achieved until 10–14 days after the second vaccination (RUMA, 2007).

If the immune system is to be stimulated and primed it needs to be in good working order. If an animal is ill, deficient in trace elements, or stressed, it may respond very poorly to a vaccine and as a consequence the vaccine may not stimulate an immune response, in effect it will not have worked. Similarly cows and heifers should not be vaccinated within 14 days of calving as the stress and the hormonal changes at that time are highly likely to compromise their immune system's response.

Vaccines are all about *acquired immunity*. Any discussion of the immune system should acknowledge that immunity can be innate as well as acquired.

Innate immunity

This is the part of the immune system that is not *specific* to any pathogen, it treats them all the same or is simply a passive defence mechanism. It includes anatomical barriers such as the skin that stops pathogens gaining access to the body, or the stomach acid that kills pathogens in the gastrointestinal tract, or non-specific defensive chemicals in the bloodstream such as *interferon* and *complement*.

Acquired immunity

This is the part of the immune system that is specific to the pathogen, that achieves recognition of the pathogen and that forms 'immunological memory' to produce the correct antibody or killer cell for that pathogen, especially for the next time it sees it – known as priming – so it is quicker to respond when re-infected.

Marker vaccines

The antibodies generated by vaccines, or at least most vaccines, those that elicit a humoral response, can cause complications when blood testing animals to see if they have been naturally infected with the disease; such tests are, after all, usually based on measuring antibodies. These diagnostic tests usually do not differentiate between antibodies produced from natural infection and those produced by vaccination. To provide a solution to this problem, manufacturers have developed vaccines called marker vaccines. Marker vaccines generate a slightly different antibody that can be distinguished from the real one.

Route of administration of vaccines

Vaccines can be administered via different routes. The majority of vaccines are injected either under the skin or intramuscularly. Some are administered orally, lungworm vaccine for example, and some are given up the nose – intranasally as it is called. Intranasal vaccines work slightly differently from those that are injected.

Intranasal vaccines

For any pathogen that infects by inhalation, that is via the respiratory route, the lining of the nasal cavity is the first barrier it encounters. This nasal lining has, as a result, evolved to be capable of challenging these pathogens. When a pathogen, or a vaccine for that matter, hits the lining of the nose, or the respiratory system generally, it generates two types of response. There is the standard response that all infections and vaccines generate, which is to trigger a whole body humoral reaction in the form of antibodies in the bloodstream (and other body tissues) but there is a more local response also. The local response is to pour out a special type of antibody onto the surface lining of the respiratory system, an antibody in the respiratory secretion rather than in the blood. This type of antibody is called immunoglobulin A (IgA) as opposed to the whole body based antibody, immunoglobulin G (IgG). This local response with IgA happens relatively quickly; immunity from intranasal infection or vaccination is established within 3–4 days rather than weeks, as is the case with whole body (systemic) infection or vaccination. While systemic IgG is prone to being interfered with by colostrum derived antibody, or, MDA, as it is more correctly called, there is little such interference with IgA – it evades the MDA by being relatively exterior to the systemic body, that is by being on the surface of the respiratory lining. Lack of MDA interference is useful; it means the vaccine can be used from a very young age. They are especially useful in calves born late in the autumn close to housing; calves that are susceptible to respiratory infections soon after hitting the ground where there is a lack of time for a course of systemic injections to work. It seems you cannot have it all though – the duration of protective immunity from intranasal vaccines is usually shorter than that from injectables. Intranasal vaccines have been used widely in the beef and dairy industries in the UK and many other countries.

Intraoral vaccines

These vaccines, given by mouth, have features in common with intranasal vaccines. While they too can generate a systemic IgG response, they can also generate a local IgA response on the lining of the intestine similar to the response in the lining of the respiratory system. As with intranasal vaccines, this relatively rapid response provides a first line defence against ingested pathogens. Examples from the human world would be the smallpox vaccine, famously given to children on a teaspoon with a sugar cube! This vaccine was so successful it is now believed that smallpox has been globally eradicated. A veterinary example of an oral vaccine would be the one for lungworm where the attenuated lungworm larvae in the vaccine trigger a local gut lining based response, as well as a systemic one.

Multivalent vaccines

Multivalent vaccines contain antigen for more than one disease or more than one strain of the same disease. Clostridial vaccines are the best example – they cover up to ten different clostridial diseases and some pneumonia and scour vaccines are also good examples, covering up to five or six different bugs or, at least, strains. Multivalent vaccines were designed for convenience so that many diseases could be protected against with just one product. There are many challenges in designing such a product as it is possible for the different specific antigens of the vaccine to interfere with each other so eliciting a suboptimal antibody response

to some or all of the antigens; a phenomenon called *immunological interference* (Sherwin and Down, 2018).

Autogenous vaccines

Autogenous vaccines are vaccines prepared by isolating a bug from an individual animal and using it to make a vaccine for administration to the same individual, to help it overcome the bug it is already infected with, and, to help reduce the excretion and spread of that bug.

Also referred to, somewhat incorrectly, as autogenous vaccines are those specifically made for animals with a disease where there is no commercially available 'readymade' vaccine. The pathogen is isolated from an animal with the disease, either a sick, live animal or from post-mortem material. The pathogen is then cultured, made safe (inactivated or attenuated) and a vaccine produced. This process is under strict control by the drug governing authorities; in the UK for example, the production of the vaccine needs to be officially approved and once the vaccine is produced it is only allowed to be used on the farm of origin, and under licence. Autogenous vaccination against *Mycoplasma* and *Papilloma* virus (warts) are the most commonly developed autogenous vaccines. Historically, and perhaps still now in some industries and in some countries, a very basic form of autogenous vaccination is the unpalatable practice of so called *feedback vaccination*. Here the bodies or body parts or infected material (for example, aborted placenta) of infected animals are fed back to the affected population in a desperate attempt to enhance group immunity. This was practised in the UK pig industry in the not too distant past.

Administration of vaccines

As a general rule, vaccines should not be administered at the same time as any other medicinal product. A gap of 14 days is either required or advised. Antibiotics, for example, could interfere with live bacterial vaccines and, similarly, anthelmintics could upset the function of lung-worm vaccine by killing the vaccine larvae. These are obvious and specific examples of interference but non-specifically any drug that generates a physiological response in an individual could distract the immune system in some way from fully responding to a vaccine. Conversely, the vaccine's effect on the immune system could, likewise, affect the physiological response of the body to some other administered drug. Just like any other medicinal products, vaccines should certainly not be mixed in the same syringe and, similarly, two vaccines or medicinal products should not be administered in the same site on the animal, even if it is a number of days apart. This is because the body may be having a local response to the product and that should either not be interfered with or, alternatively, not allowed to interfere with the next product. There are a few products produced by the same manufacturer that are approved for concurrent use. Here the data sheet guidelines must be adhered to; examples would be certain leptospirosis and BVD vaccines, and, certain pneumonia vaccines.

Vaccine failure or suboptimal response

When a vaccine fails at preventing or, at least, controlling a disease there is great disappointment all round and there is a great temptation to jump to conclusions: 'the vaccine does not work!'. There are, of course, many reasons why a vaccine may fail and all possible explanations need to be taken into account.

- **Incorrect vaccine storage**. Vaccines are usually very sensitive to temperature.
- **Exceeding the broach time**. Most vaccines need to be used within 8 hours of opening, often because air within the vial can damage the antigen through oxidation.
- **Incorrectly reconstituting the vaccine**. Some vaccines are supplied un-constituted as a powder in a bottle and a solvent in a bottle. The two need to be mixed together so as to dissolve the powder in the solvent. Scenarios have arisen

in the past where only the solvent has been administered to the animal! In other words, no antigen at all, just water!
- **Incorrect dosing**. To save money a half dose may have been used or at least a reduced dose to spread the bottle a bit further!
- **Failing to administer the second dose** of a primary course, or an annual booster. This is a common problem.
  - Poor timing of second doses or boosters. The immune system has 'memory' so exact timing of second doses and boosters is not critical but they should not be wildly out of time – not just because efficacy may be reduced but because failure to stay in line with the manufacturers guidelines would make any failure the fault of the operator not the vaccine.
- **Misdiagnosis** and vaccination against the wrong disease.
- **Incorrect route of administration**. Intramuscular instead of subcutaneous. This may not always be critical, but all elements of doubt are best avoided.
- **Excessive disease challenge**. A balance exists between immunity and challenge in any infection. Vaccine increases an animal's immunity but it can still be overcome by an even higher challenge of pathogen. An example would be high stocking rates and poor ventilation preventing the success of pneumonia vaccination, or dirty conditions spoiling scour vaccination efforts.
- **Variation in the strain of the pathogen** in the animal compared to that in the vaccine.
- **Immunosuppression** of the animal due to concurrent disease, old age, poor nutrition, trace element deficiency, giving birth or concurrent drug or vaccine administration.
- **Maternally derived antibody** (see below).

Maternally derived antibody

MDA is antibody of the IgG type that exists in a cow and is passed to the calf via her colostrum. MDA protects calves from a whole range of diseases that their dams have either been vaccinated against or been exposed to at some point in their lives. For example, calf scour vaccination programmes are designed to protect young calves from rotavirus, coronavirus and *E. coli*. The vaccine, however, is actually given to the cow, not the calf. An inactivated vaccine is administered to the cow a couple of weeks pre-calving. The cow responds with the production of antibodies against these calf scour bugs. These antibodies, in freshly stimulated high levels, end up in the colostrum; the colostrum ends up in the calf. To ensure this vaccine is effective, and represents money well spent, the cows need to be in good health to produce an adequate immune response, but there also needs to be an effective colostrum management programme to ensure the calf gets this antibody rich colostrum soon enough after birth. Interestingly it has been identified that even unabsorbed antibody in the colostrum 2–3 days after birth still provides local gut-based protection against the scour pathogens (Sherwin and Down, 2018). MDA declines over time. The rate of decline depends on how much MDA was present initially and on the calf's own individual destruction of the MDA over time – remember these proteins are not continually produced by the calf, they came from the mother, so, like any other protein, they break down, or are broken down, with time. The body has to continually produce or ingest proteins – that is why the immune system has to be kept healthy, and, to an extent, continually stimulated.

MDA is obviously a good thing, but it causes problems when we want to start vaccinating very young animals against disease. When a vaccine is administered to a young calf that already has MDA against that bug, the MDA may neutralise the vaccine. This is vaccination in reverse! Instead of the vaccine mimicking the bug to stimulate the immune system, the cow's immune system already knows the bug and the antibodies it has given to the calf then knobble the vaccine and the vaccine does not get a chance to stimulate the calf's own antibody production. Because the rate of MDA decline varies from calf to calf it is difficult to

know when it is late enough to vaccinate. Usually, there is a specification on the data sheet, somewhere between 1 and 12 weeks often, but most vaccines administered to young calves are repeated to ensure effective immunisation occurs, to ensure MDA has declined sufficiently.

Vaccines available for beef cattle

There are 14 different diseases affecting beef cattle that can be vaccinated against (see Box 26.1); more if you subdivide groups of bacteria. Do we need to vaccinate for everything? The answer is no. Deciding on what to vaccinate against involves a risk-based analysis involving the farmer and vet. The decision will depend on practicalities, objectives of the herd, biosecurity and the existing profile of disease on the farm and any immediate threats. Vaccines should be targeted at diseases whose control is likely to provide the most benefit, either economically or through improved welfare (Paton, 2013). Vaccination could be viewed as not only an insurance policy against disease but a savings account for welfare and production.

Box 26.1 Fourteen diseases that affect beef cattle for which there are commercially available vaccines

- *Histophilis somni*
- Pasteurellosis
- RSV
- Pi3
- IBR
- BVD
- Salmonellosis
- Lungworm
- Ringworm
- Leptospirosis
- *E. coli*
- Coronavirus
- Rotavirus
- Clostridial disease

Antimicrobials and antibiotics

Antimicrobials are medicines that are used to treat microbial diseases in animals. Those used to treat bacteria are called antibiotics and they form the biggest group by far. Other groups include such drugs as anticoccidials, antimalarials, antifungals, antivirals and so on. For ease of discussion the term antibiotic will often be used in this context but the term antimicrobial may at times be more appropriate. Pharmacologists classify antimicrobials as *chemotherapeutics*. That is quite a thought … antibiotics classed alongside chemotherapy. Why? Antibiotics, like chemotherapeutics, are drugs used in a very tailored way to destroy a particular target cell – a specific bacterium in the case of an antibiotic, a specific cancer cell in the case of a chemotherapeutic. A sobering thought. So, in this new era of reduced antibiotic usage it is worth remembering that just like a doctor does not prescribe chemotherapy for a headache nor should we give antibiotics to an animal simply because it does not look quite right!

Used properly, antimicrobials are used accurately and specifically to treat diagnosed infections in an individual or an infected group of individuals. Less correctly they are sometimes used to prevent microbial disease (known as prophylaxis) or at the start of an outbreak where not all individuals have yet contracted the disease but a reduction of spread is desirable (known as metaphylaxis) (for example, bacterial pneumonia in calves) (RUMA, 2015).

Antibiotics

Antibiotics are the subclass of antimicrobials that are used to treat bacterial infections. Most antibiotics originate from nature. These are the chemicals one type of bacteria produces to compete with other bacteria. That is how they were discovered. Famously, Louis Pasteur and his co-workers noticed that one 'mould' could not grow within a ring around another mould, so the story began. Nowadays, some, but still the minority of, antibiotics are synthesised but the majority are still cultured in labs from other bacteria. To understand antibiotics first involves a fuller understanding of bacteria, especially their classification.

There are several different ways of subclassifying bacteria.

Do they require oxygen to survive?

Anaerobic bacteria can live without oxygen. *Aerobic bacteria* require oxygen. *Facultative anaerobes* can grow with or without oxygen. *Microaerophilic bacteria* like some oxygen but at a lower concentration than that which exists in normal atmospheric air; *Campylobacter* spp. falls into this category. Examples of aerobic bacteria are some *E. coli* and streptococci. Examples of facultative anaerobes are other *E. coli*, staphylococcal and streptococcal species. Examples of anaerobic bacteria are the clostridial species.

If a crystal violet (gram stain) is applied to a bacterium, what colour does it adopt?

Gram-positive bacteria turn dark purple, *gram-negative* fail to take up the stain and do not turn purple. The difference between gram-negative and gram-positive bacteria is largely based on whether they have a thick or a thin cell wall structure. Gram-positive bacteria include *Clostridia* spp., staphylococci, *Listeria* spp., *Bacillus* spp., and *Corynebacterium* spp. Gram negative bacteria include *E. coli*, *Salmonella* spp. and *Pasteurella* spp.

What shape are they?

Bacteria can be rod shaped, described as bacilli, or spherical, described as cocci. They may form chains such as streptococci, clusters, such as staphylococci or pairs, such as diplococci. When bacteria are viewed using a microscope, especially after a stain is applied to them, their shape and formation help in their identification.

The antibiotics used on cattle are in most cases identical or, at least, closely related to those used in human medicine, with a few minor exceptions being certain molecules that are exclusive to the veterinary market and vice versa. Just like worms can become resistant to wormers so too can bacteria become resistant to antibiotics. Use of antimicrobials in food animals can create an important source of antimicrobial resistant bacteria in these animals that can then spread to humans through the food supply or through other forms of contact between the animals, the farms they live on and the human population. Given that there are now bacterial infections of humans that cannot be treated with antibiotics due to multiple antibiotic resistance then any likelihood of further increasing antibiotic resistance, be it in animal infecting bacteria or human infecting bacteria, is a significant threat to the human population. Human health must obviously be given priority when considering the use of antimicrobials in the animal population. The current compromise view is that antimicrobials should be used 'as little as possible and as much as necessary'. The cattle industry has developed the following practical guidelines to help mitigate the problem.

1. Identify and implement practical strategies by which the need for antimicrobials might be reduced without adversely affecting either the welfare of animals or the viability of the food producing business.
2. Provide good practical guidance on how antimicrobials can be used when they are deemed necessary for animal health and welfare.

What is imperative here is that antimicrobials are not deployed as a substitute for good husbandry, biosecurity and vaccination.

The antibiotics that are most important to human medicine have been identified by the WHO and are constantly reviewed. Antimicrobials on the list are referred to as critically important antimicrobials (CIAs). This largely dictates what antimicrobials can, from now on, be used in food producing animals so preserving the benefits of the other antimicrobials when used in people.

There are many different antibiotics. They can be classified into five groups. The antibiotics within each group differ in their chemical composition, how they work – their 'mode of action' – and, therefore, to some extent, which bacteria they kill. Vets have a working knowledge of which bacteria cause which diseases and therefore which antibiotic will be effective. The methodology of this decision making by vets is being questioned. Vets working solely on pattern recognition in terms of which disease they think it is and which antibiotic worked last time will have to be a bit more scientific in the future. The correct course of action is to obtain a sample of tissue, in the case of post-mortem situations, or a swab of a lesion, in the case of a live animal. These samples are then submitted for culture and sensitivity in a laboratory. Culture and sensitivity testing involve growing the bacteria on special culture plates in an incubator and then identifying the bacteria in question. The cultivated bacteria are then exposed to a range of antibiotic discs placed on the culture plate to see which ones kill the bacteria and worst of all which ones do not. The vet then knows exactly what the cause of the infection is (the diagnosis) and which antibiotic is likely to be effective in treating the condition. It is not always that simple though; vets still have their uses! Vets are trained to know how different antibiotics distribute themselves in the body, which ones penetrate some tissues better than others and which ones to avoid in certain situations. The ultimate choice of antibiotic will still be down to the vet.

There are limitations to this approach in practice.

- Culture and sensitivity testing take 3–5 days and often the animal requires treatment sooner than that.
- The sample for culture needs to be taken without any contamination with other bacteria from the environment. Dirty on-farm settings can make this very difficult.
- There are often large distances between farms, vets and laboratories so samples have to be sent

by post, so adding further delays and potentially sample deterioration.

- Even though an antibiotic kills a bacterium on a culture plate within a laboratory it may not be effective in the animal. As mentioned above, the antibiotic needs to be able to 'get to' the bacteria within the animal's body to be effective. The correct product needs selecting but it may not exist or if it does it may not be licensed under food production rulings.

Classification of antimicrobials

Antibiotics can be classified as *bactericidal* or *bacteriostatic*. Bactericidal antibiotics directly kill the bacteria, bacteriostatic ones inhibit the growth of the bacteria but require the animals own immune system to do the actual killing.

Antibiotics can, similarly to anthelmintics, be classified as narrow spectrum or broad spectrum. Narrow spectrum antibiotics kill only a few types of bacteria while broad-spectrum antibiotics kill a relatively large range. To reduce the rate at which resistance to antibiotics develops, narrow-spectrum products should be used so only the bacteria causing the disease are killed rather than challenging a range of other bacteria to the antibiotic which in turn would encourage resistance. It is important to acknowledge that many of these bacteria live naturally in, on or around the animal, causing no ill effect. These bacteria are essentially good bacteria, they not only do no harm, but they may even benefit the animal. For example, the gut is full of good bacteria which help with digestion and keep the bad ones out. Similarly, the skin and body orifices have good bacteria living on and in them and they preserve the harmony – again, keep the bad ones away. Killing these bacteria indiscriminately along with the infection can therefore be seen to be undesirable both for the reason of increasing the likelihood of resistance and also for removing the population of 'good guys' leaving room for the influx of 'bad guys'. To make the prescribing of a narrow antibiotic feasible the vet must be sure of exactly which bacterium is causing disease, and that requires laboratory culture and sensitivity.

Antibiotics are also classified as *concentration dependent* or *time dependent*. To understand this classification, the concept of the MIC needs first to be understood. MIC stands for Minimum Inhibitory Concentration. This is the concentration of antibiotic needed in the animal's tissue for the bacterium to be unable to survive. The efficacy of time dependant antibiotics is proportional to the time that the antibiotic level is above the MIC. The efficacy of a concentration dependent antibiotic is proportional to how much higher the level of antibiotic is at the site of the infection over and above the MIC. Knowledge in this area enables the choice of either high level short sharp shock protocols or of long courses of lower level treatment, accordingly.

Beta-lactams (penicillins and derivatives)

This group includes penicillins, amino-penicillins and cephalosporins. Their chemical structures all include a beta-lactam ring in their configuration. They are active against gram-positive bacteria with only some of them having activity against gram-negative bacteria and even then rather limited. The antibiotics in this group kill bacteria by affecting the make up of the cell wall. Gram-negative bacteria which do not have a thick cell wall fortuitously find themselves resistant to these drugs. Bacteria have developed resistance to beta-lactam antibiotics by producing an enzyme called *beta-lactamase*. One antibiotic in this group, amoxicillin, is sometimes combined with clavulanic acid. This extra ingredient blocks the effect of beta-lactamase so overcoming this mechanism of resistance. Beta-lactams are time dependant antibiotics so are typically, although not always, given as a reasonably long course, usually at least four days but in some stubborn cases, such as lung abscesses, several weeks.

Aminoglycosides

This group includes streptomycin and neomycin and is one of the oldest group of antibiotics, their discovery dating back to 1944 (Barragry, 1994). Unlike beta-lactams these drugs are particularly effective against gram-negative infections but not gram-positive. They are poorly absorbed from the gut but absorbed rapidly from intramuscular injection sites. They are not particularly penetrative, they do not get through the meningeal membranes around the brain and spinal cord so are not suitable for treating infections of the brain, such as listerioisis or spinal abscesses. Aminoglycosides are excreted by the kidneys so rely on the animal having reasonable kidney function – where this is not the case they can further damage the kidneys. They also have a reputation for damaging hearing, most notably in humans. They have a narrow safety margin which means the dose rate should be carefully calculated – overdoses are dangerous. They are concentration dependant so for some infections a single large dose may be effective as is the case when treating leptospirosis.

Macrolides

These antibiotics have a macrocyclic lactone ring as part of their chemical compositition, hence the name. The group includes tilmicosin, tylosin, gamithromycin and tulathromycin. These drugs target the protein synthesis in rapidly dividing bacteria. At low doses they are bacteriostatic becoming bactericidal at higher concentrations. They are predominantly used for gram-positive infections but they have some gram-negative capability, most notably against *Pasteurella* spp. and some mycoplasmata.

Macrolides are excreted by the liver through the bile ducts; the kidneys have a limited role in their excretion.

Macrolides concentrate in the reproductive tract, lung, liver and spleen so blood levels drop quickly. Their concentration, and persistence in the lungs make them highly useful in the treatment of bacterial pneumonia in cattle whether caused by *Pasteurella* spp., *Haemophilus* spp. or *Mycoplasma* spp.

They are time dependent so their tendency to persist in infected tissues fits nicely with this mechanism.

Tetracyclines

Oxytetracycline is the main member of this long-standing group, which was identified back in 1950 (Barragry, 1994). These drugs are very broad spectrum, being effective against gram-positive, gram-negative, intracellular (*Chlamydia* spp. and *Mycoplasma* spp.) and anaerobic organisms. After administration, tetracyclines enter the bloodstream and bind to proteins in the blood but despite this manage to become widely distributed around the body. Levels are concentrated in the liver, kidneys and lungs and the drug is excreted via the urine and faeces.

Tetracyclines do not pass through meningeal membranes so they are not useful when treating conditions such as meningitis or listeria. They do, however, cross the placenta to the foetus, are excreted in milk, and distribute into joints and peritoneal fluid (the small amount of fluid that surrounds organs within the abdomen).

Tetracyclines are used widely in cattle for their broad-spectrum activity, but widespread resistance exists so threatening their ongoing usefulness.

Fluoroquinolones

The two antibiotcs relevant to cattle in this group are marbofloxacin and enrofloxacin. Their main activity is against gram-negative aerobes; they have some gram-positive activity. They are not effective against anaerobic bacteria. They are concentration dependant; some are even licensed as a one-off dose given at four times the usual daily dose when given as a course.

This group of antibiotics is largely redundant within food producing animals as they are classified as CIAs.

Sulphonamides

Sulphonamides are not of bacterial origin, they are man made, so for that reason they are not actually classified as antibiotics. These antimicrobials are active largely against gram-negative organisms but some activity against gram-positive bacteria occurs and also some activity against protozoa such as *Coccidia* spp.

They are bacteriostatic and broad spectrum. They are excreted by the kidneys. Sulphonamides are effectively absorbed from the gut, and blood levels two hours after oral administration are the same as if the antibiotic had been administered by injection.

Sulphonamides are often combined with the antibiotic trimethoprim; they work together *synergistically*, that is, killing more bacteria together than either would kill individually (Barragry, 1994). They only work when the bacterial cells are replicating so they need to be administered early on in an infection. As the antibiotics are bacteriostatic the animal's own immune system has a responsibilty to help clear up the infection.

Anti-inflammatories

Anti-inflammatories, as the name suggests, are drugs that block, to some extent, the process of inflammation in the body. Why block inflammation? Surely inflammation is a good thing? Inflammation is the body's response to infection or a traumatic insult of some sort such as physical or chemical damage. Inflammation involves the body shunting extra bloodflow to the affected area and the internal bathing of the damaged tissue with extra fluid, structural proteins to plug holes and repair tissue and defensive chemicals that attack infection and block oxidation. This is indeed a good response, evolved over millions of years. Medicine has found, however, that inflammation has an element of the 'kill or cure' to it; sometimes the response by the immune system is so strong that the inflammatory response can be quite damaging

to the animal itself and not just the infection it is fighting. The inflammatory chemicals can raise the body temeperature dangerously high or sometimes dangerously low, the chemicals can cause too much pain. Pain is an interesting concept; an evolutionary response designed to discourage the animal from repeating whatever it did to supposedly cause the problem, for example, re-entering a handling system after a traumatic event such as a difficult calving or a poorly managed dehorning procedure. During inflammation the leaking of fluid from the bloodstream can become too great, the shunting of blood can cause a critical fall in blood pressure or circulating volume. These excessive responses can lead to self damaging states such as shock, or septic shock (*sepsis* as it is now called). Physicians and vets have found that a moderation of inflammation can, therefore, be beneficial, especially when other drugs are meanwhile being used to help the person or animal overcome the problem such as antimicrobials or intravenous fluids; inflammation is then not the only measure the patient is relying on.

Anti-inflammatories have been developed over the years to do exactly this. The earliest modes of anti-inflammatory were techniques such as cold water or ice application, or perhaps rubbing, massage or compressive bandaging to reduce swelling. As time passed, drugs were developed to achieve these effects chemically rather than physically. The drugs vary in how they do this and to what extent.

There are three categories of anti-inflammatories:

- non-steroidal anti-inflammatories
- steroids
- other.

Non-steroidal anti-inflammatory drugs

This group includes aspirin and ibuprofen in the human world, but, better known in the cattle industry are meloxicam, flunixin, ketoprofen and carprofen.

NSAIDs reduce fever (antipyretic), reduce inflammation (anti-inflammatory) and reduce pain (analgesic). Some NSAIDs also have anti-endotoxic effects – they block the effect of some toxins produced by some bacteria. NSAIDs are easy to administer by injection, by mouth or by pour-on. They have a range of duration, some last 24 hours, others up to 72 hours and some products are licensed for repeated administration. There are few side effects from the use of NSAIDS although prolonged use has anecdotally been associated with abomasal ulcers, similar in principle to the stomach ulcers they can cause in people. NSAIDs are widely used as painkillers for dystocia, trauma, surgical operations, dehorning, castration and lameness. NSAIDs are also widely used in infectious disease to reduce the animal's temperature, maintain appetite and reduce pain while still allowing the immune system to work effectively to fight off the infection. Research suggests that the outcome of treatment for a number of conditions is more favourable when an anti-inflammatory drug has been adminstered and not just an antimicrobial. This is the case for lameness, mastitis and pneumonia. In these examples there will be occasions where bacterial infection is involved, the use of antimicrobial is appropriate but still the outcome is better with the inclusion of the anti-inflammatory treatment. There will also be occasions, however, where bacterial infection is not involved, the antimicrobial is pointless but the anti-inflammatory drug is helping. This would be the case in viral infections and in pain based conditions such as certain lamenesses. Doctors prescribing aspirin for influenza aren't to be criticised after all!

Steroids (glucocorticoids)

Steroids are our natural anti-inflammatories. They are hormones produced by the adrenal glands in response to trouble. The adrenal glands release adrenaline in the face of trouble – the fight or flight response – but it is a particular class of natural steroid, *glucocorticoids*, that follow; they

provide a more sustainable response to hard times. These hormones elicit a range of changes in the body – they raise glucose levels, they trigger the burning up of fat for a sustained supply of energy, they trigger off salt retention by the kidneys to help maintain hydration and blood pressure, they encourage thirst to maintain hydration, hunger to maintain nutrition and a heightened mental state – the so called *steroid psychosis*. They also, at high prolonged levels, cause abortion which, bleakly, is a survival mechanism for the mother who is trying, herself, to survive, let alone maintain the life of the unborn.

The general consensus in the medical world is that the *steroid stress response* is useful for a while but not if it drags on too long – then it becomes *chronic stress*. Chronic stress in people and in animals has indeed been shown to be associated with a prolonged elevation of blood levels of glucocorticoids, such as cortisol, also known as cortisone. Short-term stress is probably good, it is a natural physiological response, long-term stress on the other hand probably is not – nature did not plan for a permanently stressful life, such as being a farmer!

Dexamethasone is the commonly used glucocorticoid in cattle. It has also regained fame recently as a life saving drug in the treatment of human COVID-19. In cattle it is mainly licensed for the reduction of inflammation, but also for raising glucose levels during ketosis, for the treatment of shock, and for the induction of abortion. Although glucocorticoids are broad acting anti-inflammatories they are not very good at the painkilling part. Consequently, they do not get used as analgesics but they do for unwanted swelling and bruising, including nerve damage post-dystocia and inflammatory bowel disease. For the swelling component of inflammation they are very effective unlike NSAIDs which in this respect appear to make little or no difference. Steroids should obviously be administered with care, bearing in mind their abortive potential, but also because their inhibition of the inflammatory chemical pathways is so powerful that they can be *immunosuppressive*

– so much so that steroids are actually used in people and other animals for this effect – for example, suppressing allergic reactions or treating 'auto-immune' conditions such as some anaemias. They should not, theoretically, be used alongside bacteriostatic antibiotics that rely on the immune system to clear the infection although this may be more of an academic point than a practical one.

Cleansing and disinfection

Cleansing and disinfection are essential to disease control. The cleaner the environment the less the microbial challenge to the cattle and consequently the less the chance of disease.

This is a two-step process. Cleansing prior to disinfection is the first step as most disinfectants do not work in the presence of organic material, such as faeces, urine, straw and soil. Not only does organic material inactivate most disinfectants, microbes hiding within lumps of muck and dirt are not exposed to the disinfectant and can therefore survive the process.

Cleansing agents are often more effective when used at higher temperatures and they usually require a 'contact time' to work. Pressure washers are an effective means of cleaning but may also cause bacteria to spread via an aerosol. There should be no animals within the same air space when cleaning and disinfection takes places – not

TABLE 26.2 Disinfectants and their uses (RUMA, 2015)

Active compound	Uses	Range of effectiveness	Disadvantages
Chlorhexidine	Equipment, buildings, foot baths	Ineffective against parvovirus and *Pseudomonas*	Reduced activity against certain organisms
Phenolics	Equipment, buildings, foot baths	Variety of bacteria Limited effect on fungi and viruses Poor activity against bacterial spores	Environmental concerns
Formaldehyde, other aldehydes	Equipment, buildings, foot baths	Variety of bacteria, bacterial spores, fungi and viruses	Dangerous and irritating fumes
Iodophors	Pre-cleaned equipment	Bacteria and fungi Limited effect on bacterial spores and viruses	Inactivated by organic material
Peroxides	Pre-cleaned equipment and buildings	Many bacteria, viruses, fungi and spores	Inactivated by organic material
Quaternary ammonium compounds	Pre-cleaned equipment	Variety of bacteria Limited effect on bacterial spores, fungi and viruses	Inactivated by organic material
Chlorine, hypochlorites, chloramines	Pre-cleaned equipment	Bacteria and fungi Limited effect on bacterial spores and viruses	Inactivated by organic material, may be irritant
Lime	Floors, bedding	Bacteria and viruses	Application difficult and caustic to skin (human and animal) when wet

only is the aerosol an infection risk but the chemical itself may irritate the eyes, skin and respiratory system and as we know humidity, as created by a pressure washer, is an undesirable environmental factor (see Chapters 5-7). Caked on, heavily soiled surfaces may need to be soaked for 2–3 hours with a detergent solution for an effective clean.

Surfaces should be allowed to dry before a disinfectant is applied if the disinfectant is not to be subject to excessive dilution. There are a range of disinfectants on the market all with specific uses so the right product can be tailored to the job in mind, Table 26.2. The concentration of disinfectant required may vary depending on the infectious agent being targeted. Instructions on the label should be stringently followed, including the health and safety precautions as some disinfectants can be harmful, irritant or corrosive. Pressure washers are always the best method of applying a disinfectant, a low-pressure mist is often more effective as droplets stick to the surface for longer, while high pressure can blast the product too far. Some products require a specific contact time and then need washing from the surface; others can be left in situ.

REFERENCES

Barragry, T.B. (1994) *Veterinary Drug Therapy*. Lea and Febiger, New York.

COWS (2014) Integrated parasite control on cattle farms. November. Control of Worms Sustainably, Stoneleigh.

Cresswell, E., Brennan, M.L., Barkema, H.W. and Wapenaar, W. (2014) A questionnaire-based veterinary survey on the uptake and use of cattle vaccines in the UK. *Veterinary Record Open* 1: e000042. doi: 10.1136/vropen-2014-000042.

Cresswell, L., Richens, I. and Wapenaar, W. (2019) Handling and storing medicines on beef and dairy farms. *In Practice* 41, 157–162.

Paton, N. (2013) Cattle vaccination; decision making in health planning. *In Practice* 35, 77–84.

RUMA (2007) Ruma Guidelines. Responsible use of vaccines and vaccination in dairy and beef production.

RUMA (2015) Ruma Guidelines. Responsible use of antimicrobials in cattle production.

SCOPS (2019) https://www.scops.org.uk/about/what-is-anthelmintic-resistance/ (accessed 3 June 2019).

Sherwin, G. and Down, P. (2018) Calf immunology and the role of vaccinations in dairy calves. *In Practice* 40, 102–114.

Taylor, M. (2000) Use of anthelmintics in cattle. *In Practice* 22, 290–304.

William, P.D. and Paixao, G. (2018) On-farm storage of livestock vaccines may be a risk to vaccine efficiency: a study of the performance of on-farm refrigerators to maintain the correct storage temperature. *BMC Veterinary Research* 14, 136.

FURTHER READING

Orr, J., Geraghty, T. and Ellis, K. (2014) Anti-inflammatories in cattle medicine. *Livestock* 19(6), 322–328.

Chapter 27

Advanced breeding techniques for the beef farm

Advanced breeding techniques use technologies, drugs and procedures to achieve a planned, desirable breeding outcome by interfering with the natural reproductive process in some way so as to remove the need for a natural mating and to access a choice of parent or parents that would not be otherwise easily achievable. Advanced breeding techniques to be considered here are artificial insemination (AI), embryo transfer (ET) and in vitro fertilisation (IVF).

ARTIFICIAL INSEMINATION

AI involves the deposition of previously collected semen into the reproductive tract of the female using a gun and straw (syringe and catheter) rather than relying on the bull actually mating with the female. The semen used can be freshly collected from a bull and transferred immediately into the cow or, as is much more usual, the semen collected from the bull is diluted (extended) and protected with certain additives so allowing it to be either chilled for short- to medium-term storage or, more commonly, frozen for long-term storage.

Advantages of AI

AI allows for the use of semen from bulls that would be otherwise unaffordable or inaccessible.

This access to potentially superior genetics will allow for overall genetic gain within the herd. AI is also useful in the control of the spread of certain sexually transmitted diseases (venereal diseases) which could otherwise be introduced or spread further by an infected bull used to mate the cows in the conventional manner. Campylobacteriosis would be an example.

Bulls can be dangerous so AI, in removing the presence of a bull, makes for an on-farm situation that is safer for farm staff and for other cattle and animals on the farm.

When a female has been artificially inseminated then, providing the gestation periods of both the cow and the bull are known, an accurate estimation of calving date can be made. This allows the farmer to plan ahead for the birth, provide staffing to supervise the calving and provide assistance if needed. Knowing the identity of the sire also improves family tree data and, for the customer, assurance of the breed and parentage of the meat subsequently produced.

Successful AI requires good quality semen that has been correctly extended, frozen, stored and defrosted, to then be correctly inserted through the cervix of the cow using an AI gun, into the right place in the uterus and at the right time in the cow's reproductive cycle.

Several variables affect the success of this process.

Semen quality

Bovine AI usually involves the use of frozen semen. Semen is collected from bulls either on farm for UK domestic use or in bull studs for domestic and international use. Straws can be bought and sold and moved around the world as required. The semen is collected by a procedure that involves allowing a bull to attempt to serve a restrained cow that is in oestrus but, at the moment of erection, just prior to intromission, a trained operative diverts the bull's penis away from the cow's vulva and inserts it into an artificial vagina whereupon the bull ejaculates. A typical ejaculate is 8–10 ml and can contain 10 thousand million sperm. The semen is examined microscopically and checked for abnormalities and then diluted with a solution that includes preservatives, nutrients and buffers to help the sperm survive and cope with the freezing process. The *extended semen*, as it is called, is inserted into either 0.25 ml or 0.5 ml plastic straws, each containing about 20 million sperm. After cooling, the straws can be stored frozen in liquid nitrogen (–196°C) indefinitely for subsequent defrosting and use as required.

The semen, even when frozen, is very fragile and susceptible to damage if incorrectly stored or handled. This can have a significantly detrimental effect on fertility. Semen straws can be transported and moved from tank to tank, but they must not be allowed to thaw.

A log of semen straws in the tank and their exact location is maintained so that semen can be easily and quickly accessed without removing straws out into the air. The semen is compartmentalised into mini-canisters in the tank. These canisters can be lifted up and hooked at the neck of the tank so that they are out of the liquid nitrogen but not fully out in the open; 5 seconds is the longest time allowed for this. A straw should never be completely removed from the tank and then refrozen. When thawing and preparing a straw for insemination a water bath is used and the straw is thawed at a specific temperature for a specific time. Once removed from the water bath and inserted in the AI gun

it needs to be protected so it does not cool down further and it should be inserted into the cow as soon as practically possible. For this reason, it is recommended that one straw is thawed and deposited at a time.

The level of liquid nitrogen in AI tanks needs to be monitored weekly and topped up at regular intervals depending on the tank's specifications; this is usually done every 12 weeks. Good semen storage and handling are just as important as good insemination technique.

Getting the semen in the right place

The AI straw, once loaded into the gun, is inserted into the vagina and advanced carefully towards the cervix. The cervix is manipulated by hand through the rectal wall and the AI gun is advanced gently through the cervix into the body of the uterus. The semen is expelled into the body of the uterus. The process needs to be carried out without causing damage or discomfort to the cow. It is important that this process is carried out hygienically and no faecal material is carried on the gun from the vulva into the uterus. Paper towel is used to clean the vulva accordingly. It is important that accurate records are maintained; these records to include the identity of the cow, the identity of the semen, and the date and time the insemination took place.

Inseminating at the right time

Heat detection is a vital part of the success of AI. Cows should be inseminated just after the end of standing oestrus; this time coincides with the approximate time of ovulation, that is, the release of the egg from the cow's ovary. Standing oestrus is defined as being the stage in oestrus when the cow, if mounted by another animal, agrees to stand still. The general rule is that a cow in standing oestrus in the morning should be inseminated that evening while a cow in standing oestrus in the evening should be inseminated the following morning. If a cow is still in oestrus 12 hours after insemination, she should be inseminated again. Semen will survive for a period of time in the cow's uterus if she is served too early, but this time varies between individual bulls and is usually not known so is best not relied on. That said, for this reason, a cow is better served too early than too late – the semen may wait, the egg will not.

There should be dedicated time periods when the cattle are observed for oestrus behaviour. Three times a day for at least 20 minutes is recommended; more frequent and for longer is better. Some heifers will show signs of oestrus for as little as 6 hours and 70% of cows show heat during the hours of darkness so an evening check is advisable. Oestrus observation should not take place when cattle are being fed or other management activities are taking place, the cows are less likely to show oestrus behaviours at these times.

To avoid the need for heat detection and to tighten the time period over which ovulation is likely, artificial oestrus synchronisation programmes can be used and followed up with so called *fixed time AI*. Here the cattle are all inseminated at the same set time regardless of whether oestrus has been observed or not. Their reproductive cycles will have been manipulated using hormonal drugs to ensure ovulation occurs at the same specific and predictable time.

AI should only be attempted by a vet or trained technician/stockperson. If it is not carried out correctly there are considerable welfare considerations. Figure 27.1 depicts typical on-farm AI equipment comprising an AI tank, guns, water bath and thermometer.

Sexed semen

The ability to dictate the sex of a calf at conception is possible through the use of what is described as *sexed semen*. Sexed semen was developed initially for the dairy industry to help producers maximise the number of high genetic value females being born for retention in the herd for future breeding

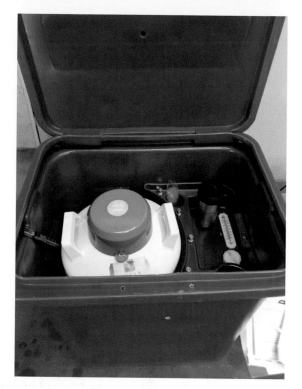

FIGURE 27.1 AI tank and equipment

and to decrease the number of low value male calves being born. Over recent years sexed semen has been developed from beef bulls also with the intention of breeding female heifer replacements for the beef herd. Sexed semen is not available for all beef breeds and the semen from some bulls does not tolerate the sorting process so sexed semen from those specific individuals cannot be produced.

The conception rates achievable from sexed semen are typically 25% lower than those from conventional semen. For this reason, sexed semen is used mainly on heifers which enjoy a slightly higher conception rate to start with. The conception rate is, fortunately, improving all the time and modern technologies are narrowing the difference between it and conventional semen. There are two reasons for the difference in conception rates. First, there is less sperm in a sexed semen straw; 2 million compared to 20 million. Second, the process of separating the male (Y) and female

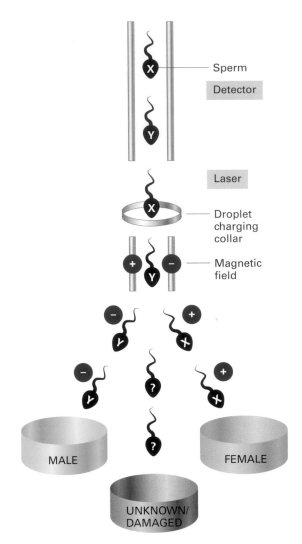

FIGURE 27.2 Semen sorting

when male calves will be born when sexed semen has been used.

The process wastes some sperm; sperm get lost in the dead space of the equipment and if sperm pass through the cell sorting process side by side they will not be evaluated. There also remains the fact that some sperm are not sex-able even if they pass through the detector in the right orientation. To make a single straw containing 2 million sperm there is sufficient wastage that 14 straws could have been made of conventional semen (Seidel, 2014). For high value bulls in great demand sexed semen is simply not a financially realistic possibility.

EMBRYO TRANSFER

ET is a procedure which makes possible an increase in the reproductive rate of a female, way in excess of that which natural reproduction would allow. Instead of a cow conceiving, being pregnant for 9 months and then calving, at best producing 1 calf, sometimes 2, a year, multiple embryos from the cow, referred to as the *donor cow*, can be harvested every few weeks. These embryos are then inserted into surrogate mothers, referred to as the *recipient cows*, for the time-consuming gestation. The recipient cow has no genetic input to the calf despite carrying it for the best part of nine months.

MOET (multiple ovulation embryo transfer) is the process behind this production of multiple embryos – to collect only one embryo at a time would be a lot of work for less gain. MOET involves using hormone injections to stimulate a cow or heifer to produce multiple eggs on her ovaries that then ovulate at the same time. These embryos are simultaneously fertilised by a *triple straw insemination* of the donor cow and the resultant embryos are lavaged from the cow's uterus via catheters inserted via the vagina through the cervix. This is referred to as *flushing*. Flushing takes place 7 days after insemination, just before the embryos would normally implant into the wall of the uterus. The embryos are either inserted immediately into recipient cows/heifers or are frozen for

(X) spermatozoa partially damages at least some of them.

The process of separating the X and Y sperm is called *semen sorting* (Figure 27.2) and it is done by a technique called *flow cytometry*. This technique relies on the difference in the amount of DNA in X and Y sperm; female sperm have 4% more. The sperm pass through the machine at a rate of 30,000 per second (Seidel, 2014). There are inaccuracies and the faster the flow rate the more the inaccuracies will occur. There are, consequently, occasions

later implantation. Pregnancy rates in the recipient females from fresh and frozen embryos are 60% and 50%, respectively. The recipients will be synchronised using hormonal implants and injections to ensure they are at the right stage of the oestrus cycle to be receptive to an embryo which will then implant in the wall of the uterus. The embryos are inserted into the uterus using a special catheter inserted through the cervix, via the vagina. Surgical techniques have been used in the past, and are still used in sheep, where embryos are injected directly through the uterine wall, usually using a laparoscope through keyhole incisions in the abdomen. Laparoscopic AI is no longer needed or practised in cattle.

IN VITRO FERTILISATION OR IN VITRO EMBRYO PRODUCTION

IVF, in vitro embryo production (IVP), involves collecting un-fertilised eggs from the ovaries of live cows by a process called *ovum pick up* (OPU) and then fertilising the eggs outside the cow in a laboratory petri dish. The eggs are collected from the ovary via the rectum; it does not require surgical access to the ovaries, instead an ultrasonographically guided needle is passed through the wall of the rectum into the follicles on the ovary and the eggs aspirated along an evacuated tube attached to the needle. The eggs are collected in a special fluid medium and transferred to the laboratory for fertilisation. The resultant embryos are incubated for seven days and are then either frozen or inserted into recipient cows. The hold rate for frozen and fresh embryos is 45% and 60%, respectively. The collection of eggs from the ovary can be done without any hormone injections, unlike in MOET. The eggs can be collected from the ovary every week, on average 12 eggs are collected per week but this ranges from 0 to over 50. On average, three viable embryos result from each collection – there is variation between cows, the number of resultant embryos can range from 1 to over 20. Eggs can be collected from the ovary when the

cows are non-pregnant and even up to week 12 of pregnancy. Another advantage for IVP is that one straw of semen can be used to fertilise multiple eggs whereas MOET requires three straws of semen per procedure which, in the case of some bulls, can be very costly.

The success of IVP largely depends on the quality of the eggs that are harvested from the ovary. The eggs that are collected are 8 weeks in the making so any stressors or nutritional change in the cow's life may affect the quality of the eggs. Cows between 3–10 years of age and with a BCS of 2.5–3 are the best candidates and preferably those with no history of dystocia, caesarean, or vaginal or uterine prolapse.

Techniques are described which involve injections prior to OPU that stimulate the ovaries to produce more eggs; this involves multiple handlings and interventions that are deemed by some to be unnecessary and a questionable challenge to the cow's welfare.

Recipient selection

Embryos, be they generated by IVP or MOET, need to be inserted and implanted into a recipient cow or heifer. Heifers are considered to have better pregnancy rates than cows in these situations, mirroring the case in natural breeding. Recipients selected should be predictably able to give birth to the calf naturally. Where a large calf is anticipated then second- or third-calving cows will be more appropriate than heifers and the cows selected should have a large birth canal and a known low dystocia score. To enter into the process expecting and planning for a caesarean birth is not ethical.

It is important to start with more recipients than will be required. There may be some that are unsuitable – they may have known reproductive problems, or they may fail to respond as expected to the hormonal injections used in the programme. All recipients should be examined by a vet and should be anatomically normal, cycling regularly and free from disease of any sort, not just reproductive. Establishing a group of heifers for the job, well in advance, helps minimise stress and fighting at a time when it is least wanted.

The background herd health status of recipients is important – they would, ideally, be home-bred rather than introduced from outwith the herd. If recipients do have to be purchased then the usual biosecurity policy should apply, that to include isolation and disease testing. Recipients may require vaccinating as part of the herd health programme. In this case all vaccines should be administered at least 6 weeks before the date of implantation so as to avoid any upsets which are known to be possible in and around the time of vaccination, irrespective of which vaccine is being used. Recipients should be in a BCS range of 2.5–3; condition score has a large influence on success rates.

REFERENCE

Seidel, G.E. (2014) Update on sexed semen technologies in cattle. *Animal* 8, 160–164.

Chapter 28

Notifiable disease and disease surveillance on the beef farm

Health and disease surveillance is defined as the systematic, ongoing, and repeated measurement, collection, collation, analysis, interpretation and timely dissemination of health-related data and information for a given population. It is essential for the planning, implementation and evaluation of risk mitigation measures in that population. In our case the population will be one of cattle – that may be a group, a herd, a region, or, of great importance a governed region or country.

Scanning surveillance is carried out in the UK to *identify new and emerging disease*. This is data collected through private vets submitting samples or carcases to surveillance laboratories for testing. Most of the time this will be routine testing for endemic disease, but occasionally something a bit different will come along which warrants further investigation and is potentially a new and emerging disease. Identification of a new disease relies on an integrated relationship between the farmer, the private vet and the laboratory.

Active surveillance, or *targeted surveillance* consists of structured testing protocols which seek to *find a specific known disease*, for example, bTB, BSE and brucellosis.

Certain diseases in the UK are classified as *notifiable*. This means there is a legal obligation for the farmer, the vet, the abattoir or the laboratory – whoever sees it first – to notify the relevant government agencies if there is a suspicion of any of the diseases listed below. Quite often the local vet will be consulted first as a 'sense check' before the reporting then goes ahead.

CRITERIA FOR NOTIFIABLE STATUS

A disease is listed as notifiable for one of a number of reasons (APHA, 2014).

- **Impact on international trade**. Live and dead animals are traded between countries and different countries have their own stipulations on health. This is akin to an individual farm having its own biosecurity plan, which may differ from the neighbouring farm. The movement of live animals or meat requires a significant amount of paperwork to be completed with a declaration signed to confirm that the animals or meat are free of certain diseases. A disease may be deemed notifiable if infection in the UK cattle population poses a significant risk to trade deals. On the same note, the UK has strict requirements that need to be met to allow animals or meat to be accepted into the country, this is to ensure that the UK remains free of certain diseases.
- **Risk to public health**. A zoonotic disease is a risk to the human population and is likely to be classified as notifiable. For example, bTB, brucellosis or rabies.

- **Animal welfare**. Some diseases have horrific consequences for the health and welfare of animals and for that reason are classified as notifiable. For example, FMD.
- **Impact on the wider population**. An animal disease may have implications for the wider human population, or the economy or adversely affect the public perception of meat and the livestock industry. BSE would be an example.

PRACTICAL CONSIDERATIONS WITH NOTIFIABLE DISEASES

All notifiable diseases are listed in statutory legislation. There is therefore a legal obligation for any suspicion of disease to be reported to a government agency. The government agency then assumes control of the confirmation of the disease, associated movement restrictions, animal slaughter and biosecurity control. Legal powers may be used if required to make this happen. Compensation is paid to the farmer in many – but not all – cases.

Some notifiable diseases are endemic in the UK, such as bTB, others are exotic, that is, they are not currently in this country, for example, at the time of writing, FMD.

KEY NOTIFIABLE DISEASES

Foot and mouth disease

The relatively recent FMD outbreak of 2001 still haunts many farmers and vets. This viral disease is often at the forefront of people's minds when they see an animal that is lame with a high temperature, and salivating with ulcers in the mouth.

This viral disease is highly contagious among cloven-hooved species and has huge animal welfare and economic consequences. The 2001 outbreak in the UK resulted in the culling of 6 million animals. Exclusion zones to stop the spread of disease effectively closed the countryside, and there was a significant financial impact on all those within the agricultural sector, rural industries and way beyond.

The 2001 outbreak started after untreated catering waste, containing the virus, was fed to pigs. By the time the disease was identified it had already spread around England – from Northumberland to Devon and Cumbria. Two crucial changes in legislation resulted from the 2001 outbreak: a ban on any food or catering waste being fed to animals and a 6 day stand-still rule for any moved stock. Now, if cattle or sheep are introduced on to a farm, then, no other cattle or sheep are allowed to move from that farm for 6 days. For pigs, the same applies, but in their case for 20 days. FMD remains a threat to UK agriculture through infected meat arriving from countries where the disease remains endemic.

Blue tongue virus

Blue tongue 'serotype 8' was last in the UK in September 2007 when it crossed over from the Continent. The disease is transmitted by the *Culicoides* midge that spreads it between animals; it is seen in months of the year when midges are present and although it affects cattle, more dramatic clinical signs are seen in sheep. Initially, it causes a fever which is followed by swelling of the head, mouth ulcers and salivation. A few days later the animal becomes lame and there is inflammation of the coronary band (the junction between the hoof and the haired skin of the leg). This disease has a similar appearance to foot and mouth disease. It can also be confused with BVD, and photosensitisation.

Blue tongue continues to circulate in Continental Europe and still poses a significant risk to the UK livestock population from the influx of infected midges across the English Channel during the summer months or via the importation of infected animals which could then infect UK midges to further pass it on.

Lumpy skin disease

Lumpy skin disease (LSD) is another viral disease transmitted by biting flies; it is yet to be identified in the UK, but it is rapidly spreading across Europe. As the name suggests, the predominant sign of disease is small lumps that form beneath the skin; they can be extensive, or few in number. There may be a discharge from the eye and nose, and salivation. The testicles and udder may be sore; bulls may become sterile; cows may abort. There is no effective treatment for LSD and although the disease rarely results in the death of an animal, there are significant welfare and economic implications from loss of production and international trade. There is, however, an effective vaccine, and along with movement restrictions this can be used in control programmes.

Anthrax

Anthrax is caused by the spore-forming bacterium *Bacillus anthracis*, which can survive for many years in the environment. Animals are typically found dead for no apparent reason, occasionally they may be seen alive.

Any sudden or unexplained death should be reported to a vet. Anthrax is a zoonosis, and can result in the loss of human life, so it should be treated very seriously. Further information is in Chapter 12.

Brucellosis

Brucellosis is a bacterial disease which causes abortion in cattle. It is a zoonosis and causes influenza-like symptoms known as 'undulant fever' in humans.

Brucellosis was eradicated from cattle in the UK in 1979, and the UK became officially recognised as brucellosis-free in 1985. There is active surveillance carried out in the UK for brucellosis through bulk milk testing of dairy herds and the testing of aborted foetuses from beef cows. There are also strict import requirements and post-import testing to prevent the re-introduction of the disease. All cases of abortion in cattle are to be reported – as per brucellosis legislation.

Bovine tuberculosis

In certain parts of the UK, testing for bTB remains part of everyday life for many vets and farmers. The disease is caused by the bacterium *Mycobacterium bovis*, which ultimately causes chronic respiratory disease in cattle, although it is rarely seen as a clinical disease. The bacterium can affect many other species such as cats, badgers, deer, goats, pigs, camelids and, of course, humans.

Human infection occurs from the ingestion of unpasteurised milk from a bTB-infected cow. This is extremely rare nowadays thanks to the introduction of pasteurisation.

Cattle can infect each other, and infection can pass from cattle to badgers and badgers to cattle. The badger link was established in the 1970s and now forms part of the bTB control policy in England and Wales with the vaccination and/or culling of badger populations.

bTB can be spread by nose-to-nose contact and indirectly through urine, faeces, saliva, contaminated feed and water, during suckling or the feeding of unpasteurised milk from infected cows to calves. Cattle can become infected by grazing in fields that have been accessed by infected badgers.

M. bovis is well-adapted to last a long time in the environment: up to 2 months in water and 3 months in soil during the winter months. The bacterium is also able to hide inside the animal and establish a long-standing chronic infection. It is not detected by the animal's immune system, so there is little antibody production until late on in the disease. For this reason, a straightforward antibody blood test, as used for other bovine diseases, cannot be used in its detection. Instead, testing relies predominantly on the single intradermal comparative cervical tuberculin test (SICCT), which can be backed up with the gamma interferon blood test. The frequency at which a herd is tested using the SICCT for the presence of bTB varies depending on geographic location and the likelihood of infection. For example, in a herd that is endemically infected, testing of all animals over 42 days will be carried out at 60 day intervals. Within a geographic area considered by government agencies to have a low incidence of bTB a herd test may occur only once every 4 years.

The bacterium is slow growing and requires specific culture techniques to be identified in a laboratory environment. If the bacterium from an infected animal can be cultured it is then possible to genotype it. Epidemiologists investigating the outbreak and its spread can then work out where it has come from. Each genotype is geographically different, for example an isolate from the south west of England is usually different from that found in Cheshire.

Other Mycobacteria exist and infect cattle, such as avian tuberculosis (*M. avium* subsp. *avium*) or the bacterium that causes JD (*M. avium* subsp. *paratuberculosis*). This causes complications when testing for bTB as infections with either bacteria can cause false negative or false positive results.

The SICCT is an internationally recognised test for bTB and can only be carried out by specifically trained individuals, who are, most often, vets. The equipment and inoculants required to perform a SICCT are shown in Figure 28.1: callipers, McLintock syringes and avian and bovine tuberculin. It involves measuring the animal's immune response to tuberculin – a complex mix of proteins extracted from cultures of *M. bovis* grown in a laboratory and killed with heat. Two types of tuberculin are injected, avian and bovine. For the test, the animal's coat is clipped at two sites on the neck, and the thickness of the skin measured (Figure 28.2). Then the injection is placed within the layers of the skin, rather than under the skin, hence the name intradermal skin test. The response to each injection is evaluated 72 hours later by measuring the change in skin thickness at both sites and comparing the reaction at both

sites. If the animal is infected with *M. bovis,* the immune system will be pre-sensitised and produce a notable response to the bovine tuberculin injection site, that is, a bigger 'lump'. The person conducting the test follows set criteria established by government agencies which dictate how large the difference in the increase of the injection sites has to be for an animal to test positive and be called a *reactor*. Avian *and* bovine tuberculin are used to minimise the number of false positive results where a reaction occurs due to a cross-reaction with the avian strain tuberculosis. Once a reactor is identified it is immediately isolated from other cattle and arrangements are made for it to be slaughtered as soon as practically possible. The slaughtered animal is examined in the abattoir for

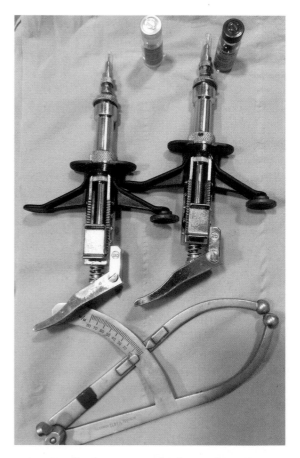

FIGURE 28.1 Equipment required to perform the SICCT: McLintock syringes precisely measure 0.1 ml of tuberculin per injection

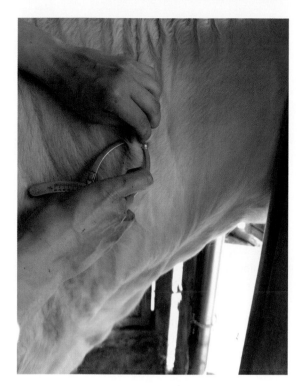

FIGURE 28.2 Measuring the thickness of the skin before injecting tuberculin

visible sign of bTB such as abscesses in the lymph nodes of the chest cavity. Samples are then taken from designated sights in the carcase for bacterial culture to see if *M. bovis* can be detected. The presence or absence of *visible lesions* and the *culture results* are the eagerly awaited extra pieces of information that follow any reactor.

No diagnostic test is perfect: the SICCT has a sensitivity of 80% (Karolemeas et al., 2012), that is, there is an 80% probability that the test will correctly identify an infected animal as positive. This means that 20% of infected animals can be missed at any one SICCT. This enforces the need for multiple tests in the case of pre- and post-movement, pre- and post-import and in a herd bTB breakdown. In contrast, the specificity of the test is high, around 99.98%, which means that a false positive result is very rare, 1 in 5000 (Goodchild et al., 2015). This means a positive is a positive in almost every case. This is an important fact to remember when an animal that tested positive using the

SICCT is found *not* to have any visible signs of the disease (visible lesions) when it is slaughtered and/ or *M. bovis* is *not* cultured from the carcase after slaughter – in other words, even if these follow up tests are negative, there is still a very high likelihood the animal was infected:

Three out of five (60%) of skin reactors do not have visible lesions present when they are examined in the abattoir after slaughter (O'Hagan et al., 2015). The meat inspector will examine the appropriate lymph nodes and the lungs, but the bTB lesions may be so small that they are not detectable with the naked eye.

- There are some subtleties in the way the immune system responds to *M. bovis* that affect the sensitivity of the SICCT. In the first 3–6 weeks of infection, *M. bovis* does not elicit a strong enough immune response to be detected by the SICCT, this is called the *pre-allergic period*.
- If a second skin test is carried out too quickly after the first, then the immune response will be subdued as the immune system needs time to recover; this is called *desensitisation*. A minimum of 60 days is required between SICCTs.
- Cattle that are in the advanced stages of *M. bovis* infection fail to respond to the SICCT, this is called *anergy*. Lesions are visible in the lymph nodes of the animal at slaughter, but they have failed to test positive on a skin test.
- Although the comparative skin test is designed to minimise the number of false positive diagnoses from cross-reaction with avian tuberculosis, there may be cases where the immune response and resulting skin lump from an avian reaction outweighs that of the response to what is actually a co-infection with bovine tuberculosis. This animal may be wrongly classified as negative when it is in fact infected with *M. bovis*. In many countries, the comparative test is not used, and they rely on injecting bovine tuberculin alone for this reason.
- The SICCT relies on a healthy immune system, if the animal is immunosuppressed in any

way, for example, through BVD infection, the animal is less likely to react to the skin test.

- The sensitivity of the skin test is greatly reduced if it is not carried out properly. It is imperative that vets carry out the procedure correctly with restrained cattle, properly identified, with well-maintained equipment at the right time. Farmers are strongly urged to help and support vets do this incredibly important job properly.

The interferon gamma (IFNγ) test is a blood test used to diagnose bTB. It is used in herds that have had a bTB breakdown to pick up positive animals that the SICCT may have missed. It has a sensitivity of 90% and a specificity of 96.5% (Schiller et al., 2009). The higher sensitivity is a benefit, fewer false negatives, but the lower specificity means that some animals that test positive on the IFNγ test are not true positives. This results in a higher false positive rate, and some animals will be slaughtered unnecessarily. The IFNγ test also detects cattle at an earlier stage of infection than the skin test, and there may not be any visible lesions at slaughter.

Enzootic bovine leucosis

Enzootic bovine leucosis (EBL) has been eradicated from the UK but remains prevalent in parts of eastern Europe. It is a viral disease featuring tumours in infected animals between 3 and 5 years of age. If the tumours affect superficial lymph nodes, then they may be visible, however, tumours can grow within internal organs such as the heart and lungs. The clinical signs vary depending on the affected organs. Tumours are more commonly identified at post-mortem examination.

Any tumour in adult cattle should be treated as a suspect EBL case until proven otherwise and the necessary authorities should be notified. There are other conditions that are not notifiable that also cause tumour-like growths associated with lymph nodes or internal organs. The younger the animal, the less likely it is to be affected by EBL, but the tumours are indistinguishable on gross appearance, hence the need for further laboratory testing.

Bovine spongiform encephalopathy

BSE, also commonly referred to as 'mad cow disease', is a fatal neurodegenerative disease of cattle. Cattle incubate the disease for a long period of time before developing signs which include weight loss, nervousness, occasional aggression directed at humans or other cattle, lack of coordination and behavioural changes.

The UK BSE epidemic started in 1986 and epidemiological studies suggested that the source of the disease was cattle feed containing BSE-infected protein from meat and bone meal. Human consumption of contaminated meat was linked to CJD in 1996. CJD is not a new disease in humans, but a new variation of the disease in young people, called *new variant CJD*, is thought to be related to human exposure to BSE.

To prevent the further transmission of disease to cattle, there was a ban on feeding ruminants with all forms of animal protein, including fish-meal. Affected animals and some cohorts and offspring were slaughtered and farmers were compensated for the loss. In the peak of the epidemic in 1992, 36,680 cases were confirmed. Since then, the number of cases has declined, with no cases reported from 2016 onwards.

The majority of cases were in the dairy herd, with only 12% of all cases within the beef suckler herd. Once the potential zoonotic implications of BSE were established, strict human food chain safety controls were enforced. Certain tissues from ruminants, such as brain and spinal cord, were banned from entry into the human food chain, these are classified as *specified risk materials* (SRM). Furthermore, between 1996 and 2005 no cattle over 30 months were allowed to enter the human food chain and farmers were compensated for this measure via the Over Thirty Months Scheme. Since 2005, cattle over 30 months are now allowed back into the human food chain, but part of the brain is still routinely removed for BSE surveillance. In addition to abattoir surveillance, any fallen stock over 48 months of age also have brain tissue removed for BSE testing.

Contagious bovine pleuro-pneumonia

Contagious bovine pleuro-pneumonia (CBPP) is a contagious bacterial disease present in Africa, caused by *Mycoplasma mycoides* subsp. *mycoides*. The disease presents as a typical BRD and is transmitted via respiratory aerosol from cattle to cattle. The presence of infectious carrier animals facilitates the transmission of disease. Although the last time CBPP was seen within the UK was 1898, imported cattle pose a risk for the re-introduction of the disease. CBPP poses no risk to human health.

REFERENCES

APHA (2014) Notifiable diseases. A guide for official veterinarians. ESO1. Rev (04/17). Available at: http://apha.defra.gov.uk/external-operations-admin/library/documents/essential_skills/ES01.pdf.

Goodchild, A.V., Downs, S.H., Upton, P., Wood, J.L.N. and de la Rua-Domenech, R. (2015) Specificity of the comparative skin test for bovine tuberculosis in Great Britain. *Vet Record* 177, 258–267.

Karolemeas, K., de la Rua-Domenech, R., Cooper, R., Goodchild, A.V., Clifton-Hadley, R.S., Conlanm, A.J.K., Mitchell, A.P., Hewinson, R.G., Donnelly, C.A., Wood, J.L.N. and McKinley, T.J. (2012) Estimation of the *relative* sensitivity of the comparative tuberculin skin test in tuberculous cattle herds subjected to depopulation. *PLOSOne* 7(8), e43217.

O'Hagan, M. J., H., Courcier, E. A., Drewe, J.A., Gordon, A. W., McNair, J., Abernethy, D.A. (2015) Risk factors for visible lesions or positive laboratory tests in bovine tuberculosis reactor cattle in Northern Ireland. *Preventative Veterinary Medicine* 120(3–4), 283–290.

Schiller, I., Waters, W.R., Vordermeier, H.M., Nonnecke, B., Welsh, M., Keck, N., Whelan, A., Sigafoose, T., Stamm, C., Palmer, M., Thacker, T., Hardegger, R., Marg-Haufe, B., Raeber, A. and Oesch, B. (2009) Optimisation of a whole-blood gamma interferon assay for detection of *Mycobacterium bovis*-infected cattle. *Clinical and Caccine Immunology* 16(8), 1196–1202.

Chapter 29

Euthanasia and post-mortem examination on the beef farm

EUTHANASIA

Euthanasia, voluntary killing on humane grounds, may be appropriate if an animal is suffering from an incurable disease, or is in pain that cannot be controlled with available means. In these cases, the animal is very rarely fit for transport without grave welfare implications. If an animal is of a significant weight such as a finishing beast, cow or bull there may be some salvage value. The question then to be asked at this stage is whether the animal is fit for human consumption. If the animal is suffering from an acute injury such as a broken leg, then emergency slaughter on farm may be an option. The animal has to be fit and well in all other respects, and sufficiently unsoiled so as to pass a pre-mortem examination. This inspection usually takes place in the abattoir but, in this case, as the animal is unable to travel, then the pre-mortem examination is the responsibility of the certifying vet on farm. A licensed slaughterman or vet then shoots the animal using a captive bolt gun and bleeds the body on farm. The carcase is then transported to the closest abattoir for processing. The cost–benefit of emergency slaughter needs to be considered. There is a cost associated with the attendance of the vet and the transportation of the carcase. There are often deductions from the value of the animal in cases of emergency slaughter where due to dirt, contamination, bruising or trauma the abattoir reduces its value in line with increased carcase trimming.

If an animal does not satisfy the requirements of emergency slaughter or it is uneconomical to do so, and if it cannot travel without breaching welfare codes, then euthanasia on farm is an alternative to treatment. This can be carried out by the farmer, vet or slaughterman using a free bullet gun, an appropriately deployed shotgun or a humane killer such as a captive bolt gun. Whoever does this must be trained and competent; mistakes could be a welfare risk to the animal and the most serious health and safety risk to the operator, other bystanders and other animals. Alternatively, a vet may choose to use a lethal injection – usually an overdose of a barbiturate anaesthetic solution administered intravenously.

A captive bolt gun or humane killer or stun gun is a device used for stunning animals, Figure 29.1.

It does not necessarily kill the animal and cannot be assumed to do so; it instead renders the animal unconscious and sends it into a severe seizure (chaotic electrical activity in what remains of the damaged brain). The gun is held against the animal's forehead and a metal pin is discharged at speed under the explosive power of a charge fired by a trigger. The metal pin or 'bolt' penetrates the skull and then retracts back into the barrel of the gun. The animal is effectively stunned and can then be fully euthanased humanely by either bleeding the animal, which involves incising the carotid artery in the neck or thoracic inlet, or by a process called pithing. Pithing involves inserting a long stick into the hole in the skull, made by the captive

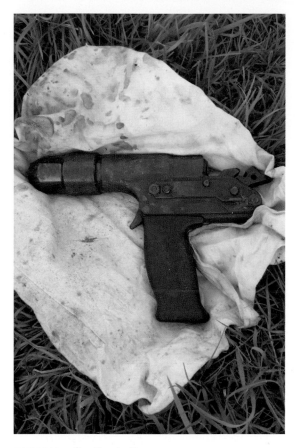

FIGURE 29.1 Captive bolt gun

bolt gun, and advancing it to the base of the brain so as to destroy so much of the brain, in particular the respiratory centre, that recovery becomes impossible. Euthanasia needs to be hygienic if the animal is for human consumption. Bleeding can go wrong in this respect; the knife can carry bacteria from dirty skin into the bloodstream – the skin and knife need to be clean. If the oesophagus is cut along with the carotid artery, then gut contents can contaminate the bloodstream and the carcase. Where a pithing rod is used then, again bacteria can be carried into the animal and also the disruption of the brain could theoretically release infectious agents into the bloodstream, of most potential concern being the *prion particles* that infect cattle with BSE.

Figure 29.2 illustrates the correct place to shoot cattle with a free bullet or captive bolt gun.

This involves aiming with a virtual cross drawn from the top of the eyes to the middle of the horn base (or where the horn base would be if there were one). The gun must be placed perpendicular to the skull (Grandin, 2019).

To ensure the process is carried out as safely and effectively as possible the operator needs to be trained and competent in the use of a captive

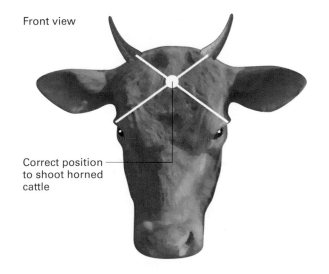

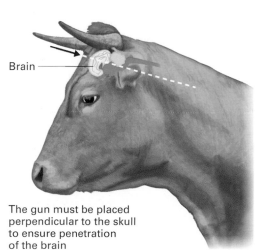

Front view

Correct position to shoot horned cattle

Side view

Brain

The gun must be placed perpendicular to the skull to ensure penetration of the brain

FIGURE 29.2 Correct position and angle of free bullet gun or captive bolt gun when used to shoot a bovine animal (a) viewed from the front and (b) viewed from the side

bolt gun, the gun needs to be well maintained and the animal needs to be well restrained. Missed shots or partial shots have serious welfare implications for the animal and huge health and safety implications for the operatives and bystanders. In the extreme situation of deploying a shotgun for euthanasia then the end of the barrel must be held 4-6 inches away from the target point on the skull. Inadvertently firing while the barrel is pressed against the skull could cause back pressure and severe injury or death to the operator. Training and competence is clearly necessary in these circumstances. Rifles have been used for euthanasia of cattle but at close range there is a high likelihood the bullet will exit the animal. Such a risk is not acceptable and rifles should therefore only be used by trained marksmen and from a distance.

POST-MORTEM EXAMINATION

A PME is an invaluable tool in helping to find out why an animal has died. A private veterinary surgeon can carry out a PME on farm, some deadstock yards can provide a vet to carry out a PME at the collection yard or the carcase can be transported to a recognised disease surveillance centre or laboratory for a PME.

A PME is a systematic examination of each body system and the gathering of evidence to build a picture of the cause of death. Sometimes the information from gross evidence is inadequate for a diagnosis so samples may be collected from the animal for further laboratory testing. To get the best out of a post-mortem examination the carcase needs to be as fresh as possible. If the PME is carried out on farm, then reasonable make-shift facilities are required. Good light is essential. The carcase should be moved to an area not accessible to other livestock and one that can be cleaned and disinfected afterwards. Any discharges from the carcase should be contained and not allowed to flow into livestock areas or water courses. The carcase needs to be accessible to the dead stock collector too. In the case of a sudden death, where anthrax (a notifiable disease) is suspected, the carcase needs to be tested and deemed clear of anthrax before a PME can take place.

The following diseases are examples that can be diagnosed on PME alone without the need for additional laboratory tests:

- wire disease (traumatic reticulo-pericarditis)
- peritonitis
- abscessation of internal organs
- metritis
- mastitis
- lungworm
- pneumonia
- twisted gut
- kidney infections
- internal haemorrhage
- ingestion of poisonous plants
- laryngeal chondritis
- there are others!

'The only good thing that can come from of a dead beast is … a post-mortem examination' – (Anon.)

REFERENCE

Grandin, T. (2019) Recommended captive bolt stunning technique for cattle. Department of Animal Science Colorado State University. Available at: https://www.grandin.com/humane/cap.bolt.tips.html (accessed 25 September 2020).

Appendix

An example of a bull pre-breeding examination report

Owners Name and Address:			
███████████████████████████████			

Place of examination:		Date of examination:	
██████		████████	

Name + ear tag number:	Species:	Breed:	Age:
██████	Bovine	Aberdeen Angus	18 months

Fertility history and reason for assessment:
Young bull

General Health Status (eyes, legs, feet, teeth, heart, lungs etc):
Good – no abnormalities detected

Condition Score (1-5):	Rectal Temperature (C): 37.6	Scrotal Circumference (cm): 31

Testes and epididymes	Right	No abnormalities detected
	Left	No abnormalities detected

Accessory glands: No abnormalities detected

	Sample 1		Sample 2		
Stimulation level for sampling (1-9)	4		4		
Penis extruded? Description	Yes – no abnormalities detected		Yes – no abnormalities detected		
Semen volume (ml)	5ml		4ml		
Semen appearance	Cloudy yellow		Cloudy yellow		
Gross motility score (Wave Motion) (grade 1-5) Target 3+	2		4		
Progressive Motility % (>30% Pass, pref 60%)	<30%		>60%		
Sperm Morphology	Tally/comments	%	Pass %	Compensable
Normal		64%	>50-70%	No
Proximal cytoplasmic droplets (PD)		24%	<20%	No
Mid piece abnormalities (MP)		1%	<30%	Yes
Tail defects and loose heads (T&H)		8%	<30%	Yes
Pyriform heads (Py)		3%	<20%	No
Knobbed acrosome (KA)		-	<30%	Yes
Vacuoles and teratoids (V&T)		-	<20%	No
Swollen acrosomes (SA)		-	<30%	Yes
Other abnormalities				

On the basis of this examination the above male has achieved a fail for the breeding soundness examination. The male is sub-fertile.

The morphology results of this sample were abnormal with a high percentage of non-compensable defects. I would advise to re-test this bull in 8 weeks time.

This report indicates likely fertility status at the time of testing and is no guarantee of the current or future status of this male. Testing for transmissible diseases (including venereal/congenital disease) is not carried out and the breeding soundness examination does not indicate freedom from these diseases. No assessment of libido or serving ability has been made during this examination.

This report is for the use of the owner only and is not a certificate that guarantees the fertility of this male.

Signature: …………………………………………   Date: ██████████

██████████████████████████████████

Cattle Purchasing Disease Checklist

Date:..No. of animals:...

Name & address of farm where cattle are to be purchased from:

....

....

....Tel:...

Vendor's vet name & address:

....

....

....Tel:...

Bovine Tuberculosis – A notifiable bacterial disease of cattle which can also affect people.

• Have the cattle to be purchased been tested recently?		☐ Yes	☐ No
• Has the source herd had a clear herd test recently?		☐ Yes	☐ No
• What is the testing frequency imposed on the source herd?	☐ Annual	☐ Biannual	☐ 4 Yearly
• Does the source herd have a history of bovine tuberculosis?		☐ Yes	☐ No

---

Johne's Disease – An invariably fatal disease of cattle with insidious onset after a long incubation period.

• Does the source herd have Johne's disease free accreditation?	☐ Yes	☐ No
• Has the source herd had any confirmed or suspect cases?	☐ Yes	☐ No
• Does the source herd vaccinate?	☐ Yes	☐ No

BVD – A viral disease of cattle that causes a multitude of clinical signs including infertility, abortions and the production of deformed or persistently infected calves. Persistently infected calves invariably die.

• What is your herd's status?	☐ Clear	☐ Vaccinated	☐ Infected
• What is the source herd's status?	☐ Clear	☐ Vaccinated	☐ Infected
• Are the animals to be purchased persistently infected?		☐ Yes	☐ No
• Are the animals to be purchased pregnant?		☐ Yes	☐ No

Leptospirosis – A bacterial disease of cattle causing reproductive failure and milk drop. It can affect people.

• What is your herd's status?	☐ Clear	☐ Vaccinated	☐ Infected
• What is the source herd's status?	☐ Clear	☐ Vaccinated	☐ Infected

---

IBR – A viral disease of cattle causing respiratory disease, reproductive failure and milk drop. A carrier status often exists following infection and apparent recovery.

• What is the status of your herd?	☐ Clear	☐ Vaccinated	☐ Infected
• Are the animals to be purchased antibody positive?		☐ Yes	☐ No
• If antibody positive, have the animals to be purchased ever been vaccinated?		☐ Yes	☐ No
• If so which vaccine was used?		☐ Conventional	☐ Marker

DairyCo

Bluetongue

- Are the cattle to be purchased being sourced from a BTV endemic area?   ☐ Yes   ☐ No
- If so, which are the relevant strains of BTV? ....
- Have the cattle to be purchased been vaccinated against BTV?   ☐ Yes   ☐ No
- If so, with which vaccine and when? ....
- Have the cattle to be purchased been tested for the bluetongue virus
  (PCR test) or for antibodies to the virus (ELISA test)?   ☐ Yes   ☐ No
- If so, when and what were the results? ....
- Have the cattle to be purchased been treated with a pour-on
  insecticide which is active against midges?   ☐ Yes   ☐ No
- If so, when and with what? ....

Campylobacter foetus venerealis – A sexually transmitted bacterial disease of cattle that can cause infertility and abortions.

- Do you use any natural service in your herd?   ☐ Yes   ☐ No
- Are the animals to be purchased virgins?   ☐ Yes   ☐ No
- If the animals to be purchased are not virgins and they
  are female, were they run with a bull?   ☐ Yes   ☐ No

Salmonella – A reportable disease with human health implications.

- Is there any evidence of salmonellosis in the source herd?   ☐ Yes   ☐ No
- If so, what? ....

Brucellosis – A disease that can affect people and which causes cattle to abort.

- Have the cattle to be purchased been imported from outside GB?   ☐ Yes   ☐ No

Neospora caninum – A protozoal parasite that can cause cattle to abort.

- Have the animals to be purchased been tested?   ☐ Yes   ☐ No

Parasites – Purchased cattle may harbour a variety of parasites including gut worms, lung worms, liver fluke, lice and mites.

- Has the parasite status of the animals to be purchased been assessed?   ☐ Yes   ☐ No
- Have the animals to be purchased been vaccinated against lungworm?   ☐ Yes   ☐ No
- Has any treatment been given to eliminate parasites?   ☐ Yes   ☐ No

Digital Dermatitis – The most common infectious cause of lameness currently affecting particularly dairy cattle in the UK.

- Is digital dermatitis present in your herd?   ☐ Yes   ☐ No
- Is digital dermatitis present in the source herd?   ☐ Yes   ☐ No
- Have the animals to be purchased had their feet lifted, cleaned, inspected and treated?   ☐ Yes   ☐ No

Mastitis – A common multifactorial disease which can cause significant economic loss.

- Are the animals to be purchased cows or maiden heifers?   ☐ Cows   ☐ Heifers
- Have the source herd's cell count and mastitis records been seen?   ☐ Yes   ☐ No
- If cows, have the cell count and mastitis records of the
  animal to be purchased been seen?   ☐ Yes   ☐ No

For further information about these, and other diseases and the threat they pose
please visit the DairyCo website at: www.dairyco.org.uk

DairyCo

Index